Praise from professionals for
SYMPTOMS: THEIR CAUSES & CURES:

"Well thought out, well balanced and well written, even appropriately funny in places. Time spent with *Symptoms: Their Causes and Cures* is time well spent in the pursuit of wellness. It can help people get well and stay well."

—Steven Jonas, M.D., professor of preventive medicine at the State University of New York at Stony Brook and author of *Take Control of Your Weight*

"The advice is quite comprehensive, quite practical and reasonable. It supplies useful, straightforward information."

—Vert Mooney, M.D., professor of orthopedic surgery at the University of California, San Diego, Medical Center

"A well-researched, practical guide to health with helpful suggestions for dealing with many common symptoms. Concise information conveys a clear picture of how the body malfunctions and allows one to recognize when a serious health problem might be occurring."

—Robert A. Weiss, M.D., assistant professor of dermatology at Johns Hopkins University School of Medicine in Baltimore

"A magnificent job of cataloging a series of symptoms, with professional advice that will be of special value to the reader."

—C. Warren Bierman, M.D., clinical professor and pediatrics chief in the Division of Allergy at the University of Washington School of Medicine in Seattle

The Bantam Library of Prevention Magazine Health Books

The Doctors Book of Home Remedies
The Doctors Book of Home Remedies II
The Doctors Book of Home Remedies for Children
The Healing Herbs
High-Speed Healing
The *Prevention* Pain-Relief System
Women's Encyclopedia of Health & Emotional Healing

**And ask your bookseller about these other
Bantam Health and Nutrition Books**

The Aspirin Handbook
The Bantam Medical Dictionary
The Best Treatment
The Herb Book
Modern Prevention
The Pill Book
The Pill Book Guide to Children's Medications
The Pill Book Guide to Everything You Need to Know
    About Prozac
The Pill Book Guide to Safe Drug Use
Symptoms
The Vitamin Book

SYMPTOMS
—THEIR—
CAUSES & CURES

HOW TO UNDERSTAND AND TREAT 265 HEALTH CONCERNS

By the Editors of
PREVENTION Magazine Health Books

Doug Dollemore • Marcia Holman • Brian Paul Kaufman
Laura Wallace-Smith • Joseph M. Wargo
Mark D. Wisniewski • Pat Wittig

Edited by Alice Feinstein

BANTAM BOOKS

NEW YORK • TORONTO • LONDON • SYDNEY • AUCKLAND

This edition contains the complete text of the original edition.
NOT ONE WORD HAS BEEN OMITTED.

SYMPTOMS: THEIR CAUSES AND CURES
A Bantam Book/published by arrangement with Rodale Press, Inc.

Publishing History
Rodale Press edition published 1994
Bantam edition/March 1996

Prevention is a registered trademark of Rodale Press, Inc.

ISBN 0-553-56989-9

Published simultaneously in the United States and Canada

Bantam Books are published by Bantam Books, a division of Bantam
Doubleday Dell Publishing Group, Inc. Its trademark, consisting of the
words "Bantam Books" and the portrayal of a rooster, is Registered in U.S.
Patent and Trademark Office and in other countries. Marca Registrada.
Bantam Books, 1540 Broadway, New York, New York 10036.

PRINTED IN THE UNITED STATES OF AMERICA

OPM   9   8

NOTICE

This book is intended as a reference volume only, not as a medical guide or manual for self-treatment. If you suspect that you have a medical problem, please seek competent medical care. The information here is designed to help you make informed choices about your health. It is not intended as a substitute for any treatment prescribed by your doctor.

SYMPTOMS: THEIR CAUSES AND CURES
EDITORIAL AND DESIGN STAFF

Editor: Alice Feinstein

Writers and Editors: Doug Dollemore, Marcia Holman, Dawn Horvath, Brian Paul Kaufman, Jeff Meade, Laura Wallace-Smith, Joe Wargo, Russell Wild, Mark D. Wisniewski, Pat Wittig

Copy Editor: Lisa D. Andruscavage

Researchers and Fact-Checkers: Susan E. Burdick, Carlotta B. Cuerdon, Christine Dreisbach, Deborah Pedron, Sally A. Reith, Sandra Salera-Lloyd, Anita Small, Bernadette Sukley

Support Staff: Roberta Mulliner, Julie Kehs, Mary Lou Stephen

PREVENTION MAGAZINE HEALTH BOOKS

Editor-in-Chief, Rodale Books: Bill Gottlieb
Executive Editor: Debora A. Tkac
Art Director: Jane Colby Knutila
Research Manager: Ann Gossy Yermish

CONTENTS

INTRODUCTION

HOW TO USE SYMPTOMS TO IMPROVE YOUR HEALTH

When your body wants to send you a message that something is wrong, it sends you a symptom. Symptoms are often painful and usually unpleasant. Do you want to get that message from your body? You bet you do!

Decoding that symptom—figuring out what your body is trying to tell you—is *vital*. Finding out what's causing that symptom often helps you correct something your body's doing wrong. If you're not eating right or getting enough exercise, if you're being exposed to something that's not good for you, your body will let you know . . . by sending you a symptom or two.

Sometimes decoding the symptom/message from your body is easy. In plain English, your "headache" message might read something like: "About that nightcap you had last night . . . If you *have* to consume alcohol before going to bed—and I would prefer that you didn't—would you kindly have something other than red wine?" Sometimes getting the message is *not* so simple, and medical science can only offer several possibilities and suggestions.

That's what this book is about: figuring out what your symptom is trying to tell you, then finding out all the possible things you can do about it.

Symptoms: Their Causes and Cures is easy to use. The symptoms are listed in alphabetical order—from A to Z—and we've used popular terms instead of medical terms. That way you won't have to know that doctors call water retention *edema*. Just look up "water retention." We realize that people in different parts of the country sometimes have different names for things, so if you don't find what you want at the first try, give a peek at the index at the back of the book.

May your body's symptoms/messages be few, and may you "read" them well and use those symptoms to find your way to good health.

Alice Feinstein
EDITOR

A

ACHE ALL OVER

- Achiness worsens or continues for more than five days.

WHAT YOUR SYMPTOM IS TELLING YOU

The windows sparkle, the walls are washed and the back porch is clean. Spring has sprung and your annual cleaning is done. You snuggle under the covers for a much-deserved and long-awaited night of sleep, ready to admire and enjoy the results of your toil and trouble in the light of a new day. But when morning breaks, you ache all over.

Overexertion is one of the more common reasons for total-body achiness. Viral infections, arthritis or other diseases could be responsible, in the absence of excessive activity, doctors say.

Anytime you do something strenuous that you're not accustomed to doing—spring cleaning, an unusually hard workout, sack-race at the family reunion—you're bound to be sore the next day. But don't be surprised if the aches don't hit until two or three days after the exertion, says Clayton W. Kersting, M.D., a family physician in Newport, Washington. Muscle soreness may take its time in appearing.

That's especially true if a fall or an accident jars the whole body, according to Anne Simons, M.D., an assistant professor of family and community medicine at the University of California in San Francisco and coauthor of *Before You Call the Doctor.* "And the soreness could grow progressively worse for a couple of days before it gets better," she says.

1

Outside of exertion or physical damage, viral infections—from a cold or flu to pneumonia—can make you feel as if you've constructed your house the day before, not just cleaned it. Invasion of your body by a virus sets off inflammation as your immune system attempts to fight back, causing the soreness in your muscles, Dr. Kersting explains.

Bites from ticks carrying Lyme disease can cause aching joints all over the body. While the threat from those little buggers has abated somewhat, it still is a problem, Dr. Kersting says. You'll get a tip-off to Lyme disease because a "bull's-eye" rash or a reddening of the skin may appear at the site of the bite or anywhere on the body. (A trip to the woods a few weeks before the achiness struck is another clue.)

Several other diseases target the joints and transfer soreness into the muscles to which they're connected, giving you a total-body achiness. Connective tissue or autoimmune disorders such as rheumatoid arthritis or (in rare cases) lupus might be the culprits, according to David R. Rudy, M.D., a professor of family medicine and chairman of the Department of Family Medicine at the University of Health Sciences/Chicago Medical School. "There are all degrees of severity with these problems," he says, "and mild forms could be mistaken for something else."

Rheumatoid arthritis pain typically is worse in the morning after you've risen from a night's worth of stillness, but it improves once you begin to move around for 30 to 60 minutes, Dr. Rudy notes. Wear-and-tear arthritis (called osteoarthritis) is usually worse toward the end of the day.

SYMPTOM RELIEF

Achiness from overactivity and most infections clear up with time. More stubborn causes require more determined treatment. Here's how to feel a bit better no matter what is causing the problem.

Go soak yourself. Twenty to 30 minutes of heat three times a day provides soothing, relaxing relief for total-body aches, Dr. Kersting says. Saunas, Jacuzzis, hot showers and long immersions in a tub filled with hot water all make you feel better. Dry heat from an electric blanket or chemical heat from one of those over-the-counter salves also feels good, Dr. Kersting says. (Warning: don't use an electric blanket or heating pad at the same time you use salves. You could be severely burned.)

Take a load off. If an accident or a viral illness is causing your aches, just take it easy for a couple of days until you feel well enough to resume your regular activities, Dr. Simons says.

Take a tablet. Aspirin or other over-the-counter anti-inflammatory medications like ibuprofen offer temporary reprieves from mild achiness, according to Dr. Simons, but they won't eliminate it unless the source is an inflammation.

For more discomforting aches, your doctor will be able to prescribe more potent drugs. Doctors prescribe antibiotics for Lyme disease and infections, and anti-inflammatories for connective tissue aches.

Move it. For aches related to overexertion or arthritis, mild exercises and stretching will make your body feel better. "Don't give into the aches," Dr. Rudy says. Choose exercises, such as swimming or light weight training, that take your muscles and joints through their full ranges of motion without overstretching the joints.

AFTERNOON SLUMP

WHEN TO SEE YOUR DOCTOR

- Afternoon slumps regularly and irresistibly overtake you, even though you're maintaining a regular sleep schedule.
- Your slumps continue well into the afternoon and even on into the night for a period of two or more weeks.
- Your afternoon slumps affect your job performance and safety (you have to drive or operate heavy equipment, for example.)

What Your Symptom Is Telling You

You rise and shine with the new day, ready to take on the world. You roll through your morning tasks like a ball of fire. And then in the afternoon, you fizzle.

What could have caused your energy and alertness to take such an extraordinary nosedive? Something serious? Not likely. This sudden slump is a normal, healthy, expected function of our circadian rhythms—the built-in biological clocks that regulate our sleep/wake systems, explains biological psychologist David F. Dinges, Ph.D., associate professor in the psychiatry department at the University of Pennsylvania School of Medicine in Philadelphia.

"In the mornings, we are refreshed after a night's sleep and our energy and alertness are at peak levels," says Dr. Dinges. "There is a dip in the middle of the afternoon when sleepiness reappears—our natural nap zone. Later in the afternoon, our alertness typically rises again."

Individuals differ in the degree to which this slump hits. Generally, the depth of the dip is a function of how sleepy you are and the amount of sleep you get at night. "If you are short on sleep and in an inactive situation, alertness will go down and you'll really feel sleepiness creep in when you're in your nap zone—usually between 1:00 and 3:00 p.m.," says Wilse B. Webb, Ph.D., professor of psychology at the University of Florida in Gainesville. "If the slump hits you extremely hard, it could just mean that you have an extremely strong nap tendency. But it could also mean that you are chronically depriving yourself of adequate restorative sleep at night."

If you're actually sleep deprived, this normally shallow dip may take on the size of the Grand Canyon. For most of us, the slump represents a few yawns and an occasional inconvenience. But if you find yourself conking out at your desk or fighting to stay awake at the wheel, it is a warning signal that the sleep you're getting is woefully inadequate. These deep, powerful slumps are usually the body's way of telling you to stop staying up so late, waking up so early and keeping such irregular hours. But for some, they may be a sign of a more serious sleep disorder that is preventing sleep's restorative powers from fully going to work. A likely suspect is sleep apnea—a serious sleep disorder that involves episodes of disrupted breathing.

Your noontime meal can also lead you into an afternoon tailspin. Bonnie J. Spring, Ph.D., professor of psychology at the University of Health Sciences/Chicago Medical School, has shown in studies that a high-carbohydrate/low-protein lunch can produce an afternoon drop in energy and alertness by elevating the brain's levels of serotonin, a substance that makes us sleepy.

SYMPTOM RELIEF

Afternoon slump may not be a priority symptom, but don't casually dismiss it. Reduced alertness can lead to poor productivity as well as traffic and industrial accidents. Here are some energy boosters you can use to recharge your battery and give the afternoon slump the slip.

Take a walk. A rapid ten-minute walk raises energy faster and to a greater degree than sweets and snacks, according to Robert Thayer, Ph.D., professor of psychology at California State University in Long Beach. "A general body arousal occurs, which activates a number of different systems in the mind and body to produce an uplifting effect for up to two hours," he says.

Take a nap. If your situation allows, heed Mother Nature's call and catch a couple of winks. "A brief nap can be quite invigorating," says Dr. Webb. "A good rule for naps is that they should never be longer than one hour and never occur after 4:00 p.m."

Get plenty of sleep the night before. "If you are sleep deprived, you're more likely to be hit hard by the circadian dip," says Dr. Dinges. Getting adequate sleep at night and maintaining regular sleep patterns can lessen its severity. For more on getting your sleep, see Insomnia on page 326.

Rearrange your schedule. Schedule more passive activities like driving, reading and paperwork for the morning and late afternoon when your alertness is high, suggests Dr.

Dinges. "Use the slump period for engaging in busier social activities like talking on the phone, interacting with co-workers and doing physical tasks," he says.

Don't skip breakfast. "Skipping breakfast creates a big energy gap that you'll feel all day, even if you eat a good lunch," says James A. Corea, Ph.D., a registered physical therapist in Moorestown, New Jersey, and former trainer with the Philadelphia Eagles professional football team. "Start with a decent-size, low-fat breakfast of cereal, fresh fruit, whole wheat toast and skim milk. You can't go wrong."

Eat a balanced lunch. The ideal lunch is a balance of proteins and carbohydrates. A good example of a slump-fighting, high-energy lunch would consist of any combination of fish, pasta, rice, baked potato, fruit salad, vegetable, lean meat or soup, according to Dr. Corea.

Avoid the lunchtime martini. Alcohol is a depressant, and like many other drugs, it can hit you like a ton of bricks.

Avoid sugary snacks. "After a brief energy surge, sugar produces increased tiredness," says Dr. Thayer. Candy bars and junk food may be convenient, but they can actually drag your slump down deeper. Fresh fruit or popcorn make a more reliable snack.

Drink coffee or soda. Caffeine is a powerful stimulant that can get you through this time period, says Philip R. Westbrook, M.D., director of the Sleep Disorders Center at Cedars-Sinai Medical Center in Los Angeles. Be careful not to overdo the coffee in the morning—the lift you get from more than four cups can send you crashing down in the early afternoon, making the dip even worse.

See also Fatigue

AGE SPOTS

WHEN TO SEE YOUR DOCTOR

- You have an age spot that bleeds, itches, tingles or changes in size.

WHAT YOUR SYMPTOM IS TELLING YOU

Age spots have little to do with aging. But they have a lot to do with the sun.

"Age spots are really sun-induced freckles," says Robert E. Clark, M.D., Ph.D., director of the Dermatologic Surgery and Cutaneous Oncology Unit at Duke University Medical Center in Durham, North Carolina. "They commonly appear on the backs of the hands.

You can also see them along the shoulders where someone has had significant sun exposure, and on the face. Age spots *are* common in older people, but someone who's had significant sun exposure can get them in their late twenties, thirties and forties."

Even a little bit of sun worshipping can cause age spots later in life. Sunlight contains ultraviolet rays that cause suntans and burns. As time goes by, tanning causes more pigment than normal to be deposited in the skin. This leads eventually to flat, brown skin lesions known as age spots. They're also known as liver spots or sun spots.

SYMPTOM RELIEF

Age spots are harmless. They're benign and they do not go on to become any type of skin cancer or premalignant skin lesion," Dr. Clark says. But because some skin cancers such as melanoma can *look* like age spots, you should ask your doctor to examine your skin during your annual checkup.

Here are a couple of ways to deal with these telltale signs of excessive sun exposure.

Bleach it out. If your age spots aren't too dark or large, over-the-counter skin-bleaching creams containing hydroquinone could help them fade away, says Marc Bauder, M.D., a family practice physician in Sun City West, Arizona. Be sure to follow the manufacturer's directions carefully when applying the cream to your skin.

Don't overexpose yourself. The best way to treat and prevent age spots is to cut the time you spend in the sun. Once you have these spots, sunlight can make them appear darker and more prominent, Dr. Bauder says. To prevent that, always wear a sun block that has a sun protection factor (SPF) of at least 15 on exposed skin. In addition, try to wear a long-sleeved shirt and a broad-brimmed hat whenever you're outdoors.

See your doctor. If you have stubborn age spots that don't fade out with over-the-counter bleaching creams, your doctor has several treatments at his disposal to make age spots disappear, says Dr. Clark. He can freeze them with liquid nitrogen, and after four or five days the spots will peel off. He can also use pulses of laser light to fade the spots.

Ask about a peel. When someone has dozens of age spots, doctors suggest a trichloroacetic acid chemical peel (TCA), says Dr. Clark. The peel, which is applied in a doctor's office, removes the top layer of skin where the spot is located.

"There is a moderately severe burning sensation, but it only lasts for about seven minutes, then the discomfort wears off," Dr. Clark says. "Over the next two to three days you'll have significant swelling and redness of the skin. After four to five days you'll begin shedding the upper layer of skin. But within a week you look like you have a sunburn, and you're ready to get back in society."

Try a slow peel. Retin-A is another option, says Dr. Clark. It's a prescription cream that you can apply directly to the age spots, causing the skin to peel. You'll probably have to put it on a couple of times a day for several months, however, before you'll notice any significant change in your skin, Dr. Clark says.

ANAL BLEEDING

WHEN TO SEE YOUR DOCTOR

- The blood is dark red or maroon.
- Bleeding occurs between bowel movements.
- You have tarlike, black or rust-colored stools.
- You're older than 50.
- Your family has a history of colon or rectal cancer.

WHAT YOUR SYMPTOM IS TELLING YOU

In most cases, bright red blood from the anus is more like an annoying car alarm than a screaming air-raid siren. Although anal bleeding is something that you should always bring to your doctor's attention, it's usually just your body's colorful and dramatic way of telling you that you have a hemorrhoid.

Just inside the anus are collections of blood vessels that act like inflatable cushions, forming a tight seal that helps prevent stool, flatus and mucus from leaking from your rectum. But if one of these vessels gets inflamed or droops out of its normal position on the rectal wall—often from intense straining during a bowel movement—it becomes a hemorrhoid. Besides itching or hurting, hemorrhoids can also bleed.

Bleeding also can be a sign of fissures (cracks in the skin surrounding the anus), ulcerative colitis or polyps. Blood that issues from your anus can also be coming from higher up in your digestive tract. That's why it's important to notify your doctor about any type of bleeding from your anus.

"About 99 percent of the time, it's just hemorrhoids, but it can be something more serious. Unfortunately, the average person just can't tell what type of bleeding is serious and what is not," says Scott Goldstein, M.D., a colon and rectal surgeon at Thomas Jefferson University Hospital in Philadelphia.

Symptom Relief

If the bleeding is bright red and only occurs immediately after you've had a bowel movement, and you've had hemorrhoids before, then there are a number of things you can try to control it, says James Harig, M.D., associate professor of medicine in the Department of Digestive and Liver Diseases at the University of Illinois College of Medicine in Chicago. But you should still let your doctor know what is going on even if these simple remedies stop your bleeding.

Bring your own roll. "I tell my patients to use plain, two-ply toilet paper, even if it means bringing their own roll to work," Dr. Harig says. "Some people use cheap types of toilet paper and rub their bottoms raw to the point of bleeding. You should always use a soft paper and pat your bottom dry. Don't rub."

Trim your fingernails. Well-manicured fingernails may make a fashion statement, but long nails can be dangerous. "Once I was called to the emergency room because a woman was bleeding quite briskly," says Juan Nogueras, M.D., a colon and rectal surgeon at the Cleveland Clinic–Florida in Fort Lauderdale. "It turned out she had accidentally nabbed a hemorrhoid with a long fingernail while wiping her bottom."

Grease is the word. Try inserting a soothing daub of petroleum jelly into the anus before a bowel movement, suggest Dr. Harig. It can help ease the passage of stools.

Watch what you eat. Chew your food carefully and be aware that what goes in, must come out, even if you can't digest it. "It doesn't happen very often, but if a person swallows a small bone, it can cause cuts, tears and bleeding when it goes through the anus," says Philip Jaffe, M.D., an assistant professor of gastroenterology at the University of Arizona College of Medicine in Tucson.

Water, water everywhere. Drink six to eight glasses of water each day. Water helps keep your stool pliable so it will slip out of your body with a minimal amount of straining. The more you strain, the greater the chance you will have anal bleeding, says Dr. Nogueras.

Bulk up on fiber. Fibrous foods, such as fruits, vegetables, beans and whole-grain cereals, increase the bulk of the stool and, like water, decrease the amount of straining needed during a bowel movement. In turn, that lessens pressure on blood vessels and helps prevent bleeding.

See also Stool, Straining at

ANAL ITCHING

WHEN TO SEE YOUR DOCTOR

- You feel a lump in the rectal area.
- You have diabetes.
- You are taking steroids.
- Your children complain of anal itching.

WHAT YOUR SYMPTOM IS TELLING YOU

Of all the places to get an itch, your anus is probably one of the most embarrassing. Face it, it's nearly impossible to look dignified while scratching your rump. Yet no matter how solemn or romantic the moment, it's hard to ignore the urgent pleas for immediate attention.

An itchy bottom usually is a signal that fecal material or body secretions are irritating nerve endings in the anus. However, the causes are numerous, and finding a specific reason for it can be elusive, doctors say.

More than likely, hemorrhoids, pinworms, fissures (cracks in the skin surrounding the anus), anal warts or allergic reactions to toilet paper or foods are responsible for your dilemma. Anal itching also can be caused by a fungal infection, which is particularly common among people with diabetes and can be one of the first signs of the disease. In rare cases, anal itching is a sign of an abscess, polyp or sexually transmitted disease.

Symptom Relief

I would be wary of using over-the-counter creams and ointments to deal with anal itching. They may do more harm than good, and frankly, there are easier ways of dealing with it," says Bruce Orkin, M.D., an assistant professor specializing in colon and rectal surgery at the George Washington University School of Medicine and Health Sciences in Washington, D.C. Here are a few suggestions on how to banish that tormenting itch from your life.

Nix citrus fruits and spicy foods. Doctors aren't sure why, but citrus fruits, such as oranges, grapefruits and tangerines, and spicy foods, like curry and hot peppers, can cause some people to develop irritating secretions at the anus, says Juan Nogueras, M.D., a colon and rectal surgeon at the Cleveland Clinic-Florida in Fort Lauderdale. Simply eliminating these foods from your diet may solve the problem, he says.

Slash your coffee drinking. Coffee beans contain oils that you can't digest. The oils irritate the skin surrounding the anus when they are excreted from the body. Simply limiting yourself to one or two six-ounce cups of coffee daily may be enough to prevent or relieve anal itching, says Scott Goldstein, M.D., a colon and rectal surgeon at Thomas Jefferson University Hospital in Philadelphia.

Tame a rebel with a gauze. Place a thin strip of gauze or cotton up against the anal opening to absorb excessive sweat and mucus and to prevent rashes and itching, says Dr. Orkin.

Make like a boxer. Loose cotton underwear is a better choice than clinging nylon or polyester because it absorbs moisture better and allows more air to pass through, keeping your bottom dry, says Dr. Orkin.

Sock it to pinworms. Pinworms generally infect young children, but other family members can attract the unwanted attention of these pests, which come out at night and cause infernal anal itching. Your doctor can prescribe an oral antiparasitic medication to relieve the problem, but you also should thoroughly wash all bedding in hot water to prevent a recurrence.

Check your medications. Some drugs can cause anal itching. Antibiotics, for example, often destroy harmless bacteria in the anus that fight off itchy yeast infections. Ask your doctor if your medications may be causing your problem.

Blow your itch away. Using a hair dryer set on low for 20 to 30 seconds after bathing or swimming is a good way to gently but thoroughly dry your bottom and prevent itching. One precaution: If you feel your skin burning, either the dryer is set too high or it is too close.

Bare your bottom to the sun. "The sun's ultraviolet light can help prevent and relieve itching and other irritations in the anal area and dry the skin. Nude sunbathing is a great way to get some of that sunlight into areas of your backside that are usually left in the dark," says Eric G. Anderson, M.D., a family practice physician in La Jolla, California. As with more modest forms of sun worshipping, you should always apply a sunscreen to exposed skin and build up your time in the sun gradually.

Don't worry. Believe it or not, if you feel anxious or are under a lot of stress, you may develop an itchy anus. Relieving your stress through yoga, progressive relaxation or exercise might end your scratching.

Wash, don't wipe. Good hygiene is crucial to preventing anal itching. If possible, after each bowel movement wash your anus with a soft cloth dipped in warm water and mild soap. Rinse and pat dry; don't rub.

Go for the plain paper. "You should stick to plain, two-ply soft toilet paper and avoid fancy stuff," Dr. Goldstein says. "You don't want anything like perfumes in those papers that may irritate the skin."

ANAL PAIN

WHEN TO SEE YOUR DOCTOR

- You are bleeding from the rectum.
- Your anus feels swollen.
- The pain persists for more than two to three days.
- You have a fever.
- You have changes in bowel habits, such as chronic diarrhea or constipation.

WHAT YOUR SYMPTOM IS TELLING YOU

Somewhere between watching a rerun of "Gilligan's Island" and being branded with a hot poker is a torment called anal pain.

Pain in your bottomside can mean that you simply have a bruise from a nasty fall or that a hemorrhoid has become clotted with blood. Fissures (cracks in the skin surrounding the anus) are another common cause of pain. "Fissures are like cold sores, only they're more painful," explains Robert Gilsdorf, M.D., a general surgeon in Phoenix.

In addition, some people have occasional muscle spasms in their rectums. These spasms, called proctalgia fugax, usually occur at night. Common among teenagers, the painful spasms tend to subside as a person ages, says James Harig, M.D., associate professor of medicine in the Department of Digestive and Liver Diseases at the University of Illinois College of Medicine in Chicago.

On the more serious side, anal pain could be a sign that you have an abscess or a sexually transmitted disease or that your rectum is slipping out of its normal position—a condition that frequently affects older women who have had several children.

SYMPTOM RELIEF

Fortunately, there are a number of easy ways to get fast relief from anal pain.

Submerge your tush. Sitting in a sitz bath—three to four inches of 110° to 115°F water—for 15 minutes two or three times a day may relieve much of your pain. (The water should be very warm, but not painfully hot to your hand.) Covering the area with towels soaked in warm water is an effective alternative.

Numb it. Applying over-the-counter medications containing benzocaine or dibucaine to the tender spot may take some of the sting out of your pain, says Dr. Harig.

Don't forget the water. Drinking six to eight glasses of water a day is a must if you want to prevent constipation and anal pain. "If you don't put enough water into your system, your stool can get hard like a sponge left out on the kitchen counter," says Bruce Orkin, M.D., an assistant professor specializing in colon and rectal surgery at the George Washington University School of Medicine and Health Sciences in Washington, D.C. A hard stool takes more effort to expel from your body, and that extra strain increases your chances of developing a painful fissure or hemorrhoid.

Eat high-fiber foods. Doctors recommend adding more raw fruits, leafy vegetables, whole-grain breads and cereals to increase the amount of fiber in your diet. Fiber increases the bulk and softness of your stool and reduces pressure on blood vessels during bowel movements.

Try laxatives. When you have problems with regularity, doctors recommend bulk-forming laxatives containing psyllium seeds to soften stools and make them easier to expel from your body. Easy evacuation lessens your chance of developing painful symptoms.

K is for Kegel. Usually used to control certain types of incontinence, Kegel exercises also can help strengthen anal muscles and prevent painful hemorrhoids, Dr. Gilsdorf says. Kegels work on the slinglike group of muscles that stretch from the pubic bone in the front to the anus and tailbone in the rear. Squeezing those muscles not only can cut off urinary flow but also can keep the rectal muscles in tone. Although it may vary according to your condition, a typical Kegel regimen might include 20 contractions of these muscles for ten seconds each, four times a day. Ask your doctor if Kegels may be right for you.

Swim like a dolphin. Exercise is an important way to help keep your bowel movements regular. When you experience anal pain, however, you should avoid exercises such as weight lifting that put a strain on anal muscles. "Swimming is good because it's a non-weight-bearing exercise. Tennis and racquetball are okay, too," Dr. Harig says. "But you want to avoid doing squats or anything that increases pressure in the anal area."

ANAL SWELLING

WHEN TO SEE YOUR DOCTOR

- You're bleeding from the anus.
- You're in severe pain.
- You have a fever.
- The swelling isn't painful, but it has persisted and gradually grown larger during the past two weeks.

WHAT YOUR SYMPTOM IS TELLING YOU

Few things can put a damper on a swell time like a swollen tush. No doubt about it, it's really hard to rumba when your rump feels as big as a rutabaga.

Anal swelling is usually caused by a hemorrhoid that has become clotted with blood. "That baby isn't subtle. It's usually a lump and can be quite painful," says James Harig, M.D., associate professor of medicine in the Department of Digestive and Liver Diseases at the University of Illinois College of Medicine in Chicago.

Swelling also can be a sign that you have fissures (cracks in the skin surrounding the anus), a cyst, an abscess or even a sexually transmitted disease.

SYMPTOM RELIEF

In most cases anal swelling will slowly subside over two to three days. But here are a few things you can do to speed the process along or prevent it from happening in the first place.

Mix a potion. Soak a cloth in equal amounts of glycerin and witch hazel and then apply it to the swollen area for about an hour, says Eugene Sullivan, M.D., a colon and rectal surgeon in Portland, Oregon. The glycerin will help relieve the swelling, and the witch hazel, an astringent that has a puckering effect, will soothe the skin. Both are available over-the-counter in most drugstores.

Cool it. "Sometimes ice is just the ticket," Dr. Sullivan says. "Ice is good for acute swelling that comes on suddenly. Heat is more for chronic swelling. Some of my patients put crushed ice into a rubber glove and apply it that way. But one woman just takes a bag of frozen peas or carrots out of her freezer and sits on it."

Sitz down and soothe it. Soaking your tush in a sitz bath—three to four inches of 110° to 115°F water—for 15 minutes two or three times a day also may help reduce swelling. Relax your legs on the sides of the tub to allow the water to get to the sore spot.

Count on hydrocortisone. Over-the-counter hydrocortisone creams and ointments can help deflate swelling. "Hydrocortisone is safe and useful for patients who apply it properly," says Eric G. Anderson, M.D., a family practice physician in La Jolla, California. However, you don't need an overwhelming amount of hydrocortisone to get the job done.

"You should try to get a product that has the least strength of hydrocortisone available and use it as directed," Dr. Anderson advises.

Leave the magazines in the living room. Sitting on the toilet reading your favorite book or newspaper may be a nice diversion, but it also puts unwanted strain on your anal muscles and leaves you vulnerable to discomfort caused by swelling.

"If the bathroom is the only place in the house where you can find privacy, and you do like to read in there, then be sure to put down the toilet seat cover and use it as a chair," says Bruce Orkin, M.D., an assistant professor of colon and rectal surgery at the George Washington University School of Medicine and Health Sciences in Washington, D.C.

Fill up on fiber. Excessive straining during a bowel movement can cause swelling. Doctors recommend regularly eating high-fiber foods such as beans, raw fruits, leafy vegetables and whole-grain breads and cereals that can help soften stools and hasten their voyage through your digestive tract.

ANKLE PAIN

WHEN TO SEE YOUR DOCTOR

- You've injured your ankle and it's so painful that you still can't put your weight on it 24 hours later.
- Your pain is not related to an injury and it lasts for more than four days.
- See your doctor immediately following an injury if, in addition to pain, you experience swelling, bruising or fever, or if the joint feels loose.

WHAT YOUR SYMPTOM IS TELLING YOU

We treat them like beasts of burden, forcing them to support heavy weight, walk great distances, twist, turn and bend in every direction. But push an ankle beyond its limitations—as we often do in sports, for example—and it will cry for help. In some cases, that cry is more like someone screaming in pain.

"The most common injury involves twisting the outer side of the ankle," says Phillip J. Marone, M.D., director of the Jefferson Sports Medicine Center at Thomas Jefferson University Hospital in Philadelphia and physician for the Philadelphia Phillies professional baseball team. "This twist can overstress the supporting ligaments, producing a sprain. Or it could tear a muscle or fracture a bone. Each of these injuries can produce significant swelling, discoloration and loss of motion as well as severe pain."

A twist isn't the only thing that can rankle an ankle. Overuse—excessive walking, standing, climbing or stooping—can lead to tendinitis, an inflammation of the tendons that connect the muscles in the legs to the ankle and foot bones. One common site is the Achilles tendon, which runs from the heel up the back of the ankle. The Achilles tendon can easily pull or tear, especially if it's not flexible enough. Overuse can also produce bursitis—a painful inflammation of the ankle's bursa (a fluid-filled sac at the back of the heel that serves as a protective cushion).

Ankles take abuse in other ways as well. "Poor-fitting, nonsupportive footwear can cause an ankle to ache from twisting or from the impact of hard surfaces," says Edward J. Resnick, M.D., professor of orthopedic surgery at Temple University Hospital in Philadelphia. "Flimsy shoes or those not designed for the task that you are giving them will put a significant strain on the joint."

There are also a few medical conditions that can cause ankle pain. Gout—an intense, throbbing pain and swelling of the joints brought on by deposits of crystallized uric acid—often strikes the ankles. Other ankle aggravators include bone spurs, loose fragments of bone or cartilage, rheumatoid arthritis, bad circulation and nerve damage.

SYMPTOM RELIEF

Ankle pain is not something to be taken lightly. Complications could arise if you delay getting proper medical treatment following an injury. Here are some suggestions for easing the pain.

Apply some RICE. Rest, ice, compression and elevation is your first line of defense for all ankle injuries . . . and most other forms of ankle pain, too.

"Rest is imperative so you don't aggravate an already angry ankle," explains Gary M. Gordon, D.P.M., director of the Running and Walking Clinic at the University of Pennsylvania Sports Medicine Center in Philadelphia. "Bed rest is best; if you have to get around, use crutches or a cane. Ice applied 15 minutes at a time several times per day brings down painful swelling, numbs sensitive nerve endings and constricts capillaries to prevent excess bleeding."

Apply compression with an elastic bandage or use a brace to immobilize the ankle. And elevate the ankle several inches with pillows to drain away fluids. Maintain RICE for three to five days.

Treat your ankle like a headache. Aspirin, ibuprofen and acetaminophen can significantly lessen the pain of a sore ankle, says Dr. Resnick.

Raise your heels. You can relieve a strained Achilles tendon by inserting a lift or pad in the heel of your shoe, according to Dr. Resnick. Half an inch should be sufficient. Pads are available in drugstores and lifts can be fitted by a shoemaker.

Prevent Problems with the Right Shoes

If you tend to injure your ankles often, you might want to take a long hard look at your shoes.

Wear the proper shoe. Are you jogging in tennis shoes? Out on the basketball court in running shoes? Tsk! Tsk! Always wear a shoe designed specifically to give the proper support and protection for your occupation or activity, advises Dr. Resnick.

Install an arch support. All shoes should have adequate support in the arch to prevent pronation—the tendency of the foot to roll inward. This is especially true for people with flat feet. Most quality shoes and sneakers have an adequate arch support already built in, while docksiders, sandals and some lesser-quality shoes do not. You can purchase arch supports to insert in shoes at most pharmacies or shoe stores.

Cushion the blow. If you are on your feet all day, cushioned innersoles, available at drugstores, absorb much of the impact of walking on hard surfaces, says Michael Rask, M.D., chairman of the American Academy of Neurological and Orthopedic Surgeons in Las Vegas.

Put old shoes to rest. Shoes lose their cushioning and support with wear. "Many people wear shoes for one to two years of heavy usage, and that's too long," says Dr. Gordon. "Most shoes only have a life of six to eight months of reliable support."

Dealing with Gout

Once you've been diagnosed with gout, there's a lot you can do to keep ankle pain at bay.

Change your diet. High-purine foods such as dairy products, kidney, liver, shellfish, sardines and nuts can contribute to high levels of uric acid and thus trigger gout attacks, says Dr. Rask. Staying away from these foods will help prevent the problem. Avoid alcohol, too, because it increases your body's production of uric acid. It also helps to drink lots of water; it helps flush uric acid out of the body.

Shed excess pounds. Simply being overweight can put excess stress on your ankles. It's common for people who have gout to be overweight. A lighter load may be all your ankles need.

Ask your doctor about these anti-inflammatory painkillers. Severe bouts with gout and arthritis pain are often brought under control with prescription oral medications like Indocin, Naprosyn and Colchicine. Extreme cases might be treated with injections of steroidal medications like cortisone.

See also Ankle Swelling; Joint Inflammation; Joint Pain; Joint Swelling

ANKLE SWELLING

WHEN TO SEE YOUR DOCTOR

- See your doctor immediately if you twist your ankle and it causes swelling, bruising and pain.
- Any unexplained swelling lasts more than 72 hours.
- The swelling seems to be getting worse, or you cannot walk following an injury.

WHAT YOUR SYMPTOM IS TELLING YOU

The human ankle is truly an astounding example of biomechanical engineering—an interactive network of bones, nerves, muscles and blood vessels working in precise harmony. But like most complex systems, if you disrupt that harmony, the whole system can suddenly go haywire.

When you severely injure an ankle, that once-quiet joint becomes a hotbed of activity, according to Gary M. Gordon, D.P.M., director of the Running and Walking Clinic at the University of Pennsylvania Sports Medicine Center in Philadelphia. "Nerves, muscles and other tissues become aggravated. Vessels and capillaries tear, leaking blood. More blood rushes to the area to begin the healing process. Fluids accumulate faster than they can be removed, and you have swelling."

The most common ankle injuries involve an inversion—or inward wrenching of the joint—resulting in a sprain (a tearing of the ligament), strain (a tearing of a muscle or tendon) or even bone fracture. All three can swell, hurt and leave an ugly bruise. Only a physician can properly diagnose which one you have.

In addition to injury, there are a number of other possible causes for a swollen ankle. And all of them are fairly common. Chronic overuse—doing too much, too soon, too fast—can lead to excess fluid accumulation and swelling. It can cause tendinitis, for example, an inflammation of the tendons. In tendinitis, stretching and repetitive action tear or irritate a tendon, causing it to swell. Underuse can also be a problem. If you're prone to water retention, just lazing around on a hot day can produce grapefruit-size ankles. So can certain medications.

Even something as commonplace as shoes can turn traitor and transform ankles into mini-replicas of the Hindenburg. "A shoe that's too loose or too tight, worn out, flimsy or inadequate for the way it's being used can swell an ankle well above it's normal size," says Michael Rask, M.D., chairman of the American Academy of Neurological and Orthopedic Surgeons in Las Vegas.

Circulatory and vascular diseases can also produce swelling. Venous insufficiency—a weakness in the valves of the veins—can cause blood to back up in the ankles, leading to an uncomfortable swelling. Swelling can also result from heart failure, which has many causes, such as high blood pressure, heart attack or anything that weakens the heart muscle.

Other common causes of chronic ankle swelling are lymphatic and kidney disease, diabetes, gout and rheumatoid arthritis.

SYMPTOM RELIEF

Athletes usually make quick recoveries from sore or swollen ankles because they are properly diagnosed as soon as possible. Take a tip from the pros: Don't take chances when your ankle puffs up following an injury; see a doctor. Your doctor will order x-rays to rule out fractures. Here are some treatments your doctor may recommend as well as a few things you can try on your own.

Serve up some RICE. It's not the "San Francisco Treat," but an acronym for the most reliable treatment of injury and noninjury related swelling: rest—taking a load off your feet; ice—15-minute applications several times a day to control bleeding and leaking of fluids; compression—using an elastic bandage or ankle brace to immobilize the joint; and elevation—propping up the ankle so gravity can pull the fluids away. Maintain RICE for three to five days.

Choose pain relievers carefully. Anti-inflammatory pain relievers, like aspirin and ibuprofen may reduce pain but must be avoided when an injury causes a swollen ankle, because they can promote bleeding, says Dr. Gordon. Acetaminophen, like Tylenol, is good for pain and does not have anti-inflammatory properties, he says.

Let your fingers do the walking. "As long as there is no pain, massaging the ankle is excellent," says Dr. Gordon. "It should be a gentle kneading with the fingers once or twice a day, pushing everything up toward the knee to force the fluids away from the joint."

Walk in the water. Strolling around in waist-deep water is an excellent and gentle means of exercising an ankle and reducing swelling, says Dr. Gordon. "The movement of water against the muscles helps pump out the fluids that accumulate."

Change your prescription. Puffy ankles are often the result of a reaction to a medication. Ask your doctor if any of your medications could be contributing to the problem and whether a different prescription or different dosage is appropriate.

Wear a running shoe. A worn, improper or poorly constructed shoe may be the culprit that caused your swelling in the first place. If you have to get around on swollen ankles, the best shoe is a quality running shoe, says Phillip J. Marone, M.D., director of the Jefferson Sports Medicine Center at Thomas Jefferson University Hospital in Philadelphia and physician for the Philadelphia Phillies professional baseball team. "It's light, comfortable and has the sole, arch and ankle support so as not to aggravate the situation."

Take a hike. Chronic swollen ankles are a way of life for the sedentary. The lack of muscle movement only causes fluids to accumulate, causing further decreases in activity. According to Dr. Gordon, a regular walking and exercise program can break this vicious cycle and bring ankles back to normal.

Go for the cold. Especially in the early stages of an injury. "Heat dilates the capillaries, but stimulates the leaking of blood and other fluids, making the swelling worse," says Dr. Gordon. Ice is much better at re-establishing a healthy blood flow, he says. Soaking your feet and ankles in cold water for 15 to 20 minutes at a time may provide some relief.

See also Ankle Pain; Water Retention

ANXIETY

WHEN TO SEE YOUR DOCTOR

- You find yourself avoiding situations, places or people in order to avoid feeling anxious.
- You have chronic symptoms, such as tension, headaches, muscle aches, bowel trouble, shortness of breath, chest discomfort, stomach problems or dizziness.
- You have panic attacks (short, unexplained periods of intense fear or discomfort).

WHAT YOUR SYMPTOM IS TELLING YOU

How could you possibly prepare for a test, meet a deadline or psych yourself up for an important event without at least a few butterflies flitting through your stomach? "Some level of anxiety is probably healthy," says Jack Maser, M.D., a psychiatrist with the National Institutes of Mental Health. "It motivates you to get up and do something."

But when the butterflies feel more like swarms of skittering bats, and you feel trapped in a cycle of uneasy fears that just won't let up—your anxiety has become a problem.

SYMPTOM RELIEF

Those bats *can* be turned back into butterflies. There are a variety of therapies, practical approaches and medical treatments to help control anxiety.

Take a motion potion. Ventilate your anxiety by taking it for a walk. A daily exercise program of at least a half-hour will help, says Bernard Vittone, M.D., a psychiatrist and director of the National Center for the Treatment of Phobias, Anxiety and Depression in Washington, D.C.

Make yours decaf. When you're anxious, drinking caffeine is like pouring gasoline on a fire, Dr. Vittone says.

Ban the bottle. Even though alcohol may seem to calm you at first, the next day you will feel much more anxious, because of the irritating effect that withdrawal from alcohol has on the brain, says Dr. Vittone.

Breathe easy. Hyperventilation, or overbreathing, is a prime suspect in anxiety and can leave you feeling light-headed, anxious and depressed, says Herbert Fensterheim, Ph.D., clinical professor of psychology in psychiatry at Cornell University Medical College in New York City.

"The main difficulty is not breathing too fast but breathing with the upper part of the chest rather than the diaphragm," Dr. Fensterheim says. Breathing more deeply can help you relax, he says. To do that, lie down and place one hand on your chest and the other on your abdomen. Breathe through your nose, letting only the hand on your abdomen rise and fall. Practicing a deep-breathing exercise such as this one will help teach you how to control your breathing when your anxiety level creeps up, says Dr. Fensterheim. Focusing on your breathing can actually help you cope with anxiety, he says.

Sit in the worry chair. One common cause of anxiety is letting yourself become overwhelmed by all your worries, says Dr. Vittone. Instead of worrying aimlessly all day, he suggests, set aside 30 minutes a day to sit and do nothing but worry. When anxiety sneaks in during the day, tell yourself, "I'm going to worry about that later, during my worry time."

Quick Fixes for Anxious Moments

Ruth Knowles Grainger, Ph.D., an advanced registered nurse practitioner and clinical director of the Therapy Research Institute in Miami, Florida, offers these tips for instant anxiety relief.

Look up. Research shows that our feelings intensify when we're looking down. Scan the ceiling.

Breathe calmly. Slow your breathing, exhale completely and mentally add a one-word soother with each exhalation, like "Calm...calm...calm."

Soften that shrug. Raised shoulders and tension go together. Lower your shoulders to ease the tension.

Slow your thinking. Think in slow, complete sentences when anxious thoughts are coming on too rapidly.

Alter your voice. Slowing, lowering and softening your voice conveys calm and control to others as well as yourself.

Move your body. Run in place or dance for a few moments when you feel your anxiety level rising.

Let your face fix it. When you smooth out your forehead and turn up the corners of your mouth, you can fool your brain into lightening up.

Be a fly on the wall. Change your perspective by imagining yourself watching a tense, anxious person (you) from another angle—the ceiling or the other side of the room.

When Anxiety Just Won't Yield

Tried everything and still shaking in the breeze? You might want to talk to your doctor about anti-anxiety medication, or ask him for a referral to a therapist.

Try the thinking therapy. Your doctor may recommend that you visit a cognitive therapist. These anxiety experts can help you change the thoughts that might be triggering your anxiety.

"There's nothing mysterious, magical or frightening about therapy," says Jerilyn Ross, psychotherapist and director of the Ross Center for Anxiety and Related Disorders in Washington, D.C. "You'll be taught various exercises and techniques to help you understand and face what's keeping you stuck."

Find help at your pharmacy. Your doctor may prescribe medication for short-term or occasional use. Effective drugs include benzodiazepines, tricyclic antidepressants and monoamine oxidase inhibitors (MAOIs). There are important dietary restrictions to follow with MAOIs, so be sure to ask your doctor for a list of foods to avoid.

What If It's a Panic Attack?

A panic attack is anxiety run amok. Some people prone to anxiety may suffer sudden, short periods of intense fear or discomfort. Symptoms can include shortness of breath, dizziness or faintness, trembling, palpitations or rapid heartbeat, sweating, choking, stomach upset, numbness or tingling, flushes or chills, chest pain or discomfort and fear of dying or going crazy.

Panic attacks are a problem that you should discuss with your doctor. There are, however, a few things that you can try on your own. Dr. Vittone offers these six steps.

1. Reassure yourself that the attack will pass, usually within five or ten minutes.
2. Remind yourself, even though you may feel terrified, that no one has ever died or gone mad from a panic attack. Tell yourself, "This *will* pass."
3. Ride with your feelings, telling yourself, "These are just feelings." Allow yourself to experience having trouble breathing, and just breathe slowly. You *are* getting sufficient oxygen.
4. Every minute or two, rate your anxiety on a scale of one to ten. You'll find that although levels fluctuate, it's gradually going down.
5. Take ten slow, deep, diaphragmatic breaths. Check your anxiety level again.
6. Focus on physical things around you. Mentally describe the room, your clothes, sounds, smells. Stay in the present, and get your attention from inside your body to outside.

Repeat these steps until the panic subsides.

APPETITE LOSS

WHEN TO SEE YOUR DOCTOR

- You lose your appetite for more than two weeks.
- You are also experiencing frequent fatigue, a change in taste sensitivity or pain anywhere in your body.

WHAT YOUR SYMPTOM IS TELLING YOU

If you're like most people, a temporarily misplaced appetite is a welcome opportunity to reduce calories. (Visions of fitting back into last year's jeans dance in your head.) But when the days stretch into weeks and treats that normally tempt you continue to turn you off, there could be cause for concern.

Undereating or a loss of appetite is a common symptom that could signal any number of conditions, many of which are no big deal.

Almost any infection could cause a loss of appetite, according to Donald S. Robertson, M.D., medical director of Southwest Bariatric Nutrition Center in Scottsdale, Arizona, and coauthor of *The Snowbird Diet*. A passing cold or flu virus could be responsible, for example. So could more serious things like tuberculosis, low thyroid function, diseases of the heart or lungs or liver problems.

"Unfortunately, one of the most common early warning signs for cancer is appetite loss, which is usually accompanied by changes in taste sensitivity," says Robin Kanarek, Ph.D., professor of psychology and physiological psychologist at Tufts University in Medford, Massachusetts.

"Appetite loss is the body's defense against ingesting anything that could slow the healing process," explains David Levitsky, Ph.D., professor of nutrition and psychology at Cornell University in Ithaca, New York.

Disease is not the only thing that can dampen the appetite, however. Sometimes things you take into your body on purpose—prescription drugs, for example—can cause problems, according to G. Michael Steelman, M.D., vice president of the American Society of Bariatric Physicians, who is in private practice in Oklahoma City. Antibiotics like erythromycin inhibit the taste buds and slow the transport of food through the intestines, prolonging the feeling of fullness after you eat, he explains. And amphetamines—which were once commonly prescribed for weight loss—dull hunger pangs, says Dr. Robertson.

Pain relievers and anti-arthritis medications can irritate the stomach, producing nausea and an aversion to food. Digitalis (a heart medication) and diuretics (taken to combat fluid retention and lower high blood pressure) can also dampen the desire to eat.

Sometimes what you *don't* put in your mouth can cause problems. Overall nutritional deficiencies can sap the vitality right out of an otherwise healthy appetite, Dr. Steelman says. Older people, in particular, may suffer from an inadequate intake of zinc, a deficiency that can deaden taste buds.

Aging itself exacts a toll on the appetite. In older people the metabolism slows down, muscle mass decreases and physical ailments impede activity, Dr. Steelman explains. On top of all this, taste sensations diminish and stomach secretions don't flow like they used to. All of these things contribute to appetite loss.

And sometimes things that are happening in your life affect your appetite. "If you've recently begun a new exercise program, you could experience appetite loss while your body adjusts to its new demands," says Dr. Levitsky.

Psychological health, in general, plays a big role in your appetite. Over the long haul, stress can send you to the fridge for the consoling comfort of food, Dr. Steelman says. But short-term pressures usually depress the appetite. Depression robs some people of their desire to eat.

And anorexia nervosa is a disorder that forces people— usually young women—to almost completely deny the need to eat. "They're obsessed with food, but they're afraid of eating for fear of getting fat," Dr. Steelman says. "For them, it's easier not to eat anything than eat rationally."

SYMPTOM RELIEF

A brief loss of appetite is no reason to worry. But if you can't remember the last time you felt like eating, you might want to try restoring your normal eating habits. Here are a few things to be aware of.

Know what's normal. What exactly *is* a healthy appetite? "It's a level of eating that maintains normal body weight," says Dr. Kanarek.

"If you have a healthy appetite, you consume a variety of foods. A hearty appetite for nothing but steak is not a healthy appetite," adds Adam Drewnowski, Ph.D., professor and director of the Human Nutrition Program at the University of Michigan School of Public Health in Ann Arbor.

"If you must constantly *force* yourself to eat, that's not a good sign," adds Dr. Levitsky.

Vitamins may revitalize. A daily multivitamin and mineral supplement seems to help stimulate a stubborn appetite, Dr. Steelman says. And the extra nutrients certainly can't hurt if your undereating has caused undernourishment. Older people can sometimes rev up their desire to eat by taking zinc supplements, says Dr. Steelman. Ask your doctor whether a zinc supplement is appropriate for you.

Review your medications. Ask your doctor about all the medications you are currently taking—both prescription and over-the-counter. He may be able to substitute drugs that don't interfere with your appetite, Dr. Steelman says.

Eat anything you want. If food has lost its appeal, try changing your diet. Determine which foods are appetizing, and concentrate on eating them. If you only want ice cream, go ahead and indulge in your favorite flavor. "I'm not advocating an unhealthy diet, but if ice cream is the only way to get necessary calories into your body then, by all means, go ahead," says Dr. Drewnowski. "The trick is to increase the pleasantness quotient."

Downsize your eating habits. Eat smaller, more frequent meals, suggests Dr. Kanarek. Your stomach will accept smaller amounts of food more readily, she explains.

Drink plenty of water. If you've started a new exercise

program, your most important nutrient is water. Dehydration can cause appetite loss, advises Dr. Levitsky. Drink a glass of water before your workout and another immediately afterward. In addition, make sure you drink six to eight eight-ounce glasses of water every day.

Doctor your appetite. If you don't find your misplaced appetite after two weeks, see your doctor for a checkup. Physical problems must first be diagnosed before any treatment begins. You might find that all you need is a course of antibiotics to knock out a low-grade infection.

Take stock of mental health. If you are depressed, antidepressant medications might be prescribed to stimulate your appetite. By bringing your mental health back to normal, you'll find yourself wanting to eat again, says Dr. Kanarek. (For other tips on dealing with depression, see page 144.)

Let the pros help. Anorexia nervosa usually doesn't lend itself to self-help remedies, and most people with the disorder need to be hospitalized. "It's tough to treat," Dr. Steelman says. "It requires intense therapy from a psychological and nutritional standpoint." Forced feeding through intravenous injections or a gastric tube may be necessary.

ARM PAIN

WHEN TO SEE YOUR DOCTOR

- Your arm hurts for more than two days.
- The pain gets worse with work or exercise.
- You lose feeling in the affected arm or hand.
- The arm also appears deformed or swollen.
- You cannot move or straighten your arm.
- Arm pain accompanied by chest pain or shortness of breath may signal a heart attack. Treat this as a medical emergency.

WHAT YOUR SYMPTOM IS TELLING YOU

The arm is an amazingly adaptable tool. You use it for everything from throwing baseballs to lugging grocery bags to waving bye-bye. But like any tool, it can only take so much abuse.

The causes of arm pain are numerous, but most often it can be traced back to one thing: muscle fatigue. What feels sore and tired today should feel better tomorrow, no problem. But if the pain comes and goes—and comes back again—without an obvious cause, it might be arthritis.

If your pain sneaks up gradually and hangs around like an annoying relative, you might have a broken bone in your forearm or upper arm. You might think that broken bones are always obvious, but it is possible to experience a fracture without realizing it. You might hit your arm or fall, for example, and not feel the pain until you increase your level of activity or put stress on the broken area.

It's also possible for injuries to your wrist to cause considerable pain in your forearm. Among the most common are so-called repetitive motion injuries caused by something like typing, hammering or lifting. "The pain gets worse and worse as the week goes on because the arm isn't rested," says Tee Guidotti, M.D., M.P.H., a professor of occupational medicine at the University of Alberta in Edmonton, Alberta. "Eventually the strain on the tissues exceeds the ability of the arm to recover." Even though the injury affects mainly the wrist, the pain can spread all the way to the elbow.

It's hard to injure the upper arm itself because it's so well muscled. One common cause of arm pain that affects the upper arm directly, however, is bicipital tendinitis, in which a tendon near the shoulder is frayed or torn, triggering a flare-up of pain in the biceps of the upper arm.

Pain from elsewhere in the body can be referred to the upper arm. Lifting heavy weights, for example, can inflame the tendons in the shoulders, which shows up as pain in the upper arm.

Severe pain radiating down the left arm is a classic sign of heart attack. It can be accompanied by nausea, shortness of breath or chest pain, but sometimes pain in the left arm is the only symptom.

SYMPTOM RELIEF

Treatment for arm pain depends on what part of the arm hurts and how badly it is injured. But here are a few rules of thumb.

Easy does it. If your pain isn't severe and there's no obvious deformity, doctors recommend starting with the most conservative treatment of all: rest. Give your arm a break from activity for a few days.

Slow but steady. If complete rest isn't possible—for example, if you have to use those aching forearms for work—cut the activity in half. Spread the task out and take frequent breaks. "It's reasonable to get people to the point where they are able to continue their activity at a level where they don't experience pain," says Andrew Tucker, M.D., a family practitioner specializing in sports medicine at the Cleveland Clinic Foundation in Ohio. "But it's unwise to work or play through significant pain. Pain is a warning sign."

Hang 'em high. Raise the arm to about the level of your chest during periods of rest. For example, if you're sitting on the couch, prop up your arm on a few fluffy pillows.

Be cool. Try running an ice cube back and forth over the painful area until the skin goes just numb to the touch, no longer than four minutes, advises Steven Bogard, lead physical therapist at the Mayo Clinic Hand Center in Rochester, Minnesota. Check the skin to make sure it isn't getting white or blue. Or use a chemical "quick-cold" pack wrapped in a wet towel, keeping it over the site for up to 20 minutes. Check the skin every 10 minutes.

Medicate. Take an over-the-counter pain reliever as needed, following the package directions, says Bogard.

Pick up the phone. If you try all these approaches and the pain is still there, call your doctor. Further treatment may include cortisone shots to reduce tissue swelling, lightweight splints and, in extreme cases, surgery to correct the underlying disorder.

ARM WEAKNESS

WHEN TO SEE YOUR DOCTOR

- You experience a loss of sensation or a feeling of numbness lasting more than a few minutes.
- If your arm simply doesn't work, treat it as a medical emergency.
- You've recently had an accident and your arm looks deformed or misshapen, or you hear a popping, clicking or grinding noise from the joints.

WHAT YOUR SYMPTOM IS TELLING YOU

While the arm is generally designed to take a lot of abuse, certain parts are vulnerable to injury. Quite often, weakness in the upper arm results from a kind of internal squeeze play. At some point between the neck and fingertips, a nerve or blood vessel may be compressed, perhaps between the muscles of the neck and shoulder. Blood flow to the affected area may be slowed to a trickle, and the nerve endings of the arm may not be able to transmit signals to the brain at full strength, creating a sensation of numbness or weakness.

These nerve injuries go by many names—thoracic outlet syndrome (if the compression is somewhere between the shoulder and neck), ulnar nerve entrapment (specifically from the elbow down) and carpal tunnel syndrome (in the wrist and hand)—but they all have one thing in common. They involve the nerves (and sometimes the arteries) that run the length of the arm from the neck down.

Another compression injury, often overlooked, is an ulnar neuropathy, which can occur where the ulnar nerve that passes under the elbow—the so-called funny bone—is injured, causing numbness and tingling in the hand as well as pain in the elbow. People who lean on hard surfaces sometimes develop this problem. Bicyclists report a similar loss of feeling in their fingers. In this case, leaning on the handlebars with their hands puts undue pressure on the ulnar nerve, a hazard known as ulnar tunnel syndrome.

These injuries are usually triggered by repetitive motions of the arm over many weeks or months, says David Rempel, M.D., an assistant professor of medicine at the University of California, San Francisco, and a biomedical engineer specializing in work-related musculoskeletal disorders. For example, electricians, who use a constant twisting motion to turn screwdrivers and wire strippers, are vulnerable to injury in the tendons of the elbow.

All of these abused tendons, ligaments and muscles have a tendency to get good and angry. They puff up and crowd in on the nearby nerve. Although these injuries occur in the elbow, wrist and shoulder, they often cause a sensation of weakness in the forearm or upper arm, says Steven Bogard, lead physical therapist for the Mayo Clinic Hand Center in Rochester, Minnesota.

SYMPTOM RELIEF

The treatment depends on the diagnosis. Restoring strength to a bum arm can be as benign as rest and as serious as surgery. Here's what to do.

Call in the experts. "If there's a nerve entrapment, the first thing is to determine how severe it is," says Dr. Rempel. "Doctors send some people to surgery right away, especially if the symptoms are persistent. But we start with conservative management: Rest until the symptoms subside, use splints, and perhaps inject cortisone to reduce the inflammation."

Put it to the test. Your doctor may order a battery of electrodiagnostic tests to determine where the nerve is compromised; other tests may measure the arm's sensitivity to pressure or temperature. Your doctor may also assess your grip strength or have you move the affected joint or limb, to determine how weak it is.

Go back to school. You may benefit from some retraining by an occupational or physical therapist to teach you ways of performing your job—or your favorite sport—with less strain on your arm. For example, sitting lower on your bike seat and wearing padded gloves may prevent ulnar tunnel syndrome. Getting special padded armrests may relieve pressure on your elbows, preventing ulnar neuropathy. But the earlier the problem is treated, the better. These injuries are nothing to fool around with. In time, an injured nerve could become damaged beyond repair, causing permanent weakness. "Even if you were to attempt to correct it with surgery later on, the recovery is frequently limited," explains Dr. Rempel. "What doctors really prefer to do is keep the problem from becoming disabling."

B

BACK STIFFNESS

- Your stiff back is interfering with your work or home activities.

WHAT YOUR SYMPTOM IS TELLING YOU

Back stiffness is often a message from the body that goes something like this: *Read my hips, spine and shoulders—no more improper movements.*

That's because improperly performed movements can cause stiffness and pain. Rearranging the living room furniture, preparing the garden for planting, roughhousing with the grandkids—any activity that you're not used to and not in shape for—can wrench back muscles or ligaments or injure spinal disks. (Disks are the rubbery, doughnut-shaped cushions located between the vertebrae of the spine.) Then the back stiffens up to protect itself from further injury.

"Improper movement is what causes most back problems," says Philip Paul Tygiel, a physical therapist who serves as a consultant for the University of Arizona University Medical Center Back Pain Clinic in Tucson. "How many people say they slowly developed back stiffness? No, they moved wrong, they bent over too quickly, they picked something up the wrong way, and now they're stiff and hurting."

Of course, improper movement isn't the *only* cause of a stiff back. Too soft or too hard a mattress or sleeping in an awkward position has also been known to create back stiffness.

38

SYMPTOM RELIEF

Your stiff back may seem like it's made of stone, but you can snap back to normal, pain-free movement by following these tips.

Imitate a cobra. Here's a simple yoga pose that can loosen your back. First, lie facedown on the floor. Place your palms on the floor directly under your shoulders. Now gently raise your torso off the ground, supporting yourself with your arms and keeping your hips on the ground. Go just to the point of tension and then come all the way back down. Relax for a moment, then repeat the exercise several times, trying to go a little further each time, says physical therapist Wayne Rath, co-director of Summit Physical Therapy and senior lecturer of the McKenzie Institute International (U.S. Headquarters) in Syracuse, New York, and clinical assistant professor in the Department of Physical Therapy at Thomas Jefferson University in Philadelphia. Do not perform the exercise if it's painful.

Take a walk. Walking balances the mechanical stress on the spine caused by bending and sitting and allows the disks the freedom to move back into their proper position, says Rath.

Untie those knots. Place your hands in the small of your back, stand up tall and carefully lean backward without bending your knees. This moves your spine in the opposite direction of nearly all your activities, helping to balance the mechanical stress on your disks, says Rath. If you work at a desk, repeat this movement twice every hour on the hour, he says.

Make it hot. In chronic back disorders, moist heat can help a stiff back. The warmth increases the flow of blood and oxygen to the injured area, which speeds healing and brings relief, says Brent V. Lovejoy, D.O., a member of the board of trustees of the American Osteopathic College of Preventive Medicine and director of the Rocky Mountain Medical Group in Denver. Soak a towel in hot water, wring it out and place it on the stiff area of your back until it cools. One caution: Don't apply heat for the first three days following an injury.

Don't be a softy. Does your bed sag when you climb into it? If it does, you might want to think about getting a new mattress. A mattress that provides firm support is usually kinder to your back and may help alleviate morning stiffness.

See also Lower Back Pain; Midback Pain; Neck Stiffness; Upper Back Pain

BAD BREATH

WHEN TO SEE YOUR DOCTOR

- Regular and thorough brushing of the teeth and tongue and flossing fail to eliminate the odor.
- A foul breath odor is accompanied by bleeding, swelling or pain in your mouth or throat.

WHAT YOUR SYMPTOM IS TELLING YOU

You have to wonder why bad breath isn't discussed more often on the talk shows. After all, if you believe TV ads, the main reason why young love is victorious and old love renewed is because the breath of the lovers was sweet as...well, as mint or cherry flavoring.

Yes, as breath sours, so sours love. But what *really* gets those violins playing is a toothbrush and floss. That's because bad breath more often than not indicates gum inflammation called gingivitis or the more damaging gum disease periodontitis.

For any number of reasons—but most often because you haven't brushed and flossed as well as you should have— bacteria accumulate in your mouth, on your teeth and on your gums like mildew in a wet corner of the shower. If you don't keep teeth and gums free of the bacterial buildup, they'll start to cause odor as the bacteria rot leftover food particles in your mouth. This bacterial buildup can also lead to gum disease, according to Timothy Durham, D.D.S., director of adult general dentistry at the University of Nebraska Medical Center in Omaha. You also may even notice some bleeding or swelling of your gums along with the bad breath, he says.

If gingivitis and plaque aren't giving you breath that could fell a flower, dry mouth could also be the culprit. While some people have chronically arid oral cavities, most of us notice this dryness when we awaken. "Overnight, saliva flow is significantly reduced," Dr. Durham says, "and saliva contains protective enzymes that help keep bacteria in the mouth low." Without saliva, it doesn't take long for bacteria counts to build up. When you awaken, you have morning breath, and the only thing you want to kiss or be kissed by is a bottle of mouthwash.

Medications can also sour your breath. "Antihistamines and many over-the-counter drugs for sinus problems can cause bad breath because they dry out the mouth along with the nose," Dr. Durham says. Certain antidepressant drugs have a similar saliva-depressing side effect.

Other producers of bad breath, dentists say, include sinus or airway tract infections, inflamed tonsils or adenoids, mouth breathing, mouth ulcers, tooth decay, tooth abscesses and diseases of the liver or lungs. People with diabetes can have a sweetly acidic scent to their breath that may be somewhat objectionable. Digestive problems in which food finds its way back up the esophagus can also create an unpleasant odor.

SYMPTOM RELIEF

Even if you have advancing gingivitis or periodontal disease, "the best thing you can do to eliminate bad breath is brush and floss and see a dentist for consultation and treatment of the gum problem," Dr. Durham says. See the chapter on gum problems (page 261) for how to brush properly, and check out these extra air fresheners.

Get cheeky. Don't forget to brush the insides of your cheeks, Dr. Durham says. "You should remove any debris and buildup there, too. You don't have to scrub," he says. "A few passes of the brush will do."

Brush your tongue. You often can eliminate bad breath simply by brushing your tongue, which holds the same plaque and bacteria found around your gums, Dr. Durham says. Try to brush your tongue as far back as possible, he suggests.

Dump mouthwash down the drain. All of those mouthwashes you see on TV and lining drugstore shelves are little better than useless in countering the true source of bad breath. "Brushing your teeth is a better solution than washing your mouth," says Michael Weisenfeld, D.D.S., spokesperson for the Academy of General Dentistry and a dental consultant with a private practice in Livonia, Michigan. "All mouthwashes do is mask the real problem, and they're not even a good way to cover it up at that. They're mostly just flavored water." The rare exceptions are available only by prescription, he says.

Dr. Durham agrees. "Using a mouthwash is like someone who doesn't take a bath for several days and then puts on lots of perfume to cover the odor," he says.

Take the pledge. If you suffer from dry mouth and choose to use mouthwash, look for a preparation that does not contain a high alcohol content, Dr. Durham says. Alcohol will dry out your mouth and enhance noxious emissions.

Wet your whistle. Keeping your mouth moist will help prevent the buildup of bacteria and plaque, dentists say. (For tips on dealing with a dry mouth, see page 415.)

Breathe on your dentist. If after scrupulous scrubbing you still have breath that would stop a steer stampede, it's time to visit the dentist because, most likely, plaque has hardened into tartar and your gingivitis is getting worse. "If you don't keep the plaque off, you have to come to one of us," Dr. Weisenfeld says, "and we have to scrape it off." If that doesn't do it, the dentist will have to look for other causes.

BALANCE PROBLEMS

WHEN TO SEE YOUR DOCTOR

- You also have a sudden change in your hearing or ringing in your ears.
- Your ears feel clogged all the time.
- You feel nauseated or lose your balance and fall.

WHAT YOUR SYMPTOM IS TELLING YOU

In your dreams, you nimbly stroll across Niagara Falls on a high wire. But in reality, you're about as steady on your feet as Woody Allen dancing *Swan Lake* in a tutu.

What's going on here? Normally, your eyes, inner ears, muscles, brain and nerves work in conjunction with each other to maintain you in an upright position as you go about your daily business. You hardly notice this finely tuned collaboration, but once it's disrupted, you experience balance problems.

A multitude of ailments can send you reeling, including ear disorders, allergies, muscle weakness, vision problems, arthritis and stroke.

SYMPTOM RELIEF

In many cases your sense of balance can be regained with a few simple adjustments.

Watch what you eat. Some foods and food additives trigger allergic reactions that can affect your sense of balance. "I have a particular sensitivity to monosodium glutamate (MSG). It causes me to have some breathing problems, but sometimes it also causes some unsteadiness," says Ronald Amedee, M.D., associate professor of head and neck surgery at Tulane University Medical Center in New Orleans. If you suspect a food allergy may be contributing to your balance problem, try eliminating that food from your diet and check with your doctor about it, advises Dr. Amedee.

Question your medications. Some drugs have balance problems as a possible side effect. Ask your physician to review any medications you may be taking—both prescription and over-the-counter types. He may be able to suggest alternatives.

Shy away from alcohol. "Alcohol creates a sensation in the inner ear similar to what astronauts feel while floating weightless in space," Dr. Amedee says. "If you drink regularly and to excess, you're going to have a problem with your balance. The easiest way to treat that problem is to cut your alcohol consumption."

Give coffee the cold shoulder. Coffee constricts blood vessels and drastically reduces blood flow to the brain. "We routinely tell our patients who have balance disorders to cut back on their coffee consumption," says Dennis O'Leary, Ph.D., director of the Balance Center at the University of Southern California University Hospital in Los Angeles. "One or two eight-ounce cups of coffee is fine; five or six is not."

Stroll away from it. Some people have difficulty maintaining their balance because they have weak muscles. "They know what they need to do to keep their balance, but they just don't have the strength to do it," says Peter Roland, M.D., an otologist at the University of Texas Southwestern Medical Center in Dallas. "Doing weight training and some form of cardiovascular exercise, such as aerobics, walking or riding a stationary bike, is terribly important for people, particularly the elderly, who want to regain their ability to maintain their balance."

Use it or lose it. Regular exercise also may help your body's balance system adapt and heal itself. "You should try to do any activity where you are moving and trying to keep your balance at the same time," says Jim Buskirk, a physical therapist at the Dizziness and Balance Center in Wilmette, Illinois. "Racquet sports like tennis are especially good because they develop hand/eye coordination and force you to focus on a moving object."

Practice walking on soft surfaces. The softer the surface that you walk on, the more difficult it is to maintain your balance, Dr. O'Leary says. If you practice walking on a piece of foam rubber, thick carpet or even a mattress, you might learn how to stand more erect or plant your feet differently so you feel more stable when walking on all types of surfaces, he says. If you attempt this, you should have a person standing by to catch you in case you fall.

Create a safe haven. Safety begins at home and that's particularly true for people with balance problems. Slick surfaces are dangerous, so remove scatter rugs and avoid polished floors, Dr. O'Leary says. Get a night-light and make sure your stairways are equipped with railings. To help keep your balance while showering, keep your eyes open.

Use your imagination. Imagery or visualization can help you learn to regain your balance, says Dennis Gersten, M.D., a San Diego psychiatrist and publisher of *Atlantis: The Imagery Newsletter*. To try it, sit in a chair and take a few deep breaths to relax. Then close your eyes and imagine that you're in a room with two poles on the floor forming a big X. Up through the middle of the X is a vertical pole that you are standing next to. "In your imagination, stand at the center of these three poles and try to maintain your balance," Dr. Gersten says. "Every time you move or fall off of center, step right back to the center and rebalance. Keep practicing this until maintaining your balance becomes an effortless task in your mind."

See also Dizziness; Walking Difficulty

BEDSORES

WHEN TO SEE YOUR DOCTOR

- You have a red, irritated bedsore that doesn't heal after two weeks of self-care.
- The skin around a bedsore ruptures or cracks.
- Your bedsores or the areas around them show signs of infection: swelling, soreness, discharge or heat.
- You also have a fever.

WHAT YOUR SYMPTOM IS TELLING YOU

Bedsores aren't so much a problem of skin against bed. They're a problem of bone against skin. When you lie in the same spot without moving for a long period of time, areas of the body where bone is close to skin can get red and start feeling sore. That's because the tender skin gets "squeezed" between bone and bed.

"Bedsores usually crop up in areas of the body where there is underlying bone that is fairly close to the surface of the skin," says Rebekah Wang-Cheng, M.D., associate professor of general internal medicine at the Medical College of Wisconsin in Milwaukee. "The pressure causes the skin to become irritated and inflamed."

Bedsores are actually a misnomer; they don't happen only to those who are bedridden. "People who are in wheelchairs also have problems because there is even more pressure on certain points, like the buttocks, when you're sitting up."

In its early stages, a bedsore—more accurately called a pressure ulcer or pressure sore—may look like a red patch that doesn't go away. If left untreated, these sores can grow. Eventually, the skin will crack and an open wound and infection will develop. In very severe cases, the tissue can even erode to the point of exposing bone or muscle.

Obviously, bedsores are common among the bedridden.

Anyone who spends a few weeks in the hospital and even a few days in bed with the flu can develop sore, red skin. "Pressure sores can begin after just an hour of pressure on the skin," Dr. Wang-Cheng says. And they can be aggravated by anything that creates friction on the skin, such as poor hygiene, wetness from incontinence, poor blood circulation, chafing caused by efforts to move about in bed—all common problems for those who are seriously ill. Bedsores most commonly develop on the back, tailbone and buttocks. But they also can form on the knees, ankles, heels and back of the head.

Bedsores are also more common among older people, because they are usually less active and their skin is thinner and less able to withstand pressure.

SYMPTOM RELIEF

The best time to treat a bedsore is before a blister forms, Dr. Wang-Cheng says. "Once there is a blister, you're in for a long wait. These sores heal very slowly," she explains. "You're going to be measuring your recovery in terms of weeks, not days."

The best thing to do is to stop them before they start. Constantly check the skin of a bedridden person for irritation. If you find bedsores developing, here's what to do.

Take a load off. Relieving pressure on the sore spot is the most important thing you can do, Dr. Wang-Cheng says. For example, move the bedridden person from side to side if the sores are on the back. If a person confined to a wheelchair is getting sores on the buttocks, get him off his bottom and into bed and on his side or stomach until the sore heals.

Keep moving. Change body positions frequently. If the person is capable of moving, be sure he shifts his weight every 15 minutes, says Dr. Wang-Cheng. If the person you're caring for is immobile, move him into a new position at least once an hour (if he's in a wheelchair) or once every two hours (if he's bedridden).

Float on air. "A lot of people try using egg crate or

sheepskin mattress coverings. But those two things don't reduce the pressure on the skin enough to prevent bedsores," Dr. Wang-Cheng says. An air mattress with a bedside pump that alternately inflates and deflates the mattress is a much better way to reduce pressure on the sores. These mattresses are available at many medical supply stores.

Keep it under wraps. Clean the bedsore with saline solution. Then cover it with a transparent film bandage that seals itself around the wound and can be left in place for up to four days. "The body is producing growth factors that help heal the wound. But if you're changing that bandage every day, those growth factors are whisked off the skin before they have a chance to work," says Kevin Welch, M.D., assistant professor of dermatology at the University of Arizona Health Sciences Center in Tucson. "An airtight dressing will help keep the growth factors in contact with the wound and promote healing." These bandages, called occlusive dressings, are available at most medical supply stores.

Be gentle. "Because of the irritating effects of stool and urine on the skin, people who are incontinent and immobile are four times more likely to develop pressure sores than those who aren't," says Katherine Jeter, Ed.D., an enterostomal therapist in Spartanburg, South Carolina, and executive director of Help for Incontinent People. "These people need intensive skin care. Use products such as spray washes and moisture barriers that are specifically made for incontinence." Most of these products are available at medical supply stores.

Eat, drink and keep your skin healthy. "Malnutrition is one of the first things we look for in people who have bedsores," Dr. Jeter says. "The skin is the body's largest organ, and just like any other organ of the body, it will suffer severe damage when it doesn't get a sufficient amount of nutrients." To keep skin nourished, drink at least eight glasses of water a day and eat a balanced diet including plenty of protein. Protein is the body's repairman and is vital for maintaining healthy skin.

Take vitamin C. "Studies suggest that taking 500 milligrams of vitamin C supplements twice a day helps reduce the size of some bedsores by as much as 84 percent," Dr. Wang-Cheng says. Before taking vitamin C therapy, however, get your doctor's approval.

BED-WETTING

WHEN TO SEE YOUR DOCTOR

- Bed-wetting persists almost nightly after the age of seven.
- Urination is painful.
- Bed-wetting is accompanied by loud snoring.

WHAT YOUR SYMPTOM IS TELLING YOU

It's not the kids' fault, plain and simple. They're not doing it to make Mom wash the sheets every day. And they're certainly not doing it to embarrass their parents—the kids are humiliated enough and don't have a desire to spread the shame.

Almost every child wets the bed. Most kids simply grow out of it, says Neil B. Kavey, M.D., director of the Sleep Disorders Center at Columbia Presbyterian Medical Center in New York City. Those who don't—and many people into their teens and twenties have not learned to control their bladders while they sleep—can be treated. "They have to know they're not a lost cause," he says.

SYMPTOM RELIEF

More boys than girls are bed-wetters, physicians who are sleep experts say. Heredity plays a strong role in determining whether the child will wet the bed and when to be concerned if he or she doesn't stop at an early age. "If the father wet the bed until he was nine," Dr. Kavey says,

"there's no need to rush to the doctor if the child is six."
Still, here are the options to consider.

Remember and confess. "The first goal is to minimize
the trauma on the family and especially on the child," Dr.
Kavey says. Kids don't enjoy waking up in the middle of the
night drenched in urine. Their humiliation can be eased
somewhat if parents explain that bed-wetting runs in the
family. "You have to look at grandfathers, grandmothers,
aunts and uncles," Dr. Kavey says. "And fathers can con-
veniently forget that they, too, wet the bed when they were
young."

Check for medical problems. Urinary tract infections
and, curiously enough, severe respiratory restrictions like
sleep apnea can cause bed-wetting. If the urinary infection
is cured, bed-wetting stops.

Many children who continue to wet the bed also snore
and appear to have significantly obstructed upper airways,
a condition known as obstructed sleep disorder, according
to Dudley J. Weider, M.D., a professor of surgery (otolaryngology) at Dartmouth-Hitchcock Medical Center in
Lebanon, New Hampshire. If tonsils and adenoids are
removed to treat the disorder, in about three-quarters of the
cases studied so far, the soaked sheets dry up.

Poor sleep patterns associated with sleep apnea and
obstructed sleep disorder prevent people from drifting into
the deepest stages of sleep, Dr. Weider explains. Only during those deepest stages are certain pituitary hormones
secreted, and one of them, a natural antidiuretic hormone,
seems to regulate the production of urine, he suspects.

As of yet, throat operations aren't performed merely to
stop bed-wetting. But for those who have serious breathing obstructions, "the difference is like night and day."

Buy an alarm. Bed pads attached to alarms that ring at
the first drop of moisture are still probably the best method
to end bed-wetting, Dr. Kavey says. But they should be used
only when the children recognize they need to help themselves in stopping. "If they see it as an imposition," he says,
"it won't be effective."

Build that bladder. Exercises can help increase bladder
capacity and the ability to hold back urination, according

to Dr. Kavey. Try encouraging your child to delay going to the bathroom for 10 to 30 minutes after he or she feels the need to urinate, he suggests. Pelvic constriction exercises like Kegels can help them gain more control over starting and stopping the urinary flow. Ask your child's pediatrician to teach your child these exercises, if appropriate.

Don't drink the water? Many pediatricians and bed-wetting experts frown on the idea of restricting fluids before going to bed, Dr. Kavey says. "But it's something to try, if you'd like, because the idea does make sense," he says.

Medicate for special occasions. A few prescription drugs, such as imipramine and DDAVP (a synthetic version of the natural pituitary hormone) can almost miraculously end bed-wetting—but only as long as they're used. "You can use them, say, when your child is going to camp or to sleep over at a friend's house," Dr. Kavey says, "but once you take away the drug, the bed-wetting usually returns."

BIRTHMARK CHANGES

WHEN TO SEE YOUR DOCTOR

- Your birthmark changes in size, shape or color.
- Your birthmark starts to itch, burn or sting or develops bumps or sores.

WHAT YOUR SYMPTOM IS TELLING YOU

It's not unusual for a newborn's peaches-and-cream complexion to have a strawberry garnish. A strawberry mark—one of the most common birthmarks—looks like a flattened version of its namesake that's been stuck on the skin.

Strawberry marks—and all other birthmarks for that matter—can either already be there when the baby enters the world or show up soon after birth, says Robert J. Friedman,

M.D., clinical assistant professor of dermatology at New York University School of Medicine in New York City.

One change you can expect from any newborn's birthmark is growth. As the child increases in size, so does the birthmark, explains Dr. Friedman. "As a person grows from infancy to adulthood, a birthmark on the face becomes eight times larger," says Robert E. Clark, M.D., Ph.D., director of the Dermatologic Surgery and Cutaneous Oncology Unit at Duke University Medical Center in Durham, North Carolina.

Here's a primer on the kinds of changes that the most common types of birthmarks can undergo.

Strawberry marks—which get their ruddy color from blood vessels at the skin's surface—very often disappear by the time a child is six years old, says William Dvorine, M.D., chief of the Section of Dermatology at St. Agnes Hospital in Baltimore and author of *A Dermatologist's Guide to Home Skin Treatment.*

Port wine stains, which are often very large, are also caused by blood vessels—in this case an extensive network. In time, port wine stains can become darker, thicker and bumpy, according to Joseph G. Morelli, M.D., associate professor in the departments of dermatology and pediatrics at the University of Colorado Health Sciences Center in Denver.

A *congenital nevus*—a brown to brownish black mark—can range in size from very tiny to (rarely) enormous, says Dr. Morelli. A small percentage of these kinds of birthmarks become cancerous in adulthood. For that reason, they must be carefully watched for changes in size, shape or color.

Cafe au lait spots are like dashes of extra melanin (a natural brown pigment) splashed across the skin. They rarely change except possibly to get a little darker, says Dr. Dvorine. And when they do change, it's no big deal.

SYMPTOM RELIEF

So suppose you notice a change in one of your birthmarks. Or suppose you want the birthmark to do a permanent disappearing act. What do you do about it?

Watch and wait. "Watching and waiting is the best technique for most strawberry marks," says Dr. Friedman. Marks that don't go away on their own can be removed by freezing, surgical excision, laser treatments or injections with a substance that collapses them.

Make stains disappear. Port wine stains were permanent—until the laser came along. "It's a wonderful development in medical science because it literally revolutionizes the lives of patients," says Dr. Clark. (Unfortunately, the treatment doesn't work as well in dark-skinned people because it can destroy pigment cells, leaving white spots.) If port wine stains show signs of growing and developing bumps, it's probably a good idea to get them removed. They aren't dangerous, but they can become increasingly unsightly.

Operate immediately. A congenital nevus that changes—a sign of a possible malignancy—is always removed surgically so it can be examined, says Dr. Dvorine. Large marks are often removed at birth as a precaution.

BLEEDING

WHEN TO SEE YOUR DOCTOR

- You bleed heavily and persistently when you get a cut or wound.
- If blood is spurting, go to an emergency room.

WHAT YOUR SYMPTOM IS TELLING YOU

Your stir-fry dinner was turned into a bedtime snack while you waited for your finger to stop bleeding after you cut *it* instead of the onion. And yesterday, you nearly missed your bus because a shaving mishap took a half-hour (and half a roll of toilet paper) before the blood was stanched.

Few of us escape our "slice of life"—whether it's from the knife in the kitchen, the razor in the bathroom or the blade in the workshop. But a lot of blood doesn't always mean a lot of damage.

"The face and scalp are heavily lined with small blood vessels and a shaving nick or a slight cut on the scalp can bleed profusely," says Kurt Kleinschmidt, M.D., director of the Emergency Medicine Program at Darnall Army Hospital in Fort Hood, Texas.

Normally, blood oozing from a minor cut soon stops by itself or with simple control measures. If bleeding seems to continue longer than usual, it may be because you've recently taken aspirin, a painkiller that also delays clotting. In fact, many stroke-prone people take aspirin to prevent abnormal clotting and to keep their blood thin and flowing. The downside is that it also keeps blood flowing from minor injuries. "Taking a single aspirin can interfere with clotting for up to two weeks," says Dr. Kleinschmidt.

You may also bleed excessively when you get a cut or wound if you're taking warfarin (an anti-clotting drug prescribed for heart problems) or vitamin E.

Other factors linked to abnormal or profuse bleeding include hormonal disorders and damage to internal blood vessels caused by an infection, an ulcer or gastritis.

SYMPTOM RELIEF

Your doctor should evaluate any heavy or persistent bleeding so he can find the cause, says Dr. Kleinschmidt. This will also help prevent iron-deficiency anemia, which can result from heavy blood loss.

For the run-of-the-mill cut or nick, here's what you can do.

Press firmly. For any bleeding, press firmly and directly over the wound, using a clean cloth. "Pressure seals off ruptured blood vessels and allows natural clots to form faster," says Dr. Kleinschmidt. But don't lift the cloth for any reason—moving it will disturb the clotting mechanism. If blood seeps through the cloth, simply place another cloth on top of the soaked one and continue to apply pressure.

Once the bleeding has stopped for ten minutes, remove the cloth, cleanse the wound with soap and water, apply a dab of antibiotic cream and cover the wound with an airtight, adhesive bandage.

Take a deep breath. "The sight of blood—especially if there is lots of it—presses the panic button in some people," says Clorinda Margolis, Ph.D., clinical professor of psychology and human behavior at Jefferson Medical College of Thomas Jefferson University in Philadelphia. Taking several slow, deep breaths can reduce your panic and may even help wounds clot quicker, she says.

Avoid aspirin before surgery. "We advise people not to take aspirin for eight to ten days before surgery or a trip to the dentist," says Robert E. Clark, M.D., Ph.D., director of the Dermatologic Surgery and Cutaneous Oncology Unit at Duke University Medical Center in Durham, North Carolina. The same holds for vitamin E and other anticoagulants. If you need to take a pain reliever, try acetaminophen. It doesn't block clotting.

Stock up on styptic pencils. Some people—such as those at risk for stroke—*must* take an anti-clotting medicine. For them, a shaving nick or nosebleed can turn into an endless leak. Styptic pencils can help save the day, says Dr. Clark. The active ingredients in these little white wands narrow blood vessels, tighten the skin and help speed the clotting of minor cuts.

Handle sharp objects with care. If you take an anti-coagulant, always keep first-aid kits or adhesive bandages wherever you use sharp utensils or tools. For prevention, wear protective gloves when using sharp objects such as hedge trimmers. "Wearing Playtex gloves may even be prudent when slicing vegetables," says Dr. Clark. And whatever you do, when you handle something sharp, *don't rush*. For example, take your time shaving your face or legs, especially when the razor rounds the jawbone or ankle bone, where nicks are more likely.

BLEEDING AFTER INTERCOURSE

WHEN TO SEE YOUR DOCTOR

- You experience bleeding after intercourse anytime other than during your menstrual period.

WHAT YOUR SYMPTOM IS TELLING YOU

Although exuberant or rough sex can cause occasional bleeding, infection is a more likely suspect. Aspirin, blood-thinning drugs or birth control pills may also cause post-sex bleeding. And you'll want to rule out the possibility that your partner is the one with the problem.

Benign cervical polyps can bleed when touched during intercourse. And rarely, bleeding can result from abnormal cell changes in the cervix, certain blood diseases or uterine cancer.

SYMPTOM RELIEF

Don't worry though; a visit to your doctor can help you to clear up the cause of those stains.

Don't wash away the evidence. Your post-sex bleeding is a symptom, not a crime. So don't douche before seeing your doctor, says Roger Smith, M.D., professor of obstetrics and gynecology at the Medical College of Georgia Hospital and Clinics in Augusta. It's important that your doctor be able to see the source of the problem.

Fine-tune your prescription. Sometimes low-dose birth control pills may cause hypoplasia—a too-thin uterine lining—which in turn may cause bleeding after sex. Missing a pill or taking one late may also trigger this bleeding, which is just a nuisance, not a danger sign, says Dr. Smith.

Your doctor may need to change your prescription to clear up the bleeding.

Eliminate the "-itis." Hormones can interact with normal genital bacteria to create cervical irritation (cervicitis). Cervicitis is the most common cause of bleeding after intercourse and may frequently cause spotting, not just after intercourse. It's generally not dangerous, says John Grossman, M.D., a gynecologist at George Washington University Hospital and Medical Center in Washington, D.C., and it can be treated with antibiotic creams. (Antibiotics can also clear up vaginitis, which sometimes causes bleeding.) For a persistent irritation, your doctor may recommend cauterization, a simple surgical procedure.

Cancel out chlamydia. If your doctor finds a chlamydial infection, you'll need either tetracycline antibiotics or a family of medicines called the fluoridated quinolones, says Dr. Grossman.

Prune the polyps. Endocervical polyps—benign grape-like growths that protrude through the cervix—may cause bleeding when they're jostled during lovemaking. Your doctor may recommend that they be surgically removed, which usually involves only a simple procedure done right in the office, says Dr. Grossman.

Update your Pap. A doctor who finds abnormal cells in your Pap smear may recommend minor surgery, either cryosurgery (which kills the cells by freezing) or cauterization (which kills the cells with heat).

BLINKING

WHEN TO SEE YOUR DOCTOR

- Your contact lenses cause persistent rapid blinking.
- Your blinking is so frequent and forceful that your face contorts.

WHAT YOUR SYMPTOM IS TELLING YOU

Blinking is like breathing: It goes on whether you're
aware of it or not. Several times a minute, your lids are
busy swishing away dust, keeping your eyes moist and
comfortable.

This slow lid action gears up to a quick flutter if your
eyes are threatened in any way—by a flying fist or a flash of
light, for example. Constant blinking, however, can be an
S.O.S. that your eyes are too dry or they've been invaded by
a foreign body that won't flush out with normal blinking.

The irritating combination of dry eyes plus contact
lenses can make you blink like a police car on the chase.
Excessive blinking may be a reaction to a buildup of debris
on the lenses.

Older people who have had a stroke or have Parkinson's
disease can have a lid spasm that causes them to frequently
squeeze their eyes shut forcefully, according to Douglas
Fredrick, M.D., clinical instructor of ophthalmology at the
University of California in San Francisco. This kind of
spasm worsens with anxiety, he says, and may be accompanied by facial contortions.

SYMPTOM RELIEF

Frequently, the key to ending excessive blinking is in
keeping your eyes moist and protecting them from irritation. Consider the following.

Use fake tears. Artificial tears that mimic your own will
help moisten eyes dried out from smoke, smog or other
causes. (For more tips on dealing with dry eyes, see page 188.)

Give your lenses a bath. Contact lens wearers can keep
their eyes moist by using a wetting agent, such as ReFresh
P.M., throughout the day, says Dr. Fredrick. Look for wetting agents—and all other lens solutions—without preservatives. Preservatives can be irritating to sensitive eyes, he
says.

Let your eyes wake up slowly. Allow your eyes to
"breathe" for an hour before inserting contacts, suggests

Mitchell H. Friedlaender, M.D., director of corneal services in the Division of Ophthalmology at the Scripps Clinic and Research Foundation in La Jolla, California, and coauthor of *20/20: A Total Guide to Improving Your Vision and Preventing Eye Disease*. This will help give your eyes time to adjust to being awake and focused and may reduce discomfort, he says.

Consider breathable lenses. Gas-permeable lenses allow more oxygen to reach the eye than more rigid lenses and are less likely to suffocate and irritate the eye. Plus, they won't readily absorb irritating mucus and particles in the lens surface, says Dr. Friedlaender.

Look into disposable lenses. You wear them 'round the clock for a week. Then you toss them and insert a fresh pair, thereby eliminating the protein buildup problem of standard soft lenses. Before inserting the new pair, however, spend a night sleeping lensless, says Eleanor Faye, M.D., ophthalmologic surgeon at the Manhattan Eye, Ear and Throat Hospital. This lets your eyeballs breathe, she says. Do not try to clean these flimsy lenses, and never reinsert disposables.

Put in eye whiteners at bedtime. As you prepare for a lensless night, use a decongestant/antihistamine eyedrop, which your doctor can prescribe. It'll reduce itchiness and swelling and control contact lens sensitivity, says Dr. Faye. If you still have a problem with contact lenses, remove them and see your doctor as soon as possible.

Medicate the muscle. If your blinking is caused by an involuntary muscle spasm from a nervous system disorder, your doctor can prescribe a medication that controls the spasm, says Dr. Fredrick.

BLISTERS

WHEN TO SEE YOUR DOCTOR

- You've just started taking a new medication (even one you've taken before without problems.)
- You are elderly or have diabetes and suddenly get blisters on your feet or ankles.
- Your blisters don't start healing after a day or two, or become pus-filled, red, hot or painful.
- You have a blister that's larger than two inches in diameter.
- You have painful blisters around your mouth.
- You don't know what's causing the blisters.

WHAT YOUR SYMPTOM IS TELLING YOU

You spend a day in the sun—perhaps hiking in new boots or rowing a canoe. Say hello to blisters.

Things like stiff shoes or rowing—if you're not used to it—can cause friction blisters. And blistery sunburn is inevitable if your unprotected skin is exposed to the sun long enough.

The causes of most blisters are obvious, says Guy F. Webster, M.D., Ph.D., assistant professor of dermatology and director of the Center for Cutaneous Pharmacology at Thomas Jefferson University in Philadelphia. "Other causes are a little more obscure, though," he says. For example, reactions to medications—including some antibiotics, diuretics and pain relievers—can raise blisters anywhere or everywhere on your body.

There are also blister-raising infectious diseases—ranging in severity from a touch of athlete's foot or herpes (fever blisters) to extensive blistering from shingles (adult chickenpox).

Finally, close encounters with substances that you're

allergic to—poison ivy, for example—can raise whole patches of itchy blisters.

No matter what the cause, blisters are all alike: "They're separations of the skin's outer layer from its inner layer," says Ellen Cohen-Sobel, D.P.M., Ph.D., associate professor of podiatric orthopedics at New York College of Podiatric Medicine in New York City. Liquid between the estranged layers forms a little water balloon.

SYMPTOM RELIEF

How you treat a blister will depend very much on how many there are and the cause. Here are a few things to be aware of.

Leave it alone if you can. Intact blisters are best left undisturbed. "By *not* popping a blister, the skin underneath can heal in a happy environment. And if it's bathed in body fluids, it's happy," says Dr. Webster.

"If you're hiking and a large blister is physically in the way, you might make an exception and drain it," says Jerold Z. Kaplan, M.D., medical director of the Alta Bates Burn Center in Berkeley, California. A doctor does this by drawing fluid out with a sterile syringe, Dr. Kaplan explains. "To doctor yourself, hold a needle under a flame or use rubbing alcohol to sterilize it. Then gently poke a hole near the edge of the blister, push the fluid out and cover the area with a bandage. Don't rip the blister's whole roof off," he instructs. (It might be a good idea to include a couple of needles in your backpack first-aid kit.)

Patch the roof. "If a blister's already rubbed open, fold the skin back in place so you have your own skin protecting the soreness," says Mark D. Sussman, D.P.M., of Wheaton, Maryland, a podiatrist and coauthor of several foot-care books, including *The Family Foot-Care Book*. Then dab it with antiseptic first-aid cream and cover it with a fabric— not plastic—bandage. Pharmacies and some sporting goods stores carry products made specifically for covering blisters as well.

Walk away from pressure. The best way to take pressure off intact foot blisters is to pad around them with adhesive felt or foam, which you can buy in a drugstore. Nonmedicated callus or corn pads work too, says Dr. Sussman. Bandage the area and change shoes to eliminate the source of friction. Make sure there is a small area of nonblistered skin around the pad so it doesn't impinge on the edges of the blister.

Protect the little ones. Protect small, ruptured blisters with something nonadherent, such as Vaseline Gauze, Dr. Kaplan suggests. Then cover the Vaseline Gauze with a plain gauze bandage. You can coat small broken blisters—like burst sunburn blisters—with Preparation H, says Dr. Kaplan. "It's not an FDA-approved use, but it will help them heal," he says.

Solve a blister mystery. Blisters from medications and most infectious diseases should be seen by a doctor. (In fact, show any blisters that you can't account for or don't go away in one week to your doctor.) Treatment may include switching medications or an antibiotic to clear up an infection.

See also Cold Sores; Foot Itching; Rashes

BLOATING

WHEN TO SEE YOUR DOCTOR

- You have persistent, unexplained bloating for more than three days.
- You also have abdominal pain.

WHAT YOUR SYMPTOM IS TELLING YOU

A single scoop of cherry vanilla ice cream; several sips of a frothy, strawberry shake; a few bites of a cream cheese omelet—as much as you love dairy foods, they don't seem to love you. Eating even modest portions makes your stomach balloon up, and you feel uncomfortably stuffed.

Doctors call the gassiness, bloating and discomfort that occurs after eating dairy foods lactose intolerance. It means your stomach is unable to digest the lactose—or milk sugar—in dairy foods.

Unfortunately, most adults have this problem to some degree, according to Jay A. Perman, M.D., associate professor and director of the Division of Gastroenterology and Nutrition in the Department of Pediatrics at Johns Hopkins University School of Medicine in Baltimore. As people age, he says, they produce less lactase—the enzyme needed to digest lactose. Without lactase, the undigested milk sugar ferments and gases form. The trapped gas makes your stomach bloat.

Other hard-to-digest foods—such as beans, nuts, seeds, fruits, brussels sprouts, oats, barley, honey and yeast—can also cause gas and an inflated stomach.

Food allergies can cause your stomach to puff out, too. But this is a reaction of the immune system involving the whole body, and usually hives and runny nose are the more prominent symptoms.

If your digestive system is the least bit sensitive—and you have what's called irritable bowel—then, milk, beans and other common problem foods may be even more intolerable. With an irritable bowel, the nerves in your intestines may overreact to irritating food and drink. This triggers spasms in the muscle wall of the large intestine. The contents can't move along, so you become constipated. This distends the bowel. As the contents ferment, gases are produced, making you bloat even more.

If you eat your food too quickly, you'll swallow air, which also stretches out the bowel.

Persistent bloating with pain could indicate a number of digestive diseases. These include obstructions in the bowel or kidney, diverticulitis, appendicitis, gallstones, ulcers or a tumor.

SYMPTOM RELIEF

Here's what to do if you're feeling bloated.

Take a post-meal stroll. Besides nudging bowel contents along, exercise may release hormones that encourage bowel activity, according to Ralph Bernstein, M.D., clinical professor of medicine at the University of California and chief of gastroenterology at Highland Hospital in Oakland.

Get rid of gas. To deflate that full feeling, try Phazyme 95. This over-the-counter medication contains simethicone, which quickly breaks up gas bubbles, says Ronald Hoffman, M.D., director of the Hoffman Center for Holistic Medicine in New York City.

Try herb tea. For on-the-spot relief, try a cup of peppermint, chamomile or fennel tea, says Dr. Hoffman. These herbs help relieve gas.

Get more fiber. Fiber softens the bowel contents and seems to help if bloating is caused by intestinal spasms. You can add fiber to your diet by eating vegetables and whole grains, says Roger Gebhard, M.D., gastroenterologist at the Veterans Administration Medical Center and professor of medicine at the Univeristy of Minnesota in Minneapolis. But wheat starch may cause bloating, he adds, so try switching to rice and potatoes, which contain starch that is more easily tolerated. Or try a tablespoon of Metamucil mixed into juice once a day. "In some people, Metamucil may cause gas, although generally this seems to be a more tolerable form of roughage," says Dr. Gebhard.

Skip the stimulants. Coffee, tea and chocolate can all overexcite the digestive tract, says Dr. Gebhard. Fat is another food that's often hard to digest and may stimulate spasms—and consequently bloating—in the bowel, he adds.

Approach milk with respect. Just because milk and dairy products cause bloating doesn't mean you have to give them up. You can drink lactose-free milk, which tastes sweeter, or add liquid lactase to your dairy products, says Dr. Perman. Both the more easily tolerated milk and the digestive enzyme are available at many supermarkets and health food stores. Nonfrozen yogurt and aged cheeses such

as Romano have only small amounts of lactose in them, so
you may be able to eat them without a problem, says Dr.
Perman.

Avoid too-hot or too-cold foods. You may be unconsciously drawing in air when tasting foods that are extreme
in temperature, says Dr. Gebhard. Bubbly beverages and
chewing gum can also make you swallow air, so it's a good
idea to avoid them as well.

Slow down; chew carefully. When you eat too fast, you
can easily trap a pint or more of air in your gut. With slow,
careful chewing, you'll take in less air and you'll drench
your food with saliva, says Dr. Hoffman. Saliva contains
enzymes that begin to break down food before it even
reaches your gut.

Take a PMS supplement. "Prior to menstruation, the
female abdomen often becomes the repository of all fluids,
much like camels' humps," says Michele Harrison, M.D.,
professor of psychiatry at the University of Pittsburgh and
author of *Self-Help for Premenstrual Syndrome*. Women
who take supplements containing the B-complex vitamins
and also magnesium and calcium seem to have fewer complaints about bloating, she says.

Keep a bloat diary. People have different reactions to
specific foods, according to Dr. Hoffman. A diary will help
you identify your own troublemakers so you can reduce
portions or eliminate them.

Get a diagnosis. Bloating can signal any of several serious digestive diseases, says Dr. Gebhard. If none of these
self-help remedies provides help, see your doctor for a thorough exam.

See also Constipation; Gas; Water Retention

BODY ODOR

WHEN TO SEE YOUR DOCTOR

- The odor occurs on a daily basis and is noticeable to others, despite judicious hygiene.
- The odor is so strong that you notice it.
- You have a sweet or fruity odor or one that varies from the traditional "locker room" smell.
- Any body odor in a prepubescent child should be brought to the attention of a doctor.

WHAT YOUR SYMPTOM IS TELLING YOU

As any subway rider can tell you, the aromatic emanations of the human body are sometimes enough to make a person seriously question just how far man has evolved as a species. B.O. may be the fragrance of choice in the animal kingdom, but in the civilized world it's not going to be confused with Chanel No. 5.

The popular notion that body odor is the smell of sweat is true . . . sort of. We actually produce two kinds of sweat: *eccrine*, a clear, odorless sweat that appears all over our bodies, performing the vital role of regulating body temperature, and *apocrine*, a thicker substance that is produced by glands in the underarm and groin areas. Apocrine sweat is a vestige of our prehistoric days and serves no apparent purpose. It, too, is odorless—until bacteria on the skin's surface act upon it. The by-product of this unholy union is what we call B.O.

"The intensity of some body odor may lead people to think that they have a serious medical problem, when in most cases they are merely the victims of bad genes or inadequate hygiene," says Selma Targovnik, M.D., staff dermatologist at Good Samaritan Medical Center in Phoenix. "Most B.O. sufferers were simply born with larger, more active apocrine glands, or else they aren't doing as good a job as they should keeping the odor-producing bacteria off their skin."

"We don't know of any illnesses that cause that locker-room, apocrine smell, but some diseases will produce other kinds of skin odors," says R. Kenneth Landow, M.D., clinical associate professor in the Department of Medicine and Dermatology at the University of Southern California in Los Angeles. "Gastrointestinal abnormalities can give the skin a very unusual smell. Diabetics and people with urinary infections will sometimes develop a sweet-smelling or fruity body odor. Diseases of the past, like the vitamin C deficiency disease scurvy and typhoid fever, were associated with strange smells."

In adolescents, B.O. is a sign of puberty, when the apocrine glands are first activated. Aging and metabolic changes can also bring on increased apocrine activity. And the smell of certain pungent foods (like garlic) can ultimately work its way through your pores and into the nostrils of others.

SYMPTOM RELIEF

The secret to combating most body odors is to inhibit the body's production of apocrine sweat, decrease the number of bacteria acting upon that sweat or remove the offender. Give these tips a try, and soon you, and those around you, will be enjoying the sweet smell of your successful war against B.O.

Wash daily with a deodorant soap. "Using an antibacterial soap like Dial or Safeguard will work well on the bacteria that are producing the odor," say Dr. Targovnik. "You don't have to scrub long or hard; the antibacterial will do all the work. Use it at least once a day, twice, if possible." If these fail, more powerful prescription soaps like pHisoHex and Hibiclens are available.

Zap it like a zit. If antibacterial soaps aren't producing results, Dr. Targovnik suggests washing the areas with an acne cleanser such as those that contain benzoyl peroxide, which has strong antibacterial properties. But be aware: Excessive use could cause drying and irritation. If these cleansers don't work, you can also try dabbing on some Neosporin or an antibacterial ointment.

Freshen up. "During the day, if you can do a quick wash of your armpits with a wet washcloth or paper towel, you can take care of some of that odorous material that has been produced as well as many of those bacteria that will produce odor in the future," says Dr. Targovnik.

Use a deodorant. "Over-the-counter underarm deodorants will work fine on all odor-producing areas," says Stephen Z. Smith, M.D., a dermatologist in private practice and clinical instructor in the Department of Dermatology at the University of Louisville School of Medicine in Kentucky. "Check your labels. The deodorant should contain antibacterial metallic salts (aluminum or zinc) to kill odor-causing bacteria. Roll-ons and sticks will provide better coverage and longer-lasting protection than sprays."

Use an antiperspirant. "Commercial antiperspirants will slow down some of the apocrine sweat production," adds Dr. Smith. "They should contain aluminum chlorohydrate as their active ingredient and are often combined with deodorants."

Powder the offensive area. "Sprinkling some baking soda, talc, baby powder or cornstarch under the arms or across the body will absorb and mask many of the odors produced," says Dr. Landow.

Get the odor out of your clothes. Wash your clothes with an odor-fighting detergent. If necessary, take a change of clothes or underwear with you to work or school.

Rub on some alcohol. "You may want to try directly applying a splash or two of some rubbing alcohol, witch hazel or hydrogen peroxide during the day just as some extra maintenance," recommends Dr. Landow. These substances help reduce the number of odor-causing bacteria. Aim your splash where bacteria hang out—under the arms, for instance.

Avoid spicy, pungent foods. Frequent consumption of foods containing garlic, curry and cumin can cause some overpowering odors to emanate from your pores—often up to 24 hours after consumption. Try cutting back on these spices and see if it helps.

Trim underarm and body hair. "Since men are the biggest offenders, they should follow the example of women and shave their armpits," says Dr. Targovnik. "The hairs trap a lot of the sweat and odor and provide hiding places for the bacteria."

BOILS

WHEN TO SEE YOUR DOCTOR

- You have a boil with redness around it.
- You have red streaks spreading from the boil.
- You also have a fever.
- You also have diabetes.
- You are taking antibiotics or cortisone medication.

WHAT YOUR SYMPTOM IS TELLING YOU

A boil is just what it looks like: a big pimple. Perhaps it's called a boil because of how it feels—hot and painful.

The angry, red swelling and pain are the result of an infection, usually an infection involving *Staphylococcus cuteus* (staph) bacteria. Staph germs love hospitals, so it's very easy to pick up boils during an extended hospital stay. Or you might have a carrier of the staph bacteria in your family or among your acquaintances. It's hard to tell who's the culprit. The people carrying the bacteria that cause boils may never develop boils of their own. The germs can hang out in the nasal passages without causing any symptoms—until they get passed on to another person.

You can also get a boil after taking antibiotics. Staph bacteria may become resistant to antibiotics, and with all their competition killed off they can spread and create problems, such as boils. Taking cortisone may decrease resistance to boils.

Doctors say you are more likely to develop a boil if you have a condition like diabetes or if your immune system is suppressed.

SYMPTOM RELIEF

There's just one home treatment uniformly recommended for boils. Beyond that, for sure and safe results, see your doctor.

Soothe it with heat. Try treating the boil with a hot compress, says J. Michael Maloney, M.D., a dermatologist in private practice in Denver. "Put a washcloth under hot water and lay it over the boil for five minutes, or sit in a hot bath if the boil is on your bottom," he says. After several days of hot compress treatments, often a boil will spontaneously rupture and drain some puslike, yellow, foul-smelling material. Afterward, you should feel much better, Dr. Maloney says.

Get it lanced. If your boil won't respond to hot compresses, you should see your doctor, who may decide to lance it, says Alan R. Shalita, M.D., professor and chairman of dermatology at the State University of New York Health Science Center at Brooklyn. "Your doctor will numb the boil, nick the center and drain out the contents," he says.

Do not lance a boil yourself, he adds, because you can spread the infection.

Cure the infection. Your doctor will most likely do a bacterial culture and treat the boil with an appropriate antibiotic, says Dr. Shalita. Often, he says, boils are treated with dicloxacillin—a penicillin derivative designed specifically for staph infection. If your boils occur over and over in the armpits and genital area, this may be related to a type of acne, not an infection. In that case, your doctor may recommend long-term antibiotics, says Libby Edwards, M.D., chief of dermatology at the Carolinas Medical Center in Charlotte, North Carolina.

For these types of boils, you'll need to take antibiotics with anti-inflammatory properties, such as tetracycline, erythromycin or minocycline, she says. Penicillin won't help clear them up.

Keep it clean. Once your boil has drained, be sure to keep the area clean with an antibacterial soap, says Dr. Maloney. Good soaps to use are pHisoHex, Dial or Safeguard.

Consider cortisone. If your doctor says your boil is actually an early acne or epidermal cyst, and the center is not yet too full of liquid, "a tiny amount of injected cortisone may tremendously improve it within a day," says Dr. Edwards.

Clean up the carriers. If boils seem to be passing around the family, your doctor can help to break the cycle, says Ralph Coskey, M.D., clinical professor of dermatology at Wayne State University School of Medicine in Detroit. "Antibiotics in the nose may prevent repeated spreading back and forth among family members," he says. Your doctor can do a simple nasal culture test to determine who is carrying the infection.

BREAST CHANGES

WHEN TO SEE YOUR DOCTOR

- You discover an unusual lump.
- You have a spontaneous nipple discharge, rough skin with enlarged pores, red patches or a bulge or dimpling in the contour of one of your breasts.

WHAT YOUR SYMPTOM IS TELLING YOU

If women were made of marble, they would have eternally firm, smooth, symmetrical breasts like the statue of Venus. Flesh-and-blood women, however, have breasts that are constantly changing.

Gaining or losing weight causes changes in the breasts. So do a woman's hormones. Prior to each menstrual period, the surge in estrogen and progesterone stimulates fluid retention and growth in breast tissue. Breasts may swell an entire bra size every month and also become tender and lumpy. Then when menopause arrives, breasts may lose their firmness.

All these breast changes are normal and shouldn't be cause for alarm, according to Kathleen Mayzel, M.D., director of the Faulkner Breast Centre in Boston. "The time for concern is if you notice any sudden or unusual changes in the shape, texture or feel of the breasts," says Dr. Mayzel.

A dimpling of the breast skin or nipple could be from the loss of elasticity in the supporting ligaments as you age. But dimpling may also be a sign that a tumor buried in the tissues is pulling on the skin or nipples. In the case of a tumor, dimpling might show up long before a lump becomes large enough to feel.

SYMPTOM RELIEF

Here are some hints to help you spot changes in your breasts that should be brought to your doctor's attention.

Use your eyes to look at all sides. Strip to your waist and stand in front of the mirror with your hands on your hips. Slowly turning from side to side, look to see if one breast has become bigger than the other. Check also for any puffiness or bulging, red or discolored patches of skin, thickened areas with big pores or clear, bloody, sticky or yellow nipple discharge.

Raise your arms behind your head. This stretches the breast tissue and makes swelling, dimpling or puckering more prominent, according to Susan Love, M.D., director of the Breast Center at the University of California in Los Angeles and author of *Dr. Susan Love's Breast Book.* You can also get a good look when you put your hands on your hips and press your shoulders forward, she adds.

Feel the entire breast. Gliding your hands over a wet, soapy breast is a quick way to check for changes, says Dr. Mayzel. Just make sure you feel the entire breast from your collarbone over to your armpit, she says. For more details on doing a breast self-exam, see Breast Lumps on page 77.

Report any unusual findings. If you've found something unusual that isn't in the other breast or you are unsure of your findings, contact your doctor. He or she will help you better learn what's normal or not and set your mind at ease, says Dr. Mayzel.

See also Breastfeeding Problems; Breast Lumps; Breast Tenderness; Nipple Discharge

BREASTFEEDING PROBLEMS

WHEN TO SEE YOUR DOCTOR

- Your breast is red, warm and sore for 24 hours and you have a fever, chills and feel achy as if you have the flu.
- You're not producing milk within a week after giving birth.

WHAT YOUR SYMPTOM IS TELLING YOU

Nursing a baby doesn't always go smoothly, especially in the first weeks after birth. "Breastfeeding takes skill that mothers have traditionally learned by watching other mothers," says Ruth Lawrence, M.D., professor of pediatrics and obstetrics and gynecology at the University of Rochester School of Medicine in New York. "The problem is that many of today's mothers don't get to witness breast-feeding firsthand to learn the correct technique."

As a result, she says, a mother may not know how to properly position her baby at the breast. Held at an awkward angle, the infant can't latch onto the nipple correctly, and the nipples become sore.

And until the mother understands the baby's needs—and her own—her breasts may not be emptied enough at each nursing. This can cause the milk to back up, creating painful engorgement and sore nipples, says Dr. Lawrence. Also, milk ducts can get plugged up in overly full breasts. And a plugged milk duct can become infected, a condition known as mastitis. You'll know you have mastitis if, in addition to having a sore, red breast, you also feel feverish and achy, as if you have the flu.

Nursing technique is not the only source of problems, however. Both stress and fatigue can interfere with milk flow.

SYMPTOM RELIEF

Most breastfeeding problems can be easily relieved with a little know-how.

Try a dab of cream. An over-the-counter breast cream like Massé helps soothe sore, cracked nipples without harming the baby, says Betty Crase, director of scientific information of La Leche League International in Chicago.

Warm your breasts. If your breasts feel full and sore, you may have a plugged milk duct. Get things moving again by leaning over a basin of warm water and immersing your breasts for five minutes, says Dr. Lawrence. Or cover your breasts with a warm, wet washcloth to encourage milk flow.

Get a bra that fits. "Anything that presses against a milk duct and interferes with the flow can lead to engorgement and possibly infection," says Karen Ogle, M.D., associate professor of family practice at Michigan State University in Lansing. Make sure your bra fits well and try not to sleep on your stomach for prolonged periods, she adds.

Use your own milk. Soothe and strengthen tender nipples between feedings by applying a thin layer of breast milk and allowing them to dry uncovered. "Breast milk has healing properties," says Dr. Lawrence. To speed the drying, use a blow dryer set on low.

Get some R and R. Rest and relaxation is absolutely essential for milk flow, says Dr. Lawrence. You need it to build your resistance and to counteract stress. Let someone else comfort the baby now and then. Let Dad do the cuddling or give the baby a bottle of pumped breast milk while you take a snooze. During breastfeeding or pumping, take the phone off the hook and remove other distractions, she adds.

Get an antibiotic. If you feel achy and feverish, see your doctor promptly. If you have infectious mastitis, your doctor will prescribe an antibiotic. You can still nurse, since it's the breast tissue, not the breast milk that is infected, says Dr. Ogle. The antibiotic that passes into the breast milk is probably fine for your baby, she adds, but you should check with your doctor to be sure. Ask your doctor about taking aspirin to relieve the discomfort while you're waiting for the antibiotic to kick in.

Get some support. If you're having a lot of breastfeeding problems and you've never been around other nursing women, it might be helpful to review your nursing technique. Ask your doctor to recommend someone who can show you the ropes. There are women's breastfeeding support groups, such as La Leche League International, that can provide detailed information and answer any questions that you may have.

Getting Off to a Good Start

Learning proper nursing technique before you ever put your baby to the breast will go a long way toward preventing problems. Here are a few things to be aware of.

Keep baby close after birth. A Swedish study found that when newborns are taken away from their mothers for measuring and dressing within the first 20 minutes following birth, they do not latch onto the breast as well as babies who are allowed to rest naked on their mothers' abdomens for an hour. "Don't hesitate to let the delivery room staff know that you wish to keep your baby on your tummy for a short while following birth," says Dr. Lawrence.

Assume the right position for nursing. The baby should be squarely facing the breast with his tummy touching yours, says Dr. Lawrence. Make a V with your fingers around the nipple to angle it up slightly. (If the breasts are so full that the nipple has flattened out, hand-pump a little milk to soften it.) Stroke the baby's cheek to make him open his mouth, then pull him in rapidly, thrusting the entire nipple and 1/4 to 1/2 inch of the areola (darkened area around the nipple) into his mouth.

Easy does it. When the baby is finished feeding, insert your finger in the corner of his mouth. This breaks the suction of the baby's mouth around the nipple and prevents soreness.

Trust your baby's cues. Within a day or so after birth, breast milk will naturally "let down" into the breasts, replacing the initial yellowish secretions. As a rule of thumb, use both breasts during a feeding and let your baby suckle as much or as little as he wants. "Don't worry about underfeeding," says Dr. Lawrence. "Worry can lead to reduced milk. Breastfeeding is a baby-led phenomenon. The breast makes what the baby takes. If you have six soaked diapers a day during the first few weeks and the baby is gaining weight, you're making enough milk."

Try it on your side. Breastfeeding in various positions, such as lying on your side with the baby placed on the bed, helps evenly distribute the stress on the nipples and relieves soreness, says Crase.

BREAST LUMPS

WHEN TO SEE YOUR DOCTOR

- You find any unusual lump, swelling, bulge or dimpling in one of your breasts.

WHAT YOUR SYMPTOM IS TELLING YOU

When it comes to breasts, there's a lot that fits under the umbrella of "normal"—big, little, pear-shaped, downward drooping. Women's breasts look different, and they can *feel* different.

In a lot of women, the tissue at the base of each breast is thick and ridgy, giving it a bumpy or lumpy feel. For many women a certain amount of lumpiness is perfectly normal. In fact, it's quite common for women beyond age 40 to complain of lumpy breasts.

A woman's breasts can feel lumpier just before her menstrual period. At this time of the month, she experiences a surge in female hormones—estrogen, progesterone and prolactin. These hormones stimulate fibrous breast tissue to grow and retain fluid. Once her period starts, her body reabsorbs the excess tissue and fluid. But as a woman ages, a certain amount of excess fibrous tissue remains behind, making breasts feel lumpy. This lumpiness is often called fibrocystic breast disease, but many doctors are now saying it's wrong to refer to these lumps as a disease. They may, after all, simply be a natural part of an older woman's breasts.

Why all this talk about normal lumps? The answer is simple. Because breast cancer first announces itself in the form of a lump (unless it's detected early by mammography), women tend to panic when they find one. In fact, the vast majority of lumps are not cancerous.

A squishy, movable lump that feels like a grape and stands out from the general lumpiness is probably a cyst.

These fluid-filled sacs are caused when milk ducts become plugged and do not drain. Cysts may be painful, but they do not cause cancer. And they usually disappear when your period arrives.

A lump that doesn't move and feels hard like a dried bean or pea is cause for concern. Hard, nonmovable lumps *can* (but don't always) contain cancerous cells.

Movable, marblelike lumps are probably noncancerous swellings known as fibroadenomas. Firm, irregular clumps of breast tissue are probably caused by a breast injury or a boil near the breast's surface. And a swollen wedge-shaped area near the nipple is probably an infected milk duct.

SYMPTOM RELIEF

When it comes to lumps, don't second-guess yourself. If you find a lump that concerns you—or anything else about your breasts doesn't feel right—ask your doctor to examine it. Here are some things you should be aware of.

Have an expert educate your fingers. The best way to become familiar with the normal terrain of your breasts is to have a health professional examine your breasts along with you the first time, says Kerry McGinn, R.N., nurse coordinator at the Breast Care Center of the University of California, San Francisco, and author of *The Informed Woman's Guide to Breast Health*.

"Guidance from a doctor or nurse has saved many a woman from panicking when she discovers a large, hard lump—which happens to be a tip of a rib," she says.

Stick to a monthly schedule. This makes it easier to remember what your breasts felt like last month. The best time to perform a breast self-exam is a week to ten days from the first day of your period when your breasts are less tender and feel less lumpy, according to Rosalind Benedet, R.N., nurse practitioner with the Breast Health Center at the California Pacific Medical Center in San Francisco. If you no longer menstruate or you're taking hormone replacement therapy, do your breast exam on the first day of the month. No matter which method of self-examination you choose, it's a good idea to use it consistently. That way you'll be able to recognize any changes that occur.

Get flat on your back. Smaller lumps may be easier to detect—especially in large breasts—if you're lying down with one arm raised above your head. Using the pads of your fingers of the other hand, press firmly on your breast following a pattern of concentric circles outward from the nipple until you've examined the entire breast including the nipple and areola. You should also examine the area above the breast up to the collarbone and the underarm area. If you've gained or lost weight, you may encounter lumpiness that you never felt before. (A firm ridge in the lower curve of each breast is normal.)

Schedule a mammogram. Breast x-rays can find a lump two years sooner than you or your doctor can, studies show. Three-fourths of lumps that show up on mammograms turn out to be cysts, clumps of tissue or calcium deposits. The American Cancer Society recommends having the first mammogram at age 40, then having one every one to two years until age 50. After that you should have one annually.

Try the needle test. If you have a blisterlike cyst, your doctor may want to drain it with a needle in a simple office procedure. If it deflates—as is most likely—then you know that it's not cancerous, according to Robinson Baker, M.D., professor of surgery and oncology at Johns Hopkins University School of Medicine in Baltimore.

Prepare for further diagnostic tests. If the cyst doesn't drain, you may be sent for a mammogram or ultrasound, which will help determine the shape and size of the lump. Your doctor may then perform a needle biopsy—surgical removal of a tissue sample—to analyze your breast cells for any abnormalities.

"A biopsy is the only definitive way to diagnose a lump," says Dr. Baker. If the lump is small, the surgeon may remove the whole thing during a biopsy. If it's a large lump, only a section is removed for analysis. If cancer is found, then you and your doctor can decide between a lumpectomy—which removes the lump plus the surrounding mar-

gins of healthy tissue and underarm lymph nodes—or a
mastectomy—removal of all or part of the breast.

Plan to Stay Lump-Free

By limiting factors that influence excess estrogen production, you may be able to prevent lumpiness. Here are some
tips.

Swear off high-fat foods. Fats promote breast growth
and fluid retention, according to Susan Lark, M.D., director of the PMS and Menopause Self-Help Clinic in Los
Altos, California, and author of *Premenstrual Syndrome
Self-Help Book* and *Menopause Self-Help Book*. "Fat converts to estrogen, a tissue promoter in the breast and also
increases fluid and salt retention, worsening cysts," she
notes. She recommends adopting a diet based on whole
grains, fruits and vegetables to help prevent lumpiness.

Make friends with bran flakes. Boosting your intake of
fiber-rich foods can help absorb excess estrogen and move
it out of the body. "If estrogen is not eliminated and
remains in high levels in the body, it will promote fluid
retention and stimulate the development of breast lumps,"
explains Dr. Lark. Again, the ideal diet consists mainly of
whole grains, fruits and vegetables.

Lose excess pounds. "Try to maintain your ideal weight
for your height," says Robert London, M.D., assistant clinical professor of obstetrics and gynecology at Johns
Hopkins University School of Medicine in Baltimore.
Obesity is linked with higher blood estrogen levels, he says,
and also places you at a greater vulnerability to breast cancer.

BREAST TENDERNESS

WHEN TO SEE YOUR DOCTOR

- The pain is severe or persists for two months or more.
- You are taking hormone replacement therapy.

WHAT YOUR SYMPTOM IS TELLING YOU

Forget the calendar. Like many women, you chart your menstrual cycle by consulting your breasts. A week or two before your period, your breasts start to hurt. Then once your period begins, the discomfort subsides...only to start up again next month.

No one has pinned down the exact cause of monthly breast pain. Many doctors believe that it's caused by excess female hormones—too much estrogen, progesterone or prolactin. An imbalance in these hormones is another possibility. In any case, the monthly change in hormones causes fluid retention in the breasts, which makes them feel swollen and tender.

For some women, breast pain may be at its worst during the decade prior to menopause, according to Susan Lark, M.D., director of the PMS and Menopause Self-Help Center in Los Altos, California, and author of *Premenstrual Syndrome Self-Help Book* and *Menopause Self-Help Book*. "This is when female hormones are in greatest flux," says Dr. Lark.

No matter what a woman's age, the discomfort seems to escalate with emotional stress or prolonged inactivity. Excessive amounts of salt, fat and caffeine also seem to have a negative impact.

Breast tenderness that doesn't disappear in two weeks could be a sign of pregnancy. It could also be from an injury or arthritis of the neck.

SYMPTOM RELIEF

If you're experiencing monthly breast pain, you don't have to wait until menopause to get relief. Here are some things you can do now.

Go for a walk. Breast pain is likely to be worse if you're a benchwarmer, according to Boston gynecologist Robert Shirley, M.D., past director of the Breast Clinic for the Boston Hospital for Women. "A half-hour to an hour daily walk or bike ride could begin to make a real difference in your monthly breast discomfort," he says.

Give your breasts full support. Wearing a good support bra while exercising and even to bed can help take strain off tender tissues, according to Kerry McGinn, R.N., nurse coordinator at the Breast Care Center of the University of California, San Francisco, and author of *The Informed Woman's Guide to Breast Health*.

Pad your bra. Try placing some lamb's wool inside your regular bra. The soft material sends a comfort message to your brain and crowds out the pain message, says McGinn.

Take a pain reliever. Taking two ibuprofen or other over-the-counter anti-inflammatory tablets three times daily may be all it takes to keep breast pain at bay during the week before your period, says Lois Jovanovic-Peterson, M.D., endocrinologist with the Sansum Medical Research Foundation in Santa Barbara and coauthor of *Hormones: The Woman's Answer Book*.

Chill your chest. Many women find that ice packs help quell the throbbing pain, says McGinn. Place a cloth-covered plastic bag filled with ice cubes against your breasts for 10 to 15 minutes and see if it brings some relief.

Imagine your breasts resting in warm sand. A simple visualization exercise can help you unwind, dissipate daily stress and program your mind to relieve pain, says McGinn. To begin, sit in a comfortable chair, close your eyes and breathe slowly and deeply. Then relax every muscle in your body, starting with your toes and working up to your forehead. Now, visualize warm sand enveloping your breasts. Hold the image for approximately ten minutes. If you find that it helps, you can practice this visualization as often as you like.

Have your hormones adjusted. If you're taking hormone replacement therapy and your breasts ache, tell your doctor. "The problem can usually be solved by prescribing progestin (synthetic progesterone) in lower doses to be taken for more days," says Dr. Jovanovic-Peterson.

Diet for Pain-Free Breasts

Here are a few dietary remedies that may help defend you against breast pain.

Forget about butter. Research shows that a low-fat diet can help relieve breast pain by reducing estrogen levels, according to David P. Rose, D.Sc., M.D., Ph.D., chief of the Division of Nutrition and Endocrinology at the American Health Foundation. "The women in our study reported that when they reduced their fat to 20 percent of their total calories, they also reduced their breast pain," says Dr. Rose. A low-fat diet bonus: It may also help you decrease your breast cancer risk. You can reduce the amount of fat in your diet by eating more fruits, vegetables and whole grains and cutting back on meat and dairy products.

Start your day with a high-fiber cereal. Dietary fiber helps keep estrogen from overstimulating breast tissue, says Dr. Shirley. Fiber may also help rid the body of excess estrogen. Bran cereals are great fiber sources. So are fruits and vegetables—especially those still wearing their skins, such as whole apples, peaches and pears.

Forgo that jolt of java. In a study done by researchers at Duke University Medical Center in Durham, North Carolina, 61 percent of women with breast pain experienced reduced tenderness when they eliminated caffeine from their diets. While the study was not conclusive, it certainly wouldn't hurt to try cutting back on caffeinated beverages like coffee, tea and cola, says Duke researcher Linda Russell, R.N., family nurse practitioner with the Department of Surgery.

Give up chocolate. Researchers at the State University of New York at Buffalo asked 102 women to keep track of their intake of substances containing methylxanthine, which is found in such things as chocolate, coffee, tea, aspirin and some cold and asthma medications. They found that the women who had the highest intake of methylxanthine also reported the most breast pain. This doesn't surprise Dr. Shirley. "I've been impressed by the improvements in my patients who have eliminated methylxanthines," he says.

Slash your salt intake. Salt promotes fluid retention and can boost pain, according to Dr. Shirley. This means stay away from processed foods. Also, read labels and avoid foods containing more than 300 milligrams per serving.

Flush out the fluid. Sarsaparilla, buchu and uva-ursi are all herbal diuretics that can help prevent fluid retention, says Dr. Lark. "I recommend that women take two dropperfuls of tincture of sarsaparilla dissolved in warm water twice daily when swelling and pain are at their worst," she says. You can purchase all these herbs as teas in most health food stores. Ditto for tincture of sarsaparilla. A number of foods also have helpful diuretic properties, she says. These include parsley, celery and cucumbers.

Take a multivitamin/mineral supplement. Your brand should include vitamin A, the B-complex vitamins, vitamin E, iodine and selenium. In research trials, all have been shown to have some beneficial effect on breast pain and lumps, even though some of the evidence is inconclusive, says Dr. Shirley. The B vitamins, for example, may function to help the liver metabolize estrogen, he says.

BREATH, SHORTNESS OF

WHEN TO SEE YOUR DOCTOR

- You're short of breath but cannot breathe more rapidly to compensate.
- You also have chest pain, swollen feet or legs or a history of heart problems.
- You have not been previously diagnosed with asthma or another breathing disorder.
- Shortness of breath is accompanied by wheezing, rapid breathing or coughing up phlegm.

WHAT YOUR SYMPTOM IS TELLING YOU

Being a little winded is entirely natural and harmless if you've exerted yourself. The shortness of breath simply reflects the increased oxygen demand that you've placed on your body. But there's a difference between a brisk walk around the block and walking upstairs.

If you pant at the top of the stairs, it could simply mean that you're unfit, says Henry Gong, Jr., M.D., a professor of medicine in the Pulmonary Division of the University of California at Los Angeles Medical Center. But it could also mean that you're unwell.

A person could be short of breath because of any number of lung problems. Any lung infection—from a mild cold or case of bronchitis to pneumonia and tuberculosis—can turn breathing into a chore.

Three chronic respiratory diseases—asthma, chronic bronchitis and emphysema—all cause shortness of breath and frequently, wheezing.

A collapsed lung—a problem in people with emphysema and other lung diseases and (for reasons not understood) in tall, young men—is another cause of shortness of breath.

In addition to feeling a sudden onset of shortness of breath, a person with a collapsed lung will probably also feel pain on the affected side of the chest, Dr. Gong says.

In several serious neurologic conditions—multiple sclerosis, Lou Gehrig's disease and myasthenia gravis—a person gradually loses the ability to breathe because of progressive muscle weakening, says Michael S. Sherman, M.D., an assistant professor and medical director of the Department of Pulmonary Services in the Division of Allergy, Critical Care and Pulmonary Medicine at Hahneman University Hospital in Philadelphia.

But there are also a couple of emergency situations that can produce sudden, severe shortness of breath. Botulism (a rare but potentially fatal form of food poisoning) and lead poisoning both block messages from the nervous system to the breathing muscles, leaving a person unable to breathe more deeply even though they feel it is necessary, according to Mark J. Rumbak, M.D., an assistant professor of pulmonary medicine at the University of South Florida College of Medicine in Tampa.

Symptom Relief

Relief for shortness of breath typically involves helping you get the most use out of your available lung capacity with exercises, drugs or surgery. Asthma is often reversible, doctors say, and most other conditions are at least treatable to some extent. Here are a few things you should be aware of.

Nix the sticks. Cigarette smoking causes many of the conditions that lead to shortness of breath. It goes without saying, but don't smoke. Talk to your doctor about quitting. He can recommend medication or a stop-smoking program.

Be fit to breathe. If you're overweight or sedentary, all you may need to eliminate your shortness of breath is a fitness program to get your heart and lungs in better condition, Dr. Gong says. Brisk walking is a good choice. Your goal should be a minimum of 20 minutes of brisk walking three times a week.

Breathe from your belly. Abdominal breathing with your diaphragm uses more lung capacity more efficiently, enabling you to breathe deeply instead of rapidly, Dr. Sherman says. Inhale through your nose and allow your stomach, not your upper chest, to move outward. That permits air to reach to the bottoms of your lungs, filling them completely.

Kiss the air. People with cardiopulmonary problems can breathe better if they exhale through pursed lips, Dr. Sherman says. Just pucker up after inhaling and slowly let the air out from your mouth, not your nose.

Be the Arnold Schwarzenegger of air. Increase the strength of your diaphragm and other muscles used in breathing with the help of a resister—a device that is available through either your doctor or medical supply stores. "There are several on the market. Some look like a kazoo with an adjustable hole in one end," Dr. Sherman says. You perform several sets of breathing exercises through the resister every day. In succeeding weeks, you increase the resistance, which forces your diaphragm and other breathing muscles to work harder. "That increases the strength of your diaphragm, and you may be able to breathe more powerfully. However, the effectiveness of these devices is controversial," he says.

Inhale before you exercise. Even if strenuous exercise causes exercise-induced asthma, you don't have to shy away from physical fitness, says Susan R. Wynn, M.D., an allergist in private practice with Fort Worth Allergy and Asthma Associates in Texas. Take a couple of draws on your bronchodilator about 20 minutes before working out, and make sure you warm up for at least ten minutes.

Take the plunge. For anyone troubled by shortness of breath, but particularly for people with asthma, swimming is an ideal exercise, according to Dr. Wynn. "You're breathing humid air, which is easier on your lungs," she explains.

Prop up your bed. If breathing is impaired when you lie down at night, put several books beneath the legs of your bed's headboard, raising it between 30 and 45 degrees, Dr. Sherman says. You also could purchase a foam wedge to lie on from a medical supply store.

Consider medications. Doctors treat asthma with corticosteroids to reduce lung inflammation. For asthma and many other respiratory conditions, doctors also prescribe bronchodilators—oral medications and inhaled sprays that help to open airways. "Some patients with severe asthma may benefit from receiving bronchodilators using a home nebulizer," says Dr. Sherman.

Get treatment for a collapsed lung. If only a small area of the lung has collapsed, it may reinflate on its own. Usually, though, doctors have to quite literally inflate it like a balloon with oxygen treatments or insert a needle into the chest to suck out the air pocket compressing the lung.

Breathe in unison. Pulmonary rehabilitation programs allow you to interact with other people who share your lung problems, while at the same time teaching you a variety of breathing and relaxation therapies to make your life easier, Dr. Gong says. Call a hospital or the local chapter of the American Lung Association for more information.

See also Wheezing

BREATHING RAPIDLY

WHEN TO SEE YOUR DOCTOR

- The onset of rapid breathing is sudden and severe, and there is *no* numbness or tingling around your mouth or in your hands. (Such numbness and tingling is a symptom of hyperventilation, which is usually not serious.)
- You also feel shortness of breath, pain in your chest or your feet or legs are swollen.
- Recurrent rapid breathing is not in response to a physical activity.

What Your Symptom Is Telling You

If you just crossed the finish line of a potato-sack race, you have a good reason to huff and puff: You put a big demand on your body and it needed more air.

But if you're sprawled out on the sofa watching TV and you begin to pant like a dog on an August afternoon, you don't have a good reason—or at least not a healthy one—for your rapid respiration.

Most people breathe between 8 and 15 times a minute at rest, says Henry Gong, Jr., M.D., professor of medicine in the Pulmonary Division of the University of California at Los Angeles Medical Center. But, he explains, that rate can go up (or down), depending on your level of physical fitness, your emotions and how much stress you're experiencing.

That third factor—stress—is perhaps the most common cause of lungs going into fifth gear. People who spend their days feeling nervous and tense are more likely to suffer bouts of rapid breathing that doctors call hyperventilation. And once you start hyperventilating, you'll feel even *more* hyper: That fast breathing disturbs the body's balance of blood gases, numbing the mouth and hands and depriving the brain of oxygen. Yellow alert turns to red alert, and the emotions go into overdrive: You're having what's known as a panic attack and breathe even *faster*. Luckily, none of this causes physical damage. But the emotional cost—the disruption and scariness of the attack and the added anxiety and nervousness about having more panic attacks—is quite high.

Rapid breathing isn't always caused by emotions. Sometimes it has a physical cause: a problem in your lungs. "Asthma, chronic bronchitis, emphysema, pneumonia, tuberculosis—anything that affects the lungs can cause a rise in respiration," says Mark J. Rumbak, M.D., an assistant professor of pulmonary medicine at the University of South Florida College of Medicine in Tampa.

Occasionally, rapid breathing is a symptom of nervous system disorders and brain problems that scramble the messages to the lungs.

And rapid breathing can also mean you should move rapidly to the emergency room: Along with chest pain, it's an early warning sign of a heart attack and other serious heart malfunctions.

SYMPTOM RELIEF

A doctor should treat a serious lung disorder. But hyperventilation—though it certainly *seems* serious when it's happening—can be treated at home. Here are three ways to convince your lungs to calm down.

Brown-bag it. Breathing into a paper bag to balance your blood gases is the standard short-term treatment for hyperventilation, says Dr. Rumbak. Here's the technique: Scrunch the opening of the bag closed with one hand; with your other hand, stick a finger into the opening to create a small hole; now take out your finger and hold the bag to your mouth and breathe slowly and evenly for four or five minutes, inhaling your exhaled air from the bag. If your hyperventilation doesn't let up, get to a doctor or the emergency room, says Dr. Rumbak.

Pay attention to your stress level. You can put an episode of hyperventilation in a brown bag, but there's a landfill's worth of stress that's behind this symptom. One way to cope with the stress, says Dr. Gong, is with breathing exercises.

Many stress experts recommend "diaphragmatic" breathing to help you unwind. To practice this form of breathing, sit up straight in a chair or lie flat on the floor. Place one palm on your chest and the other palm on your abdomen. Now inhale through your nose for a slow count of five. Your hand on your stomach will feel like it's being pushed out with the air that's going deep into your lungs. Make sure your hand on your chest stays perfectly still. Then exhale through your nose to a slow count of five. Repeat the deep breath three times, rest for a moment then repeat it three more times.

If your hyperventilation and panic attacks are frequent, consider seeing a doctor or psychologist for help.

Go with the flow meter. Asthmatics sometimes can't tell the difference between hyperventilation and a full-fledged asthma attack (and those attacks can kill). Needless to say, this causes even more anxiety, which can push a hyperventilating asthmatic over the edge into a panic attack. That's why Susan R. Wynn, M.D., an allergist in private practice with the Fort Worth Allergy and Asthma Associates in Texas, suggests that asthmatics use a device called a peak flow meter. This device measures the strength of your exhalations. If the meter shows your normal maximum exhalation, you're hyperventilating. If the meter shows less than your normal maximum, you're having an asthma attack. "People find it reassuring to know if it's hyperventilation or an asthma attack," says Dr. Wynn. (You can buy a meter from medical supply stores or your doctor can order one for you.)

See also Anxiety; Wheezing

BRUISES

WHEN TO SEE YOUR DOCTOR

- Bruises appear easily and frequently.
- Bruises typically take longer than a week to disappear.
- You're suddenly getting more unexplained bruises than usual.

WHAT YOUR SYMPTOM IS TELLING YOU

Ice skating with your niece was loads of fun—you only took one spill. But it was a doozy. The next day, the bluish purple marks on your shins and hip made you look like you tumbled down two flights of stairs.

Unless you live in a bubble, you're bound to bump into something—whether it's an ice-covered rink or the edge of a desk—or something is bound to bump into you. When a blow occurs, blood vessels rupture under your skin and blood spills into the surrounding area. The spilled blood shows through the skin as a darkened bruise.

Once the vessels are ruptured, the area swells as scavenger cells flood in to cart off injured cells. The swelling cuts off oxygen, making the hemoglobin in the blood turn blue. Later, as the hemoglobin breaks down, the bruise turns yellowish green and then brown.

"The size and shape of your bruise depends on the force of the blow as well as where your body is hit," says Jerome Z. Litt, M.D., assistant clinical professor of dermatology at Case Western Reserve University School of Medicine in Cleveland. If you lightly bump your forearm on a doorknob, he says, a minor number of blood vessels may be damaged and the resulting bruise is barely noticeable. On the other hand, if the furniture mover knocks into your hip full-force with a 50-pound table, many blood vessels will be crushed. You'll wind up with a nasty bruise the size of a hockey puck.

And if a blow occurs over a bone where the skin is thinner—around your eye, for instance—the bruise and swelling are likely to be more even prominent.

Women generally have skin that is more easily bruised than men. One reason is that their skin is thinner, possibly because the female hormone estrogen softens the blood vessels and affects the supporting network of collagen beneath the skin.

Another reason may be that one in ten women has a mild platelet defect (platelets are blood cells that play a role in clotting). "This doesn't pose a noticeable problem unless they take an aspirin-containing product," says Sandor Shapiro, M.D., director of hematology at Jefferson Medical College of Thomas Jefferson University in Philadelphia. "Aspirin interferes with platelet function for several days. This means that if you take one aspirin today, it can still interfere with clotting five to six days later."

Bumping into a desk corner during that time can make

you look like you got in the way of a champion kick-boxer. Aspirin may also contribute to bruising in men.

Both sexes are more prone to bruising once they hit middle age, when the protective tissue and supporting fibers of the blood vessels beneath the skin naturally begin to break down. Plus, a lifetime exposure to the penetrating rays of the sun weakens the collagen and other elastic fibers. This makes the vessels in the upper skin layers vulnerable, especially in sun-exposed areas such as the backs of the hands and arms. The vessels in these areas can rupture at the slightest tap.

Easy bruising may also be a side effect of birth control pills, arthritis medications and some diuretics (medications that flush excess water from the body). Corticosteroids (cortisone-like drugs) may also contribute to easy bruising. These powerful anti-inflammatory agents relieve swelling in asthma, rheumatoid arthritis and itchy skin rashes.

In rare cases, unexplained bruising can signal a clotting disorder or immune problem.

SYMPTOM RELIEF

Here's how to minimize the bumps and bruises you're bound to get along the road of life.

Apply icy pressure, pronto. If you've just bumped into something and you *know* it's going to cause a bruise, immediately press the area with ice wrapped in a washcloth for seven minutes or so. "This keeps blood from leaking out of vessels and will minimize the black-and-blue marks," says Robert E. Clark, M.D., Ph.D., director of the Dermatologic Surgery and Cutaneous Oncology Unit at Duke University Medical Center in Durham, North Carolina. Ice also helps deaden the pain, he adds.

Give a lift to a just-bumped limb. Raising a bruised arm or leg above the level of your heart will keep blood from pooling in the injured area.

Try warm compresses. Applying a warm washcloth a day or two after an injury helps disperse the extra red blood cells into the tissues. Hold the warm cloth in place for about 20 minutes. The dark area may fade more quickly, says Dr. Litt.

Apply a dab of zinc oxide. "Never bandage a bruise," says Dr. Litt. But covering the bruise with a coating of zinc oxide—a common ingredient in many first-aid creams—before going to bed provides a protective shield and may nudge healing in some way, he says. Both topical and oral zinc play an important role in wound healing.

Try a little arnica. The American Indians knew what they were doing when they smeared the juice of the arnica bush on bruises, according to Varro E. Tyler, Ph.D., a plant-drug specialist and professor of pharmacognosy at Purdue University in West Lafayette, Indiana. "Several years ago, a German study found two substances in this herb that produce anti-inflammatory and painkilling effects," says Dr. Tyler. Health food stores sell ready-made arnica ointments such as Antiflora, which may help bruises disappear. They should contain at least 10 percent arnica to be effective, says Dr. Tyler.

Reach for vitamin C skin cream. The latest "miracle" ingredient to show up in skin cosmetics is vitamin C. This one seems to have some merit. "Vitamin C penetrates the skin deeply and may help build up the skin's support structure of collagen," says Dr. Clark. "This may reduce your vulnerability to bruising."

Vitamin C also helps toughen up older skin, protecting against fragility and bruising. "Preliminary studies have shown that when vitamin C is applied to fresh bruises in older people, the discoloration is minimized," says Douglas Darr, Ph.D., assistant research professor at Duke University Medical Center. Dr. Darr's own research has found that topical vitamin C helps prevent damage from past overexposure to sunlight and inactivates harmful substances that corrode the cells and further age the skin. A few of these products are now available; ask your dermatologist.

Swallow vitamin C, too. "Taking 500 to 1,000 milligrams of vitamin C daily may help enhance skin collagen formation and make blood vessels less brittle," says Dr. Clark. Taking vitamin C may be especially important if you also take aspirin or corticosteroids for arthritis. During a study, British researchers observed that arthritis inflammation robs the body of vitamin C, and aspirin and steroids used to combat the disease also tend to drain the body of this nutrient, weakening the capillaries. When people were given 500 milligrams of vitamin C daily, their bruises showed rapid improvement. Before taking large doses of any vitamin, including vitamin C, you should get the consent of your doctor.

Become an oyster lover. Shellfish as well as beef and chicken is an excellent source of zinc. This mineral may help keep blood cells from leaking out of the blood vessels following injury, according to Joseph Bark, M.D., chairman of the Department of Dermatology at St. Joseph's Hospital in Lexington, Kentucky. You may also want to take a daily multivitamin/mineral supplement that contains zinc.

Switch to acetaminophen. Unlike aspirin and ibuprofen, this painkiller does not affect platelet function, says Dr. Shapiro.

Go easy on rash cream. If you are using an over-the-counter hydrocortisone cream for an itchy skin condition, don't use it for more than one to two weeks. "These products have the potential to thin the skin and make you more prone to bruising," says Dr. Clark. Be especially careful not to overuse these products in moist areas, such as the armpit and groin, where they can more easily penetrate the skin, he adds.

Check your medications. Make a list of all medications you're taking—both prescription and over-the-counter drugs—and show it to your doctor. Your doctor may be able to suggest changes that will help prevent excess bruising.

BUNIONS

WHAT YOUR SYMPTOM IS TELLING YOU

This is the story of Paul Bunion—not the massive, axe-wielding lumberjack of literary legend (actually spelled Bunyan), but the large bump on your big toe joint.

Mr. Bunion has probably been with you from birth—many doctors say the propensity toward bunions is inherited. The reason he suddenly (it seems) came out swinging: You've been wearing shoes that are too tight.

As you get older, tight shoes can actually cause extra bone growth and the development of a fluid-filled sac on the toe joints on either side of your foot. And that's enough to make the joints bulge and ache, cause erosion of the surrounding cartilage or even put painful pressure on the rest of your toes, says Michael Coughlin, M.D., past president of the American Orthopedic Foot and Ankle Society and an orthopedic surgeon in Boise, Idaho.

SYMPTOM RELIEF

To beat bunions, try these tips.

Stretch those shoes. If your favorite pair of shoes is causing or irritating the bunion, take them to a shoe repair store and have them stretched, or do it yourself with a device that's available for under $10 at most drugstores, says Myles Schneider, D.P.M., an Annandale, Virginia, podiatrist and coauthor of the book *How to Doctor Your Feet without a Doctor*.

Slip into some sandals. If your dress code is more relaxed, consider wearing sandals or even going barefoot, says Steve Guida, D.P.M., a Fort Lauderdale, Florida, podiatrist who's treated hundreds of older patients. A more open shoe means less binding and, as a result, less opportunity for bunion discomfort, he says.

Shield yourself. Pads called bunion shields can serve as a comfortable barrier between you and your shoes, Dr. Guida says. After the shield has been placed directly on the bunion, adhesive on the back keeps it in place. For long-term use, try bunion shields made of silicone, says Dr. Guida. Both kinds are available at drugstores.

Shine those shoes. Some shoe polishes applied once a week can soften shoe leather, which may help your favorite pair relax to the shape of your bunion rather than press against it, says Dr. Schneider.

Exercise those bunions. The following exercise helps loosen the stiffness that often accompanies bunions, says Dr. Schneider. Using a 1-inch-by-18-inch piece of cotton cloth or a thin rope, tie a loop and place one end around each big toe. While keeping your heels on a flat surface with the cloth or rope extended between the feet, gently pull the toes apart and hold for five seconds. Repeat 10 times, says Dr. Schneider. Increase this routine by one repetition each day until you can do 25.

Give orthotics a try. Custom-made arch supports called orthotics may also help relieve the pain by reducing the amount of foot motion in the shoe. Expect to pay $50 for one made of hard rubber and $350 and up for one made of graphite, says Dr. Coughlin.

Customize your footwear. Shoes made with your bunion in mind should never bind or irritate that delicate area, says Dr. Guida. Pedorthists—skilled craftspeople who specialize in making shoes for folks with foot problems—charge from $300 to $500 for a pair, according to Dr. Guida. Before beginning their work, pedorthists take a plaster impression of your foot and then build a shoe around it, says Charley Simpson, a certified pedorthist and former owner of Simpson Shoes in Boston.

Consider a bunionectomy. If the pain continues despite your best efforts, you might want to consider a bunionectomy. During this procedure, the doctor may remove some of the bone that's causing the discomfort and tighten the joint—or even replace it. Surgery should always be the last resort, says Dr. Coughlin.

BURPING

WHAT YOUR SYMPTOM IS TELLING YOU

After polishing off a particularly palatable plate of bratwurst, you uncork a belch that seems to bounce off the Bavarian Alps. Your host's reaction: an invitation to next year's polka party. Your stomach's: Thanks for letting me blow off a little steam—or at least a little trapped air.

While you're chewing and sipping, air routinely makes its way into your mouth, stealing a ride down your esophagus when you swallow. From there, one of two things happens: The air is either pushed into your stomach or sits at the bottom of your esophagus waiting for the next elevator up. Then, like a bubble at the bottom of a water cooler, the air suddenly drifts back up your throat and out of your mouth—sometimes on cue.

"You could fill someone's stomach with air and there's no guarantee that he'll burp," says James Cooper, M.D., professor of medicine at Georgetown University in Washington D.C., and a spokesman for the American Association of Gastroenterologists. "But if he has air trapped in his esophagus, he's a prime candidate."

"Swallowing air is probably one of the most common causes of burping," says Wendell Clarkston, M.D., an assistant professor and director of the Fellowship Training Program in Gastroenterology and Hepatology at Saint Louis University School of Medicine.

Food allergies and sensitivity to milk can also contribute to burping, as can a deficiency of stomach acid.

SYMPTOM RELIEF

While burping isn't considered a health problem, it can be a little hard on your pride—particularly when you're in public. Here's how to keep your decorum.

Eat less air. Although there's no evidence that chewing

with your mouth closed will help stop burping, chewing more slowly and carefully should, says Dr. Clarkston. It also enhances digestion, helping cut down on gas and stomach upset.

Nix nervousness. Some people fidget with their fingers or tap their toes when they're nervous. Others gulp literally gallons of air as they try to soothe a dry mouth and throat, says Dr. Cooper. Try finding other outlets for your nervous energy. Stand up and stretch or go for a walk around the block.

Forgo the fizz. Carbonated beverages taste great on the way down. What's less satisfying is the way the pressurized air sometimes forces its way back out, says Alan R. Gaby, M.D., a Baltimore physician and president of the American Holistic Medical Association. If you'd like to squelch that belch until *after* the dinner party—you might be wise to select a noncarbonated beverage instead.

Get rid of gum. Chewing gum helps create saliva that's later swallowed along with air, says Dr. Clarkston.

Sip from a glass. Drinking from straws and water fountains allows still more air to mix in with water, says Dr. Cooper. Drink directly from a glass or cup instead.

Go light on airy foods. Whipped foods like milk shakes and soufflés tend to have air in them, increasing your chance of burping, says Dr. Cooper.

Do the elimination diet. If none of the previous tips seem to help curb excess burping, a food allergy or sensitivity to milk may be to blame. Carefully eliminating some foods from your diet may give you some insight into the problem. Some of the most common culprits are milk, eggs, wheat, corn, soy, peanuts, citrus fruits, colas and chocolate.

"Many people have food allergies, and when they get off the food, their symptoms miraculously go away," says Dr. Gaby. If you stop drinking milk for several days, for example, and your belching stops, you may have found the problem. Just to be sure, have some more milk: If your belching resumes, you may have to find another source of calcium, he says.

Take a test. If you've investigated several causes of excessive burping and still don't have a clue, have your doctor perform a Heidelberg test. This quick office procedure checks the acid level of your stomach. While extra acid can lead to ulcers, low acid can slow digestion, causing burping, says Dr. Gaby.

Add some acid. If you're a touch low on stomach acid, you may need to add some with the first few bites of your meal. Hydrochloric acid tablets are available at most health food stores, says Dr. Gaby.

C

CALF PAIN

- You experience a cramping pain that comes on with exercise and is immediately relieved with rest.
- You experience aching or throbbing at night.
- You've injured yourself and pain, discoloration and swelling are still there after 24 hours.
- You have unexplained pain that lasts more than three days.
- You notice any tender lumps beneath the skin.

WHAT YOUR SYMPTOM IS TELLING YOU

Usually they're as quiet as a cow. Suddenly they're as angry as a bull. When calf pain strikes, it can strike hard, leaving your otherwise docile calves feeling like tenderized veal cutlets. And there's a whole herd of possible causes.

Any acute or overuse injury in the calf area can feel like a swift chop from a meat cleaver. Climb a ladder all day—or overreach just once for a low backhand in tennis—and you can easily strain or tear a muscle or tendon.

Frequently, however, calf pain has nothing to do with wear and tear. The calf muscles are hot spots for circulatory problems. Sudden pains that show up during physical activity, such as walking, are usually a sign of what doctors call arterial insufficiency. That means the arteries aren't able to supply the calf muscles with enough blood and oxygen to meet their needs. This usually arises from atherosclerosis—hardening of the arteries.

On the other hand, pain and swelling while at rest could mean venous insufficiency. In this case, blood doesn't pump *away* from the calf muscles efficiently, so it backs up and causes pain.

Of the two, arterial insufficiency is the more common, and it is usually seen in the form of intermittent claudication. In this condition the painful cramping quickly comes and goes. It's always preceded by exercise, when the muscle demands more blood, and it's completely relieved within five to ten minutes of stopping the exertion that produced the pain.

"Think of claudication as a heart attack of the lower leg," explains Joseph M. Giordano, M.D., professor and chief of surgery at George Washington University Hospital in Washington, D.C. "If blood flow is obstructed, the increased needs of the muscle aren't being met, and the attack occurs. With immediate rest, the muscle's blood demands return to normal, and the pain goes away."

"Intermittent claudication is a relatively benign and manageable condition, but people with more advanced arterial insufficiency can experience what is known as rest pain," says Richard F. Kempczinski, M.D., chief of vascular surgery at the University of Cincinnati College of Medicine. "The blood flow is so restricted that pain now comes on at rest or while sleeping. At its worst, the condition can produce painful, slow-healing ulcers or even gangrene."

The backup of blood arising from venous insufficiency can lead to the development of thrombophlebitis—an inflammation and clotting in the veins. The superficial variety, visible below the skin as a tender, reddish, varicose vein, is not too worrisome. But deep-vein thrombophlebitis can produce greater pain and a greater health risk if a clot should break away and move elsewhere in the body. Both produce tenderness, throbbing and heaviness.

SYMPTOM RELIEF

If you have recurring or ongoing calf pain, it's important for you to see your doctor. But here are a few remedies you can try.

Feed your calf some RICE. The best recipe for an injured calf muscle is RICE: rest, ice applied intermittently throughout the day, compression with an elastic bandage and elevation of the feet with pillows. Bedrest and elevation will also alleviate the swelling and heaviness associated with thrombophlebitis, says Robert Ginsburg, M.D., director of the Cardiovascular Intervention Unit at the University of Colorado Health Science Center in Denver.

Try an OTC pain reliever. Over-the-counter anti-inflammatories like aspirin and ibuprofen will lessen the pain and swelling associated with a muscle injury or with thrombophlebitis, says Lyle Micheli, M.D., director of the Sports Medicine Division at Boston Children's Hospital and associate clinical professor of orthopedic surgery at Harvard Medical School.

Hoof it till it hurts. Though walking brings on intermittent claudication, a walking program is the first step in treating it. "You should walk until you reach your level of pain tolerance," says Dr. Giordano. "When you reach the point where you can't stand the pain anymore, stop. Push yourself a little more each day, keep increasing the distance, and gradually the condition will become less prevalent."

Stop smoking. People who have intermittent claudication should kick the habit, says Dr. Ginsburg. Smoking is a leading contributor to the atherosclerosis that decreases blood flow, he says.

Apply heat. A warm, not hot, heating pad or blanket can alleviate superficial pain from thrombophlebitis, says Dr. Ginsburg. (Don't use heat on a recent injury, however. It will make the swelling worse and interfere with healing.)

Step into support hose. Department store hosiery can constrict your circulation, but compression support stockings prescribed by a physician can greatly improve blood flow and relieve pain from venous insufficiency, says Dr. Kempczinski.

Consider surgery. Stripping and removing damaged veins can relieve severe venous insufficiency, says Dr. Ginsburg. Anticoagulants can also be helpful, he says. Rest pain and severe arterial insufficiencies may require such procedures as a balloon angioplasty or bypass surgery.

CALLUSES

WHEN TO SEE YOUR DOCTOR

- Your callus is painful.
- You have diabetes or circulatory problems and need to have your callus pared down.
- A callused area is red and hot.
- Your callus splits open or cracks and bleeds.
- Your callus has a bluish color.

WHAT YOUR SYMPTOM IS TELLING YOU

A callus is your skin's self-generated shield, a way to defend itself from too much pressure. And that shield does a good job, says Ellen Cohen-Sobel, D.P.M., Ph.D., associate professor of podiatric orthopedics at the New York College of Podiatric Medicine in New York City. Think of how the fingertips of a professional guitar player or the palms of an Olympic gymnast would feel if they weren't guarded by thick calluses. They'd *hurt*. In fact, they'd probably bleed.

Similarly, a few thin, well-placed calluses on your feet can offer a little bit of protection when you're walking barefoot on the beach. But those calluses aren't only caused by pressure on your feet. You have your parents to blame.

"The underlying cause of callused feet is hereditary," says Mark D. Sussman, D.P.M., a podiatrist in private practice in Wheaton, Maryland, and coauthor of *The Family Foot-Care Book*. Parents pass on instabilities in the feet, he explains. "If you inherit poor foot mechanics, your foot moves around instead of being stable when it hits the ground." That constant friction causes calluses.

Calluses like those on the feet that cover a wide area are sometimes irritating but rarely painful, says Dr. Cohen-Sobel. The major exception tends to be a smaller, deeper callus with precisely defined edges (a plantar keratosis), which is usually painful. It often has a deep, white area in its center with a clear area around it that looks almost like a moat, says Dr. Cohen-Sobel.

SYMPTOM RELIEF

"If you've been living with your calluses for many years and they don't bother you, don't do anything to them," says Dr. Cohen-Sobel. Thin calluses spread over the bottoms of the feet are not a health problem, says Howard Dananberg, D.P.M., a podiatrist and medical director of The Walking Clinic in Bedford, New Hampshire. "When calluses become focused at one site, that's a different story, especially if they become painful," Dr. Dananberg says. The body tries to protect the site by making yet more hard, protective skin. To break this cycle, the callus has to go. Here's what to do.

Sand it. You can keep calluses under control at home by carefully sanding them down, says Dr. Sussman. First, wash your feet. Then soak them for 20 minutes in a basin of clean, warm water with two tablespoons mild dishwashing liquid added. Then rub the callus with cooking oil until it feels moist and soft, usually about one minute. Finally, sand the callus with a pumice stone, fine sandpaper, sandstone or a callus file. "Stop sanding before the area becomes tender—one to two minutes," says Dr. Cohen-Sobel.

Protect it. To take pressure off callus-prone areas, cut a slightly-larger-than-callus-size hole in a piece of adhesive moleskin, which is available at pharmacies. Position the doughnut-shaped pad around the filed callus and fill the hole with petroleum jelly, says Dr. Sussman. Then cover the area with gauze. Just make sure your podiatrist knows you're using this method and approves.

Avoid acids. "Over-the-counter callus removers contain acids that can burn your skin," says Dr. Dananberg. Dr. Sussman agrees, warning that they can also cause infections.

If the shoe fits, wear it. Poorly fitting shoes don't cause calluses, but they can aggravate them, says Dr. Sussman.

"Feet get larger as you get older, especially in women who've had children," he explains. "So don't just squeeze into the size you wore last year. And if the shoes hurt after wearing them at home for a few hours, return them."

Put your feet in a doctor's hands. The only person who should remove or trim your calluses with a sharp instrument is a podiatrist—not you and not a beautician—says Dr. Cohen-Sobel. *Never* take a razor or scissors to a callus, she warns. "You can *easily* cause an infection or worse."

A severe callus—such as a plantar keratosis—might need monthly or bimonthly medical attention. In many cases, the doctor may arrange to see you less often by fitting you with an in-shoe device that redistributes your weight, says Dr. Sussman. As a last resort, severe calluses can be corrected surgically. Be sure to get a second opinion before having this done, he adds.

CANKER SORES

WHEN TO SEE YOUR DOCTOR

- A sore in your mouth does not heal within two weeks.
- You develop a painless sore in your mouth.

WHAT YOUR SYMPTOM IS TELLING YOU

*C*anker. Even the name sounds decidedly unhealthy and a little disgusting. But these painful little sores actually are quite harmless. Their evil twin, herpes-caused cold sores or fever blisters, are the highly contagious ulcerations that you have to be more concerned about.

Both kinds of ulcers look a lot alike—they're round, red and possibly pus-filled. Canker sores usually don't grow together like herpes blisters, though, and they typically erupt on the movable, flexible parts of the mouth, such as the tongue and tissue below it, the cheeks and the upper soft palate. When you have a canker sore, you probably won't feel the tingling or burning that signals the onset of a herpes cold sore.

Doctors don't really know why some people get canker sores, which are technically known as aphthous ulcers. Heredity appears to play a role, says Eric Z. Shapira, D.D.S., a trustee on the national board of the Academy of General Dentistry and a dentist in private practice in Half Moon Bay, California. Some people are just more sensitive to the *Streptococcus sanguis* bacteria that cause the eruptions. If you get canker sores once, you're likely to get them again.

Women are much more vulnerable to outbreaks of canker sores, dentists say, especially during pregnancy and during parts of their menstrual cycles. Stress might also encourage a sore to appear, as can food allergies, Dr. Shapira says. Denture wearers can get them from the pressure and rubbing of their false teeth on their gums. Bites and abrasions also can lead to an eruption in people prone to developing canker sores.

SYMPTOM RELIEF

Canker sores can really sting. In very vulnerable people, they'll hurt like heck. They will go away on their own in 10 to 14 days. But you probably don't want to live with pain for that long, so here's what you can do.

Cover it with hydrocortisone. A prescription gel or paste containing hydrocortisone will seal off the canker sore and make you feel better and usually speed the healing, says D'Anne Kleinsmith, M.D., a dermatologist in private practice in West Bloomfield, Michigan.

Rub some salve on the sore. Over-the-counter ointments, such as Zilactin or Blistex, will coat the sore and sterilize it to some extent, Dr. Shapira says. Ointments will at least numb the pain so you can eat more easily.

Try a Kaopectate quencher. For a canker sore or any other minor mouth pain, mix equal parts of Kaopectate with Benadryl elixir, both of which you can find at pharmacies, says Louis M. Abbey, D.M.D., a professor of oral pathology at Virginia Commonwealth University/ Medical College of Virginia School of Dentistry in Richmond. Swish the concoction in your mouth for at least a minute before eating, to soothe your mouth. The Benadryl numbs the pain, while the Kaopectate helps the anesthetic stick to the inside of your mouth, he explains.

Soothe it with saline. Rinsing your mouth with some salt water several times a day will help ease the pain from a canker sore, Dr. Shapira says. Mix a teaspoon of salt in an eight-ounce glass of warm water and swish it around in your mouth.

Don't eat the acid. Spicy or highly acidic foods like tomatoes and citrus juices will burn and irritate the ulceration. Avoid them until the sore heals, Dr. Shapira says.

Lysine gets the red out? Several years ago, researchers showed some interest in treating canker sores with supplements of the amino acid lysine. "It works for some people and doesn't work for others," Dr. Shapira says. Check with your doctor before taking any supplements on your own.

Handle with care. Because your hand can slip while you're vigorously or hastily brushing your teeth, take your time and gently go through your oral hygiene routines, dentists say.

See also Cold Sores

CHEEK AND TONGUE BITING

WHEN TO SEE YOUR DOCTOR

- You frequently bite your cheek or tongue while chewing or speaking.
- Blood flow from a cheek or tongue bite doesn't stop within ten minutes or so.

WHAT YOUR SYMPTOM IS TELLING YOU

When you bite your cheek or tongue, you create a small wound that's exactly the same as a canker sore. It may or may not bleed, depending on the bite's severity. But the amount of blood doesn't indicate the severity of the bite, for even a few drops mixed with some saliva can create a gory mess.

Fortunately, most such bites *aren't* severe. Unless you fall or are hit hard enough to bite yourself deeply, cheek and tongue bites are usually harmless little nips that sting for just a bit. But—in just the same way that 1 mosquito bite is an annoyance while 50 mosquito bites are intensely uncomfortable—these cheek and tongue bites can become a real nuisance if they're frequent. And that can happen if you have problems with your dentures or the alignment of your real teeth.

False teeth that slip and shift can cause you to miss your mark and bite your tongue, says JoAnne Allen, D.D.S., a dentist in private practice in Albuquerque. And if your real teeth are crooked or otherwise not properly placed, they too can make you chomp on your cheek.

So can poor table manners. "Think about it," Dr. Allen says. "What are you almost always doing when you bite your tongue? You're talking and eating at the same time. Your mother told you not to do that for a reason."

Nipping on your cheek can also be a nervous habit. "You create a little white line on the inside of your cheek called hyperkeratosis. It's like a callus," says Michael W. Dodds, Ph.D., who holds a bachelor of dental surgery and is an assistant professor in the Department of Community Dentistry at the University of Texas Health Science Center in San Antonio. "Although it's not a big deal, you should stop the habit, if at all possible."

SYMPTOM RELIEF

The sting from a cheek or tongue bite probably will fade soon after you stop thinking about it. For relief, you can try any of the treatments mentioned in Canker Sores on page 106.

Let Jack Frost nip on your bite. If the bite has drawn blood, suck on an ice cube or hold cold water in your mouth until the bleeding slows, says J. Frank Collins, D.D.S., a dentist in private practice in Jacksonville, Florida.

Clean it up. Swish an antiseptic mouthwash around the wound to prevent any chance of infection, Dr. Collins recommends. Listerine is a good choice.

Go to a mouth pro. If the bleeding doesn't stop after ten minutes, Dr. Collins suggests, call your dentist, who may want to suture the wound.

Check your bite. Mention repeated cheek or tongue biting to your dentist, who will check the fit of your dentures or the alignment of your teeth. If misaligned teeth are the problem, braces may be in order—even for adults.

CHEST PAIN

WHEN TO SEE YOUR DOCTOR

- See your doctor for any chest pain.
- Consider it a medical emergency if the pain is severe and radiates from the chest to the shoulders, neck, arms or jaw or is accompanied by dizziness, fainting, sweating, nausea or breathlessness.

WHAT YOUR SYMPTOM IS TELLING YOU

Suddenly, you're having chest pains, and a wave of fear overtakes you. You've seen enough episodes of "General Hospital," "St. Elsewhere" and "Marcus Welby, M.D." to know what that means: the Big One.

Before you go into a panic, consider one thing first: While TV chest pains are always heart attacks, the causes of real life chest pains are not always so dramatic.

"Though we must always consider the worst, there are over 50 possible causes of chest pain, many of which have nothing to do with the heart and are not at all life threatening," says Charles E. Chambers, M.D., assistant professor of medicine at Pennsylvania State University and a cardiologist at the Milton S. Hershey Medical Center in Hershey. "In general, a sudden jab of pain, a dull, lingering ache, a burning feeling or a sensation that changes when you shift your upper body is not cause for panic. In those instances, doctors can usually rule out a heart disease problem or one that needs immediate emergency treatment."

How can you recognize what are probably true heart-related pains? Picture this: You're walking or exercising and suddenly you experience a pressure, tightness or squeezing directly behind or slightly to the left of your breastbone, possibly radiating up and down your arms, back, neck and jaw. You sit down, catch your breath and the discomfort subsides in 5 to 15 minutes. Heart attack? More likely it's what cardiologists call angina pectoris or just plain angina. (If you experience an episode like this, don't assume it is angina; see your doctor for a diagnosis.) With angina, fatty deposits accumulate inside the coronary arteries, narrowing the channels, slowing the blood flow to the heart muscle and depriving it of much-needed oxygen.

"Angina typically occurs during exertion or moments of excitement when the heart works harder and requires more oxygen-rich blood," says Marvin Moser, M.D., clinical professor of medicine at the Yale University School of Medicine and author of *Week by Week to a Strong Heart*. "It's the heart's way of signaling that it needs more oxygen, just as your calf muscle does when you develop a cramp."

A number of lifestyle factors, such as smoking, stress and lack of exercise, can make the coronary blockage worse and, therefore, makes the potential for pain greater.

Angina is not a medical emergency, but it may be a warning of one to come. Suppose one of those arteries is severely narrowed or a blood clot completely cuts off blood supply to a portion of the heart. A portion of the heart muscle can actually die.

When that happens, it *is* a heart attack, and in most cases the heart will let you know in no uncertain terms. The resulting pain can resemble angina, but typically lasts longer, is more severe and is often accompanied by dizziness, nausea, shortness of breath and sweating. When these symptoms occur, you don't sit around hoping that it will go away. You get immediate emergency medical treatment to prevent further destruction of heart tissue.

Heart pain isn't always coronary artery disease, however. Consider *pericarditis*, an inflammation of the tissue sac surrounding the heart. It's usually caused by a virus. This common condition can produce a constant sharp pain that worsens with each breath or when you lie down. Rips in the heart's artery or diseases of the heart's valves can lead to a wide variety of chest pain symptoms, and all are usually different from those of angina or heart attacks.

There are also chest pains that don't originate in the heart. "A great number of them are stress related," says

John Cantwell, M.D., director of preventive medicine and cardiac rehabilitation at Georgia Baptist Hospital in Atlanta. "Anxiety attacks and stress can produce tension in the chest muscles or cause the heart to beat a bit erratically. People who suffer from anxiety often hyperventilate, and their rapid breathing can lead to chest discomfort in addition to tingling and numbness of the lips and extremities."

For many people, the pain can be traced to relatively benign gastrointestinal causes like gas, heartburn, hiatal hernia (which is actually a small portion of the stomach that has slipped through an opening in the diaphragm) or the regurgitation of stomach acid. Usually this kind of pain is in the lower chest and produces sensations ranging from burning to a dull ache.

Any sharpness that worsens when you inhale could be a sign of *pleurisy*, an inflammation of the lining of the lungs. Or it could mean pneumonia or some other lung condition. Another possibility is any kind of injury—a strained chest muscle or cartilage or bruised or broken ribs.

SYMPTOM RELIEF

Chest pain does not always mean a visit to the emergency room. Still, when it occurs, be safe and let a doctor check it out. Here's how you and your doctor can keep angina and other chest pains under control.

Make an immediate pit stop. "Don't try to walk off a sudden chest pain," says Dr. Cantwell. "If the pain is from angina, it should go away with a few minutes of rest. If it doesn't, or if it gets worse, get to a doctor."

Blast the pain with nitro. A prescription nitroglycerin tablet dissolved under the tongue safely relieves most angina attacks in minutes by acting as a vasodilator. That means it causes the blood vessels to relax so more oxygen-rich blood can pass through. "Today you can get nitroglycerin in a skin patch, but many people find that the patches lose their effectiveness over the long term. There are long-acting tablets available that can be taken two to four times a day," says Dr. Moser.

Ask your doctor about medications. Other vasodilating medications for angina and other heart conditions include calcium channel blockers (nifedipine or diltiazem, for example). They increase the heart's oxygen supply. Beta blocker drugs (atenolol, propranolol) decrease the heart's need for oxygen by reducing the heart's workload.

Take aspirin. Aspirin can be a big help for injury-related pain as well as the inflammation that comes with pericarditis, says Dr. Moser. Also, people with angina may help lower their risk of heart attack by taking aspirin every day (with their physician's consent). A baby aspirin or half of a full aspirin is all that is necessary, he says. And if someone is suffering a heart attack, swallowing an aspirin on the way to the hospital may help to prevent clotting, says Dr. Moser.

Settle your stomach. Take an antacid tablet or a spoonful of Maalox, gulp some water, eat a cracker—anything to cool down your raging heartburn. And avoid those foods that tend to anger your gastrointestinal system.

Let one rip. Take a big gulp of club soda, open your mouth and let out a loud belch. It may be rude, but if the pain is from gas or a large meal, you'll feel a lot better than if you mind your manners. (For more tips on getting rid of gas, see page 246.)

Prop yourself up. Some chest pain, like that caused by pericarditis, comes on while lying down. Dr. Chambers recommends propping yourself up with pillows to prevent and alleviate this discomfort.

Uncoil yourself. Loosen up. Relax. Meditate. Take a vacation. Or seek professional counseling. Stress and anxiety buildup may create chest pain, which only makes you more stressed and anxious.

Avoid activities that bring on the pain. Although exercise is important, angina pain may be more prevalent with certain aerobic activities like running or shoveling snow. Find less strenuous workouts like walking or swimming to keep yourself fit.

Kick the habit. Smoking constricts the blood vessels and makes the heart work harder. People who have angina often see a marked reduction in chest pains within weeks of quitting.

Imbibe with caution. One too many highballs can go to your heart as well as your head. Excessive alcohol consumption produces many heart irregularities, including chest pains.

Curtail your coffee consumption. Ditto for colas and other beverages containing caffeine or other stimulants.

See also Heartburn; Muscle Pain; Stomach Cramps

CHILLS

WHEN TO SEE YOUR DOCTOR

- A child who has chills and is also irritable or lethargic should see a doctor immediately—this could be a medical emergency.
- Your chills are so severe that your teeth are chattering.
- You have severe chills for more than an hour or the chills are recurring.
- You also have pain or discomfort anywhere.
- You have a heart valve abnormality and recently had either dental work done or an infection.
- You have a condition that compromises your immune system, such as diabetes.
- You have been taking oral steroids or are being treated for cancer.

WHAT YOUR SYMPTOM IS TELLING YOU

When you dash out into a frosty winter morning in your pajamas to fetch the newspaper, a quick shiver is your body's natural response. A home thermostat set too low might produce the same reaction: Brrrrr, I'm cold!

Other than when you're simply *chilly*, a chill is most likely to be your body's signal that a fever is on the way.

When viruses or bacteria invade, your trusty white blood cells release proteins that send a message to your brain's temperature control center. To fight off the infection, this control center begins to raise your temperature by constricting your blood vessels and making you shiver. As you shiver, the increased muscle activity produces heat, and the blood vessels in your skin contract to prevent heat loss.

When you have a chill, your skin may *feel* colder, but as blood is diverted from the skin to deeper inside your body, the temperature at the core of your body is actually on the rise. Most chills last for no more than 15 minutes before the fever becomes truly obvious, doctors say.

The flu bug or some other virus most often cues your chills, but any infection is a possibility—from pelvic or urinary tract infections to pneumonia. If your chills are bad enough that you feel like you're shaking all over, suspect an infection that has spread throughout your bloodstream. And if you've recently traveled in the tropics, it could be malaria.

SYMPTOM RELIEF

When you shake, rattle and roll and there's no music playing, here's comfort and cure.

Treat the fever. The over-the-counter medicines you normally use for fever will also blunt the chill response, says Harry Greene, M.D., chief of general medicine at the University of Arizona College of Medicine in Tucson. Acetaminophen and ibuprofen are both effective. (For a complete discussion of how to deal with a fever, see page 219.)

Hydrate and rest. The basics of virus care are the same for chills, Dr. Greene says. Be sure to increase your intake of liquids and get plenty of rest, he advises.

Use comfort strategies. Try these steps when a chill hits, suggests John C. Rogers, M.D., M.P.H., vice chairman of the Department of Family Medicine at Baylor College of Medicine in Houston. "During the chill, pile on the blankets. In a while, you'll get a fever," he says. "Then take your Tylenol and sit in a tub of body-temperature water. Use a washcloth to rub your skin, which will dilate blood vessels, and as the water slowly evaporates, you'll cool off."

Avoid alcohol rubdowns. Don't use alcohol as a body rub, Dr. Rogers says. Rubbing alcohol on your skin will evaporate quickly but add to your discomfort. "You don't need to bring your temperature down that quickly, and if you're having chills, your skin will feel even colder," he says.

Dismiss the Saint Bernard. You may feel like reaching for the brandy when a chill hits, but don't, says Dr. Rogers. "Alcohol will affect your mental abilities and may mask more dangerous symptoms you need to be alert for," he says. "When the fever comes, alcohol may also cause fainting and a fall in the tub."

See the doctor. When chills and fever are really persistent, your doctor will need to evaluate any other symptoms you may have, such as pain or a cough. If you have respiratory symptoms, he may want a sample of your sputum to test for bacteria that may be responsible. If a treatable infection is diagnosed, your doctor will prescribe antibiotics, says Dr. Greene. In the unlikely event that you have malaria, a variety of antimalarial drugs is available.

CLUMSINESS

WHEN TO SEE YOUR DOCTOR

- You suddenly become clumsy for unexplained reasons.
- You have difficulty seeing clearly.
- You have numbness, tingling or loss of feeling in your hands or feet.

WHAT YOUR SYMPTOM IS TELLING YOU

Somewhere in all of us, a klutz lurks.

"We're all clumsy to some extent. It just varies from person to person," says Robert Slater, M.D., an assistant professor of clinical neurology at the University of Pennsylvania School of Medicine in Philadelphia. "For the average person, a normal amount of clumsiness might be one or two awkward incidents a day. You might tip over a glass or bump into a doorway on any given day," Dr. Slater says. "On the other hand, if you bump into the doorway half the time you try to go through it or you knock the same glass over three times in a row in quick sequence, that may be cause for concern."

If you find yourself being more clumsy than you normally are, it could simply be a symptom of fatigue, premenstrual syndrome or anxiety. But it also could be a warning sign of a stroke, multiple sclerosis or a tumor.

SYMPTOM RELIEF

While a sudden increase in clumsiness should be brought to the attention of your doctor, there also are a number of quick, easy remedies for those occasional times when things near you seem to go bump, crash and rattle.

Don't dwell on it. "People who notice they're clumsy invariably become more clumsy," Dr. Slater says. "In reality, they may have been this clumsy all of their lives and suddenly, for some reason, often stress or fatigue, they become more aware of it."

Take a nap. You may be a bit more clumsy because you're tired. "If you know that you've been missing sleep, and you've been fumbling things around, then the first thing to do is to get some rest," says Dr. Slater.

Take time to relax. Some people who are prone to stress or are suffering from anxiety can become more fumble-fingered, Dr. Slater says. Stress-reduction techniques such as biofeedback or meditation may help.

Tennis, anyone? Exercises requiring hand/eye coordination can improve your reflexes and make you less clumsy, says Jim Buskirk, a physical therapist at the Dizziness and Balance Center in Wilmette, Illinois. "Activities like tennis and Ping-Pong are particularly good for hand/eye coordination," he says. "Just taking a paddle with a ball on a string and bouncing that for one or two minutes twice a day can help. We also have people hold two round sticks in their hands and we put a third stick on top so it forms an H. Then we ask them to roll the sideways stick back and forth."

Imagine your worst nightmare. Imagery can help you overcome your clumsiness, says Dennis Gersten, M.D., a San Diego psychiatrist and publisher of *Atlantis: The Imagery Newsletter*. To try it, close your eyes and imagine that you're in a shop full of china or glass figurines. Then imagine that you're the clumsiest person in the world. In your klutziness, you stumble and fall into all sorts of precious objects. Now let go and have a good laugh because the world did not fall apart.

"Many people walk on pins and needles so they avoid some imagined catastrophe. But actually imagining the worst-case scenario often takes the bite out of that fear of klutziness," Dr. Gersten says. Practice this imagery for five to ten minutes a day.

Bring out the animal in you. Animals are another image that helps people become less clumsy. "What is the most graceful animal that you can think of? A cheetah? An eagle?" Dr. Gersten asks. "Imagine yourself as that animal. Feel yourself as that animal. Feel how every muscle in your body works together. Feel the wind in your face as you run or soar through the air in perfect balance with yourself and with nature." Practice this imagery for five to ten minutes whenever your self-esteem is low because of an episode of clumsiness.

COLD SORES

WHEN TO SEE YOUR DOCTOR

- The first sore or any subsequent sore is accompanied by fever, swollen glands or flu symptoms.
- You get four or more eruptions in a year.
- The pain interferes with eating or daily living.

WHAT YOUR SYMPTOM IS TELLING YOU

A cold sore sounds so benign, like a little inconvenience you get along with the sniffles. You probably think of it as an innocuous nuisance that won't bother anyone and will go away soon enough.

Well, it'll go away, but it's far from innocuous. What we call cold sores or fever blisters actually are highly infectious mouth sores that affect about one-third of all Americans.

Cold sores are usually caused by the herpes simplex Type I virus, a variant virtually indistinguishable from the herpes simplex Type II strain, which normally affects the genitals, according to Eric Z. Shapira, D.D.S., a trustee on the national board of the Academy of General Dentistry and a dentist in private practice in Half Moon Bay, California. Once you get the virus, you have it for life and any subsequent eruptions will appear in exactly the same spot, he says.

A variety of environmental and physiological factors can coax a cold sore to reappear, including spicy food, sunlight, menstrual cycles, rainy days, stress and a fever.

Cold sore infections are quite common. You get one through contact with people who already have the virus, either by kissing them or touching them where they have an active, open lesion. Some 40 percent of the people with oral sores actually have the strain of the virus that usually affects the genitals, according to JoAnne Allen, D.D.S., a dentist in private practice in Albuquerque. And about 60 percent of the herpes virus found on genitals comes from the Type I strain most commonly found in the mouth.

As opposed to canker sores, which target the fleshy parts on the inside of the mouth, cold sores almost always erupt on or around the lips, says D'Anne Kleinsmith, M.D., a dermatologist in private practice in West Bloomfield, Michigan. Though they appear less frequently on the inside of the mouth, they can hit the parts that don't move—the gums and the roof of the mouth and occasionally the nostrils, fingers and even the eyelids.

The very first time you get a cold sore will probably be the most painful, Dr. Kleinsmith says. You'll also probably run a temperature and feel as though you've come down with the flu. In subsequent eruptions, you'll notice a tender, tingling sensation 36 to 48 hours before the cold sore appears. Usually, several round, reddish, pus-filled sores sprout in a cluster, often eventually forming one big ulceration that burns and swells until it breaks open, forms a yellow crust and fades away—all within a week to ten days—without scarring.

After the first one, subsequent cold sore eruptions inevitably—and unpredictably—occur every few months or so, sometimes at whim, sometimes because of factors like stress, fatigue, illness or cold weather. "There's no way to predict when or how frequently they erupt," Dr. Shapira says. "It depends on the person."

SYMPTOM RELIEF

When cold sores appear, here's what to do.

Keep it to yourself. The open ulceration is extremely infectious, Dr. Allen cautions. So be careful if you touch it, and don't touch anyone else after you've touched it. That means no kissing and no oral sex until the sore disappears. And no sharing towels, toothbrushes or cups, either.

"Since it can be so easily passed on to other mucous membranes," she says, "don't touch the sore and then rub your eyes or your nose or your genitals. If it gets in your eyes, it could cause blindness." (This is extremely rare but certainly possible.) You also can transfer the virus and the sores anywhere there's an open wound, like a cut on your finger, Dr. Shapira adds.

Wait for the scab. Even after a scab has formed, you can still transfer the virus to someone else or to some other part of your body. "I'd wait a week or two after the scab comes off before you resume kissing or any other contact," Dr. Shapira says.

Ask for acyclovir. Only one prescription drug, acyclovir, is used to treat all strains of herpes, whether on the mouth or the genitals, according to Dr. Shapira. He recommends a two-pronged approach—applying acyclovir ointment topically to the area as soon as you feel a cold sore coming on and taking the pill version orally.

Acyclovir prevents the virus from reproducing, Dr. Shapira says, and it should prevent a sore from forming if you catch it soon enough. If one or two small blisters appear, they'll probably last only a few days, he says. Without the drug, you might have a crusted ulcer that lasts two weeks. The pain, at least, usually will subside in 24 hours, he says.

Anesthetic might ease the pain. Over-the-counter ointments containing benzocaine can be applied directly to the herpes sore to numb it enough so you can eat comfortably, Dr. Allen says, but they won't speed healing.

Dull your diet. Spicy or acidic foods will aggravate the sore and produce a lot of pain, Dr. Shapira says. So take it easy on the tomatoes, jalapeño peppers and orange juice.

See also Canker Sores

COLD SWEATS

WHEN TO SEE YOUR DOCTOR

- Your cold sweats happen repeatedly during the night, night after night.
- You suspect that anxiety is causing your cold sweats.
- You also have sickle cell disease or a condition that impairs your immune system.
- If your cold sweats accompany overexposure to sun or heat, treat it as a medical emergency.

WHAT YOUR SYMPTOM IS TELLING YOU

You're an ice cube with the jitters, a snowman on a vibrating bed. You're wet, you're shivering, you're cold—and you're probably miserable.

More likely, a virus like the flu or mononucleosis has made your body its playground. Other, more serious infections, like tuberculosis and AIDS, can also cause cold sweats.

But maybe you're not under the weather—just under too much stress or feeling very anxious, two other causes of cold sweats.

Besides intense emotions, intense pain—like the pain of a migraine headache—can cause cold sweats. A surge of pain-sparked adrenaline can force open your sweat glands and shut down the blood vessels in your skin, making you sweaty and cold.

Adrenaline isn't the only hormone involved in cold sweats. Estrogen—or the lack of it—also plays a role. If you're a woman nearing menopause, you might sleep through a hot flash and wake up during the aftermath wrapped in clammy sheets. In fact, for some women, nighttime cold sweats are the only sign of hot flashes.

But the hormones aren't done yet—there's also insulin. If you're diabetic—a problem of too little insulin—you can experience cold sweats when your blood sugar drops.

Finally, cold sweats sometimes signal a medical emergency. They might be the sign of a severe heart or circulatory problem, though you'd probably notice chest pain first. (In a few rare cases cold sweats are the first sign of a heart attack.) Cold sweats might also indicate lowered blood pressure because of shock from loss of blood, perhaps from internal bleeding like a ruptured blood vessel.

SYMPTOM RELIEF

Because cold sweats are almost always linked to another condition, they don't really need separate treatment doctors say. They will go away when the underlying problem is treated. Here's a brief look at a few ways to deal with those problems.

Get tested. If your doctor thinks that an infection is causing your cold sweats, medical tests will show which microbe is responsible, says Adel Mahmoud, M.D., Ph.D. chairman of medicine at Case Western Reserve University School of Medicine in Cleveland. Your doctor will then prescribe an antibiotic to knock out the offending bacteria.

If the verdict is mononucleosis, you'll be advised to take fluids, eat a balanced diet and avoid exhausting exercise says Oliver Cooper, M.D., professor of family and community medicine at Texas A & M University Health Science Center College of Medicine in College Station. You'll also need to boycott contact sports when you're on the mend (to avoid rupturing your mono-swollen liver or spleen).

Ease your anxiety. If you suspect your cold sweats are caused by anxiety, don't hesitate to ask your doctor for help, says Robert Wesselhoeft III, M.D., director of family medicine at Tufts University School of Medicine in Boston (For other ways to cope with anxiety, see page 25.)

Relieve a migraine. When over-the-counter remedies like aspirin, acetaminophen or ibuprofen don't ease the pain your doctor can prescribe medicines to ease migraines and prevent further attacks, says John C. Rogers, M.D., M.P.H. vice chairman of the Department of Family Medicine at Baylor College of Medicine in Houston.

Evaluate your estrogen. If you think hot flashes may be causing those clammy sweats, ask your doctor what treatments may be appropriate, says David Losh, M.D., associate professor of family practice at the University of Washington School of Medicine in Seattle. Hormone replacement therapy is one possible option. (For other coping techniques, see Hot Flashes on page 315.)

CONGESTION

WHEN TO SEE YOUR DOCTOR

- You're also coughing or wheezing, your sputum is discolored and you have chills and a fever.
- You also have chest pain, irregular heartbeat, swelling in your ankles or a history of heart disease.
- You're short of breath or find it difficult to breathe.

WHAT YOUR SYMPTOM IS TELLING YOU

It's rush hour in your lungs. Your bronchial highways are packed tightly with bumper-to-bumper congestion, and you're honking and hacking. Every inhalation is a fight for an exit ramp off that breathing bottleneck.

Congestion means different things to different people. Some use the term to describe a tightness in their lungs, as if a wide strap were affixed firmly across the chest, says Richard L. Sheldon, M.D., a pulmonologist and internist at Beaver Medical Clinic in Banning, California. They also may find it difficult to breathe or feel short of breath.

If by congestion you mean a tightness in the chest, it's likely that you have asthma. If this is the case, you may notice a dry cough or wheezing as your constricted and swollen bronchial passages try to move air in and out.

Tightness and congestion also could indicate heart trou-

ble. The lungs fill with fluid because the heart isn't pumpin
properly. Clues to look out for include swollen ankle
shortness of breath, awakening at night with difficult
breathing, chest pain and palpitations (or irregular hear
beat) as well as a history of heart problems.

When other people complain of congestion, "the
describe a lot of soupy stuff down there in their lungs," say
Dr. Sheldon. "They're usually coughing up a lot of tha
soupy stuff, too."

If you feel as if there's burning in your windpipe or lik
you're trying to breathe through the froth of a tall glass o
root beer, chances are you have some sort of respirator
irritation or infection. Something is harassing you
bronchial tubes enough to force them to counterattack b
increasing the production of mucus, according to Anne I
Davis, M.D., associate professor of clinical medicine in th
Division of Pulmonary and Critical Care Medicine at Nev
York University Medical Center and assistant to the direc
tor of chest service at Bellevue Hospital Center in Nev
York City.

An irritant in the air—such as pollution, dust, poller
smoke or chemicals—may be responsible, says Dr. Davis
If it is, the congestion may be fleeting, leaving soon afte
you've escaped the irritant. But sometimes there can be
lag time of six to eight hours.

If your congestion is caused by an infection, you'll prob
ably know it, says Charles P. Felton, M.D., chief of pu
monary medicine at Harlem Hospital Center and a clinica
professor of medicine at Columbia University College o
Physicians and Surgeons in New York City. The phlegm
that you cough up will be yellow, green or brown. You'
also have a fever or the chills, and you won't feel very wel
The infection could be anything from a mild cold to sever
bronchitis or pneumonia, says Dr. Felton. Latent chroni
bronchitis or emphysema also could be stirred from it
slumber by a milder bug, he says.

SYMPTOM RELIEF

As with traffic on the way home from work, you may have to tolerate the congestion until it clears. But here are a few shortcuts to try and some snarls to avoid.

Love those liquids. Drink more water and juices to loosen up and liquefy the increased mucus that's stuck down in your lungs, Dr. Felton says.

Go full steam. Holing up in the bathroom and turning on the hot water may provide some relief if you have an infection, Dr. Davis says. The hot, moist air may make you feel better. "But some people feel worse after exposing themselves to steam," she notes. "It's a matter of trial and error."

Try some tea. Have something warm to help loosen lung secretions, Dr. Davis recommends. Enjoy some tea with a little honey and lemon, for example. "It's also soothing on your irritated throat," she says. In addition, caffeine in tea or coffee may help open up your air passages.

Take something for your cough. Over-the-counter cough syrups containing guaifenesin help thin out the mucus lodged in your lungs, making it easier to cough up, says Dr. Felton.

Suppress the suppressants. If your lungs feel clogged with mucus and you're already hacking, leave cough suppressants on the shelf, Dr. Sheldon advises. You're *supposed* to cough and get rid of that gunk.

Widen the bronchial highway. If your physician diagnoses your congestion as asthma, Dr. Sheldon says you'll be given bronchodilating inhalers or pills to help you breathe easier.

Don't play doctor. One of the most counterproductive self-treatment steps is to rummage through the medicine cabinet and take a few old antibiotics from infections gone by. "Those antibiotics have made whatever bug you have down there stronger," Dr. Sheldon says. "The last time you took that drug, the bugs were warned that it was in the environment and they built up their defenses against it. You have to go after those bugs with something the little devils don't expect." And Dr. Sheldon also urges you to take the antibiotics your doctor prescribes for the full course of treatment: seven to ten days. Stopping earlier—even if you feel better—means you won't kill all the bugs.

See also Coughing; Wheezing

CONSTIPATION

WHEN TO SEE YOUR DOCTOR

- You're uncomfortable from not having a bowel movement.
- Your bowel habits suddenly change.
- You're also suffering from abdominal pain or vomiting.

WHAT YOUR SYMPTOM IS TELLING YOU

Let's see now: Once a week you do your laundry, water your plants and go to the grocery store. Not a bad schedule. But if your bowel movements have suddenly joined this list of weekly activities, and you're feeling bloated and uncomfortable, you're probably constipated.

"Generally speaking, your comfort level is probably the best indicator of constipation," says Barry Jaffin, M.D., a motility disorder specialist and clinical instructor in the Department of Gastroenterology at Mount Sinai Hospital in New York City. "But if you've gone from making a trip to the bathroom once a day to once a week, that's a pretty sure sign also." Other symptoms of constipation, according to Dr. Jaffin: Straining, small hard stools and hemorrhoids.

A lot of everyday things can turn down the volume on nature's call—certain medications, lack of fiber or water, lack of exercise and too much iron. But a number of digestive problems can also cause constipation. These range in severity from irritable bowel syndrome to more serious conditions like colon cancer, colitis, Crohn's disease, diverticulitis and ischemia (decreased blood flow to the colon). One digestive disease, *colonic inertia*, can keep a person from having a bowel movement for more than two weeks. In colonic inertia, the colon fails to squeeze properly.

Just don't try to blame constipation on aging. As far as doctors can tell, with a little care your digestive system is built to perform for the life of your chassis.

"There's no evidence that the bowel stops working as you get older," says Nicholas J. Talley, M.D., an associate professor of medicine at the Mayo Clinic Medical School in Rochester, Minnesota. "In fact, it probably works just as well whether you're old or young."

SYMPTOM RELIEF

If you're not suffering from abdominal pain, you can probably treat your constipation yourself. Try these tips.

Fill up on fiber. Fiber—the nondigestible bulk found in whole-grain products, fruits and vegetables—works in at least two important ways to help prevent constipation, says Peter Holt, M.D., chief of the Division of Gastroenterology at St. Luke's–Roosevelt Hospital Center and professor of medicine at Columbia University College of Physicians and Surgeons in New York City. Instead of immediately turning into soup during digestion, fiber acts like a sponge, sopping up liquid in your intestines and colon, resulting in firmer stool, says Dr. Holt.

But fiber's benefits don't stop there: Fiber's arrival gives your colon the green light to contract. And because the colon is the last stop on your meal's digestive tour, you'll soon get the signal that it's time to find a bathroom.

So how much fiber is enough? Aim for about 25 grams a day, he says. "If you were to adhere to the recommendation of 5, one-ounce servings of fruits and vegetables a day, then you should have more than enough fiber in your diet," he adds.

Add an OTC fiber product. If you're unwilling or unable to crunch through all that fiber, you can occasionally add one of several over-the-counter fiber products like Metamucil, Citrucel or Perdiem to your diet. But use them carefully: If you don't add them to enough fluid, you could end up more constipated than when you started, says Dr. Talley. That's why it's important to follow directions on the label carefully.

Don't forget fluids. Whether you prefer juice or water, most doctors recommend that you drink between six and ten eight-ounce glasses of fluids a day to prevent constipation, says Dr. Jaffin.

Avoid artificial laxatives. Are you using stimulant laxatives once a week to keep yourself regular? Be careful—there's evidence that you could be damaging your colon, says Dr. Talley. "Sustained use of these products—if you were to use one daily for a year or more, for example—is one of the worst things you can do in the long run," he says.

Get some exercise. Here's yet another reason to put on your walking shoes: Exercise can help prevent constipation by stimulating the colon, says Dr. Holt.

Keep your eye on iron. While iron is an important mineral—especially for women—too much can cause constipation. Unless you're under doctor's orders, you can probably meet your iron needs with a good multivitamin rather than taking a separate iron supplement, says Dr. Jaffin.

Check medications. Certain drugs can cause constipation by blocking the creation of a chemical that helps push waste through your bowel, says Dr. Jaffin. These include medications to relieve high blood pressure, antipsychotic drugs and even some over-the-counter antihistamines and pain relievers. If you're taking any over-the-counter remedies, give them a rest and see if that makes a difference. Before going off any prescription drugs, however, see your doctor.

Try an enema. Stubborn causes of constipation may require an enema—an over-the-counter product containing fluid that's inserted in the rectum and causes the colon to contract, thereby inducing a bowel movement. Use only occasionally and as directed, says Dr. Holt.

See your doctor. If you're faithfully following dietary

guidelines and not taking any drugs that may cause constipation and are still having trouble, ask your doctor to perform a sigmoidoscopy or other tests to look at the colon. This simple office procedure will allow your doctor to get a closer look at your colon and anything in it that might be causing a problem, says Dr. Jaffin.

CORNS

WHAT YOUR SYMPTOM IS TELLING YOU

What causes corns—those small, yellowish gray, wartlike protuberances on your toes? "Constant pressure and friction between skin and shoe," says Richard Abdo, M.D., director of the Foot and Ankle Clinic at the Lahey Clinic in Burlington, Massachusetts.

As your shoes rub the tops of your toes, the skin thickens and hardens to absorb the punishment. Over the years, the dead skin is molded into a mound called a hard corn, which may be painful, Dr. Abdo says.

If you have more than one hard corn, you may have hammertoe, which is a contraction that pulls the toe upward into a flexed position, forcing it to rub against your shoes.

Soft corns, which develop between toes, are caused when small bone spurs are forced to rub together. The forcing is done by—you guessed it—tight shoes.

SYMPTOM RELIEF

If you'd rather keep your corn in the cupboard, try these treatments.

Shed those shoes. You obviously can't stop wearing shoes entirely, but you can go shoeless as often as possible.

"It certainly would keep you from having any discomfort," says Steve Guida, D.P.M., a Fort Lauderdale, Florida, podiatrist.

Buy shoes that fit. Make sure that your shoe has what's called a high toebox—which means enough room from the sole of the shoe to the top of the shoe so that your toes are comfortably accommodated, including any corns or hammertoes that you already have. "As long as there is no direct pressure to the top of the foot, you're not going to have any problems with irritations or corns," says Dr. Abdo.

Throw your corn a lifesaver. You can temporarily relieve corn pain by using doughnut-shaped corn pads. Available at any drugstore, most of the nonmedicated pads have an adhesive backing and a hole in the middle that fits directly over the middle of the corn. "The pad takes the pressure off the corn, or at least spreads it out," says Dr. Abdo.

Soak 'em and pumice 'em. After soaking your feet in lukewarm water for 20 to 25 minutes and applying some baby oil directly to the corn, take a pumice stone or an emery board and gently rub off several layers of the corn. Do not use a razor blade! Remember, you're not trying to remove the corn completely, you're just making some room between your corn and your shoe, says Myles Schneider, D.P.M., an Annandale, Virginia, podiatrist and coauthor of *How to Doctor Your Feet without a Doctor.* Apply a corn pad after the procedure.

Watch that acid wash. Topical acids and plaster treatments purchased over-the-counter to treat corns aren't recommended by the American Podiatric Society, says Dr. Schneider. Many podiatrists feel that these are not safe, as they can cause infections. People with diabetes or circulation problems should not use them at all. But if you do use one, follow the directions carefully—using too much of the acid or using it improperly can burn the healthy skin.

See your doctor. If you're reluctant to wield your own pumice stone, your doctor or podiatrist can soak your feet briefly in a whirlpool to soften the corns and then shave them for you, says Dr. Guida.

COUGHING

WHEN TO SEE YOUR DOCTOR

- The cough persists for more than two weeks and doesn't seem to be getting better.
- You're coughing up a lot of discolored phlegm or what appears to be blood.
- You also have chest pain, fever, chills or night sweats.

WHAT YOUR SYMPTOM IS TELLING YOU

Is that the dog barking its head off at some rabbit out in the yard? Is it the neighborhood automatic weapons expert playing with his new machine gun? Or is it just your husband having another coughing fit?

Virtually *anything* could be responsible for that big hack attack, which is the lungs' reflexive response to some sort of irritation—much like a tap on the kneecap with a mallet makes the leg bounce. The key to understanding your cough and choosing its cure is what (if anything) comes up with it—whether it's a dry, unproductive cough or a wet, phlegm-producing cough.

Any irritant in the environment can spark a dry cough, according to Anne L. Davis, M.D., associate professor of clinical medicine in the Division of Pulmonary and Critical Care Medicine at New York University Medical Center and assistant to the director of chest service at Bellevue Hospital Center in New York City. "If you have an allergy, a cough can be a major manifestation of it," she says. Smoke, chemicals, noxious fumes, pollen, dust and animal dander all can irritate the lungs' bronchial tubes, prompting a cough as an attempt to get rid of the offender. "If you're sensitive, even moving into a new office or getting a new carpet might make you cough," she says.

Asthma often produces a dry cough instead of the traditional wheeze, according to Richard L. Sheldon, M.D., a pulmonologist and internist at Beaver Medical Clinic in Banning, California. "In fact, asthma is the most common cause of an undiagnosed cough, especially if you're coughing at night," he says.

Postnasal drip and a digestive problem called gastric reflux are two other frequent and relatively harmless sources of coughing, says Sally E. Wenzel, M.D., assistant professor of medicine at the National Jewish Center for Immunology and Respiratory Medicine in Denver. If the drip trips your cough, you'll usually feel it trickling down and tickling your throat. In reflux, a malfunctioning valve separating your stomach from your esophagus allows digesting food and stomach acid to defy gravity and seep up into your throat, giving you a sour taste in your mouth along with the cough.

Bacterial, viral and fungal infections—from a simple cold to bronchitis and pneumonia—inflame the respiratory tract and can trigger a cough, Dr. Sheldon says. All of these illnesses frequently start with an arid, raspy cough and, as the lungs manufacture more mucus, progress to a sputum-filled hack.

Besides possible fever, chest pain, congestion and a general feeling of the blahs, Dr. Sheldon says, you'll know you have an infection if your phlegm is any color other than clear or white.

Don't worry too much if a cough lingers on after the rest of your cold goes away. "That's just some residual congestion in the outer areas of the lungs that you'll get, especially after a viral cold," Dr. Sheldon says. "It doesn't mean you have asthma or anything like that, just some swelling that the lung senses and wants to cough out."

Smoking, of course, is an obvious source of a lingering cough, especially in a longtime smoker. In response to the irritant, the lungs create many more mucus-secreting cells. But you may not notice the extra phlegm. The muck can't get up the throat easily because the smoke paralyzes the hairlike cilia that line the bronchial tubes, Dr. Sheldon explains. That's why smokers often awaken in the morning with a gagging, sputum-laden cough that stops after they've had a couple of butts.

More seriously, a nagging, constant cough could be chronic bronchitis or emphysema, in which the lungs try to cough out trapped air that can't escape through restricted passages, Dr. Sheldon says. People with these conditions also experience shortness of breath and difficulty in breathing.

Most seriously, the cough could be a sign of a tumor or lung cancer. "Lung cancer is now the most common cancer in both men and women," says Dr. Sheldon, "and it presents itself mostly as a cough."

SYMPTOM RELIEF

You certainly don't have to go to the doctor every time you get a little tickle in the back of your throat, or even if you pick up a little barking bug. "They come and go," Dr. Sheldon says. "You know what it is. You had it a year ago. Your wife had it two weeks ago. It'll resolve itself in a few days."

If it doesn't, see your doctor. And, if you feel sharp pain when you cough—or you cough up what looks like blood—or that hack persists unabated for a couple of weeks, you'd better visit your doctor. In the meantime, though, don't sit by idly, sputtering and spitting like an old jalopy. Try these cough controllers.

Drown that hack. If you have a phlegm-producing cough, you need to thin the phlegm so you can more easily expel it from your lungs. "Probably the best way to liquefy sputum so it comes up easily is to keep yourself well hydrated," Dr. Sheldon says. So drink as much water as you can stand. (You also want to stay well hydrated if you have a dry cough, which will be much more tolerable if it's drenched with drink.)

Go for guaifenesin. Over-the-counter cough syrups containing guaifenesin help to water down thick mucus, according to Dr. Sheldon.

Don't muzzle your bark. You're coughing because your reflexes are attempting to eliminate an irritation, so stifling the hack with cough suppressants will be counterproductive, especially if your lungs are working overtime on the phlegm assembly line. "You usually want to get that stuff out of there," Dr. Sheldon says. "If you turn that mechanism off, that stuff is going to puddle and pool down there."

Silence it for some sleep. If you have an incessant, naggy, noisy cough that's keeping you and everybody else in the house awake at night, you can consider some *judicious* use of an over-the-counter cough suppressant. "If you have a bad cough and your ribs hurt and you're losing sleep, you can just shut it off for a while with a cough medication," Dr. Sheldon says. With a phlegm-producing hack, "you have to recognize that you'll have some puddling of mucus down there. But you can accept that so you can get some relief."

The best over-the-counter cough suppressants contain dextromethorphan. A prescription syrup most likely will contain codeine. Both tend to make you drowsy.

Soothe it with salt. If you're coughing a lot, your throat probably is sore and scratchy, and that irritation will only make your cough worse. For relief, gargle frequently with salt water, Dr. Wenzel suggests. Just stir 1/2 teaspoon salt into one cup warm water. Don't swallow, especially if you're on a salt-restricted diet.

Banish the butts. It goes without saying, but it's worth emphasizing: Smoking causes and aggravates any cough you might have. If you can't quit on your own, ask your doctor to recommend a program that can help you quit.

Be a broncho buster. To tackle that lingering hack, ask your doctor for a bronchodilator. "It accelerates the clearing, and the cough will be gone," says Dr. Sheldon.

Get a whiff of water. Dry air will irritate your lungs and make your cough worse, says Dr. Wenzel. Using a humidifier in your home will moisten the air and make it easier going for your respiratory tract. But keep the humidifier clean, she cautions. They tend to grow mold, which, if you're sensitive to it, will aggravate your cough.

COUGHING UP BLOOD

WHEN TO SEE YOUR DOCTOR

- In the absence of a cold or the flu, you notice small spots or streaks of red in your phlegm.
- You also have a fever, pain in the chest and shortness of breath.
- Your phlegm is very red or you cough up what seems to be blood more than once.

WHAT YOUR SYMPTOM IS TELLING YOU

At the very least, it might be a nosebleed. At the very worst, it might be a serious lung problem. Either way (and anywhere in between), coughing up blood should be taken seriously, even though it may *not* be.

The presence of blood in your sputum or phlegm usually indicates at least a little bleeding in your respiratory tract somewhere between your nose and the bottom of your lungs. An innocuous nosebleed, for example, might cause some red postnasal drip that you cough up, according to Richard L. Sheldon, M.D., a pulmonologist and internist at Beaver Medical Clinic in Banning, California. But bleeding from anywhere other than your nose is more problematic. A harsh coughing spell, for example, could have ruptured a blood vessel in your lung, according to Charles P. Felton, M.D., chief of pulmonary medicine at Harlem Hospital Center and a clinical professor of medicine at Columbia University College of Physicians and Surgeons in New York City. "Many times you'll also see blood in early viral infections," he says.

Bronchitis and certain strains of pneumonia may cause blood vessels in the lungs to bleed, Dr. Sheldon says. So can blood clots and swelling of lung tissue caused by heart problems. At the worst, tuberculosis and lung cancer could produce bloody phlegm, Dr. Sheldon says.

The source of the blood isn't always confined to the respiratory tract. You could also be bleeding in your stomach and coughing it up, Dr. Sheldon says.

If the blood is a fresh bright red, you're still bleeding. If it's a darker red, or perhaps brown or rust-colored, the blood has dried or clotted. In less serious cases, the blood will appear as small red dots or flecks in the mucus, says Dr. Felton. In more serious cases, the blood may appear as streaks or clots, or it could just well up in the mouth, Dr. Sheldon says.

SYMPTOM RELIEF

You can't put a tourniquet on bloody sputum. Either the blood disappears harmlessly soon after it appears, or you continue to cough it up, and you're on your way to the doctor's office. In either case, here's what you need to do.

Keep an eye on it. If you have a bad cold or a viral infection and you notice a few spots of blood in your mucus, Dr. Felton says to stay vigilant: Watch out to see if it happens again or gets worse. If it does, see your doctor.

Don't block the blood. Don't take an over-the-counter cough suppressant to stifle your blood-tinged sputum, cautions Sally E. Wenzel, M.D., an assistant professor of medicine at the National Jewish Center for Immunology and Respiratory Medicine in Denver. By treating yourself, you might be allowing blood to pool somewhere inside your body, and you could be masking a sign of a serious problem. Your doctor may decide you need a cough suppressant so you don't aggravate whatever might be producing the blood, but let that be his or her option.

Cough into a container. If you cough up blood more than once or are worried enough by what you see to go to the doctor, make sure you take along a sample of the phlegm for testing, says Dr. Wenzel. If it's an infection, the test will ensure that you get the right antibiotic.

D

DANDRUFF

WHEN TO SEE YOUR DOCTOR

- You also have itchy red patches on your scalp.

WHAT YOUR SYMPTOM IS TELLING YOU

The first flakes fluttering from the sky usually confirm that winter has arrived. Flakes falling from your head—dandruff—are usually a tip-off that an annoying yet common yeast called *Pityrosporon ovale* has set up a snow-making machine on your scalp.

There's no need to catch the next sleigh out of town, however. *Pityrosporon* lives on *everyone*. In about 20 percent of the population, the yeast inflames the skin of the scalp, which makes it shed and flake faster than normal—a condition doctors call seborrheic dermatitis. This condition turns the light dusting on your shoulder—which happens imperceptibly to everyone, everyday—into a whitish blizzard.

It may just be a cold day in you know where before doctors know what transforms this mild-mannered yeast into a dermatological demon. One theory suggests that the immune system, which normally guards your skin, stages a slowdown, allowing the freeloading yeast free reign.

"It might be that the immune response of the skin—the checks and balances, so to speak—for some reason suddenly allows the proliferation of bacteria and fungi on our skin, which may aggravate the dandruff," says Maria Hordinsky, M.D., associate professor of dermatology at the University of Minnesota in Minneapolis. Heredity may also play a role.

Skin conditions like psoriasis, characterized by bright red patches on elbows and knees, can also start with what seems to be a bad case of dandruff, says Jerome Shupack, M.D., professor of clinical dermatology at New York University Medical Center in New York City. These more severe types of dandruff should receive medical attention.

SYMPTOM RELIEF

Once you've had dandruff, its return is as inevitable as fresh powder on your driveway after a day at the shovel.

There's simply no cure. But you can manage your scalp's flaking and itching by killing the yeast that causes it. "That's your whole goal," says Albert Kligman, M.D., Ph.D., professor of dermatology at the University of Pennsylvania in Philadelphia, who was once dubbed the King of Dandruff for his work in the field. "When you suppress that yeast, dandruff disappears."

If dandruff has your dander up, try these remedies.

Work yourself into a lather. If you're suffering from only a few errant flakes, just washing your hair more often (at least once a day) with a standard shampoo may be enough to do the trick, says Dr. Shupack.

Choose your weapon. If the flakes persist, it's time to move to a more aggressive treatment. Over-the-counter shampoos containing selenium sulfide are the best at battling dandruff, says Dr. Kligman. "It's great stuff—knocks the heck out of it in two to three weeks," he says. Next on Dr. Kligman's list: shampoos made with pyrithione zinc, coal tar and salicylic acid, in that order. "Coal tar and salicylic acid aren't as good because they're messy, they smell lousy and they just aren't as effective," he says.

Take turns with your treatment. "I've found that if you have people rotate their shampoos, they get an even better response," says Dr. Hordinsky. "When you shampoo on a daily basis with a particular shampoo, all of a sudden you perceive a plateau—the shampoo doesn't do any good any more." For best results, says Dr. Hordinsky, buy a couple different dandruff shampoos and use them in rotation.

Shampooing twice is nice. That line on the dandruff shampoo bottle urging you to lather your hair twice isn't just a line to get you to buy more shampoo, says Dr. Shupack. "Dandruff shampoo has two elements to it, the soap or detergent action to degrease the hair, and the medicinal quality delivered the second time around," he says. "You'd probably have a little better penetration of the medicine when you have a degreased scalp."

Subdue stress. "Certainly the three conditions that are the most common causes of dandruff are all known to be influenced by stress or aggravated by stress," says Dr. Shupack. "If you could reduce that, it would probably help."

Put some sunlight on the subject. If your hair is thinning and you have dandruff, some exposure to sun may help temper the yeast, says Dr. Shupack.

All's well with oil—when it's not too hot. "Applying oil to the scalp will often help loosen and dissolve dandruff. But oil, when it's too hot, can damage the hair shaft and cause breakage of the hair," says Dr. Shupack. Rather than buying a hot-oil treatment, simply put a few drops of olive oil on your scalp after shampooing at night, cover your head with a shower cap and shampoo again in the morning. "That's an excellent home remedy," he says.

Hunt down some hydrocortisone lotion. Available without a prescription, 1 percent hydrocortisone lotion helps relieve the inflammation that contributes to dandruff, says Dr. Shupack. The only drawback: Hydrocortisone can mask a serious fungal infection until treatment is stopped—allowing it to reappear with a vengeance, he says. Apply several drops after shampooing and work it into the scalp. A stronger hydrocortisone cream is also available by prescription; see your doctor.

Make your dandruff miserable—with Nizoral. This highly touted antifungal shampoo is available by prescription only, but it works well on stubborn cases, says Dr. Shupack. Ask your doctor.

See also Scalp Itching

DELIRIUM

WHEN TO SEE YOUR DOCTOR

- Anyone experiencing delirium needs immediate medical attention.

WHAT YOUR SYMPTOM IS TELLING YOU

Delirium comes on like a dense fog rising out of the cool night air. It envelops your mind in a shroud of confusion, where everyone seems like a stranger. You don't know where you are or what day it is.

Scary? You bet. Perplexing? No doubt. But there's an excellent chance of quickly re-establishing a link with reality with prompt medical care.

Delirium develops within minutes and can last for days, disrupting the workings of the brain in ways that are still unclear to medical researchers, says Larry Westreich, M.D., a psychiatrist at Bellevue Hospital Center in New York City. Even during the worst attack of delirium, a person can have moments of rational thought before suddenly falling back into never-never land.

Many things can cause delirium, including high fever, alcohol abuse, illegal drugs such as marijuana and cocaine or even a knock on the head. Sometimes delirium comes as a side effect of certain medications, such as cimetidine, used for ulcers, or corticosteroids, used for inflammation. Delirium can also be a sign of serious disease such as appendicitis, epilepsy, diabetes, heart disease or stroke.

SYMPTOM RELIEF

Delirium can signal a potentially life-threatening ailment, and you should seek medical care immediately," Dr. Westreich says.

While help is on the way, here are a few things you can

do to make a delirious person more comfortable and help doctors make the right diagnosis.

Let nothing past the lips. Don't let a delirious person eat or drink anything, advises Steven Mandel, M.D., clinical professor of neurology at Jefferson Medical College and an attending physician at Thomas Jefferson University Hospital in Philadelphia. Doctors may also have to pump the person's stomach to remove drugs that may be causing the delirium. In addition, if the delirium is caused by appendicitis or some other ailment that requires surgery, food or drink may complicate the procedure, Dr. Westreich says.

Nab the culprit. Scan the area near the person who is delirious for prescription medications, illegal drugs and drug paraphernalia such as pipes or needles. If you find any, make sure that a doctor, nurse or emergency medical technician knows about it.

Be on guard. Never leave a delirious person alone, says Peter Roy-Byrne, M.D., professor of psychiatry at the University of Washington and chief of psychiatry at Harborview Medical Center in Seattle. "You shouldn't assume that a delirious person is capable of taking care of themselves," he says. "If the person says, 'Leave me alone. I just need to go outside and get some air,' don't let him. He may lapse back into delirium and wander out into the street."

Speak softly. "As a person becomes delirious, they often get frightened," says Alan Unis, M.D., assistant professor of psychiatry and behavioral sciences at the University of Washington School of Medicine in Seattle. "Talk to the person in a calm voice. Let the person know where he is, assure him that you won't leave him alone and tell him that help is on the way."

Keep it one-on-one. The delirious person might become more frightened and confused if several people are talking to him, says Dr. Westreich. He suggests one person do all the talking.

DEPRESSION

WHEN TO SEE YOUR DOCTOR

- You feel a sad, worried or "empty" feeling that never goes away.
- You're thinking of suicide.
- Relationships and activities you once enjoyed have lost the "joy." Even sex has lost its savor.
- You can't sleep, you're sleeping too much or you're waking too early in the morning.
- You're feeling down and you're having trouble concentrating, remembering or making decisions.
- You're feeling down and you're drinking more than usual.
- You're experiencing crying spells.

WHAT YOUR SYMPTOM IS TELLING YOU

Remember that black cloud hanging over Joe Btfsplk's head in the comic strip "Li'l Abner"? No one needed a caption to know what it meant. Readers of all ages instinctively recognized Joe's pessimistic mood. Like the Sunday comics that appeal to us because of their universal humor, there's a universal sad side to life, too.

The pain of grief and the lingering sadness you feel after the loss of someone you love are part of the human package. So are personal disasters like a divorce or losing a job. Depression under these circumstances (even depression lasting several months) can be perfectly normal, says Paul Wender, M.D., distinguished professor of psychiatry at the University of Utah School of Medicine in Salt Lake City.

If you have low self-esteem or are easily overwhelmed by stress, you may also be prone to depression. And depression can have a physical cause, too. Researchers have found that many people with major depression often have an imbalance of certain chemicals in the brain.

SYMPTOM RELIEF

No matter what the cause, there are many effective ways to lighten your own shade of blue.

Put guilt in perspective. If your depression springs from a sense of wrongdoing, beating yourself up over it won't help, says Heather Andersen, a registered nurse with a master's in nursing and a lecturer in the School of Social Work at the University of Washington in Seattle. "It's important to take some kind of action," she says. "Guilt actually deals with the mistake, but toxic guilt or shame says 'I *am* the mistake.'"

Lighten the load with regular routine. "Regularize your sleep/wake cycle," suggests Ellen Leibenluft, M.D., a Bethesda, Maryland, psychiatrist. "Cut out the naps. That will make it easier for you to regulate your sleep cycle and structure your time. You'll get more work done, which boosts your self-esteem and makes you feel better. But if your schedule asks you to be in three places at once, cut it back—you're overstressed."

Put down your morning picker-upper. That sweetened cup of coffee may pack a double depressant, says Larry Christensen, Ph.D., a psychologist at Texas A & M University in College Station. "Sugar and caffeine can be tremendous contributors to depression." Many people who eliminate them feel the difference within four or five days to a week, Dr. Christensen says.

Designate drinking—to others. A low period is a good time to forgo alcohol, says David Dunner, M.D., professor of psychiatry and co-director of the Center for Anxiety and Depression at the University of Washington in Seattle. Despite its short-term numbing effects on your feelings, alcohol is a potent depressant.

Exercise the blues away. "Many people find that exercise has an antidepressant effect," says Dr. Leibenluft. Exercise regularly, within the bounds of what's okay for you medically.

Arm yourself with education. Read a good book about depression, recommends Dr. Dunner. His top titles? *The Good News about Depression* by Mark Gold, *Feeling*

Good by David Burns and *Moodswing* by Ronald Fieve. Or contact the D/ART (Depression Awareness, Recognition and Treatment) Program for information. Write to D/ART, National Institutes of Mental Health, 5600 Fishers Lane, Room 10-85, Rockville, MD 20857.

Turn off the tube. Watching TV is seductive and can be closely tied to depression, says Robert Kubey, Ph.D., a psychologist and associate professor of communication at Rutgers University in New Brunswick, New Jersey. "One of the primary symptoms of depression is lethargy, lack of zest and lack of energy," he says. "Heavy TV use can make it more difficult for some people to break out of the depression." Dr. Kubey is also coauthor of *Television and the Quality of Life*.

Kick the habit. Smoking is another habit linked to depression, but if you're deep in the blues, you'll need more help to quit. "You may need to seek professional help," says Naomi Breslau, Ph.D., director of psychiatry research at Henry Ford Hospital in Detroit. "It takes many tries, so don't give up!"

Go easy on yourself. "Don't make major decisions when you're depressed," says Dr. Dunner. Changing jobs or getting married or divorced ought to be seriously considered only *after* the depression has lifted. Feeling better takes time, so don't expect too much from yourself too soon.

Treat your senses to scents. Research has shown that there is a direct and powerful connection between smell and emotions. Even subliminal amounts of scent can change brain waves, say researchers at the Smell and Taste Treatment and Research Foundation in Chicago. The odor of jasmine may actually improve a depressed person's level of energy, for example, according to Alan R. Hirsch, M.D., neurologic director of the foundation. Buy some jasmine oil at a health food store and try his suggestion: "Take a little and put it on your arm or hand and just sniff when you feel your energy level is low."

When Depression Lingers

Tried everything and still buried in the blues? When depression just won't budge, there are still more sources of relief. Your doctor can help you decide which of these approaches may work best for you.

Review your Rx. Certain prescriptions, including blood pressure medications, antihistamines and steroids prescribed for asthma, can trigger depression. An over- or underfunctioning endocrine gland, such as the thyroid, can also bring on the symptoms. Talk to your doctor about these possible effects of your prescription medications.

Consider counseling. A trusted therapist can offer tremendous insight into your problems. Interpersonal therapists focus on the disturbed relationships that can cause or intensify your depression. Cognitive or behavioral therapists can help you change the negative styles of thinking and behaving that often accompany the blues.

Change your chemistry. Your doctor may prescribe an antidepressant medication. Antidepressants have a proven track record and are not habit-forming. Two traditional types are tricyclics and monoamine oxidase inhibitors (MAOIs). You might ask your doctor about fluoxetine and bupropion, two antidepressants that generally lack the side effects sometimes associated with the traditional drugs.

Bolster your Bs. New research suggests that increased levels of the B vitamins thiamine, riboflavin and B6 may make tricyclic antidepressants work better in elderly people, according to researcher Iris Bell, M.D., Ph.D., a psychiatrist at the University of Arizona Health Science Center in Tucson. But as with all medications, take vitamins only in consultation with your doctor. Vitamin B6 can be toxic when taken in high amounts.

DIARRHEA

WHEN TO SEE YOUR DOCTOR

- You have diarrhea for more than one week.
- You're also losing weight.

WHAT YOUR SYMPTOM IS TELLING YOU

Diarrhea may very well be the thunderstorm of stomach problems—a painful, sometimes embarrassing display of both sound and fury. But you have to really search to find a silver lining behind this dark digestive cloud. In fact, doctors say the best you can do is to learn how to weather the storm or avoid it altogether.

Why the weather analogy? Consider the crucial role water plays in your discomfort. Including both what you drink and the liquid contained in the food you eat, three to four gallons of fluid reach your intestines each day. If all goes well (pardon the pun), no more than eight ounces or less of fluid a day is supposed to come out when you visit the bathroom, says William B. Ruderman, M.D., chairperson of the Department of Gastroenterology at the Cleveland Clinic–Florida in Fort Lauderdale.

And when you get liquid when you were expecting solids? That's diarrhea, says Barry Jaffin, M.D., a motility disorder specialist and clinical instructor in the Department of Gastroenterology at Mount Sinai Hospital in New York City. "Whether you're talking about three times a day or five times a day—if your stool is basically watery and of increased frequency compared to the normal amount, then that's defined as diarrhea," says Dr. Jaffin.

Sorting out the causes of your distress is a little bit trickier than defining it, says Dr. Ruderman.

If your stomach lacks an enzyme needed to properly digest the sugar in milk—a condition called lactose intolerance—nonabsorbed fluid will continue to build up in your colon as long as you eat dairy products, says Dr. Jaffin.

Excess magnesium, found in most antacids, can also cause fluid in the colon, says Dr. Jaffin, as can sorbitol, an artificial sweetener found in some diet products. Many antibiotics, such as penicillin, which are prescribed for common infections, have also been known to cause diarrhea, says Dr. Jaffin.

And if you've been infected by a parasite or bacteria, the organism can actually cause your gut to secrete fluid until the bug is dead, says Dr. Jaffin. Ordinarily, none of these should cause your distress to last more than a week. But here's where diarrhea gets tricky.

Other bugs, like those caught during a trip overseas, for example, seem to hang on like a palm tree in a hurricane. The result: Some forms of diarrhea can last more than two weeks.

Other causes of chronic diarrhea include everything from a malfunctioning pancreas and bacterial overgrowth to inflammatory bowel disease and thyroid disease. "There are hundreds of different causes of diarrhea," says Dr. Ruderman. "But if you've had diarrhea for over one week, you need to see your doctor."

SYMPTOM RELIEF

While doctors says it's best to try to ride out a case of diarrhea, there are a few things that may make life more pleasant. Try these.

Drink up. Even not-so-severe diarrhea can cause dehydration, which often leads to weakness and dizziness, says Dr. Jaffin. Drinking clear liquids during a particularly nasty bout helps prevent dehydration, but sports drinks like Gatorade are even better because they replace glucose and potassium—nutrients vital to good health. "A lot of people have the misconception that if they drink, they're going to cause more diarrhea, and that's just not true," says Dr. Jaffin. "You have to replace that fluid that you're losing every time you go to the bathroom or you're going to end up in the hospital."

Cut the caffeine. Because caffeine stimulates the intestine, it can worsen your diarrhea. You'll want to avoid drinks high in caffeine, such as coffee, tea and caffeinated sodas, while you're suffering with diarrhea, says Dr. Ruderman. In addition, caffeine causes you to urinate, worsening the dehydration.

Eliminate your trouble. You may be able to dump noninfectious diarrhea by eliminating the foods that could be causing the problem, says Dr. Jaffin. If you're suffering from lactose intolerance, for example, removing milk products from your diet may end the problem. Also, try eliminating sorbitol and see if that helps.

Ease back into eating. Instead of trying to make up for lost meals, ease back into eating after your symptoms begin to subside by sticking with bland fare, says Dr. Ruderman. Among the best: bananas, broth or soup, toast, juices and Jell-O, he says. When you can tolerate this lighter fare, try more solid bland food, like chicken or baked fish.

Say yes to yogurt. To have any effect at all on noninfectious diarrhea, you need yogurt that still contains lactobacilli. These are active yogurt cultures that may balance out bacteria in your colon and may help in reducing lactose intolerance, says Peter Holt, M.D., chief of the Division of Gastroenterology at St. Luke's–Roosevelt Hospital Center and professor of medicine Columbia University College of Physicians and Surgeons in New York City. "Although there's not a lot of scientific data to back this up, people over the years have reported good results," he says. You may have to do a little label reading, but you should be able to find yogurt with live cultures. If you can't find it in the supermarket, try the local health food store.

Try Pepto-Bismol. Some doctors recommend Pepto-Bismol for travelers' diarrhea, says Nicholas J. Talley, M.D., associate professor of medicine at the Mayo Clinic Medical School in Rochester, Minnesota.

See your doctor. If you suspect you've been infected during your travels, ask your doctor about several prescription antibiotics that are extremely effective, says Dr. Talley. Among them are Cipro and Bactrim.

Review your medications. List all the medications you

are currently taking—prescription and over-the-counter drugs—and ask your doctor whether any of them could be contributing to the problem. Your doctor may be able to make helpful substitutions.

DISORIENTATION

WHEN TO SEE YOUR DOCTOR

- Any feeling of disorientation should be discussed with your physician.

WHAT YOUR SYMPTOM IS TELLING YOU

Sure, it's annoying when you walk out of the grocery store and momentarily can't remember where you parked your car. Yes, it's frustrating when you get lost driving in a strange city. But imagine how terrifying it must feel to be sitting in your own living room and suddenly not have a clue where you are, or even if it's day or night.

This kind of disorientation can be a sign that you're having a panic attack. Other causes include low blood sugar, poor blood circulation or anemia, a seizure, Alzheimer's disease, a tumor, a stroke or a transient ischemic attack—a mini-stroke that can cause temporary stroke-like symptoms such as speech difficulties and memory loss.

SYMPTOM RELIEF

Disorientation isn't a symptom that you should fool around with. This is a serious symptom that should be investigated by your doctor promptly," says Maurice Hanson, M.D., a neurologist at the Cleveland Clinic–Florida in Fort Lauderdale.

If your doctor determines that your disorientation isn't caused by a serious medical condition, then you might consider these possibilities.

Investigate your drugs. Disorientation is a side effect of some drugs. Mention all medications you are currently taking—both prescription and over-the-counter—to your doctor.

Learn to relax. "One-third of young people who complain about disorientation are actually suffering from anxiety or panic attacks," says Robert Slater, M.D., an assistant professor of clinical neurology at the University of Pennsylvania School of Medicine in Philadelphia. Practicing stress-reduction techniques such as progressive relaxation, yoga or deep breathing may help relieve your symptoms.

DIZZINESS

WHEN TO SEE YOUR DOCTOR

- Your dizziness is unexplained, severe, recurrent or persistent.
- You also have ringing in your ears or a sudden loss of hearing.
- Your vision also suddenly gets worse or you have double vision.
- You have a severe headache.
- You have a family history of dizziness.

WHAT YOUR SYMPTOM IS TELLING YOU

The world seems to rise up to the very tip-top of the horizon and then cascade down into an endless swirl. That sensation might be okay if you're riding on a roller coaster, but it's disconcerting, to say the least, if you happen to be standing on your patio.

At one time or another, we all feel dizzy—a sensation that you or the world around you is spinning. Many people feel it when they look down from a tall building or after riding on a merry-go-round. Even astronauts can be overcome by dizzy spells while traveling through space.

About 70 percent of the time, dizziness is a sign that your inner ears—which act like gyroscopes to keep you standing upright—aren't working right. But dizziness also is an elusive symptom that can be caused by more than 350 ailments, including colds, flu, allergies, poor dietary habits, stress, certain drugs, viral infection, high blood pressure, diabetes, internal bleeding, heart disease or an impending stroke.

SYMPTOM RELIEF

There are things that people can do to cope with their dizziness. But if you experience an unexplained dizzy spell, see your doctor, because you can't be sure if it's a trivial problem or a symptom of a serious illness," says Robert Slater, M.D., an assistant professor of clinical neurology at the University of Pennsylvania School of Medicine in Philadelphia.

Here are some suggestions you might use at home to stop the spinning.

Turn off your ears. Along with your inner ears, your feet and eyes help you maintain your balance. Just sitting in a chair with your feet on the ground, holding the chair with your arms and staring at a stationary object for a few minutes may help subdue your dizziness. That's because your brain will learn to ignore the faulty messages coming from your inner ears, says Jim Buskirk, a physical therapist at the Dizziness and Balance Center in Wilmette, Illinois. He cautions, however, that this technique should not be overused. If you have persistent dizziness, see your doctor.

Go slow, but steady. "The name of the game when you're really dizzy is to move as slow as a turtle," says Diran Mikaelian, M.D., professor of otolaryngology at

Thomas Jefferson University in Philadelphia. Avoid rapid changes in head position, especially when standing up or lying down. Instead, move in stages. When getting out of bed, for example, sit on the edge of the mattress for at least 30 seconds before standing.

Check your medications. Many over-the-counter and prescription drugs, particularly those used to control blood pressure, can cause dizziness as a side effect. Ask your doctor if it would be appropriate to make changes in any of your medications.

Shake the salt habit. Too much salt in the diet causes the body to retain fluid, which can disrupt the workings of the inner ear. Avoid cheese, bacon and canned foods and limit your overall salt consumption to less than 2,000 milligrams a day (about one teaspoon), says Ronald Amedee, M.D., associate professor of head and neck surgery at Tulane University Medical Center in New Orleans. That's about the amount of sodium in one cheeseburger and a small chef's salad.

Say sayonara to stimulants. Avoid coffee and tobacco, because they heighten your body's sensitivity to motion, doctors say. If you insist on drinking coffee, limit your consumption to one or two cups a day. But herbal teas that don't contain caffeine are a better choice.

Banish the booze. Even modest amounts of alcohol—in some cases, just three sips of beer—can trigger violent dizzy spells in some people, Dr. Slater says. If you notice that alcohol makes you dizzy, cut back or cut it out altogether.

Find a stress buster. People who are under stress or feel anxious, particularly people who have hard-driving Type-A personalities, are prone to dizziness, Dr. Amedee says. Relaxation exercises such as deep breathing, yoga or biofeedback might help.

Watch out for allergies. Dizziness may be a symptom of allergies caused by pollen, pets or even foods. "I had a patient who got dizzy every time he ate hot dogs," says Peter Roland, M.D., an otologist at the University of Texas Southwestern Medical Center in Dallas. "It's rare, but food allergies can do that." If something you eat leaves you spinning, eliminate it from your diet.

Take a pill. Some over-the-counter motion sickness drugs containing dimenhydrinate or meclizine reduce the sensitivity of the inner ear to motion and may suppress your dizziness. But in severe cases, stronger prescription drugs may be needed.

Drugs are usually a last resort reserved for people who have the most serious forms of dizziness, says Dr. Slater. That's because over time the brain has a remarkable ability to compensate for most types of dizziness.

Exercise Your Dizziness Away

"Keeping active is actually one of the best treatments for dizziness caused by an inner ear problem," Dr. Slater says. "Any exercise that involves a lot of head and body movement such as walking, swimming, jogging, even karate will help the brain overcome it. If you keep turning and moving, it will work." Here are a couple of suggestions to get you going.

Start slow if you have to. For some people with severe dizziness, just standing up and walking across a room can cause dizziness. But you can gradually overcome this by moving into a position where you just begin feeling dizzy, then returning to your chair. If that means you can take only three steps before you feel dizzy, that's fine. It's still a good start, Dr. Slater says. "The exercise—moving, feeling dizzy, sitting down—should be done several times a day. The optimum would be three times every day for 2 to 15 minutes a session," he says. "But in the beginning, if you can only do it for 20 seconds at a time without feeling dizzy, that's okay. Twenty seconds of exercise is better than nothing."

Swing your partner. "Dancing is a fantastic exercise for dizzy people because it involves a lot of turns and swinging around," Dr. Slater says. "If you're really dizzy, you can start out making slow 90-degree turns. Then, as your body adapts, you can work your way up to fancy spins."

See also Balance Problems; Walking Difficulty

DOUBLE VISION

- Any instance of double vision should be brought to the attention of your doctor.

WHAT YOUR SYMPTOM IS TELLING YOU

Andy Capp—the comic strip Cockney with an overfondness for beer—knows he's stayed at the saloon too long when he comes home and sees two wives standing at the doorway. But double vision is no laughing matter.

"Some people who report double vision are actually seeing a fainter, ghost image or overlapping shadow vision, rather than two distinct images," says George Sanborn, M.D., associate clinical professor of ophthalmology at the Virginia Commonwealth University/ Medical College of Virginia in Richmond. This is often an early sign of cataracts, he says.

If you see two totally separate images, it means that your two eyes are not pointed at the same target. This misalignment can be from an abnormality in the muscles or nerves that control the eyes' movement. Graves' disease, for example, is a thyroid condition that gradually thickens the eye muscles so that they no longer move properly. And if you're seeing double and also feel dizzy, there's a chance that a stroke is affecting the nerves that control your eye alignment.

You may also begin to suddenly see double if you receive a blow to the head.

SYMPTOM RELIEF

No matter what the cause, if you're seeing double, see your doctor on the double. "Double vision is a natural warning bell that something may be seriously wrong," says Dr. Sanborn. Depending on the cause of your problem, you may require either eyeglasses or surgery to help re-align the eye muscles. As for shadow images, they will generally vanish once cataracts are surgically removed and special glasses are prescribed.

DROOLING

WHAT YOUR SYMPTOM IS TELLING YOU

Drooling is one of those medically benign (yet socially suicidal) symptoms that doctors just can't figure out. They don't know how to stem the flow.

But if drooling is your problem, knowing that doctors don't know what to do about it is no big help. You may, though, find some comfort in knowing *why* your faucets won't turn off.

Some women notice a pronounced saliva increase shortly after they become pregnant, says Maureen Van Dinter, R.N., a senior clinical nurse specialist in the Department of Family Medicine and Practice at the University of Wisconsin in Madison. The increased salivary flow causes a maddening difficulty in swallowing and speaking until the delivery, when the flow returns to normal as mysteriously as it increased.

"Their cheeks puff up like a chipmunk's because of swollen salivary glands, and the insides of their mouths become very red and irritated," she says. An especially nasty taste often develops, and the women must almost constantly wipe their mouths to prevent saliva from dribbling down their chins.

Little attention has been given to the problem, and over the years, most doctors have dismissed it as psychosomatic, says Van Dinter. "A lot of distress has been caused by telling these women they're crazy, that it's all in their heads," she says. "But it's not in their heads. It's in their mouths."

Excessive spittle can occur after you quit taking certain medications. A whole host of drugs can, as a side effect, dry out your mouth, according to Louis M. Abbey, D.M.D., a professor of oral pathology at Virginia Commonwealth University/Medical College of Virginia School of Dentistry in Richmond. "Once you're off the drug, your saliva flow returns to normal, but you *feel* like your mouth is dripping and gushing," he says.

People who get dentures or a partial for the first time also notice an upturn in their saliva flow, Dr. Abbey says. "The presence of anything in your mouth stimulates saliva production, and some people who receive a complete or partial denture for the first time have the sensation that they're almost drowning in saliva."

Conditions that affect brain-to-body impulses—such as Bell's palsy, Parkinson's disease or a stroke—may impede people's ability to swallow correctly or to keep their upper and lower lips sealed, says Michael W. Dodds, Ph.D., who has a bachelor of dental surgery and is an assistant professor in the Department of Community Dentistry at the University of Texas Health Science Center in San Antonio.

SYMPTOM RELIEF

Many techniques have been tried to slow the flow of saliva, but few actually work, Van Dinter says. With surgery, doctors can redirect the salivary ducts so they drain straight down the throat, but, says Dr. Dodds, "I wouldn't recommend it." Here are some less drastic measures.

Sip or suck. Pregnant women have experimented with all sorts of remedies—lozenges, frequent sips of water, frequent small meals—to handle the excess saliva, eliminate the foul taste and help them swallow. Sometimes they work, but usually they don't, Van Dinter says. Give all of them a try and see if any work for you.

Don't dry out with drugs. Excess saliva isn't serious enough to "cure" with drugs that have dry mouth as a side effect—and that caution goes triple for pregnant women, since the drugs could harm the fetus.

DROWSINESS

WHEN TO SEE YOUR DOCTOR

- You experience repeated episodes of drowsiness for a week or more but are getting adequate (six to eight hours) sleep every night.
- Drowsiness affects your alertness or puts you and others in physical danger, such as when driving.
- You also snore excessively or experience frequent interruptions in your sleep.
- Sleep overtakes you so suddenly that you collapse.

WHAT YOUR SYMPTOM IS TELLING YOU

Feeling drowsy all the time? Join the crowd! America is a nation of sleep-starved yawners fighting a daily battle against the sandman. We increasingly live in a world where people drive themselves on a relentless schedule that never lets up. Something has to be pushed aside, and for far too many of us, it's our sleep time. No wonder so many people are rubbing their eyes and nodding out at inappropriate times!

Irregular sleep patterns are just as likely to cause drowsiness as lack of adequate sleep. Jet lag, shift work, inconsistent bedtimes and weekend partying can all disturb our natural sleep/wake cycles, says Charles Pollak, M.D., director of the Sleep-Wake Disorders Center at the New York Hospital–Cornell Medical Center in White Plains. "Too often people try to function when their brains and bodies are in the sleep mode," he says.

In addition to reflecting how much and when you are sleeping, drowsiness can also be a sign of the quality of your sleep. Millions of Americans, especially snorers, may suffer from a potentially life-threatening sleep disorder called obstructive sleep apnea, in which closures in the upper airway cause breathing to periodically stop for 30 to

60 seconds or even longer. The brain, sensing a lack of breathing, will trigger a snorting or gasping reflex that partially reawakens the individual and restarts normal breathing.

These events can occur hundreds of times a night, preventing you from enjoying the restorative benefits of uninterrupted deep sleep. People with chronic sleep apnea also run an increased risk of high blood pressure, heart disease and stroke. And the drowsiness associated with sleep apnea is the suspected cause of thousands of industrial and highway accidents every year. (For more information on sleep apnea, see Snoring on page 573.)

Sleep factors are not the only thing that can cause drowsiness, however. Virtually any virus, allergy or illness can interfere with sleep, leaving you drowsy and craving more than 40 winks. Among the most common offenders are the flu and the common cold. And some of the medications used to fight these ailments—especially antihistamines—can leave you positively struggling to keep your eyes open. Many medications have drowsiness as a side effect.

Alcohol, of course, can leave you in a drowsy stupor. And so can the *withdrawal* of caffeine.

In addition, narcolepsy is a relatively rare neurological condition that causes extreme drowsiness and severe, recurrent sleep attacks.

SYMPTOM RELIEF

Tired of feeling like a zombie? Ready to face the world with a glimmer in your eye and a spring in your step? Here are some tips to chase away that lousy, drowsy feeling.

Get more quality sleep. More likely than not, you need to catch more Zs. But how much is enough? "It differs from person to person, but for most of us it's eight hours or more," says biological psychologist David F. Dinges, Ph.D., associate professor in the psychiatry department at the University of Pennsylvania School of Medicine in

Philadelphia. "We tend to devalue sleep by living with less. There is a cumulative sleep debt that develops from living that way, and the body will come to collect its due if we don't pay it back." If you've been depriving yourself of sleep, Dr. Dinges recommends getting at least one more hour of shut-eye every night to pay back your sleep debt. Once you've determined your optimal night's sleep, get that same amount of sleep every night in the same time period. Depending on your sleep debt, it could take a day or two to repay. (For other tips about getting a good night's sleep, see Insomnia on page 326.)

Take naps. Napping is a great way to make up for lost sleep and to rejuvenate yourself when drowsiness hits, says Wilse B. Webb, Ph.D., professor of psychology at the University of Florida in Gainesville. Up to 45 minutes in the early afternoon will do the job nicely. Naps are especially helpful to people who have narcolepsy.

Try a cup of java. "Caffeine is a powerful stimulant that can be very helpful," says Philip R. Westbrook, M.D., director of the Sleep Disorders Center at Cedars-Sinai Medical Center in Los Angeles. One to two cups of coffee in the morning and then one cup at lunch is sufficient in a day. More than that could lead to a caffeine crash in the afternoon. That's worse than the drowsiness you're trying to reduce.

Keep active. "If you are in a low-demand situation like driving or reading, you can get drowsy," says Dr. Webb. "By contrast, no one ever went to sleep playing tennis. Continuing to do active, busy things like walking and talking will interfere with the urge to sleep."

Light up your life. Bright lights or a walk in the sunshine may erase some of your drowsiness, according to recent studies. Light may have a stimulating effect on the central nervous system, resets your biological clock and suppresses the production of melatonin—a hormone thought to induce drowsiness.

Get the sensation. A hot shower, a cold breeze, loud rock music, physical contact or any stimulus that jars the senses can activate and increase your alertness, says Dr. Westbrook.

Review your medications. List every medication you're currently taking—both prescription and over-the-counter—and show the list to your doctor. Your doctor may be able to suggest alternatives that won't cause drowsiness.

See also Afternoon Slump; Fatigue; Insomnia

DRY HEAVES

WHEN TO SEE YOUR DOCTOR

- Your dry heaves continue for more than two hours.

WHAT YOUR SYMPTOM IS TELLING YOU

The good news is that your vomiting has stopped. The bad news is that your body hasn't stopped trying to vomit—and now you're panting from the pain of dry heaves.

The area of your brain that controls vomiting—your vomit center—is still in high gear even though the food in your stomach is long gone. Don't panic: It may take a while for your system to calm down. "Think of it as a kind of an overdrive of the nausea center—continued stimulation without anything being in the stomach," says William B. Ruderman, M.D., chairperson of the Department of Gastroenterology at the Cleveland Clinic–Florida in Fort Lauderdale.

SYMPTOM RELIEF

Although you're uncomfortable, there's a good chance that your dry heaves will go away a short time after they've started. "In a lot of cases, particularly food poisoning and things like that, it won't be long until you're feeling better," says Jorge Herrera, M.D., assistant professor of medicine at the University of South Alabama College of Medicine in Mobile and member of the American Gastroenterological Association and the American College of Gastroenterology. Here are a few things you can try.

Check out Dramamine. Although traditionally used for motion sickness, the over-the-counter medication Dramamine may help end dry heaves.

Call your doctor. Because you may need a prescription antinauseant to bring your dry heaves to a halt, you may want to give your doctor a call, says Dr. Ruderman. "If someone is at home and they keep vomiting, I will prescribe a drug, in suppository form, to calm the vomit center," he says. In fact, any techniques that put an end to vomiting should also prove helpful in banishing the heaves. A doctor can also give you a shot to eliminate dry heaves if your case is persistent enough, says Dr. Herrera.

See also Vomiting

E

EARACHE

- Your ear pain lasts more than a week.

WHAT YOUR SYMPTOM IS TELLING YOU

Once you've stayed up half the night with a child who has an earache, you learn to respect this symptom. Adults get earaches, too, although less often, and it's just as likely they'll be kept awake by the pain.

The microbes that cause earaches usually show up first as a respiratory infection in your nose or throat. All it takes is a little push—you blow your nose, you lie down—and the viruses or bacteria move into your eustachian tubes. These are tiny channels that connect your nasal passages to your inner ears. From there, it's a short trip to the middle ear and your eardrum, which is laced with sensitive nerve endings. The infection creates pus, which pushes against your eardrum, causing pain. It can even make the eardrum burst.

Children get more earaches because they have more respiratory infections and because their eustachian tubes are immature and unable to handle even a small infection.

Other causes of earache include swimmer's ear, which can happen when excess water is trapped in the ear canal. Earaches can also be triggered by hair and other objects that get stuck in the ear.

SYMPTOM RELIEF

Try these tips to take the ache out of your ear.

Warm up to olive oil. A few drops of olive oil or mineral oil can provide temporary relief, says Clough Shelton, M.D., an associate clinical professor of otolaryngology at the University of California, Los Angeles, and a member of the House Ear Institute at the University of Southern California. Warm it up like a baby's bottle under hot tap water for a few minutes. Test the oil first (it should be about body temperature) and apply it with an ear dropper. Make sure to use only enough to coat the inner lining of the ear, he says.

Turn on the heat. There are two approaches for using heat to help relieve the pain of an earache. You can try setting a heating pad on medium and placing it on top of the sore ear. Or you can turn a hair dryer on the lowest warm setting and direct the warm air down the ear canal, holding the dryer 6 to 12 inches from your ear. Do not use the hair dryer for more than three to five minutes.

Prop yourself up. You're better off sitting up in bed than lying flat on your back, says David Marty, M.D., a Jefferson, Missouri, otolaryngologist and author of *The Ear Book*. Sitting up actually allows blood to drain away from the head so there's less congestion in the eustachian tube, he says. "That's why kids with an earache will quit crying when you pick them up and start crying again when you lay them down," he says. "It's not that they want to be held, it's just that they feel better with their heads up."

Fill up on fluids. Drinking lots of water and juice not only helps soothe the symptoms, but repeated swallowing can also help clear your eustachian tubes, says Charles P. Kimmelman, M.D., professor of otolaryngology at Manhattan Eye, Ear and Throat Hospital. Chewing and yawning are also good for clearing your eustachian tubes, he says.

Try a vasoconstrictor. Over-the-counter nasal sprays like Neo-Synephrine contain the ingredient phenylephrine, which helps return your eustachian tube to normal functioning, says Dr. Kimmelman. "The spray shrinks down the lining of the nose and hopefully the region around the entrance of the eustachian tubes, allowing the tube to function better. If the eustachian tube returns to normal, you'll feel better," he explains. Don't use phenylephrine-containing nosedrops for more than a few days, and make sure you don't exceed the daily dosage recommended on the label. Overuse of nasal sprays can actually make the problem worse.

Opt for a painkiller. Another possible temporary remedy for ear pain: an over-the-counter analgesic like Advil or Tylenol, says W. Steven Pray, Ph.D., professor of pharmaceutics, School of Pharmacy, at Southwestern Oklahoma State University in Weatherford. "Just don't fall into the trap of taking an analgesic and thinking because your ear doesn't hurt anymore, you don't need an antibiotic," he says. "The analgesic doesn't kill the organisms—it just controls the pain."

Ask about antibiotics. Because a bacterial infection is one of the most common causes of earache, most doctors recommend taking antibiotics like Amoxil and Ceclor to beat the bug, stresses Dr. Pray.

Beaching Swimmer's Ear

It's great to take a dip in the pool on a hot summer's day—what's not so great is when you bring some of the water home with you in your ear. Consider these tips for beaching swimmer's ear.

Be careful with your cleaning. Cleaning your ears a day or so before a swim may actually rob your ears of the protection they need to prevent swimmer's ear, says Dr. Pray. "You need to keep the wax inside to protect and lubricate," he explains. "It's just as if you put wax on your finger and then put your finger in water—you know it's not going to get wet." When you do clean your ears, don't dig for wax; simply wipe the outer ear with a clean washcloth, he says.

Try alcohol. A drop or two of isopropyl alcohol in the ear may cause any water that remains in the ear to evaporate, says Dr. Pray.

Dry it out. Made with isopropyl alcohol and glycerin, Swim-Ear is one of several products on the market designed to evaporate any water that may remain in the ear, says Dr. Pray.

EAR DISCHARGE

WHEN TO SEE YOUR DOCTOR

- You experience any ear discharge other than earwax.
- See your doctor immediately if you experience a discharge following a blow to the head.

WHAT YOUR SYMPTOM IS TELLING YOU

Fluid oozing from inside your ear may seem scary, but there's no need to panic. In fact, if you take the right action, your ear could heal in just a few days. Respiratory infections often work their way into the tiny canals—called eustachian tubes—that run from the back of your nose to your ears, says John K. Niparko, M.D., associate professor in the Department of Otolaryngology at Johns Hopkins University in Baltimore. Clogged eustachian tubes are the ideal environment for bacteria to grow and multiply, creating a buildup of mucus and pus that presses on the delicate skin of the eardrum, often causing an earache.

In a very small number of cases, the pressure from the infection is so great that the eardrum pops like a balloon. This sounds gruesome, but the opening allows fluid buildup to drain from your ear, relieving the pain. The eardrum almost always grows back, but it should be assessed by an ear specialist to rule out any complications.

Repeated ear discharge, like frequent sinus infections, is often a sign that your immune system is losing the battle with bacteria in your ear and needs help from an antibiotic, says C. Warren Bierman, M.D., clinical professor and pediatrics chief in the Division of Allergy at the University of Washington School of Medicine in Seattle.

Infection is not the only thing that can cause discharge, however. In addition, swimmer's ear sometimes results in a milky, watery discharge that can make you feel like giving up the backstroke. And a sudden brownish tan flow can be the harmless discharge of earwax that has been building up for a while in the inner ear, says Dr. Bierman.

A severe head injury like a skull fracture can result in an ear discharge of spinal fluid—a colorless liquid that usually looks like water but can sometimes be mixed with blood. And while extremely rare, a tumor of the ear canal could also cause a watery discharge, says Charles P. Kimmelman, M.D., professor of otolaryngology at Manhattan Eye, Ear and Throat Hospital.

SYMPTOM RELIEF

If you have any kind of discharge from your ear—aside from earwax—it's important to see your doctor. Here's what your doctor might do as well as what you can do for yourself.

Opt for antibiotics. "The drainage is really a signal that you need to do something about an ear infection," says Dr. Niparko. "With the right antibiotics you could have it under control in 48 hours." Your doctor will prescribe the appropriate antibiotic.

Children need extra care. Ear infections in children sometimes are more stubborn to cure. Because children's eustachian tubes often don't ventilate or drain the ear properly until the children are six or seven, sometimes doctors must surgically insert what's called a tympanostomy tube in their eardrums, says Margaretha Casselbrant, M.D., Ph.D., associate professor of otolaryngology at the University of Pittsburgh School of Medicine and director of clinical research in the Department of Pediatric Otolaryngology at Children's Hospital of Pittsburgh. The tube prevents fluid buildup by allowing the ear to ventilate and thus enabling it to drain.

Pick some cotton. A cottonball placed just inside the ear will absorb discharge while allowing it to flow unrestricted from the ear canal, says Dr. Casselbrant. Don't use anything but cotton, and don't insert it deep into the ear.

A wipe or two will do. Using a washcloth or a cotton swab dipped in alcohol, you can wipe the outer ear to get rid of any discharge that's accumulated, says Dr. Niparko. Just don't venture inside the ear canal. "You run a significant risk of scratching the ear canal, which can then set you up for an ear canal infection," he says.

Wear a bathing cap. If you're plagued by swimmer's ear, it's a good idea to keep your ears covered while you're in the water.

See also Earache

EAR ITCHING

WHEN TO SEE YOUR DOCTOR

- You are also experiencing drainage (bad-smelling, pus-filled discharge), fever and pain.
- You have a reddened area around your ear opening.

WHAT YOUR SYMPTOM IS TELLING YOU

All kinds of things can start an ear itch, says C. Warren Bierman, M.D., clinical professor and pediatrics chief in the Division of Allergy at the University of Washington School of Medicine in Seattle. Topping the list are skin conditions, like eczema, psoriasis and seborrheic dermatitis (the same troublemaker responsible for dandruff).

Having any of these skin conditions elsewhere on your body is a clue that it could be responsible for the ear itch, according to Kenneth Brookler, M.D., attending otolaryngologist at Lenox Hill Hospital in New York City. Check especially your elbows, eyebrows and scalp.

A bug looking for a warm home during the winter can treat your ear like a motel and check in, causing an itch, says Charles P. Kimmelman, M.D., professor of otolaryngology at Manhattan Eye, Ear and Throat Hospital. "This is fairly common in colder climates and poorer areas," he says.

Moisture caused by earwax buildup can also make for itching ears, while too little earwax can do the same, says Dr. Bierman. Itching is also a common reaction to the rubber in some bathing caps, he says. Fungal infections in the ear canal—which can appear in the outer ear as redness and inflammation—have also been known to cause ear itching, but these infections are rare.

SYMPTOM RELIEF

When that itch starts screaming for attention, here's what to do.

Don't try to scratch it. Sticking a cotton swab—or if you're really foolish, a house key or paper clip—in your ear could damage your eardrum, says Margaretha Casselbrant, M.D., Ph.D., associate professor of otolaryngology at the University of Pittsburgh School of Medicine and director of clinical research in the Department of Pediatric Otolaryngology at Children's Hospital of Pittsburgh. It could also set you up for earwax buildup. "Doctors have an old saying: *Never stick anything smaller than your elbow in your ear.* And we mean it," says Dr. Casselbrant.

Oil that itch. A drop or two of mineral oil, olive oil or some other vegetable oil can soothe an itchy ear instantly. Have a friend or spouse use a dropper to put the oil in while you're lying down, itchy ear up, says Stephen Harner, M.D., associate professor in the Department of Otolaryngology at the Mayo Clinic in Rochester, Minnesota.

Give bugs the boot. You can evict errant bugs from your ear canal by gently squirting them with warm water from a rubber bulb syringe, says Dr. Kimmelman. A couple of drops of mineral oil will kill any insect that resists your efforts, he says. Or simply drown the little guy by putting alcohol in your ear with an ear dropper. (The bug should float to the surface, but if it doesn't, have your doctor remove it).

Go after earwax. You can remove stubborn earwax buildup by lying with your ear on a warm hot-water bottle. The heat will soften the wax and allow it to flow out, making it easier to wipe away, says David Marty, M.D., a Jefferson, Missouri, otolaryngologist and author of *The Ear Book*. Don't feel like you have to get *all* of it out, however. A little earwax actually helps *prevent* itching.

Counter with an OTC. Half-percent strength over-the-counter hydrocortisone lotion should also soothe most itching, says Dr. Bierman. Apply just a dab *carefully* with the twisted end of a handkerchief, he advises. If the OTC version doesn't work, prescription-strength hydrocortisone solution can help soothe the itch of eczema, psoriasis or other forms of contact dermatitis, says Dr. Brookler.

See your doctor. Because it's difficult to see many of the causes of itching—like a fungal infection—you may benefit from consulting with your doctor if the itching persists for more than a few days, says Dr. Brookler.

EAR NOISES

WHEN TO SEE YOUR DOCTOR

- The noise is accompanied by dizziness or pain.

WHAT YOUR SYMPTOM IS TELLING YOU

You hear constant ringing in your ears, and it's definitely not your Aunt Mildred calling long distance from Des

Moines. If it's any consolation, you're not alone. More than 34 million Americans suffer from tinnitus—a hearing disorder that can subject you to all sorts of bizarre ear noises. The most common source of the commotion: Nerves and special nerve endings inside your inner ear simply wear out with age and overexposure to loud noise. That means your inner ear may be sending phantom—or fake—sounds to your brain.

"You can have pulsations from blood vessels in the ear or you can have twitching of muscles in the ear, and they will make a fluttering sound or pulsating sound or a clicking sound," says Jack Vernon, Ph.D., professor of otolaryngology and director of the Oregon Hearing Research Center at the Oregon Health Sciences Center in Portland. "People will come in and describe ringing or buzzing, or they'll compare the sound to cicadas or crickets."

An earache, a bacterial infection, fluid in the middle ear, a hole in the eardrum or a big plug of wax can cause tinnitus. Menière's disease, a somewhat rare and mysterious ailment that attacks the inner ear, has also been known to cause tinnitus. In a tiny fraction of cases, the problem could be the result of a tumor on the auditory nerve of the inner ear.

SYMPTOM RELIEF

Your doctor can clear up an infection with a course of antibiotics, but in most instances tinnitus is simply not treatable. But you can cut some of the annoying noise with the following techniques.

Avoid too much aspirin. Arthritis sufferers take note: Megadoses of aspirin can make your tinnitus worse—although doctors aren't sure why. "One or two aspirin aren't going to do it, but if you're taking eight to ten aspirin every day, that could be part of the problem," says David Marty, M.D., a Jefferson, Missouri, otolaryngologist and author of *The Ear Book*.

Stop smoking. Here's yet another reason to quit: The nicotine in cigarettes acts as a stimulant, forcing the auditory nerve in your inner ear to fire. If you're suffering from tinnitus, that's roughly the equivalent of someone banging garbage can lids together inside your brain, says Dr. Marty.

Halt the extra salt. Excess salt causes fluid retention within the ear, which can result in swelling and pressure against the hearing organs. And that can contribute to tinnitus, hearing loss and dizziness, says Dr. Marty.

Cut back on caffeine. A stimulant, caffeine also aggravates tinnitus, says Dr. Marty.

Avoid loud sounds. "Loud sounds can exacerbate tinnitus, so it's best to avoid them," says Dr. Vernon. If you can't avoid the racket, at least wear earplugs.

Drown out the sound. Many people who have tinnitus report that they don't notice their symptoms when they're in the shower. "We have some of the cleanest patients around," says Dr. Vernon. "The noise of the water apparently covers the sound."

Because the sound of water works so well, some doctors also recommend that their patients record the sound of water pouring out of the faucet and play it just before they go to sleep or whenever they need relief, says Dr. Vernon.

Try biofeedback. During a study at the House Ear Clinic, 80 percent of people who received 12 biofeedback training sessions over a six-week period actually suffered 80 percent less ringing in their ears, says Clough Shelton, M.D., an associate clinical professor of otolaryngology at the University of California, Los Angeles, and a member of the House Ear Institute at the University of Southern California. Those who participated in the study learned through biofeedback how to relax the muscles in their foreheads—muscles that are commonly tightened when you're under stress. "Exactly why, we don't know—but there's a common connection between stress and increased tinnitus," says Dr. Shelton. "Biofeedback isn't effective on everyone, but on some it's a good treatment." During biofeedback, electronic sensors placed on your body measure your stress reactions like heart rate, perspiration and muscular tension. Using relaxation techniques taught during your biofeedback training, you may be able to lower those reactions, and in this case reduce your tinnitus, says Dr.

Shelton. Ask your doctor to recommend someone who can give you biofeedback training.

Buy a masking device. Several electronics manufacturers sell inexpensive units that help mask tinnitus by producing white noise. If you don't want to lay out the extra cash, you can get somewhat the same effect by tuning an FM radio to pick up static, says Dr. Vernon.

Banish earwax. If a buildup of earwax is causing the problem, you can put an end to all that racket with an over-the-counter product like Auro Ear Drops or Murine Ear Wax Removal System designed to unplug earwax, says W. Steven Pray, Ph.D., professor of pharmaceutics, School of Pharmacy, at Southwestern Oklahoma State University in Weatherford. It might be a good idea to check with your doctor first, just to make sure that you don't have an infection. (For other tips on eliminating earwax buildup, see page 178.)

Explore an anti-anxiety drug. During tests, 76 percent of those suffering from tinnitus who used the prescription drug Xanax reported relief, says Dr. Vernon. "I don't know of any drug that has that good an effect."

EAR REDNESS

WHEN TO SEE YOUR DOCTOR

- The redness does not diminish after 24 hours.
- A sharp blow to your ear causes it to swell and turn red.
- You have an infected sore that is larger than 1/4 inch in diameter.
- The redness follows frostbite.

What Your Symptom Is Telling You

A red flag usually signals a warning. And a red ear can serve as your warning flag for a minor ear problem.

Some of the most common causes of red, inflamed ears are skin conditions like eczema and psoriasis, says C. Warren Bierman, M.D., clinical professor and pediatrics chief in the Division of Allergy at the University of Washington School of Medicine in Seattle.

The other big cause of redness is an ear infection.

Scratching your ears with any kind of object—like a key or paper clip—can cause the infection, says Charles P. Kimmelman, M.D., professor of otolaryngology at Manhattan Eye, Ear and Throat Hospital. And your earlobe can become infected after you've had your ears pierced. (It's also possible to have an allergic reaction to the metal in your earrings, which turns your earlobes red.) A boil-like infection near the ear canal can also be a source of swelling and redness, says Dr. Bierman.

Extremes of heat and cold can paint your ears red. Ears are a prime target for sunburn. And after briefly debuting in white, a frostbitten ear turns bright red and can be painful, says Dr. Kimmelman.

Finally, a sharp blow to the ear can make it turn red. (If it also swells, you can eventually get what's known as cauliflower ear.)

Symptom Relief

Keeping your ears out of the red and in the pink is easy if you follow these recommendations.

Eliminate that infection. If you've scratched your ear and started an infection, dab the sore area with a cotton swab dipped in alcohol and then apply an over-the-counter antibiotic ointment like bacitracin, says Dr. Kimmelman. If the sore is larger than 1/4 inch in diameter or fails to improve, see your doctor for further treatment, he says.

Screen yourself. You should wear sunscreen anytime you're out in the sun for more than a half-hour. And remember to put some on your ears. "The number one thing you can do to avoid sunburned ears is to use sunscreen that really blocks out the sun—SPF 30 or higher. Some people even use zinc oxide on their ears," says Dr. Bierman. Zinc oxide is a skin protectant that allows little or no sun to reach the skin.

Keep 'em covered. Follow the same rules for your ears in the winter that you do in the summer. Protect them from exposure to the elements.

Warm the bite out of frostbite. To help save your ear after frostbite, place a warm washcloth over your ear and see your doctor immediately, says Dr. Kimmelman. Warmth helps keep the tissues alive by increasing circulation, he says.

Go for the gold. If you've experienced what looks like an allergic reaction to your pierced earrings—redness and swelling around the piercing holes—try switching to gold or silver posts. Most allergic reactions come from exposure to nickel or chromium posts.

Get attention for injury. If you receive a sharp blow to the ear that causes redness *and* swelling, see your doctor for treatment. A cauliflower ear, left untreated, can become permanent.

See also Ear Itching

EAR SWELLING

WHEN TO SEE YOUR DOCTOR

- Your ear swells following a blow to the head.

WHAT YOUR SYMPTOM IS TELLING YOU

When world champion Killer Kowalski removed one of Yukon Eric's ears during a pro wrestling match years ago, his reputation took on a menacing new meaning. It's likely, however, that the damage had less to do with Kowalski's savagery than the poor condition of his opponent's ear.

According to Kowalski, Yukon Eric had an advanced case of cauliflower (or boxer's) ear. As a result, one boot to the head sent Yukon Eric to the hospital—ear in hand. ("All that was left was his earlobe," says Kowalski, who now runs a pro wrestling school in Reading, Massachusetts.)

You might think that only boxers and wrestlers get cauliflower ear. But the fact is that one sharp blow to the head may be all it takes—unless the injury is treated immediately.

"A blood clot develops in the cartilage," explains John K. Niparko, M.D., associate professor in the Department of Otolaryngology at Johns Hopkins University in Baltimore. "If it's not removed, scar tissue will begin to form, causing the ear to thicken."

A number of things besides injury can cause ear swelling. Having your ears pierced can lead to infection and swelling in the earlobes. And it's possible to have an allergic reaction to certain metals—notably nickel or chromium—in earrings, says Margaretha Casselbrant, M.D., Ph.D., associate professor of otolaryngology at the University of Pittsburgh School of Medicine and director of clinical research in the Department of Pediatric Otolaryngology at Children's Hospital of Pittsburgh.

Yet another cause of ear swelling: a boil-like infection near the ear canal in people who have a tendency toward acne, says C. Warren Bierman, M.D., clinical professor and pediatrics chief in the Division of Allergy at the University of Washington School of Medicine in Seattle.

Finally, swimmer's ear—a cause of ear pain and discharge—can sometimes result in swelling that can actually close the ear canal, says Stephen Harner, M.D., associate professor in the Department of Otolaryngology at the Mayo Clinic in Rochester, Minnesota.

Symptom Relief

Because a blow to the ear that causes bleeding and swelling can lead to permanent damage, you should see your doctor for treatment right away. If there's a blood clot, it should be removed, as it can cause destruction of the cartilage, says Dr. Casselbrant. If your ear swells for any other reason, you can try these techniques.

Go soak. If you have an infection on your ear, add three tablespoons Epsom salts to a quart of warm water. Dip a clean washcloth into the solution and place it over the swollen area until the washcloth cools. Repeat this procedure four times a day.

Upgrade your jewelry. If your earrings seem to be causing an allergic reaction, try switching to silver or gold posts.

Put on some protection. If you engage in amateur wrestling or boxing, insist on protective headgear. "The use of headgear has dramatically cut the amount of cauliflower ear in young wrestlers," says Pretty Boy Larry Sharpe, a former pro wrestler who runs wrestling schools in Clementon, New Jersey; Baltimore and Tampa.

EARWAX BUILDUP

WHEN TO SEE YOUR DOCTOR

- You are also experiencing pain or hearing loss.

What Your Symptom Is Telling You

Forget aesthetics: Earwax buildup in your outer ear is a healthy sign that your body has been busy making the right stuff to fend off ear canal invaders like bugs, infection and dirt.

Earwax buildup in your inner ear, however, has a different meaning: In most cases you've actually taken all that healthy earwax and stuffed it back into your ear with things like cotton swabs or earplugs.

"It's like putting a cork down in a bottle—messing up the whole process of the wax moving outward in a fluid motion," says W. Steven Pray, Ph.D., professor of pharmaceutics, School of Pharmacy, at Southwestern Oklahoma State University in Weatherford. "The wax begins to build up until you have a real nice plug in your ear close to the eardrum. The longer it's there before you get it taken care of, the harder and the thicker this plug gets."

How do know if you've developed earwax buildup in your inner ear? You may experience itching, dryness, slight pain or hearing loss, says Dr. Pray.

You may also experience earwax buildup if you were born with something called twisted ear canal. In that case, your ear canal has a gentle bend in it, making it more difficult for the wax to flow out, says Dr. Pray.

SYMPTOM RELIEF

Beating earwax buildup is simply a matter of learning how to clean your ears properly. Try these techniques.

Don't stick anything in your ear. Rather than jamming your ear canal with cotton swabs, try this technique: Drape a damp washcloth over the end of your finger and wipe the entire outer ear, and *only* the outer ear. Earwax is fair game for removal only after it migrates out of the ear canal and into easy reach of your washcloth, says Dr. Pray. "Going deep into the ear is not something that should be done," he says. Make sure the washcloth isn't too wet or soapy—both water and soap in the ear canal can cause ear irritation or even an earache, says David Marty, M.D., a Jefferson, Missouri, otolaryngologist and author of *The Ear Book*.

Turn on the heat. The heat from an appropriately placed hot-water bottle can also help remove earwax, says Dr. Marty. Simply fill a hot-water bottle with warm water and lie on it, placing the affected ear right against the bottle. "In a short time, the wax begins to melt, allowing it to come out a little easier," says Dr. Marty.

Try an over-the-counter dissolver. Available at any drugstore, over-the-counter products like Auro, Debrox, E-R-O and Murine Ear Drops all contain carbamide peroxide, the active ingredient that helps dissolve earwax plugs, says Dr. Pray. Murine Ear Wax Removal System comes with an easy-to-use syringe that simplifies putting the drops in your ear, he says. Use the product as directed. If you don't get good results after using any of these products for about five days, see your doctor.

Advanced Earwax Busters

You can't do these on your own, but you can ask your doctor about the following techniques for removing earwax.

Use hydraulics. Some ear doctors and nurses use a Water-Pik-like device that shoots a thin stream of water to clean out earwax, says Charles P. Kimmelman, M.D., professor of otolaryngology at Manhattan Eye, Ear and Throat Hospital. But don't try this at home using your own Water Pik. "I've actually seen perforations of the eardrum from that," he says.

Get the scoop. Some doctors use a small, specially designed scoop to remove stubborn earwax, says Dr. Pray.

Have a Hoover. If the plug still persists, you may ask your doctor to use a tiny medical vacuum to remove it. "It's a very mild device designed to gently pull the earwax out without damaging the eardrum," says Dr. Pray.

EYE BULGING

WHEN TO SEE YOUR DOCTOR

- You should always go to a doctor if your eyes begin to bulge.

WHAT YOUR SYMPTOM IS TELLING YOU

If you have a permanently startled look, it can be a sign that you have a thyroid disorder known as Graves' disease.

The thyroid gland in people who have Graves' may be producing too much hormone. The body's immune system reacts by producing immune cells that attack the tissues and muscles of the eye. The tissues in the eye socket swell, pushing the eye forward and exposing the white. Then the muscles that move the eyes begin to thicken, which may throw the eyes out of alignment. The result is double vision.

With Graves' disease bulging may appear in one or both of your eyes. And because the lids don't completely cover the bulging eyeballs, your eyes can dry out, becoming scratchy and red, and they can be sensitive to bright light.

Other causes of bulging eyes include infections inside the eyeball, enlargement of blood vessels behind the eye and tumors.

SYMPTOM RELIEF

Bulging of the eyes is a symptom that must be evaluated and treated by a doctor. If you have Graves' disease, you may need to take anti-thyroid medication until the disease goes into remission. As the disease is treated, the bulging will eventually recede, according to Thomas Hedges, M.D., director of neuro-ophthalmology at the New England Eye Center at the New England Medical Center in Boston. This could take a year or two. In the meantime, here's how to ease the problem.

Moisten your eyeballs. With more of your eye area exposed, you'll need to use over-the-counter artificial tears during the day, says Dr. Hedges. Use an ophthalmic eye ointment (available at pharmacies) at bedtime, covered with a homemade "moisture chamber." A small patch of plastic wrap placed over each eye works nicely, says Nancy Patterson, Ph.D., executive director of the National Graves Disease Foundation in Jacksonville, Florida. (For other hints on keeping your eyes moist, see Eye Dryness on page 188.) If these simple measures do not relieve the dryness and if the bulging is severe, a surgeon may be able to stitch the corners of your eyelids so they won't open all the way.

Don't abuse red-out eyedrops. While artificial tears are fine, eyedrops to take the redness out are not, cautions Dr. Hedges. These commercial drops eliminate redness by constricting blood vessels in the eye. Overuse—say for more than three days—can make the vessels overreact and give you rebound redness, says Dr. Hedges.

View the world through tinted glasses. They'll camouflage the protrusions and provide a shield from bright light and wind, says Dr. Hedges. (See Light Sensitivity on page 372.)

Raise your bed. If your bulging eyes are mild and your main complaint is swollen eyelids, you can put the head of your bed up on six-inch blocks. "This reduces the accumulation of fluid in the eyelids during the night," says Mitchell H. Friedlaender, M.D., director of corneal services in the Division of Ophthalmology at the Scripps Clinic and Research Foundation in La Jolla, California, and coauthor of *20/20: A Total Guide to Improving Your Vision and Preventing Eye Disease.*

Lay off the saltshaker. Decreasing your intake of salt may help reduce fluid pressure, says Dr. Hedges. But don't take diuretics unless advised by your doctor, he adds.

EYE BURNING

WHEN TO SEE YOUR DOCTOR

- You have persistent burning or stinging.
- If you have a chemical burn, seek medical care immediately.

WHAT YOUR SYMPTOM IS TELLING YOU

You may encounter "the sting" anywhere, anytime. And we're not talking about the Paul Newman movie. This kind of sting involves your eyes and a run-in with an irritating substance such as smog or sunscreen trickling down from a sweaty forehead. These substances can temporarily irritate the delicate membrane over your eyeballs, making your eyes smart.

A more serious eye burn can occur after doing something as seemingly innocent as skiing or sunning yourself on a tropical beach. You can sunburn your eyes just as you can sunburn your skin, according to Hunter Little, M.D., clinical professor of ophthalmology at Stanford University School of Medicine in Palo Alto, California. "Over-exposure to the sun's ultraviolet (UV) rays can burn the cells on the eye's surface," says Dr. Little. "Hours later, you'll awake with searing pain and a sand-in-your-eye feeling."

Any number of household chemicals, including insecticides, battery acid and bleach, can cause a potentially sight-damaging eye burn if they splash into your eye.

SYMPTOM RELIEF

Blinking vigorously is likely to stop the smart of a mild eye burn, says Dr. Little. But if that doesn't do the trick, here's how to quell the pain.

Flush, flush, then rush to the doctor. A chemical burn is an emergency. "Speed is what counts," says Jason Slakter,

M.D., attending surgeon in the Department of
Ophthalmology at the Manhattan Eye, Ear and Throat
Hospital. Immediately flood the eye with water, using your
fingers to keep the eye open as wide as possible. Hold your
head under a faucet or garden hose or pour water into the
eye (*any* clean container is okay in this case) for at least 15
minutes, continuously and gently. Roll the eyeball as much
as possible to wash out the eye. Then seek medical help
immediately. If you take this swift action, the doctor may
only need to apply a patch and prescribe antibiotic drops
(to prevent infection), and your burned eye will heal on its
own. More serious damage may require surgical repair.

Cool down sunburned orbs. Cover your eyes with a cool
washcloth and take a pain reliever such as aspirin or
ibuprofen, says Dr. Little. If the sting doesn't subside in a
day or two, see the doctor.

Never stare directly at the sun. Not even if there's a solar
eclipse, reminds Dr. Little. "Staring at the sun can burn
your retina like sun directed through a magnifying glass
burns paper," he says.

Try artificial tears. To control chronic burning from dry
indoor heating, for example, try a drop or two of lubricating artificial tears, says Kenneth Kauvar, M.D., assistant
clinical professor of ophthalmology at the University of
Colorado School of Medicine in Denver and author of *Eyes
Only*. Tear products come in thick or thin viscosity, and the
first drop may sting a bit, he says. The second drop is more
soothing.

Banish Common Eye Burns

Here's how to avoid accidental eye burns.

Apply lip balm on your brows. A waxy lip balm applied
on the eyebrows or upper lids provides a waterproof barrier that blocks sunscreen from trickling into your eyes
when you sweat, says David Harris, M.D., clinical professor of dermatology at Stanford University School of
Medicine. Avoid menthol types, he adds. The vapors can
sting your eyes.

Wear cotton before you dye. A cotton headband absorbs
dripping hair dye or permanent-wave solution.

Use grease shields on frying pans. This prevents accidental food splatters.

Spritz and sprint. Close your eyes before using hair spray, then leave the area quickly.

Aim nozzles that-a-way. Direct nozzles away from your face when using any household sprayers, toxic or otherwise. Always work in a well-ventilated room when using caustic household chemicals. And when you open a container filled with a caustic substance—or even one that can release volatile fumes, like ammonia—turn your head away.

Store goggles near the jumper cables. "Jump-starting a dead battery can release caustic battery acid fumes and splashes. That's why you should learn the correct way to handle a battery and put on eye goggles and gloves before you ever touch one," says Dr. Slakter.

Don watertight goggles before the plunge. They protect against chlorine-caused eye burns in swimming pools.

Prevent Sunburned Eyes

"Sunglasses that block out 99 percent or more of the UV rays should be standard outdoor wear, especially if you live, play or work near sand, snow or water," says Dr. Little. Long-term exposure to the sun's radiation may cause cataracts, retina damage or other eye problems.

Here are specific ways to protect yourself.

Wear them in the tropics and mountains. The UV rays are extra-intense and potentially more damaging at high elevations or near the equator.

Wear them when taking sun-sensitive drugs. Photosensitizing drugs such as tetracycline that make your skin more sensitive to light can also make your eyes more sensitive to UV rays.

Wear them if you've had cataract surgery. Or make sure that your intraocular lens or post-surgery contact lenses are the UV-absorbent type.

Choose close-fitting wraparounds. Studies show that harmful UV damage can occur from rays that enter under, over and around the sides of ordinary frames.

Wear "amber-tinted" or "polarized" sunglasses for boating. Amber-tinted UV-absorbent lenses block the harmful "blue rays" of the sun. And polarized lenses cut reflected glare bouncing off pavement, water or snow. Both types are ideal for fishing or skiing, says Dr. Little.

Sport a wide-brimmed hat, too. This will help protect your face, lips and eyes from the sun's damaging rays, which can predispose you to skin cancer, wrinkles and age spots, says Dr. Little.

EYE DISCHARGE

WHEN TO SEE YOUR DOCTOR

- The discharge is yellowish, crusty or persistent.
- Your eyelid is swollen, red or painful.

WHAT YOUR SYMPTOM IS TELLING YOU

The morning alarm is ringing, but your eyes refuse to rise and shine. They're so swollen shut with sticky, crusty discharge, it feels like the sandman pasted your lids with glue.

"It can be alarming to have to pry open your eyes in the morning, but eye discharge is rarely harmful and is simply part of your body's natural defense system," says Walter I. Fried, M.D., Ph.D., clinical assistant professor of ophthalmology at University of Health Sciences/Chicago Medical School.

In most cases, waking up with oozy, crusty, red-rimmed eyes means your eyes have been invaded by bacteria from contaminated eye makeup, for example, or from extra-oily skin. A bacterial invasion can lead to blepharitis, an inflammation at the base of the eyelashes that produces thick, yellowish pus filled with bacteria-fighting white blood cells.

A sticky, yellowish discharge that seals your eyes shut is also your body's natural response to pinkeye, a bacteria or virus-caused infection that attacks the transparent membrane covering the eyeball.

Another type of sticky discharge—thinner, clear and noncrusty—can mean you have a cold, an allergy to pollen, dried-out eyes from gusty winds or an eyelash touching your eyeball. "This sticky, watery discharge usually goes away once the irritating factors are removed," says Dr. Fried.

SYMPTOM RELIEF

Oozy eyelids that are also swollen means you have an infection that requires antibiotic eyedrops and possibly oral antibiotics, too," says Dr. Fried. Here are more ways to deal with discharge.

Come unglued. If your eyes are glued shut, loosen the crusts with a warm, wrung-out washcloth.

Wash your lids. Next, dip a cottonball in a solution made with 1/2 teaspoon of salt dissolved in a teaspoon of warm water and rub it along the lash line. You can also apply a commercial eyelid scrub.

Get the oil out. If blepharitis is a problem, it helps to remove excess oil from your eyelids, says Mitchell H. Friedlaender, M.D., director of corneal services in the Division of Ophthalmology at the Scripps Clinic and Research Foundation in La Jolla, California, and coauthor of *20/20: A Total Guide to Improving Your Vision and Preventing Eye Disease*. To remove excess oil from eyelids, you may cleanse the lashes and lid margins with baby shampoo or another mild detergent. Also, gently massage the lids using a downward motion as if "squeezing toothpaste out of a tube," he says. Then massage the upper lid and pat off the oil with a tissue. Do this every night for a week or two. If you have chronic blepharitis, you should make cleaning and massaging your eyelids a regular habit "like brushing your teeth," says Dr. Friedlaender.

Don't share your washcloth. Viral or bacterial discharge is loaded with germs that can be passed on to others (or back to yourself), says Dr. Fried. Nondisposable objects— including your hands—that have touched your tears should be washed in hot water.

Give your old mascara the heave-ho. Contaminated cos-metics are prime suspects in eye infections. Toss any eye cosmetics that you used while you were infected and any that are more than six months old. Otherwise, you may be reapplying bacteria, says Dr. Fried.

EYE DRYNESS

WHEN TO SEE YOUR DOCTOR

- Your eyes are also extremely irritated, gritty, red, itchy, burning or sometimes tear excessively.
- You also have rheumatoid arthritis and dry mouth.
- You have increased sensitivity to light.

WHAT YOUR SYMPTOM IS TELLING YOU

Blinking spreads a three-layered film of water, oil and mucus over your eyes like wiper fluid washing over a car's windshield. But once you reach age 40, the tear glands begin to slow down and you have less of this soothing eye fluid, according to George Sanborn, M.D., associate clinical professor of ophthalmology at the Virginia Commonwealth University/Medical College of Virginia in Richmond. Probably because of hormonal shifts that dry up secretions, women at or past menopause expe-rience more severe tear turn-off than men or younger women, says Dr. Sanborn.

No matter what your age, you may develop a case of dry eyes if you're taking secretion-drying antihistamine/decon-gestant medications, antidepressants, diuretics or beta blockers. (See your doctor if such medications seem to be irritating your eyes.) Other things that can dry up eye moisture include sitting in a dry aircraft cabin, being outdoors on a windy day, air conditioning and home heating. Your eyes' waterworks can also dry up if you are extremely fatigued or have diabetes or a severe vitamin A deficiency (which is very rare in America) says Dr. Sanborn.

In any case, without sufficient lubricating tears to coat your eyes and swish away sand, pollen and infectious microbes, your eyes become dry and tender. This can make wearing contact lenses as uncomfortable as hiking with a pebble in your shoe. Worse, in severe cases, dry eye can lead to vision-robbing bacterial, viral or fungal infections.

SYMPTOM RELIEF

Whether your eyes are slightly dry or as arid as the Sahara, it's possible to get tears flowing again.

Blanket your eyes with a warm washcloth. If your eyes become dry only now and then, try placing a warm compress on your eyelids for five to ten minutes two or three times a day, suggests Eric Donnenfeld, M.D., an ophthalmologist in private practice in Manhassett, New York. "A warm compress is sometimes all it takes to stimulate tear flow," he says.

Blink, blink, blink. Sewing, watching TV or typing at a computer are all activities during which people tend to forget to blink. As a result of staring, eye moisture evaporates, according to Paul Michelson, M.D., senior staff ophthalmologist at the Mericos Eye Institute in La Jolla, California. Taking frequent blink breaks replenishes the tear film, he says.

Reach for fake tears. For a chronic dry eye problem, over-the-counter artificial tears can soothe tender, gritty eyes. These products contain saline and a film-forming substance, such as polyvinyl alcohol or synthetic cellulose. They may be used as often as necessary. You'll need to experiment with different products to see what works best for you, says Dr. Michelson. Thinner brands, for example, need to be inserted more often but are less likely to blur vision or leave a residue on eyelashes. To insert eyedrops gently pull down the lower lid and squeeze a drop into the corner of the eye near the nose. Hold your eyes closed for a minute. "Blinking pumps out the drops," explains Dr. Michelson.

Use preservative-free products. If you're using drops more than four times daily, look for brands that say preservative-free, advises Mitchell H. Friedlaender, M.D., director of corneal services in the Division of Ophthalmology at the Scripps Clinic and Research Foundation in La Jolla, California, and coauthor of *20/20: A Total Guide to Improving Your Vision and Preventing Eye Disease.* Preservatives such as thimerosal can build up to toxic concentrations and may damage the surface of the eye, he says. If your eyes do not respond to lubricants after using them for a week, see your doctor.

Make gooey-gooey eyes at night. If you wake up feeling like the Sandman left too much sand in your eyes, inserting a tear-replacement/moisture-sealing ointment at bedtime can cease your misery, says Dr. Michelson. These extra-thick ocular ointments contain white petrolatum and mineral oil and last longer than drops.

Wear an eye moisture chamber while you sleep. Specially designed moisture shields can be worn at bedtime to help prevent moisture evaporation from your eyes.

Have your tear drains plugged. If your dry eyes do not respond to artificial tears, your doctor can insert a tiny collagen plug in your tear drainage canal, says Dr. Sanborn. The plug remains in place for about six months and helps conserve the tears you do produce and keeps artificial tears in your eyes longer. (Or your doctor can permanently seal the tear duct with surgery.)

Prevent Arid Orbs

If you have borderline dry eye, certain environmental factors can worsen your problem and may cause extreme discomfort. Here's how to keep your eyes' waterworks in working order.

Moisturize the night air. Switching on a humidifier or placing a pan of water on the radiator in the bedroom can keep eyes from drying out while you sleep, says Dr. Friedlaender.

Wear wraparound shades outdoors. Sunglasses with lenses that extend past the sides of your eyes or side shields on your regular glasses help keep out drying sun and wind, says Dr. Michelson.

Aim the air nozzle that-a-way. Hair dryers and home air vents blowing on your eyes can worsen dry eye, says Dr. Friedlaender. It's especially important to aim overhead air nozzles away from eyes on airplanes, where the atmosphere is very drying anyway, he says.

EYE IRRITATION

WHEN TO SEE YOUR DOCTOR

- There's something embedded in your eyeball.
- The irritation is accompanied by redness or a discharge.

WHAT YOUR SYMPTOM IS TELLING YOU

A long with popcorn between your teeth and sand in your swimsuit, a speck in your eye ranks among life's more annoying sensations.

Dust particles or a bit of eye makeup floating on your eye are common irritants that can usually be worked out by batting your eyelids several times. But eyes can be red and irritated from overly dry eyes, pollen, air pollution or infection.

SYMPTOM RELIEF

W hen batting an eye won't do, here's what to do.
Squirt it out. Maybe you once used eyecups or home-

made boric acid solutions to flush out a speck, but they're a poor choice because they can be contaminated, according to Walter I. Fried, M.D., Ph.D., clinical assistant professor of ophthalmology at University of Health Sciences/Chicago Medical School. "You're better off using a few drops of non-prescription, artificial tears," he says. If you don't have commercial tears on hand, splash a little tap water on your eyes. If the particle remains or discomfort persists, see your doctor.

Bat it out. If you can feel the speck but you can't see it, it's possible that the speck has worked its way beneath your upper eyelid. If so, try lifting the upper lid over the lower lid. This enables the lower eyelashes to brush the speck off the inside of the upper lid. Then blink a few times. If the particle floats to the corner of your eye, use a cloth handkerchief to remove it.

Try the flip-over technique. Grasp your upper eyelash and bend the lid back over a cotton-tipped applicator. Now you can flick out the particle with a cloth handkerchief or flush it out with water.

Blow your nose. Blowing your nose may jostle the particle and move it to a better position for removal, says Kenneth Kauvar, M.D., assistant clinical professor of ophthalmology at the University of Colorado School of Medicine in Denver and author of *Eyes Only*.

Take lots of blink breaks. If your eyes are as dry as the Mojave Desert, artificial tears used throughout the day can be an oasis. Also, if you're staring for long hours at a computer screen, remember to blink frequently to spread the natural tear film and keep your eyes comfortable.

Defend your eyes from ragweed. If your eyes are sensitive to airborne pollen, a stroll in the woods can feel like someone kicked sand in your eyes: They feel gritty, they're red and they may sting like crazy. An over-the-counter antihistamine tablet can erase the discomfort, says Mitchell H. Friedlaender, M.D., director of corneal services in the Division of Ophthalmology at the Scripps Clinic and Research Foundation in La Jolla, California, and coauthor of *20/20: A Total Guide to Improving Your Vision and Preventing Eye Disease*.

Opt for antibiotics. If you have a discharge from your

eyes, you probably have an infection and will have to see your doctor for an antibiotic to clear it up.

End Eye Makeup Irritation

Use makeup properly to avoid the problem.

Don't go for the glitter. Ground oyster shells or tinsel used in frosted, pearlized, iridescent or other glittery eye-shadow can be harmful to any eye, but can be especially damaging if a particle finds its way under a contact lens.

Choose pencils over liquid. Eyeliner pencils are less likely to flake off. Don't apply eyeliner to the inner edge of the lower lid where it can clog oil glands and cause irritation or infection.

Avoid lash-building mascara. These products may contain nylon fibers that can fall into the eyes.

Wait until all signals are clear. "Never apply eye makeup if your eyes are irritated," says Dr. Fried.

See also Eye Dryness; Eye Redness

EYELID DROOPING

WHEN TO SEE YOUR DOCTOR

- Your upper lid dips into your line of vision or your lower lid pulls away from your eye.

WHAT YOUR SYMPTOM IS TELLING YOU

Drooping upper eyelids, known as ptosis, are caused when the eyelid's "lifting" muscles begin to sag. It's a condition you can be born with, or it can develop from aging, after cataract surgery or from an injury. Other conditions that can cause drooping eyelids include diabetes, a tumor or Bell's palsy—a viral infection that causes temporary facial paralysis. One or both lids may droop down far enough to curtain your line of sight.

When lower lids become lax from normal aging, the muscles pull away from the lids, so the lids turn out. This causes the lubricating tears that are normally spread by blinking to instead spill down your cheeks. The result: Your eyes become dry and vulnerable to light and wind.

SYMPTOM RELIEF

Tipping your head back or raising your eyebrows to see out from under droopy lids takes great effort. Here are some far more effective lid-lifting measures.

Tape your eyes open. A piece of see-through, hypo-allergenic bandage tape (available at pharmacies) can help pull the drooping eyelid skin slightly taut and lift it out of your line of vision. First, place your index finger at the outside corner of your upper eyelid and gently push the sagging skin up a bit toward your eyebrow. Use 1/4 inch of tape to hold the eyelid skin in place. Make sure you've allowed room for eyelid movement. "The trick is to keep the tape loose enough so you can still blink and lubricate your eyes," says Howard Eggers, M.D., associate professor of clinical ophthalmology at Columbia-Presbyterian Medical Center in New York City.

Wear custom-made glasses. Your optometrist or optician can solder a padded wire on the inside frames of your eyeglasses to hold up a fold of skin, says Dr. Eggers. It's flexible enough to move when you blink, he adds.

Try a lid tuck. As a last resort, your doctor can surgically shorten the lid-lifting muscles, says Douglas Fredrick, M.D., clinical instructor of ophthalmology at the University of California in San Francisco. You may be temporarily unable to fully close your eye after surgery, however. If so, keep your eyes moist—with artificial tears during the day and ointments while sleeping—until your lids can close, says Dr. Fredrick.

EYE PAIN

WHEN TO SEE YOUR DOCTOR

- You have something embedded in your eye.
- You've received a blow to the eye.
- You have a dull ache around your eyes that persists for more than two days.
- You have a sudden or piercing pain deep in your eyes.
- Your eye pain is accompanied by a change in your vision, headaches, nausea or sensitivity to light.

WHAT YOUR SYMPTOM IS TELLING YOU

The eyes have been called the most sensitive organs in the human body. That's because they're honeycombed with pain receptors—extremely sensitive, finely tuned nerve endings that help protect these vital organs.

This means that the slightest insult to the surface—a blast of cold, dry air or an inward-growing eyelash, for example—can stimulate these nerves, firing a pain signal to your brain. The result: Your eyes smart or feel scratchy.

Other factors inside your body can also excite your eye's hypersensitive receptors. A sinus infection can inflame the adjacent muscles, for example, and trigger a throbbing, sometimes sharp, pain behind the eye socket. A simple act like rolling your eyes can hurt.

Ironically, keeping your eyes too still for too long can strain the muscles that move your eyes into their proper position. That's why you feel a dull ache around your eyes after staring at spreadsheets on your computer screen for hours or reading page after page of that three-inch-thick novel. If the reading light is dim or the overhead lighting is too harsh, your orbs may ache even more.

In addition, wearing ill-fitting glasses or trying to see through outdated prescription lenses can also strain surrounding muscles.

Sometimes, the pain you feel in your eyes orginates else-where in your body. "What feels like eye pain is often actu-ally a headache or pain in the facial muscles caused by tension," says Robert E. Kalina, M.D., chairman of oph-thalmology at the University of Washington in Seattle.

But if the pain is severe, your eyes are red and your vision's blurry, the likely culprit is uveitis—an inflamma-tion involving the pigmented areas in the eye. It's often brought on by an infection elsewhere in the body. Severe pain with other symptoms—most notably nausea and haloes around lights—is a sign of glaucoma, a buildup of pressure around the eye that can lead to blindness if left untreated.

SYMPTOM RELIEF

Any kind of persistent eye soreness or sudden eye pain requires a doctor's evaluation and possibly medical treatment. If it turns out that you have uveitis, for instance, you will need to take an anti-inflammatory medication to reduce the swollen tissues that are pressing on the nerves. For glaucoma, you'll need antipressure drops. Once the pressure has been controlled, you may need laser surgery to prevent fluid buildup.

For run-of-the-mill soreness caused by overuse or sinus infection, here's what you can do.

Don't let the drops drain away. If your doctor has pre-scribed medicated eyedrops to relieve pain from infection or some other cause, you need to make sure the medicine stays in your eyes and doesn't roll down your cheeks, says Mitchell H. Friedlaender, M.D., director of corneal services in the Division of Ophthalmology at the Scripps Clinic and Research Foundation in La Jolla, California, and coauthor of *20/20: A Total Guide to Improving Your Vision and Preventing Eye Disease*. The correct way to apply eyedrops: Tilt your head back and squeeze a drop or two inside your lower eyelid. Keep your eyes closed for a good two minutes. Or, you can use your finger and press in the inside corner of your eye. "This allows the drops to penetrate into the eye and prevents them from getting into the bloodstream," says Dr. Friedlaender.

Try artificial tears for scratchiness. Home remedies such as over-the-counter artificial tears can relieve mild eye discomfort caused by dryness, cold air or smog, according to Kenneth Kauvar, M.D., assistant clinical professor of ophthalmology at the University of Colorado School of Medicine in Denver and author of *Eyes Only*. If after two days of using these drops your eyes still smart, see your doctor.

Take two aspirin and relax. If you're experiencing a dull ache in or around your eyes, it may be headache-related. If so, one or two aspirin every six to eight hours should relieve the problem, says Dr. Kalina. If the pain is still there after two days, see your doctor.

Give your eyes a break. Taking a brief rest from prolonged reading or other close work may be enough to relieve eye strain, says Dr. Kauvar. Look up from the page or computer screen and gaze off into the distance every ten minutes or so. Or let your eyes unfocus every so often.

Do pencil push-ups. Simple eye exercises can limber up tired eye muscles that have been fixed on a computer screen for hours, according to James L. Cox, O.D., behavioral optometrist with the College of Optometrists in Vision Development in Bellflower, California. Try focusing your eyes on a pencil as you slowly move it in toward your nose and then back out again. Repeat for a full minute every 20 minutes, says Dr. Cox.

Use soft overall lighting plus spotlights. Dim lighting or glare strains eyes as your muscles keep trying to move your eyes into a position to obtain the most light, says Dr. Kauvar. The best illumination, he says, is soft overall background lighting with a light aimed at what you're reading.

Take your specs in for a checkup. "Glasses that slide down your nose can make your eyes ache as the muscles on the side of your eyes try to move your eyes to compensate for an abnormal eye deviation," says Dr. Kauvar. Your glasses should fit properly, he says. An outdated eyeglass prescription can also strain your eyes. So be sure to

have your eyes checked for any vision changes at least once
a year.

See also Eye Irritation

EYE PUFFINESS

WHEN TO SEE YOUR DOCTOR

- Puffiness persists for a week or more.
- Your eyes are also red or painful.

WHAT YOUR SYMPTOM IS TELLING YOU

You board the early-bird flight to the coast looking like
you're carrying the bulk of your baggage under your
eyes. It may look gruesome, but it merely means that body
fluids have pooled overnight in the eye area, according to
Mary Stefanyszyn, M.D., associate surgeon in ophthalmology at Wills Eye Hospital in Philadelphia.

Generally, you can trace early-morning puffiness to your
activities of the previous day: You drank fluids at bedtime,
ate salty foods, spent all day with your head bent over a
garden or stayed up half the night, says Dr. Stefanyszyn.
The worst of the swelling subsides a few hours after rising,
as the fluid is re-absorbed by your body.

You may also have puffy eyes as part of an allergic reaction—from eating strawberries, for example, or from sleeping on feather pillows. Hormonal changes during
menstruation can puff up eyes, too.

A more permanent kind of puffiness can occur from
saggy skin caused by normal aging, according to Paul
Lazar, M.D., professor of clinical dermatology at
Northwestern University in Chicago and author of *The*

Look You Like. The skin around the eyes becomes thinner and less elastic with age, he says. Then underlying fat causes the skin to bulge out.

Roundish pouches or bags rather than puffiness may be a sign of a thyroid condition known as Graves' disease or an indication of a kidney problem.

SYMPTOM RELIEF

You may be tempted to don sunglasses first thing in the morning as a cover-up, but take heart, there are ways to deflate puffiness.

Start with a bracing splash. A splash of cold water on your face gets the circulation moving, according to Fredric Haberman, M.D., clinical instructor of dermatology at Albert Einstein College of Medicine in New York City and author of *The Doctor's Beauty Hotline.*

Tap into relief. Lightly tapping your upper and lower lids helps nudge fluids away from eyes, says Dr. Haberman. With a very light touch, and using fingertips only, gently tap puffy areas on upper and lower lids.

Mask the problem. Refrigerate a gel-filled eye mask and place it over your closed eyes for a few minutes after waking. If you don't have a mask, chilled teaspoons will work, says Dr. Haberman.

Try tea bags. Moisten two tea bags with cold water and rest with them on your closed eyes for 15 minutes. The tannin in the tea may help pull the skin taut and reduce the puffiness. "The main factor is the coolness, which reduces swelling," says Dr. Stefanyszyn.

Take a diuretic. If you're retaining water before your period, an over-the-counter product such as Midol may help reduce eye puffiness, says Dr. Stefanyszyn.

Try an antihistamine. If your puffy eyes are also red, itchy and scratchy, you may be having an allergic reaction. If that's the case, an antihistamine may help shrink the swelling, says Dr. Lazar.

Cover with a concealer. To minimize upper lid puffiness, apply a darker shade of makeup on your upper lid, from just below the brow to the crease. Then stroke a lighter shade on the lid from the crease to the lashes. Puffiness is less noticeable when you highlight the lower portion of the lid, says Dr. Haberman. For under-eye bags, use a slightly darker shade over your regular foundation.

Keeping Bags Away

Here's how to avoid puffiness tomorrow.

Raise the head of the bed. Six-inch wooden blocks placed under the headboard will elevate your head and help keep fluid from pooling around your eyes.

Skip the water at bedtime. Or restrict yourself to a few sips.

Cut out overly salty foods. And if you have Chinese food for dinner, tell the waiter to hold the monosodium gluta-mate (MSG). "Eating sodium-loaded Chinese food at dinner always gives me puffy eyes the next day," says Dr. Stefanyszyn.

Skip wrinkle removers. An eye cream designed for plumping up wrinkles may be doing its job too well, says Dr. Haberman. These products can backfire and give you bags by puffing up the surrounding eye area.

Switch to gel-type makeup. Water-based makeup and gels are lighter than oil-based and less likely to irritate delicate under-eye skin.

Forgo the feather comforter. If you suspect that you are allergic to feathers—waking up every morning with puffy eyes is a clue—try switching to quilts and pillows filled with synthetic material.

EYE REDNESS

WHEN TO SEE YOUR DOCTOR

- The redness persists for more than two days.
- The redness persists for more than two hours after removing contact lenses.
- You also have yellow or thick eye discharge.
- You also have piercing, throbbing pain, blurred vision or sensitivity to light.

WHAT YOUR SYMPTOM IS TELLING YOU

Forget Bette Davis eyes! You've got Rand McNally eyes: orbs lined like road maps (and you haven't even left town). Perhaps you were swimming in a chlorinated pool, had one beer too many at the barbecue or rubbed your eyes a bit too vigorously. Any one of these factors can dilate the tiny blood vessels within the whites of your eyes, making them red.

Pinkeye, for example (the common name for red eyes accompanied by a yellowish, crusty discharge), is a highly contagious infection that can circulate in classrooms faster than crib notes. Red eyes with a clear, watery discharge and a sore throat often indicate the onset of a cold.

But redness comes in all shapes and sizes—for instance, a little red blob that appears suddenly on the white of one eye. It may look frightening, but it's usually harmless, according to Mitchell H. Friedlaender, M.D., director of corneal services in the Division of Ophthalmology at the Scripps Clinic and Research Foundation in La Jolla, California, and coauthor of *20/20: A Total Guide to Improving Your Vision and Preventing Eye Disease*. These red blobs are blood vessels that burst during a bout of sudden pressure, like a powerful sneeze or while straining to lift the sofa. They're common among older people and usually fade in a week or so.

The most serious cause of red eyes is *keratitis*, an inflammation of the cornea that's usually caused by a contaminated contact lens.

SYMPTOM RELIEF

The rule is, if your eyes are red, don't rub," says Jason Slakter, M.D., attending surgeon in the Department of Ophthalmology at the Manhattan Eye, Ear and Throat Hospital. If the problem is an allergen like pollen, rubbing could trigger the release of more histamine—the allergen-sparked chemical that caused your eyes to redden in the first place. And remember, no matter what the cause, your eyes are red because they're irritated. Rubbing only irritates them more.

Here's what to do instead.

Play it cool. A cool compress can provide relief for redness from a cold virus or allergen, says Dr. Slakter. Soak a clean washcloth in cold water and relax for ten minutes with the cloth over your closed eyes.

Fumigate your shopping list. To help relieve red, weepy, itchy eyes, try using only unscented tissues, cosmetics, soaps and laundry detergents. You may have an allergy to the perfumes in these items.

Fake it. Over-the-counter artificial tears can soothe red eyes caused by dry air or smoke-filled rooms.

"Decongest" your eyes. For bloodshot eyes from pollution or pollen, look for "eye decongestant" drops that constrict blood vessels (vasoconstrictors) and remove the red. (Some brands include an antihistamine that counteracts allergic itchiness and swelling.) But using vasoconstrictors longer than three days could give you "rebound redness," because the blood vessels react to the drug by overdilating. "You may wind up with redder eyes than ever," says Dr. Friedlaender. If your eyes are still bloodshot after a day or two of using decongestants or you have excessive discharge, see the doctor.

Take your antibiotic faithfully. If you have pinkeye, you need to use antibiotic eyedrops for a week to ten days to kill the bacteria, according to Kenneth Kauvar, M.D., assistant clinical professor of ophthalmology at the University of Colorado School of Medicine in Denver and author of *Eyes Only*. To insert the drops, pull the lower lid down gently, look up and place a drop in the space between the lower lid and the eyeball. Close the lid for a few seconds.

Don't spread it around. If you have pinkeye, wash your hands frequently. "You could easily spread the infection to the other eye or to another person," says Dr. Kauvar. Also, change your towels, washcloths and pillowcases every few days. And buy fresh eye makeup.

Take out your lenses. "A contact lens left in a red eye provides the perfect incubator for bacteria," says Dr. Slakter. If redness remains after removing your contacts, see your doctor.

Practice good lens hygiene. To avoid keratitis, you should clean and disinfect your lenses every time you remove them, using fresh solutions, says Scott MacRae, M.D., associate professor of ophthalmology at the Oregon Health Sciences University School of Medicine in Portland. Use only the commercial contact lens preparations recommended for your hard or soft lenses. Clean the lens cases, too. And never use homemade solutions or saliva on lenses.

Air your eyeballs overnight. Contacts worn continuously (even the extended-wear type) rub away the cornea, causing rips that invite infection, says Dr. Friedlaender. Contacts are also a barrier to oxygen and encourage bacterial growth. "Removing lenses overnight reduces the time a foreign body is on your eyes and cuts your chance of infection," he says.

Spray and paint before inserting. In the morning, use hairspray *before* inserting your lenses. (And to further cut the chance of infection, use only water-based, nongreasy cosmetics.) In the evening, remove, clean and store your lenses before removing your makeup.

EYE WATERING

WHEN TO SEE YOUR DOCTOR

- Your eyes water persistently for more than two days and do not respond to home remedies.

WHAT YOUR SYMPTOM IS TELLING YOU

Watery eyes are too much of a good thing. Lubricating tears bathe your eyeballs each time you blink, but an irritation involving your eye or head can turn that bath into a flood. Eyes can well up from a headache, a sinus infection, smoke, wind, an eyelash grazing your eyeball, a problem with your contact lens or overworking your eyes at the computer.

You can also get teary-eyed from eating tongue-torching chili or stubbing your toe on the sidewalk. "Excessive tears are part of a nervous system reflex triggered by various assaults to the body," says Christopher Rapuano, M.D., assistant professor of ophthalmology at Thomas Jefferson University Hospital in Philadelphia. If you've scorched your tongue or scraped your toe, he says, your eyes tear up as part of your body's pain response to injury. There's some research to suggest that these tears may even help speed the healing process in some way.

Excessive tears—along with redness and itchiness—are also classic signs of an allergy. If you're allergic to cats, for example, and walk into a room where cat dander permeates the air, your eyes may begin to flow like a broken dam. These are part of your body's response to the release of irritating chemicals known as histamines that are triggered by allergens.

Ironically enough, too few tears can also trigger watery eyes. When normal tear secretions dry up from age-related changes, the eye surface burns and feels scratchy. Like a fireman at a fire, your eye responds by turning on the hose.

Another age-related problem is that the lower eyelid can become lax as skin begins to sag. This pulls the tear drainage canal in the lower eyelid away from the eyeball. Without this natural exit, the tears well up and spill down the cheeks. (Lupus, a painful disease that affects the skin, can also cause the lower eyelids to droop and spill tears).

In addition, a blow to the eye or infection in the eyelid can swell the tissues of the inner eye, blocking the tear drainage canal.

SYMPTOM RELIEF

Besides avoiding jalapeño peppers, here are some other ways to prevent watery eyes.

Try an antihistamine plus artificial tears. If allergies are triggering your tears, an oral antihistamine could stem the flow. Keep in mind that this is a secretion-drying medication, and could dry out your eye *too* much, says Dr. Rapuano. The rule: Use artificial tears every few hours when taking an antihistamine.

Wear head-hugging sunglasses. They'll keep eyes from crying in gusty weather. The best eye protectors have side shields with frames that hug the side of your head so that very little air sneaks in, says Dr. Rapuano.

Switch from contacts to glasses in dusty areas. Dust specks can get caught under a contact and scrape your eye, according to Scott MacRae, M.D., associate professor of ophthalmology at the Oregon Health Sciences University School of Medicine in Portland. Also, avoid wearing contacts on smoggy, high-pollen days. These irritants can trigger red, watery eyes even if you're not wearing contacts. Wearing them makes the problem even worse.

See your doctor about a blocked tear duct. If those suggestions don't cure a case of spillover tears, your problem may be a bit more serious: infected, swollen tissues blocking the tear canal. Your doctor can prescribe an antibiotic to help deflate the tissues and reopen the tears' natural exit route. If this doesn't do the trick, your ophthalmologist can surgically dilate the opening in a simple office procedure.

See also Eye Redness

EYES, CROSSED

- You suddenly have double vision and one or both of your eyes turns in, out, up or down.

WHAT YOUR SYMPTOM IS TELLING YOU

So, okay, Mom was wrong. Reading in the dark doesn't dim your vision. And staring at your nose didn't make your eyes get stuck in the crossed position.

Chances are, if one or both of your eyes quite noticeably turns in, out, up or down, you were born with misaligned eyes that were never corrected. No one knows for sure, but doctors suspect that eye misalignment (technically called strabismus) may be caused by an imbalance in the nerve signals to the muscles controlling the two eyes. This forces them to point off in different directions, "like two cameras aimed at different spots," says Newton Wesley, M.D., O.D., chairman of the National Eye Research Foundation in Chicago. The reason you don't see "simulcast" images, however, is that your childhood brain turned off the weaker camera, he says. Generally, your stronger eye compensated and became the dominant, vision-retaining one.

It's also possible for eyes that have been in perfect tandem throughout life to suddenly or gradually veer off. This could be from an injury, cataract, diabetes, a disease or stroke. Adult brains can't ignore the image from the turned eye, however, so you see double.

Misalignment may also cause words to blur and run together when you're reading. If you have a tendency to be cross-eyed, just trying to thread a needle can give you a walloping headache and major eyestrain. If only one eye wanders out, dimness of vision (amblyopia) may result.

These misalignment problems may bother you all the time, or just when you are ill or tired. By the way, if you notice that one eye turns in or out slightly after removing your glasses, it simply means your eyes are releasing control of the proper alignment they had with the lenses, according to Eleanor Faye, M.D., an ophthalmologic surgeon at the Manhattan Eye, Ear and Throat Hospital. This is no cause for concern.

SYMPTOM RELIEF

You'll need to see your doctor for diagnosis and treatment. There are also a few things you can do under your doctor's supervision to get your eyes working as a team.

Patch it up. When children have crossed eyes, the doctor may have them wear a patch over the stronger eye for six weeks to six months. "They're bound to get a few stares, but it's a good way to help strengthen and improve vision in the weaker eye," says Douglas Fredrick, M.D., clinical instructor of ophthalmology at the University of California in San Francisco.

Try pencil push-ups. Special eye exercises called orthopics help stimulate your brain to use both eyes together, which often eliminates double vision, according to Dr. Fredrick. They are most effective when practiced regularly under the guidance of a trained doctor, he says.

One exercise that can help your eyes focus and fuse on a single image involves holding a pencil at arm's length and bringing it gradually toward your nose. If you have a problem with crossed eyes, you'll see double at eight inches away, says Dr. Fredrick. Practice keeping both eyes focused on the pencil as you gradually bring it toward you. Eventually, your eyes will learn to fuse the two images into one at about two inches.

Wear special specs. Some prescription lenses either stimulate or inhibit the movement of certain eye muscles, says Dr. Wesley. Glasses with built-in prisms can help redirect the line of sight and may help correct two images into one.

Get yourself in stitches. To reposition the misaligned eye, your doctor may suggest an operation involving adjustable stitches, says Dr. Fredrick. A bow-knot suture is left trailing out of the eye muscle so the doctor can tug on the muscle and fine-tune the alignment while you are actually looking at objects.

Do the penlight test. The earlier you treat a misaligned eye, the more likely you'll save the sight in the weaker eye, says Dr. Fredrick. It's not always easy to tell if babies have crossed eyes, however. They all have wide, flat noses and an extra fold of skin at the inner eyelid, creating a crossed-eye appearance.

True crossed eyes will reveal an off-center reflection in one of the pupils when you hold a penlight in front of a baby's eyes. If this happens, make an appointment with an ophthalmologist.

EYES, DARK CIRCLES

WHAT YOUR SYMPTOM IS TELLING YOU

If you have dark circles under your eyes, it's a good bet that your father, mother and siblings have dark circles under their eyes, too.

"The most common type of under-eye circles are usually an inherited trait like varicose veins and have nothing to do with underlying disease or how much sleep you get," says Paul Lazar, M.D., professor of clinical dermatology at Northwestern University in Chicago and author of *The Look You Like*.

The skin under the eye is very thin, he says. In fair-skinned people, blood that passes through the large veins close to the surface shows through the skin, producing a bluish tint. The more transparent your skin, the darker the circles. In both fair and dark-skinned people, dark circles under the eyes can also be from a higher-than-normal amount of skin pigmentation in this area.

The paleness that occurs with fatigue, a cold or sinus

infection or during menstruation or pregnancy may accentuate the circles even more, adds Dr. Lazar. And with age, the under-eye circles are likely to become more pronounced and permanent. Aside from inheriting circles, if you're allergy-prone, you may develop shadowy under-eye smudges in hay fever season. Substances that you are sensitive to can dilate the blood vessels in the delicate under-eye area, says Dr. Lazar. The blood then shows through the skin, he explains.

Dark circles can also develop if you have eczema, an itchy skin condition, under your eyes. Inflammation and rubbing your eyes can thicken and darken the skin.

SYMPTOM RELIEF

You can't totally eliminate dark circles any more than you can banish freckles. But here are a few ways to make them less noticeable.

Go the camouflage route. For women, color-correcting underbases worn under foundation makeup can improve unattractive skin tones, according to Fredric Haberman, M.D., clinical instructor of dermatology at Albert Einstein College of Medicine in New York City and author of *The Doctor's Beauty Hotline*. For bluish circles, apply a pale yellow underbase before applying your regular foundation, he says. Use a pale blue or mauve underbase for brown circles.

Mix your own. Commercial concealer makeups are fine, but stay away from too-light ones or you'll look like a raccoon in reverse. You can custom-blend your own concealer by mixing a bit of moisturizer with a drop of foundation, says Dr. Haberman.

Don't bleach or peel. "Chemical skin lighteners or peels remove only the topmost layer of skin and are practically ineffective at permanently removing dark circles," says Dr. Lazar.

Wear tinted lenses. A pale rose tint on the bottom third of your eyeglasses will help disguise dark circles, says Dr. Lazar. Your optician can add a flattering tint to your glasses.

Reach for an antihistamine. If allergies are causing your dark circles, a combination antihistamine/decongestant may be of some help. Staying indoors in air-conditioned rooms during hay fever season may also deter dark circles, says Minneapolis allergist Malcolm Blumenthal, M.D.

Get treatment for your itch. Prescription steroid skin creams can help reduce the thickness in under-eye skin that causes eczema-related dark circles. Ask your doctor whether this medication is appropriate for you.

F

FACE PAIN

- You also have pain in your eyes.
- You have a fever, develop a rash on your face or your face feels swollen.
- You also feel pain, tingling or numbness in your hands or feet.

WHAT YOUR SYMPTOM IS TELLING YOU

Doctors know that pain in the face means that you probably have a problem somewhere else—like your head, jaw, neck or even your teeth. Finding the "where" can sometimes take a little detective work.

The face, head and neck have nerves that communicate together. If a nerve in your neck is pinched or irritated, the hurt can travel up that nerve and cause pain in your face, says Steven Mandel, M.D., clinical professor of neurology at Jefferson Medical College and an attending physician at Thomas Jefferson University Hospital in Philadelphia.

Lots of conditions can cause facial pain. People who get migraines or cluster headaches can get it. Sinus, ear and eye infections can cause it. A toothache can make your face hurt. And arthritis in the neck can cause discomfort in the face. A controversial and hard-to-diagnose jaw condition called temporomandibular joint disorder (also known as TMD) can sometimes cause facial pain, although you're likely to experience other symptoms as well, such as a "clicking" sound in the jaw or headaches.

Sharp facial pain is the major symptom of a condition called tic douloureux, a nerve disorder. In those who have the disease, it can be triggered by cold drafts, drinking cold liquids, washing the face, shaving, chewing or even talking.

"Tic douloureux is an intermittent, shocklike pain," says John Loeser, M.D., director of the Multidisciplinary Pain Center at the University of Washington School of Medicine in Seattle. "The mechanism that produces this pain in the face isn't fully understood," he adds. "But we do know that when the pain occurs, there is absolutely nothing else wrong."

Facial pain is also a rare but possible sign of a stroke, although you're likely to experience other symptoms as well, such as numbness or trouble with your vision.

Symptom Relief

Since facial pain is usually caused by an underlying problem, treating that problem—be it toothache, headache or TMD—will make the facial pain go away. (You'll find solutions for treating toothache on page 645 and headache on page 280; see Jaw Problems on page 338 for help with TMD.)

If you have tic douloureux, here are a few things you should know.

Take medication for control. Doctors have found that the best way to control the pain of tic douloureux is through drug therapy. Anticonvulsants or similar medications, such as carbamazepine, that directly affect the nerves are often prescribed.

Consider surgery when medications fail. A minor operation using a special needle inserted into the nerve through the cheek can stop the pain. The downside is that there is some loss of feeling in the area of the nerve.

FAINTING

WHEN TO SEE YOUR DOCTOR

- You've suffered a recent injury to your head.
- You have two or more fainting spells within 24 hours.
- You faint without warning symptoms, such as light-headedness.
- You have a previous history of heart disease, stroke or seizures.
- You have a memory lapse or lose control of your bowels.
- You're taking medication.
- You work around machinery or in a high-risk occupation and your fainting could endanger you or your co-workers.

WHAT YOUR SYMPTOM IS TELLING YOU

There is no diplomatic way to faint. Former President George Bush found that out the hard way when he collapsed at a formal dinner in Japan a couple of years ago. Unlike Bush, most of us don't have TV cameras pointing at us when we faint. But fainting can still be an embarrassment. It's also a cause for concern.

Fainting (it's also called swooning, passing out or blacking out) occurs when the heart isn't pumping efficiently enough to maintain adequate blood flow to the brain. As a result, you lose consciousness and faint, says Gerald Rogan, M.D., a family practice physician in Walnut Creek, California.

Just before fainting, a person might feel weak, nauseated, dizzy or light-headed; experience blurred vision or sweat profusely.

Among the many causes of fainting are poor blood circulation, pain, stress, the sight of blood, drug or alcohol use, dehydration, sleep deprivation, head injury, seizure,

heart disease and stroke. Excessive dieting or mineral deficiencies, particularly of potassium, can make a person
black out. And there are a number of medications that can
cause fainting as a side effect.

In some rare instances, urination, vomiting and intense
coughing or laughing can cause fainting by stimulating the
vagus nerve, one of the main nerves in the body that relays
instructions from the brain to the heart, says Eric G.
Anderson, M.D., a family practice physician in La Jolla,
California. When the vagus nerve is stimulated, the brain
senses that the heart is beating too fast and orders it to slow
down. Normally, that's good. But when some people have a
severe coughing spell, for example, the vagus nerve erro-
neously signals the brain that the heart is working too hard.
As a result, the heart slows down when it doesn't have to,
blood flow to the brain is reduced and the person faints.

SYMPTOM RELIEF

Although dramatic, most faints last only 10 to 15 seconds and usually aren't a sign of a serious illness. Still,
you should let your doctor know about any fainting spell.
In most cases, fainting can be prevented or relieved with
commonsense remedies, doctors say. Here are a few that
may help you fight off fainting.

Make gravity work for you. The worse thing you can do
is to remain seated or standing when you start feeling faint,
Dr. Rogan says. "You need to lie down and elevate your
legs to stimulate blood flow to the brain," he says. "If you
do that, there's a good chance you won't faint."

Don't search for the perfect spot. If you feel faint, drop to
the ground right where you are, even if it is in middle of a
crowded restaurant. "You have about five seconds between
the time you start to feel faint and actually do," Dr. Rogan
says. "A lot of people will try to make it to someplace soft
or inconspicuous before they pass out, but they seldom
make it. My advice is to lie down right where you are and
put your feet up. Then after a minute or two, try to slowly
get up and get to the bed or wherever else you were going."

Breathe deep. Take 10 to 12 deep breaths a minute until you stop feeling faint, Dr. Rogan suggests. Deep breathing helps draw blood in your arms and legs back to your heart. But take no more than 1 deep breath every five seconds, because overbreathing can cause hyperventilation.

Eyeball your drugs. Some prescription drugs, particularly diuretics, sedatives and blood pressure medications, can cause fainting. Ask your doctor or pharmacist if the drugs you're taking may be contributing to your problem and if you should stop using them.

Make time for snoozing. Lack of sleep can contribute to fainting, so be sure to get at least six to eight hours of sleep each day, says Dr. Rogan. (For some good tips to assure that you get an adequate night's sleep, see Insomnia on page 326.)

Walk away from it. Exercise helps strengthen blood vessels and maintain adequate blood flow, says Dr. Anderson. Walking briskly for about 20 minutes three times a week may be all you need to do to lower your risk of fainting.

Get your minerals. "In almost all cases, you're much better off eating a well-balanced diet," says Dr. Rogan. "If you're on some kind of unusual diet, like an all-liquid diet, you could create a mineral imbalance in your body that could cause fainting.

Don't forget the water. Dehydration may make you feel faint. Drinking at least eight eight-ounce glasses of water a day will prevent that, Dr. Rogan says. If you do feel dehydrated, avoid alcohol, because drinking alcohol will only make you more dehydrated. Instead, try quenching your thirst with a sports drink that will replenish your body's supply of important minerals, including potassium and magnesium.

Be a good detective. "Medicine is a lot like detective work," says Dr. Anderson, "and guess who the best detective is? You. So if you faint more than once, it would be worthwhile for you to begin keeping a diary. Where were you when you fainted? What was your body position? Were you sitting, standing or bending over? This sort of detective work may help your doctor determine the underlying cause."

FATIGUE

- You have unexplained feelings of lethargy and energy loss that last for two or more weeks.
- Your fatigue is accompanied by muscle aches, pain, nausea, fever, depression or mood swings.

WHAT YOUR SYMPTOM IS TELLING YOU

You feel like you just ran the Boston Marathon—only you just got out of bed. You're completely drained. Washed out. Running on empty. Not just today, but every day.

Call it fatigue, exhaustion—whatever. If you have it, you're not alone. "Fatigue is second only to pain as the most common symptom doctors see in patients," says David S. Bell, M.D., a chronic fatigue researcher at Harvard Medical School and the Cambridge Hospital in Massachusetts. "One-fourth of all Americans will have long episodes of lethargy and tiredness. This could be because of anything from a case of the 'blahs' to overexertion to a more serious illness."

The most common energy eaters are usually related to a person's lifestyle, says D. W. Edington, Ph.D., director of the Fitness Research Center at the University of Michigan in Ann Arbor. "Poor eating habits, obesity, crash diets, lack of rest and exercise, smoking, drinking—all take heavy tolls on the body," he says. "Stress, job pressures and depression can all build up until they simply wear you down." Even something like not drinking enough water can be a factor.

Virtually any illness can leave you tapped out, even weeks after it goes away. The viral infection mononucleosis, the liver condition hepatitis and the flu are notorious strength sappers. You could also have a hormonal disorder like Addison's disease or an underactive thyroid gland.

Anemia, hypoglycemia and low blood pressure can also leave you weak as a newborn kitten. So might the medications used to treat these illnesses.

Of course, there's always the possibility that you have chronic fatigue syndrome (CFS). It's possible but not as likely as you might imagine, given how much has been written about it in the popular press over the past few years.

CFS—sometimes called the yuppie flu—is a debilitating disorder that leaves people immobile and inactive for months, even years. This illness usually manifests itself after a bout with the flu or some infection. For years CFS was assumed to be caused by the Epstein-Barr virus. Today, doctors admit that they just don't know what causes it.

"It probably doesn't have a single cause but is a combination of viral infections, an altered immune system and other factors," says Nelson Gantz, M.D., chairman of the Department of Medicine and chief of the Infectious Diseases Division at the Polyclinic Medical Center in Harrisburg, Pennsylvania, and clinical professor of medicine at the Pennsylvania State University College of Medicine in Hershey.

CFS is an illness that leaves you chronically fatigued. Just because you feel tired all the time, however, does not necessarily mean that you have CFS. The Centers for Disease Control and Prevention in Atlanta have established criteria that doctors use to determine whether someone has CFS. A person with CFS:

- Was previously healthy.
- Has experienced a 50 percent reduction in activity for at least six months and has no other illnesses that cause fatigue.
- Has a mild fever, sore throat, painful lymph glands, head and muscle aches, joint aches and restless sleep.

CFS has no cure, but eventually it runs its course and some people who have it recover fully. Others have persistent symptoms that wax and wane.

Symptom Relief

Get back your get-up-and-go with these fatigue fighters.

Get plenty of rest. Insufficient and irregular bedrest can drain anybody's body.

Start an exercise program. A body at rest tends to stay at rest. Moderate exercise, even a simple 10-minute walk, can be quite energizing. An aerobic exercise program can help banish fatigue and keep it at bay, says Dr. Edington. That means 20 minutes of something like brisk walking, swimming, running or bicycling at least three times a week. Add stretching and strength-building exercises to your exercise program as your energy builds, he advises.

Eat right. Dieting? Be advised that skipping meals can deprive you of needed energy. Women should shoot for about 1,500 calories a day; men need 2,000. What you eat is at least as important as how much. Nutritional deficiencies can also lead to fatigue, according to James A. Corea, Ph.D., a registered physical therapist in Moorestown, New Jersey, and former trainer with the Philadelphia Eagles professional football team.

The major portion of your meals should consist of whole grains, fruits and vegetables, says Dr. Corea. He recommends the following meal plan.

Breakfast—cereal, fresh fruit, whole wheat toast and skim milk.
Lunch—any combination of fish, pasta, rice, baked potato, fruit salad, vegetable, lean meat or soup.
Dinner—a light meal of soup, cereal, salad and fruit.

Drink water. Fatigue often results from dehydration. Try to drink at least eight glasses of water per day, says Dr. Edington.

Liven yourself up. "It is often useful to indulge in pleasant mood-lifting activities like listening to music or watching a good movie," says Dr. Bell. So be nice to yourself: Take a vacation, buy yourself a new outfit or indulge in a hobby—anything to give your attitude a boost.

Organize and prioritize. Most people's lives are full of tasks, burdens and responsibilities. As projects and obligations mount, just *thinking* about them can make you tired. A good strategy is to divide and conquer, says Dr. Edington. Break your workload into little subdivisions and attack one problem at a time.

See the doctor. If your fatigue hangs on for two weeks or more, it's time to pay your doctor a visit to find out whether you have an illness that may be causing the problem. Treatments might include antibiotics, antidepressants or some other medications.

Review your medications. Fatigue is a side effect of many medications. List all the medications you are taking—both prescription and over-the-counter drugs—and show the list to your doctor. If appropriate, your doctor may suggest some alternatives.

See also Insomnia; Malaise

FEVER

WHEN TO SEE YOUR DOCTOR

- You have a fever higher than 103°F or more.
- Your fever persists for more than 72 hours.
- You also have a severe headache or stiff neck, you're coughing up discolored phlegm or you have pain while urinating.
- You have a history of heart disease, diabetes or other chronic illness.
- Seek immediate medical care for any infant less than three months old who has a fever.

WHAT YOUR SYMPTOM IS TELLING YOU

Believe it or not, fever is your friend.

And like any close friend, fever tells you a couple of things that you may not like but that you need to know. First, fever is an early warning sign that a viral or bacterial infection has invaded your body. Second, it lets you know your body's defenses are vigorously resisting that invasion.

But more important, fever itself is part of that defensive struggle. When a virus or bacterial infection sneaks into your body, your white blood cells release substances called endogenous pyrogens. These pyrogens stimulate a part of the brain called the hypothalamus, which raises your body's internal temperature, causing a fever. That fever may speed your recovery.

"By heating itself up, the body slows down the growth of invading organisms," explains John C. Rogers, M.D., M.P.H., vice chairman of the Department of Family Medicine at Baylor College of Medicine in Houston. "That makes it easier for the immune system to track down and kill these invaders."

In most cases, fever is caused by minor ailments such as cold or flu. But any infection and an armada of other conditions and diseases can induce a fever.

SYMPTOM RELIEF

High fevers of 103°F or more should be evaluated by a doctor. But if you have a fever of less than 103°F and you don't feel too uncomfortable, Dr. Rogers recommends letting the fever break naturally without treatment.

"Most fevers are less than 103°F and aren't going to harm you," Dr. Rogers says. "I probably wouldn't even consider treating a person unless their fever was 101°F or higher. Even then, I would only do it to make him more comfortable."

Here are a few ideas for coping with fever on your own.

Keep those drinks coming. Get plenty of water, but also make sure you drink teas, juices, sports drinks and chicken and beef broth, says Gerald Rogan, M.D., a family practice physician in Walnut Creek, California. "You can get dehydrated when you have a fever, so it's important to drink lots of fluids, particularly something like a sports drink, which will restore your body's supply of vital minerals," he says.

Eat only if you want to. "That saying about feeding a fever is just a myth," Dr. Rogers says. "If you feel hungry, eat. Otherwise, don't force yourself to eat, because all of us have adequate stores of fat to go a day or two without food. It's more important to drink an adequate amount of fluids."

Cool off. "Soak in tepid water—water that is neither hot nor cold to the touch—and sponge the skin," Dr. Rogers suggests. "As the water evaporates off your body, it cools the skin and the blood vessels underneath it, which in turn may reduce your fever." Repeat the bath every two hours, if necessary.

Take aspirin, but don't give it to the kids. Two aspirin tablets every four hours may help adults keep a fever in check. But never give aspirin to children under 21, Dr. Rogers warns. Aspirin can cause feverish children to develop Reye's syndrome—a potentially fatal illness that affects the brain and liver. Instead, give your children acetaminophen in the dosage recommended by the manufacturer.

Know your medications. Drug allergies can cause fevers. Some of the prime suspects include antibiotics such as penicillin and high blood pressure drugs like methyldopa. Even ibuprofen and aspirin can cause fevers in a few people. "There isn't a rip-roaring epidemic of drug-induced fever, but people can be allergic to almost anything," says Philip Mackowiak, M.D., associate chairman of the Department of Medicine at the University of Maryland School of Medicine. If you suspect a drug reaction is causing your fever, ask your physician to prescribe another medication.

Find your normal. Determining whether you have a fever, or when it's over, is not all that cut and dried. To be prepared for dealing with fever, it helps to know your normal temperature.

Just because you have a temperature other than 98.6°F doesn't mean you have an abnormal temperature. In a study of 148 healthy men and women ages 18 to 40, researchers at the University of Maryland found that normal temperatures for the group ranged from 96° to 99.9°F. "Based on our study, we consider fever as anything greater than 99.9°F. But an individual might be able to refine that considerably if he knew his own normal temperature," says Dr. Mackowiak, an author of the study. To determine your normal temperature, record your temperature every four hours while you're awake for three days. This should give you a reasonable indication of your particular range of normal temperatures.

FINGER DEFORMITY

WHEN TO SEE YOUR DOCTOR

- See your doctor as soon as you perceive that your fingers are beginning to look twisted and out of shape.

WHAT YOUR SYMPTOM IS TELLING YOU

Those bumpy, knobby knuckles are just a sign of time passing—and of the osteoarthritis that inevitably comes to aging joints.

Osteoarthritis is often called wear-and-tear arthritis and is often simply the result of years and years of microinjuries. Usually, these gnarly bumps won't prevent you from carrying out your normal activities, though they may hurt from time to time, doctors say.

If your hands begin to feel distorted and quite painful as early as your thirties, however, you may be showing signs of rheumatoid arthritis—a potentially debilitating form of the disease that may require ongoing medical treatment. The joints are held together by ligaments, which become stretched out when rheumatoid inflammation fills the joints with fluid. Gradually, the ligaments may deteriorate to the point that they can no longer hold the finger joints stable. The fingers may then start to "drift" out of position, sometimes quite severely.

For reasons no one yet understands, rheumatoid arthritis tends to strike more women than men, usually between the ages of 35 and 45.

Symptom Relief

Nothing, short of surgery, is going to untie the knots or smooth out the bumps once fingers have become gnarled. But you can reduce the pain.

Start with OTCs. If osteoarthritis hurts, take over-the-counter pain relievers. Try acetaminophen first, then enteric-coated aspirin or ibuprofen, suggests Sidney Block, M.D., a rheumatologist in private practice in Bangor, Maine.

Get help from your doctor. A variety of prescription medicines can help to control the damage that rheumatoid arthritis causes, says Earl Marmar, M.D., an orthopedic surgeon at Einstein Medical Center, director of the Einstein/Moss Joint Replacement Center and assistant clinical professor of orthopedic surgery at Temple University in Philadelphia. The first line of defense is anti-inflammatory drugs, followed by gold, methotrexate and steroids, he says.

Try a wax bath. Your favorite offering from a physical therapist is likely to be the paraffin bath, Dr. Marmar says. Your hand is placed in very warm paraffin, which soothes your joints wonderfully as it dries.

Consider surgery. If your rheumatoid deformities are so severe that you feel disabled, don't despair. Advances in reconstructive surgery can restore a great deal of function, says Dr. Marmar. A reconstructive hand surgeon can rebalance joints, remove inflamed tissues, repair destroyed tendons and even insert rubber spacers to support the joints. Often the surgery is a combination of procedures and may include treatment of the wrist joints, where arthritic changes may have contributed to deformity in the fingers.

See also Joint Inflammation; Joint Pain

FLUSHING

WHEN TO SEE YOUR DOCTOR

- Your flushing is recurrent.
- You've been overexposed to the sun and are also experiencing muscle cramps.
- You are also feeling dizzy or have a fever or severe chills.

WHAT YOUR SYMPTOM IS TELLING YOU

You were around 12, daydreaming through Latin class, happily doodling the name of that special someone on the back of your notebook. Then you looked up—to find the object of your affections reading over your shoulder.

Remember that sensation? Your cheeks flamed and your best friend loudly informed you that you were red as a beet.

Well, some of the same feelings that made you blush at 12 can produce a flush in adulthood. Stress, embarrassment or anxiety can produce a sudden rise in temperature that your body tries to lower by dilating all the blood vessels near the surface of the skin. The result: that rosy flush.

It's also perfectly normal to look and feel flushed after exercise or sex, doctors say. Ditto, after too many alcoholic drinks or a meal that's highly spiced or seasoned with monosodium glutamate (MSG).

If you're a woman, you may have special reasons for flushing. During pregnancy, your body's changing hormones and increased blood volume may cause occasional flushing. Later in life, during menopause, dwindling estrogen may announce itself with hot flashes that involve severe bouts of flushing, according to John E. Midling, M.D., chairman of the Department of Family and Community Medicine at the Medical College of Wisconsin in Milwaukee.

Any cause of high temperature can produce flushing.

Fever from an infection, heat exposure, sunburn or dehydration can all cause your internal thermostat to produce a flush.

In addition, any chronic condition that affects circulation—from diabetes to heart problems—can produce flushing, doctors say. An overactive thyroid can also produce a flush.

Certain medications, particularly some that are taken to reduce high blood pressure or cholesterol levels may cause flushing as a side effect. And flushing is a common reaction to safe but high doses of the B vitamin niacin, taken in the form of nicotinic acid.

SYMPTOM RELIEF

Whether you're prone to a rose-petal blush or to flushing that looks more like a ripe tomato, here's help.

Watch what you eat and drink. Alcohol, strong spices and MSG are the prime dietary causes of flushing, says Robert Wesselhoeft III, M.D., director of family medicine at Tufts University School of Medicine in Boston. Skip cocktails, weed the curry and ginger out of your spice cabinet and read labels to detect MSG in prepared foods, he suggests.

Evaluate your estrogen. If you're nearing the age of menopause, ask your doctor to test your estrogen levels, suggests Oliver Cooper, M.D., professor of family and community medicine at Texas A & M University Health Science Center College of Medicine in College Station. Ask whether you are a candidate for hormone replacement therapy, which can help halt hormonal swings and stop flushing.

Handle the heat. If you've been overdoing everything under the sun, here's how to handle heat exhaustion, says Harry Greene, M.D., chief of general medicine at the University of Arizona College of Medicine in Tucson. "Get in the shade and cool off with a fan or cool water. Drinking cold beverages won't hurt, but take it slowly. Too much may make you vomit," he says.

Review your medications. It would be wise to review with your doctor any medications—prescription or over-the-counter—you may be taking, says Dr. Greene. You may be experiencing flushing as a side effect.

If you take niacin to control high blood cholesterol or for any other reason, your doctor may suggest that you take an aspirin up to an hour before taking the supplement, says Dr. Greene. Aspirin will block the production of prostaglandins, hormones that contribute to the flushing response.

Get help from your doctor. There are many causes for repeated episodes of flushing. Your doctor should prescribe appropriate medical treatment. If you have an overactive thyroid, for example, your doctor can prescribe medications to cut back its production of hormones.

See also Hot Flashes

FOOD CRAVINGS

WHEN TO SEE YOUR DOCTOR

- Food cravings dominate your thinking—you become so obsessed that satisfying cravings interferes with your normal lifestyle.
- *You* think your cravings are a problem.

WHAT YOUR SYMPTOM IS TELLING YOU

Ever fill up on chocolate chip cookies while watching the late show? Or maybe you've munched through a jumbo bag of potato chips...until you ate the whole thing?

Everyone knows what it's like to have such an intense taste for a certain food that it must be satisfied *immediately*. But overdoing it on a routine basis is something else. In other words, there are food cravings that are annoying little nuisances. And there are food cravings that go beyond the norm and signal that all is not right with mind and body.

Not surprisingly, the most frequently craved foods are high in sugar and fat. "People want these foods not because of any nutritive value, but because they are easy to consume and instantly satisfy their 'needs,' " adds David Levitsky, Ph.D., professor of nutrition and psychology at Cornell University in Ithaca, New York. And what might those "needs" be? Sometimes their origin is partly psychological. Possible need-inducing culprits include depression, stress and seasonal affective disorder (SAD). People who have SAD respond to decreased exposure to light during the winter months by becoming irritable and depressed.

While cravings may reflect your state of mind, they can also indicate that your body is experiencing a change worthy of medical attention. For example, people with diabetes often crave carbohydrates, explains Dr. Levitsky. And some nutritional deficiencies, such as a lack of iron, can set up cravings.

Some people are more susceptible to food cravings than others. People who are battling eating disorders are particularly vulnerable, according to Adam Drewnowski, Ph.D., professor and director of the Human Nutrition Program at the University of Michigan School of Public Health in Ann Arbor.

And women are much more likely than men to decide they simply *have to* eat certain foods. Women who experience premenstrual syndrome (PMS) describe irrational tastes for certain foods—predominately chocolate—just before they get their periods. These cravings could be attributed to monthly changes in taste sensitivity, says Robin Kanarek, Ph.D., professor of psychology and physiological psychologist at Tufts University in Medford, Massachusetts.

What about pregnancy-induced cravings—like the infamous pickles and ice cream? Because nausea often accompanies the onset of pregnancy, Dr. Levitsky explains, a woman's digestive system will only tolerate certain foods.

She's likely to reach for the things she finds particularly soothing or comforting.

SYMPTOM RELIEF

In most cases food cravings are temporary and will disappear. But if you need to curb regular feeding frenzies, here are some things you should be aware of.

Exercise your options. Cravings can attack when you're bored or depressed, so keep yourself busy. Find a hobby, read a good book or, better yet, exercise. Not only will you keep your mind away from food, but you'll burn unwanted calories! (For other ways of dealing with depression, see page 144.)

Eat regularly and take a multivitamin. Eat well-balanced meals regularly. If you're on a diet, don't let yourself get to the point where you're so hungry you'll eat anything, because you will. Whether you're on a diet or not, a daily multivitamin supplement will help ensure that you get all the vitamins and minerals you need. The B vitamins are especially important in controlling cravings, says Dr. Levitsky.

Chart your PMS flow. Keep track of your cravings for several months to see if any patterns develop, says Dr. Kanarek. Knowing that the real reason you want that chocolate bar is that your period is due in two days may help you understand your cravings.

Be human. Succumbing to an occasional craving means that you're human. Perpetual denial will only put you in a bad mood and will make you eat more in the long run, advises Dr. Levitsky. If your craving for a chocolate sundae is a rare event—go ahead, indulge.

See the light. If you think you're suffering from SAD, your doctor could prescribe light therapy. Controlled exposure to light could chase away the winter feeding doldrums, says Laurie Humphries, M.D., professor of psychiatry at the University of Kentucky Chandler Medical Center in Lexington.

Ask for help. If you think your cravings are out of control, check with your doctor for a professional medical assessment. If there's a history of diabetes or high blood pressure in your family, have your doctor test your blood pressure and glucose levels. Getting these serious conditions under control will help eliminate food cravings.

FOOT ITCHING

WHAT YOUR SYMPTOM IS TELLING YOU

Stuffed inside those ancient, well-used (oh-so-comfortable) tennis shoes, your feet are so moist and hot you could start your own swamp. Is it any wonder the fungus that makes your feet itch has taken up residence?

Like mold on bread, *Trichophytonrubrum* thrives in the sweat and heat generated by improper footwear and excessive sweating, and as it and other fungi multiply, it causes athlete's foot—also called ringworm of the feet.

"Most people who work have to keep their feet in a dark, warm, moist environment—their shoes—most of the time," says Myles Schneider, D.P.M., an Annandale, Virginia, podiatrist and coauthor of *How to Doctor Your Feet without a Doctor*. "And that's the very thing that causes athlete's foot."

And once athlete's foot breaks out, scratching the maddeningly itchy irritations between the toes can cause a break in the skin, allowing a second, even more painful bacterial infection to develop, says Roy Corbin, D.P.M., president of the American Academy of Podiatric Sports Medicine.

Itchy feet can also be caused by dry skin or contact dermatitis—an allergic reaction to something that touches the feet.

Symptom Relief

While it's best not to scratch that itch, you don't have to suffer. Try these treatments for athlete's foot.

Take an antihistamine. It doesn't get at the cause, but an over-the-counter antihistamine can quell the overwhelming need to scratch. "If I had itching and it was driving me up a wall, I wouldn't hesitate to use them," says Dr. Schneider. Take as directed, he says.

Wet it and dry it. Wet some gauze in an over-the-counter astringent solution like Domeboro, swab the infected area and leave the gauze pad on. As the gauze dries, it will draw moisture from the skin, aiding in the fight against infection, says James Christina, D.P.M., president of the Maryland Podiatric Association.

Toast those tootsies. After bathing, dry carefully between toes using a towel or even a hair dryer on a low heat setting, says Dr. Christina.

Get creamed. When the feet are totally dry, it's time to carefully apply an antifungal cream like Tinactin or Lotrimin to them, says Dr. Schneider. Make sure to also apply the cream before you go to bed, says Dr. Schneider.

Dust those dogs. Take a few minutes twice a day to sprinkle antifungal powder like Tinactin or Lotrimin on your feet and in your shoes, says Dr. Schneider. Continue applying powder to shoes and feet until two weeks *after* symptoms disappear, he says.

Switch socks. If sweaty feet are a problem, take several pairs of socks with you to work and change them throughout the day, says Dr. Christina.

Take a shoe break. Instead of wearing the same shoes every day—to the office or to work out—give them a 48-hour break to allow them to dry out, says Dr. Corbin. "You might even leave them in the sun to help dry them out completely," he says. While your shoes are on a break—and even on days when they're not—dust them with an over-the-counter antifungal powder that contains an antifungal agent such as tolnaftate to kill any bacteria living inside the shoes, says Dr. Schneider.

Try acrylic socks. Acrylic socks seem to wick away

slightly more moisture from sweating feet than cotton. In either case, choose white when you can, says Dr. Christina. (The dyes in colored socks can also be irritating.)

Go natural. Wear shoes made only from natural materials like leather. Weatherproof and plastic shoes don't "breathe," creating the ideal environment for hostile fungi, says Dr. Schneider. Rubber shower shoes are fine, however, and may actually prevent you from catching athlete's foot.

Disconnect Contact Dermatitis

Another cause of itching feet may be contact dermatitis, an allergic reaction to certain irritants. These irritants include dyes in shoes and socks and glue used in shoes, says Dr. Corbin.

Test yourself. If you suspect something you're wearing or using to wash your shoes and socks is causing you to itch, switch to a different pair or new detergent for a few days. If you feel better soon after, you may have found the culprit, says Dr. Christina.

Hydrate Dry Feet

The good news if you have dry feet: You probably don't have athlete's foot. The bad news is that dry feet can cause itching, too. Try these techniques to stop the itching associated with dry feet.

Create a soothing cream. Mix together a tablespoon of solid Crisco and a tablespoon of petroleum jelly. Apply the cream to the feet at bedtime and cover each with a plastic bag, says Dr. Schneider.

See about E. Vitamin E cream, available in most drugstores, works wonders when massaged each day into dry feet, says Dr. Schneider.

Ask about urea. You may be able to find urea in lotions. But if not, ask the pharmacist to help you locate a lotion containing this super-moisturizing ingredient, says Dr. Schneider. "Rubbed on twice a day, this stuff can have a dramatic effect on dryness," he says.

FOOT ODOR

WHAT YOUR SYMPTOM IS TELLING YOU

It has wrecked marriages. (She said she would rather repair the transmission on the family Buick than touch his socks.) It could inspire rap music. ("Dog Killa" by Stink E.) And your foot odor is so bad it could be cited as an environmental hazard.

But for all its unpleasantness, foot odor is nothing serious. It's merely a sign of overactive sweat glands. Excessive sweating creates the environment for excessive bacteria and fungus. And all that extra bacteria and fungus causes the overwhelming odor.

"We're not sure why, but in some people, the sweat glands excrete more sweat than they should," says James Christina, D.P.M., president of the Maryland Podiatric Association. "And because sweat propagates bacterial and fungal growth, you get the associated bacterial and fungal infections that cause the odor."

SYMPTOM RELIEF

Before you run afoul of your friends because of foot odor, try these tips.

Make a change. Frequently changing shoes and socks gives odor-causing bacteria and fungus less of a chance to breed. "That may mean you have to take a couple of pairs of socks with you to work and maybe two sets of shoes, then change shoes and socks sometime during the day," says Dr. Christina.

Spread some dust. A light, twice-a-day dusting with a foot powder like Tinactin—available at pharmacies—can also help kill odor-causing fungus. "Powders are helpful as long as your feet aren't already sweaty," says Dr. Christina. "If your foot is already sweaty, the powder will tend to cake, reducing its effectiveness."

Select synthetic socks. Cotton may be king for clothing, but synthetic socks reign when it comes to keeping foot odor at bay. "They're just more absorbent," says Steve Guida, D.P.M., a Fort Lauderdale, Florida, podiatrist. And less moisture means fewer bacteria, he says.

Insert an odor controller. Charcoal inserts that are placed in the shoes can help absorb odor, but make sure you're using them with synthetic socks—otherwise you're just masking the odor. "You really need to get at the sweating more than having something in there to absorb the sweat," says Dr. Christina. "But if you have a good synthetic sock that's wicking away moisture and then you have a charcoal insert—that would be a helpful combination." You can purchase charcoal shoe inserts at pharmacies.

Cedar is sweeter. Inserts made with sweet-smelling cedar can help freshen shoes while they're not in use, says Dr. Christina.

Go au naturel. Shoes made with natural materials like leather breathe better than man-made materials like plastic, allowing heat to escape, says Dr. Guida.

Watch what you eat. Got a taste for jalapeños and other hot stuff? In certain people, eating spicy foods can cause the odor by making feet sweat, says John Grady, D.P.M., an adjunct clinical professor at the Scholl College of Podiatric Medicine in Chicago and assistant professor of sports medicine at Chicago Osteopathic College. If you do indulge in your fiery favorites and want to avoid the odor, make sure to carefully wash your feet as soon as possible.

Throw a tea party. Tannic acid, a substance found in tea, can help eliminate foot odor. To put tannic acid to work for you, make a pot of tea and, without adding sugar or lemon, pour it into a foot-size tub. Wait until the tea has cooled, then soak your feet. For best results leave them in for ten minutes. Soap and water should remove any stain the tea leaves on your feet, says Myles Schneider, D.P.M., an Annandale, Virginia, podiatrist and coauthor of *How to Doctor Your Feet without a Doctor.*

Dunk them in Domeboro. Bathing feet twice a week in a solution made with a packet of Domeboro and warm water is a time-honored foot odor remedy, says Dr. Guida.

Wear lamb's wool. For truly excessive sweating, you can wrap your toes with small pieces of lamb's wool, an item that's available in most drugstores, according to Sally Rudicel, M.D., associate chair of the Department of Orthopaedics at Albert Einstein Medical Center in Philadelphia. "It will act like a wick that can absorb the moisture," she says. "But you have to change it a couple times a day."

Slap on some antiperspirant. Because foot odor is primarily caused by sweat, it makes sense to apply an antiperspirant. "I've found if it's not too severe a case, using an antiperspirant spray on your feet after a shower really works well," says Dr. Christina.

Defeat severe foot odor with Drysol. For severe cases, consider asking your doctor about Drysol, a prescription anti-sweating medication that contains aluminum chloride. "The idea is to actually plug some of the sweat glands," says Dr. Christina. For best results, on the first night that you use Drysol, cover your feet with plastic wrap after applying the product. Then simply use Drysol once a week without the wrap, he says.

Bring in the big gun. If your foot odor is really bad and none of these other techniques provides relief, consider a blast of Formalyde-10 spray. Formalyde is a prescription spray that contains both formaldehyde and mint and is designed to reform even the foulest-smelling feet. "This stuff is definitely for the most severe cases, and it works," says Dr. Christina. Ask your doctor about it.

FOOT PAIN

WHEN TO SEE YOUR DOCTOR

- A sore on your foot takes more than one week to heal.
- You also have increasing redness, continual prickling, weakness or a change of sensation in your foot.
- Your feet feel cold or hot all the time.

WHAT YOUR SYMPTOM IS TELLING YOU

There are lots of medical mysteries. The cure for the common cold. Why doctors always wear those funny white smocks. But the cause of foot pain isn't one of them. In many cases, feet hurt because they've been stuffed into shoes that are of unnatural shape and that don't fit.

Hard to believe? Consider this study of 356 women conducted by the American Orthopedic Foot and Ankle Society: 313 of the women were found to be wearing shoes smaller than their feet. It's not surprising that 285 of the women complained of foot pain. "Narrow, pointed shoes cram the toes and the rest of the foot," says Sally Rudicel, M.D., associate chair of the Department of Orthopaedics at Albert Einstein Medical Center in Philadelphia and chair of the Council on Women's Footwear, which conducted the study. "If you're wearing tight shoes *and* there's a genetic propensity for a foot problem, you're definitely in trouble."

And trouble can manifest itself in many ways, including bunions and corns, heel spurs, ingrown toenails and Morton's neuroma—a shooting pain between the third and fourth toe caused by an inflamed pinched nerve. Morton's neuroma can be confused with bursitis or metatarsalgia—an achy, burning sensation on the ball of the foot.

If you're overweight or on your feet a lot or have a high arch, you may be familiar with plantar fasciitis—pain under the heel and arch. Plantar fasciitis is caused by overusing the tissue that runs from your heel to the ball of your foot (the fascia). "The forces of walking and running put a lot of stress on that area," says Roy Corbin, D.P.M., president of the American Academy of Podiatric Sports Medicine. "Some- times that leads to calcium deposits and inflammation at the attachment to the heel bone."

Another cause of foot discomfort is a plantar wart—a wart on the bottom of your foot that's caused by a viral infection. Plantar warts are often confused with calluses. But here's what gives them away: small black dots on the top and some mild pain when you squeeze them, according to John Grady, D.P.M., an adjunct clinical professor at the Scholl College of Podiatric Medicine in Chicago and assistant professor of sports medicine at Chicago Osteopathic College. Stress fractures are a common cause of foot pain, especially in walkers, says Dr. Corbin. Suspect stress fractures if there's swelling on the top of the foot right behind the toes.

Other causes of foot pain include an allergic reaction to the dyes or fabrics used in footwear, constricted circulation and a severe case of athlete's foot, says Myles Schneider, D.P.M., an Annandale, Virginia, podiatrist and coauthor of *How to Doctor Your Feet without a Doctor.*

SYMPTOM RELIEF

When your feet hurt, you feel lousy all over. Here are a number of ways to banish foot pain.

Shed those shoes. Give your feet a break by going without shoes, or just wearing slippers, whenever you can, says Dr. Corbin. (Keep your shoes on if you have diabetes.)

Elevate your feet. At the end of the day, prop those dogs up, says Dr. Grady. "When you put your feet up for any length of time, fluids leave your feet and you reduce sometimes painful swelling and pressure almost immediately," he says.

Pull the old switcheroo. Switching shoes during the day disperses the pressure throughout your foot. Whenever possible, wear athletic-type shoes and carry your less-comfortable fashion shoes, says Dr. Corbin.

Some dyes and fabrics used in shoes and socks have been known to cause contact dermatitis—a condition with symptoms that can include itching, redness and burning. If you suspect the problem may be caused by something you're wearing, switch shoes and socks for a few days and check the results, says Dr. Schneider.

Go soak. Daily 20-minute foot soaks are fine, if you don't suffer from diabetes. (Soaking may make the skin of your feet drier and, if you have decreased feeling, may cause a severe burn if the water is too hot, says Dr. Corbin.) There are a number of commercial foot soaks that you can add. Make sure you moisturize your feet with cream afterward, says Dr. Corbin. Small, store-bought foot basins can also be effective at soothing dog-tired dogs, he says.

Get rubbed. Daily foot rubs with creams containing moisturizers like lanolin can do wonders for folks who spend the day on their feet, says Dr. Corbin. Ask a friend for a five-minute massage or do the job yourself. Either way, you'll love it, he says.

Get shoe smart. When you buy shoes, insist on a good fit. Here, from Dr. Corbin, is what to look for: a deep toe area (about 1/2 inch of space between your longest toe and the front of the shoe), a firm heel counter (that's the area at the back of the shoe) and a low heel. It's also a good idea to get shoes with laces. Try both shoes on with the same kind of hosiery that you're going to be wearing with the shoes. The widest part of your foot should be at the widest part of the shoe. Do your shoe shopping late in the day. Your feet actually swell in the afternoon, says Dr. Grady.

Think big. If you have Morton's neuroma–type symptoms, try wearing wide shoes or using a metatarsal arch support. (You can buy them by shoe size in drugstores.) For severe and constant pain your doctor may suggest a cortisone injection or, as a last resort, a surgical procedure to release or snip the pinched nerve, Dr. Corbin says.

Healing Heel Pain

If your heel is bothering you, you probably have plantar fascitis or heel spurs. Here's what to do.

Stretch that fascia. Roll a tennis ball or rolling pin under your feet a few times a day when you're sitting down. This soothes and stretches the fascia, making it less likely to become irritated, says Dr. Schneider.

Get some support. Over-the-counter arch supports are an inexpensive way of taking stress off the fascia, says Dr. Corbin.

Get chilled. A paper cup of ice rubbed on the heel for 20 minutes a day is a refreshing way to soothe pain, says Dr. Schneider.

Stretch those calves. Tight calves can cause pain in your Achilles tendon and fascia, says Dr. Rudicel. To avoid it, slowly stretch your calves using this technique: Stand about two feet from a wall and place your hands on the wall at about shoulder height. Step forward with your left leg. While keeping your right knee straight, lean against the wall for a count of 30 and until you feel the stretch in your right calf. Switch legs and repeat.

Pull the Plug on Plantar Warts

Once planted, a single plantar wart could cause a crop to sprout on the feet of your entire family—they're that contagious, says Dr. Corbin. Here's what to do.

Adopt a hands-off policy. Once you have the virus, you can spread a plantar wart to other parts of your feet by picking it, says Dr. Corbin.

Wear flip-flops. Shower shoes can prevent you from giving the virus to someone who's not infected (and from getting it again), says Dr. Corbin.

See your doctor. While several over-the-counter treatments purport to burn off plantar warts, you really need a stronger dose to get the job done. Rather than risk deadening the nerves around the wart with an over-the-counter acid treatment, see your doctor. Some doctors are using lasers to remove warts quickly and easily, says Dr. Grady.

Get into Circulation

If you think your burning feet are caused by poor circulation, here are a couple of ways to get your blood flowing again.

Take a midnight stroll. When the burning sensation occurs at night, instead of counting sheep, take a short walk—around the house if you like. The exercise should put your mind and feet at ease until morning, says Dr. Schneider.

Exercise your feet. Simple exercises, like circling your toes for ten repetitions, can sometimes help get the blood flowing through a burning foot, says Dr. Schneider.

FORESKIN PROBLEMS

WHEN TO SEE YOUR DOCTOR

- You've retracted the foreskin, but it is too tight to return to its original position and the head of your penis begins to swell.
- The foreskin is so tight that it restricts or prevents urination.

WHAT YOUR SYMPTOM IS TELLING YOU

This vestige of early man that evolution forgot is more useless than your tonsils and more problematic than your appendix. Usually, your foreskin behaves itself and you hardly know it's there, but it can create a few problems—and a few of those problems are potentially dangerous.

Because bacteria and germs thrive in the warm, moist fold of skin that envelops the head of the penis, males with intact foreskins are ten times more likely to develop kidney and bladder infections and sexually transmitted diseases than their circumcised peers, according to Lt. Col. Thomas E. Wiswell, M.D., chief of the Neonatology Department at Walter Reed Army Medical Center in Washington, D.C.

When it comes to foreskins, cleanliness is next to nothingness in keeping bacteria at bay. No matter how meticulously and diligently you clean that fold of flesh, it still makes you much more susceptible to urological inconveniences, says Dr. Wiswell, who was once a staunch opponent of circumcision. He has since changed his mind. "I'm obviously a proponent of good hygiene," he says. "But there's no good data saying hygiene will minimize the risk for these complications as much as or more than circumcision."

The recurrent infections cause tissue scarring that makes the foreskin lose its elasticity, a condition called *balanitis*, says Irwin Goldstein, M.D., a professor of urology at Boston University School of Medicine. Men with diabetes are particularly vulnerable.

The foreskin can close off around the head of the penis, impeding urine flow, which is known as *phimosis*. And if the too-tight sheath is retracted over and behind the head of the penis, the head begins to swell and the foreskin cannot be returned to its normal position. That phenomenon, called *paraphimosis,* is a surgical emergency and "can be dangerous," Dr. Goldstein says. "I've seen the head of the penis amputated because of this."

SYMPTOM RELIEF

With hygiene almost ineffective against infections and their complications, what recourse exists to keep your foreskin healthy and problem-free? Here's what doctors recommend.

Do keep it clean. Whether it reduces the chance of infection or not, you should keep the foreskin as clean as possible. "Wash the penis as you would any other area of the body," Dr. Wiswell says. "Then gently retract it and wash in and around it with soap and warm water. Then dry it carefully." For the infections that inevitably crop up, physicians prescribe antibiotics, he says.

Don't force the tissue. In cleaning or making love, never attempt to forcefully open the foreskin or pull it back over and behind the head of the penis, doctors say. In men, the foreskin will retract naturally as they get an erection, according to Dr. Goldstein. In children, the foreskin cannot be retracted to expose the head of the penis until the age of two or three, Dr. Wiswell says.

If you can't return the foreskin to its original position, see a doctor immediately. An incision called a dorsal slit will be made in the foreskin to allow it to move more easily over the head of the penis, Dr. Wiswell says.

Consider a circumcision. Not all doctors will recommend that circumcisions be performed, but many recognize that the benefits outweigh the risks, Dr. Wiswell says. It is, after all, the only real way to virtually guarantee prevention of the relatively rare cancer of the penis. (Interestingly, of some 60,000 reported cases of penile cancer since 1930, only 10 of the men have been circumcised.)

More and more uncircumcised males are having the procedure done later in life. "It's not entirely risk-free," Dr. Wiswell says. "The risks are there, but they're low." Possibilities to discuss with your doctor if you consider a circumcision include infection from the surgery, trauma to the head of the penis, bleeding and, although it's extremely rare, abnormal healing.

FORGETFULNESS

WHEN TO SEE YOUR DOCTOR

- You become suddenly confused or are in a familiar place and suddenly don't know where you are.
- You have difficulty remembering what month or year it is.

WHAT YOUR SYMPTOM IS TELLING YOU

You spent Sunday at your daughter's wedding, meeting a stream of her charming young friends (and maybe a few who reminded you of people you met in a nightmare last winter when you had the electric blanket turned up too high). Okay, so you never expected to remember *all* of their names. But you did spend a fascinating hour at the reception talking with one young person who made a particular impression on you. She was bright, friendly and personable, and you found her delightful. When you got home, though, you were unsettled by your inability to remember her name.

Is this a serious memory problem? Not at all, says Alfred Kaszniak, Ph.D., a psychologist at the University of Arizona in Tucson. It's normal aging. If you forgot ever having attended the wedding, though, you'd be in more troublesome territory.

Everyone finds increasing difficulty remembering certain kinds of detail as they age, says Dr. Kaszniak. While old friends' names or the ingredients in a favorite recipe may come automatically, the details we tend to lose most are those that relate to time or space—like forgetting to take along your glasses when you'll need them or losing track of your car keys or where you parked the car. No question—it's aggravating.

But the good news about forgetfulness more than offsets the bad, says Tom Crook, Ph.D., a psychologist and director of Advanced Psychometrics Corporation in Scottsdale, Arizona. For one thing, age-related memory loss does not mean your brain is in decline. In fact, many of the most important mental abilities (like decision making and creativity) actually *increase* with age. Also, memory loss is *rarely* an ominous signal of impending Alzheimer's disease. If you're 73 and can't remember names, says Dr. Crook, the odds are 99 to 1 that you have a *normal* memory loss.

SYMPTOM RELIEF

If memory slips are bothering you, there's a lot you can do about them.

Deal with depression. Your memory may play tricks if you're feeling blue or listless or are under a lot of stress, says David Masur, Ph.D., a neuropsychologist with the Albert Einstein College of Medicine in New York City. Though memory is very vulnerable to emotions, you'll retrieve the lost information once the depression or anxiety are treated, he says. (See Depression on page 144 and Anxiety on page 25.)

Assert your right to a slower pace. There's no need to be apologetic or secretive about the fact that your memory isn't what it used to be, says Glenn Smith, Ph.D., a psychologist at the Mayo Clinic in Rochester, Minnesota. One strategy he suggests for meeting a group of people and learning their names is to ask for those names more slowly. How? Try, "Hang on there, let's see, your name is Bob, yours is Mary and this is Charles, right?" Dr. Smith says, "People who are advancing in age have a right to have information presented at a pace at which they can learn it."

Leave yourself visual reminders. Rain in the forecast for tonight? As soon as you hear about it, go put your umbrella with your briefcase.

"When a thought occurs to you, go as far as you can toward accomplishing that act right away," says Dr. Crook. "If you think, 'I have to drop off the dry cleaning on the way to work,' hang it on the front door or take it out to the car *right away.*"

Choose your cues. Plant cues all around you of things you don't want to forget, says neurologist Louis Kirby, M.D., chief of staff at Thunderbird Samaritan Hospital in Glendale, Arizona. Choose places for your notes that you'll be sure to spot—the bathroom mirror, the refrigerator door, the inside of the front door, the car dashboard.

The index card is one of Dr. Kirby's favorite memory tools. "I keep them in my pocket, with a task on each one, and when I'm done with the task, I throw the card away. I like them better than a list I'm scratching on all day."

Make the essentials easier. Plan careful ploys for recalling the things you *really* need to remember, suggests Joan Minninger, Ph.D., San Francisco memory therapist and author of *Total Recall: How to Boost Your Memory Power.*

Have one regular place inside the house where you keep your keys, for example. And back yourself up with an outside stash. "I have a friend in New York who keeps an extra set on top of an air conditioner in another apartment building," she says. If you can't find your wallet because you transfer it from one pocket or bag to another, create a wallet terminal—an attractive basket where you empty your pockets or purse as you come in and gather up essential items on the way out.

Get the picture. Image association is a powerful tool for memory enhancement, says Danielle Lapp, memory researcher at Stanford University in California, and author of *(Nearly) Total Recall: A Guide to a Better Memory at Any Age*. If you're worried about forgetting or getting lost, use your senses to become aware of your environment. Parked your car in a busy spot? As you leave, pause, *turn around* and look at your car's location from the direction from which you will return. Are there memorable smells? Gas fumes from an intersection? The aroma of food from a nearby restaurant? Is there music anywhere? Use these sensory cues to deliberately orient yourself.

Talk to yourself. Dr. Lapp suggests an inner monologue to help increase your awareness, for example: "I am entering the department store through the men's clothing section" or "I am locking the door now. I am writing the check and putting it in an envelope." Foolish? Not at all. You are doing something consciously to record what you want to remember. You are paying attention, concentrating and getting organized—the basic tools of memory training, says Dr. Lapp.

Bolster your brain food. If you're low on certain nutrients, your memory may lose its edge. Studies suggest that a daily diet rich in the B vitamin riboflavin, iron and zinc may be helpful. Ready your plate with riboflavin from low-fat dairy products, such as skim milk and low-fat yogurt. To beef up your iron levels, cook potatoes, legumes and acidic foods (like tomato sauce) in an iron skillet. And for memory zest from zinc, enjoy more seafood and meat.

Program your memory with an exercise program. A study conducted at Utah State University suggests that aerobic exercise may sharpen your short-term recall. That daily walk or swim heightens your brain's oxygen efficiency and *increases* glucose metabolism, which may play a role in improving memory, says Richard Gordin, Ph.D., professor of health, physical education and recreation at Utah State in Logan. So enjoy regular exercise for healthy memories.

G

GAS

WHEN TO SEE YOUR DOCTOR

- You have gas and stomach or abdominal pain for more than three days.
- You have gas and unexplained weight loss.
- If your pain is more severe than any that you've had before, see your doctor immediately.

WHAT YOUR SYMPTOM IS TELLING YOU

The next time you break wind several times in one day and someone calls you Mr. Methane, thank him—and tell him you're just doing what comes naturally for someone on a healthy diet.

If you're eating lots of whole grains, fruits and vegetables—and you should be—it's likely that your digestive system is churning out a healthy amount of gas. That's because foods like beans, oats and potatoes contain large amounts of indigestible carbohydrates—fiber. These carbohydrates serve as nourishment for microscopic bacteria that live in your stomach and intestines, explains Thomas A. Gossel, R.Ph., Ph.D., professor of pharmacology and toxicology and associate dean of the College of Pharmacy at Ohio Northern University in Ada. As the bacteria enjoy the feast, they release gases like hydrogen, carbon dioxide, nitrogen and methane. "And those gases don't have anywhere to go but out," says Dr. Gossel.

There's really no need to be concerned if your flatulence is particularly smelly—it simply means that small quantities of methane gas (the one with the offensive odor) have been produced during the process.

A certain amount of flatulence is perfectly natural, but people who switch to a healthy diet sometimes worry unnecessarily that they're producing too much.

There are, however, several conditions that *do* produce excessive flatulence. These include peptic ulcers, stomach infections, gallstones, irritable bowel syndrome (a combination of stomach pain, gas, bloating and irregular bowel movements), lactose intolerance (inability to digest milk) and food allergies. Also, swallowing too much air while chewing can make you pass gas.

SYMPTOM RELIEF

If you'd rather pass on gas and you're not in pain, try these tips.

A drop or two may do. A drop of peppermint, cinnamon or ginger extract mixed in a cup of water has been used for years as a home remedy for gas, says Dr. Gossel. "It's been around for years and years," he says, adding that the chemicals in the extracts presumably relax the muscles of the esophagus, allowing trapped gas to escape. You can buy any of these extracts at most health food stores.

Don't fear fiber. If you're improving your diet with food like apples, apricots, bananas, beans, brussels sprouts, cabbage, citrus fruits, celery, eggplant, onions, potatoes, prunes, radishes and raisins, you may have found that you're getting more bang for your buck than you bargained for—literally. But don't let a little noise keep you from eating these important, healthy foods. Just be aware that gas comes with the territory, says Dr. Gossel. As your body gets used to digesting more fiber, gas will become less of a problem.

Cut needless flatulence foods. While you *never* want to sacrifice nutrients, some foods do cause more gas than others. Here, from Dr. Gossel, are some of the more prolific gas producers (many of which are not nutritional necessities): bacon, bagels, bran, corn chips, fruit juice, gelatin desserts, graham crackers, pastries, pretzels, popcorn, potato chips and wheat germ.

Eat like a bird. Eating frequent small meals rather than a

few large ones apparently also reduces the amount of bac
teria in the stomach, creating less gas, says Dr. Gossel.

Make Lactaid your aid. If you're lactose intolerant, th
sugar in milk is difficult for you to digest. If that's the case
Dr. Gossel says to try products made specifically for the lac
tose intolerant that have a special enzyme to break dow
the sugar. You can, however, add yogurt and hard cheeses
Yogurt contains beneficial bacteria that assist digestion
and hard cheeses, such as cheddar, are low in lactose.

Break out the pink stuff. A tablespoon of Pepto-Bismo
immediately after a meal may help reduce intestinal gas
says George Wu, M.D., professor of medicine and physiol
ogy and chief of the Division of Gastroenterology and
Hepatology at the University of Connecticut School o
Medicine in Farmington.

Check out activated charcoal. Available in most health
food stores, activated charcoal is a detoxifier that contain
an ingredient that helps prevent gas from forming, say
Alan R. Gaby, M.D., a Baltimore physician and presiden
of the American Holistic Medical Association. "You'll have
to experiment whether to take it before meals or after, bu
it has worked well for our patients," he says. Don't use i
for more than two weeks unless you're under medica
supervision.

Try simethicone. An ingredient in many over-the
counter anti-gas products available in most drugstores
simethicone helps draw smaller irritating gas bubbles from
the folds of the stomach and intestines into larger bubble
that can either be belched or passed as flatulence, says Dr
Gossel. "It's safe, it's effective—there is really no reason fo
people not to purchase this kind of product," he says. Take
as directed.

Pass the Beano. There's no need to fear the effects o
beans with this product on the market, says Dr. Gossel
Beano is a liquid enzyme, a chemical that digests. Putting a
few drops on your beans before you eat them helps break
down their fiber, preventing excess gas.

Write it down. If you're concerned about the amount o
gas you're having, keep track of the problem by writing
down each occurrence and the meal that preceded it. If you

e a pattern, eliminate one of the foods that may be caus-
ng the problem for a few days and see if it makes a differ-
nce, says Dr. Gossel.

See your doctor. If you have gas *and* abdominal pain or
weight loss, you may have a condition that needs medical
attention—such as an ulcer or gallstones.

GENITAL IRRITATION

WHEN TO SEE YOUR DOCTOR

A rash or discoloration of skin on or near the genitals
lasts more than one week.
A wartlike protuberance or pimply rash appears anywhere on your genitals.

WHAT YOUR SYMPTOM IS TELLING YOU

Skin is skin, whether it's the tip of your nose or the tip of
your penis, the lips on your face or the lips of your
vagina. "It's just like the rest of your body," says Alfred L.
Tranger, M.D., an associate professor of obstetrics/gynecol-
ogy at the Medical College of Wisconsin in Milwaukee.
"From rashes to allergic reactions to abrasions and pimples, genital skin is subject to all the diseases that skin anywhere else is."

But because of what we do with our genitals and where
we put them, they're exposed to a few conditions different
from what the skin on the rest of our body normally comes
into contact with. And because the tissue there is so sensitive and brimming with nerve endings, small eruptions we
otherwise might dismiss elsewhere become particularly
bothersome.

Hair follicles on your genitals, for example, can clog and
form pimples just as they do on your face—maybe even
more so, given the extra chafing and sweating down there

and the oily ointments and lubricants sometimes used
Genital warts are sexually transmitted, but they're caused
by the same critter that produces those ugly protuberances
on your fingers and feet. (No, not toads—the human papilloma virus.) Soaps and hygiene products can cause an allergic rash on your genitals as easily as they can on your arm

SYMPTOM RELIEF

So what do you do? Do you pop a pimple on your genitals the same way you pop a pimple on your chin? Can
you use the same wart remover you apply on your finger
What might be causing that odd rash down there? Here's a
round-up of remedies for some of the more common genital complaints.

Be Wary with Warts

Whether they appear alone or in a cauliflower-like cluster
warts are easy to acquire—all you need is to come in contact with one, says William Dvorine, M.D., chief of the
Section of Dermatology at St. Agnes Hospital in Baltimore
and author of *A Dermatologist's Guide to Home Skin
Treatment*. Usually painless, genital warts can be flat or
raised, skin-colored, white or gray, large or small. Once you
contract any of the nearly 60 strains of the wart virus, you
have it for life, and warts will tend to recur.

Don't look for a cure over-the-counter. No, you can't
melt those warts away with Compound W. Warts must be
treated by a physician before they spread. Medications you
pick up at the pharmacy without a prescription won't
remove genital warts, according to Dr. Dvorine. "Those
medications are too irritating to the skin," he says.

The topically applied prescription drug Condylox usually is used to treat genital warts, although physicians can
also surgically remove them, Dr. Dvorine says.

Be very wary if you're a woman. Except for being
unsightly and easily passed on to others, genital warts pose
no real health danger to men, but in women they are associated with a greater risk of cervical cancer, Dr. Dvorine

ays. The threat is all the more grave because women may
not notice warts inside the vagina. That's one *more* reason
for women to have a routine annual pelvic exam.

A Pimple Is Not Simple

Pimples that occur on the genitals shouldn't be popped or
played with. Instead, here's what doctors recommend.

Nix the zit creams. Don't ever reach for a benzoyl peroxide preparation to treat genital pimples, Dr. Dvorine
warns. "You'll fly through the roof," he says. "It's that irri-
ating on your genitals."

Let the doctor do it. Physicians normally prescribe a gentle topical medication or an antibiotic for genital pimples,
Dr. Franger says. Or they might soak the inflammation
with a hot compress before opening and draining it.

Beware of bumps. Sometimes an acnelike condition
called *Molluscum contagiosum* erupts on the genitals,
according to Dr. Franger. These collections of pinkish,
shiny, smooth bumps can be distinguished from pimples by
indentions in their centers. You definitely can't treat this
like acne on the face—molluscum is highly contagious, so
don't touch it. It's easy to treat with a simple surgical procedure, Dr. Franger says.

Don't Be Rash with a Rash

Plain old contact dermatitis can be the cause of rashes on
the genitals, according to Jack L. Lesher, Jr., M.D., associate professor of dermatology at the Medical College of
Georgia School of Medicine in Augusta. Give the techniques listed below a try, but if you don't get the red out
within a week, schedule a visit with the doctor. And if sores
or blisters are present, see a doctor right away.

Eliminate the obvious. The only way to figure out if
your rash is contact dermatitis is through a process of elimination, getting rid of any new products or clothing that
may come into contact with your genitals, Dr. Lesher says.
New laundry detergents or bath soaps may have prompted
the allergic reaction. Hygiene sprays and creams for women
also occasionally produce a rash.

Consider the condom. Latex condoms are a little more obscure source of contact dermatitis, but they can provoke a red, itchy rash, Dr. Lesher says. You might try switching to sheepskin condoms, but you should be aware that only latex offers the best protection from the virus that causes AIDS.

Better safe than syphilis. The sexually transmitted disease syphilis often is called the great imitator because its main symptoms in certain stages can be scaly or reddish rashes, according to Mary Ellen Brademas, M.D., chief of dermatology at St. Vincent Hospital in New York City. While a rash probably is benign if you practice safe sex, the possibility of syphilis is grave enough to warrant an appointment with the doctor, she says.

GENITAL ITCHING

WHEN TO SEE YOUR DOCTOR

- Your itching has lasted for more than a week without relief.
- Itching is accompanied by or causes severe redness, sores or oozing.
- Itching precedes formation of a blister or sore.
- Your genitals are maddeningly itchy and the sensation seems to have spread to other parts of the body.

WHAT YOUR SYMPTOM IS TELLING YOU

You don't have to be an athlete—you don't even have to wear a jock—to contract itchy genitals.

Friction and fungus are the two primary causes of genital itching. Skin rubbing against skin generates heat and sweat to produce tender, red, itchy patches, says William Dvorine, M.D., chief of the Section of Dermatology at St

Agnes Hospital in Baltimore and author of *Dermatologist's Guide to Home Skin Treatment.* People who are physically active or obese are especially susceptible. The itch may appear as a little bit of redness anywhere on the genitals but can advance to more serious inflammation, with scabs and scaling or tender, moist spots where skin has peeled away.

If caused by fungus, the itch and redness will appear more gradually, says Dr. Dvorine. The patches of scaly skin will have defined, ringlike borders—hence the medical name *Tinea cruris,* or ringworm of the groin.

Fungus-caused jock itch predominates in the summer, says Jack L. Lesher, Jr., M.D., associate professor of dermatology at the Medical College of Georgia School of Medicine in Augusta. "Fungus kind of likes warm, damp places to grow," he says, "but you don't need a fungal infection to get jock itch."

Insanely itchy private parts could be caused by scabies or pubic lice. In a woman, itching also can be the first sign of a yeast infection, especially if she is taking antibiotics. And for both sexes, severe itching, as well as pain, can precede the outbreak of herpes blisters.

Symptom Relief

You can treat plain old jock itch at home, perhaps after a trip to the drugstore—but do it before the area becomes inflamed and possibly infected. More serious scratch attacks probably will require a visit to the doctor for a prescription itch eraser. Here's how to stop the itch before it becomes a serious problem.

Powder to the people. To reduce chafing that naturally occurs when you walk around, try powdering yourself with cornstarch, Dr. Dvorine says. "It can act as a good buffer to reduce abrasion." Talcum powder also can be effective, but women should be cautious of how frequently they use it. "In women, using talcum powder on a daily basis may lead to other problems," he says. Some studies show an association with cancer of the ovaries.

Ointments salve the day. Over-the-counter creams effectively treat jock itch, dermatologists say. But in order to select the right product, it's important to know what's causing the problem. "Chafing can be aggravated by fungal medications, because those preparations do nothing to reduce the friction," Dr. Dvorine says.

Ointments containing zinc oxide or hydrocortisone work well for jock itch brought on by chafing. On the other hand, if you have jock itch caused by fungus, opt for salves made with miconazole or clotrimazole. They should be used at the first inkling of an itch.

Keep it clean. Sweat harbors bacteria that cause or further irritate itchy genitals, Dr. Dvorine says. If you work up a sweat on the job or during workouts, make sure to bathe as soon as you can. And pack a clean, dry change of clothes if you're showering away from home.

Keep it dry, keep it loose. Dry yourself thoroughly after washing, using a hair dryer, if necessary, set on low, Dr. Dvorine says. And don't squeeze yourself into tight or ill-fitting clothes that might chafe against the skin between your legs or prevent air from flowing.

Ice is nice. If you already have jock itch, soothe your savaged skin with cool compresses, Dr. Lesher says. Wrap a few ice cubes in a towel, or soak a washcloth in cool tap water, he says. "Just make sure you dry off really well when you're done."

Take a load off. While the skin is healing, stay off your feet. "Walking just generates more friction," Dr. Lesher says.

Go naked. Why waste a reason to lounge about in the buff? Providing an opportunity to let jock itch heal is a good excuse to sport your birthday suit. "Try leaving your clothes off," Dr. Lesher says. "You'll aerate the inflamed skin and give it more of a chance to dry out."

How to Get Rid of What's Bugging You

If jock-itch treatments don't seem to work or if the irritation produces an uncontrollable urge to scratch frantically, your genitals may be infested with either lice or scabies, two rather common critters.

Fight the mite. Scabies are microscopic mites that burrow into the skin and infest not only the genitals but other areas of your body—breasts, waist, armpits, hands. Besides itching, they produce skin lesions that can become infected. "We see a lot of scabies cases," Dr. Lesher says. "Any close contact with someone who's infested—it doesn't have to be sex—can give them to you."

Only a prescription drug, such as Elimite or Kwell, can eliminate them, he says, but the whole body, not just the genitals, must be treated.

Force lice to flee. In contrast to scabies, pubic lice are very visible. "You can see those little rascals crawling around down there," Dr. Lesher says. "If you have them, you'll know you have them." They look like tiny white flakes of skin or dandruff, but they move.

An over-the-counter medication called Rid is effective in destroying them, according to Dr. Lesher. If Rid doesn't do the trick within a week, see your doctor for a prescription drug.

See also Genital Sores; Vaginal Itching

GENITAL SORES

WHEN TO SEE YOUR DOCTOR

- A blister or sore appears anywhere on your genitals, whether or not it is painful.
- Sores are accompanied by swollen pelvic lymph glands, headache or a fever.

WHAT YOUR SYMPTOM IS TELLING YOU

If you get a blister on your finger or foot from a hard day of hoeing or a few hours on the jogging track, it's no big

deal. It stings a little, sure, but you wash it, put a bandage
on it, favor it a bit and forget about it.

But get a blister on your genitals and matters are much
more complicated. If it hurts, it's going to hurt like heck. It
may take a long while to heal and very likely will reappear
if not treated properly. And because it almost invariably
signals a sexually transmitted disease, it represents a health
threat not only to you but to anyone with whom you are
intimate.

The only way you'll know absolutely that a genital sore
is not herpes or syphilis is to have your doctor run some
blood tests. Even to trained eyes, oozy rashes or blisters
may be indistinguishable from, say, a bad case of jock itch.
Genital sores come in many shapes and sizes, according to
Dale Kay, director of the Centers for Disease Control and
Prevention National Sexually Transmitted Disease Hotline
in Research Park, North Carolina. They may be as big as a
dime or as small as a pinhead. They could be filled with
fluid or appear dry. Sores might sprout on their own or
cluster into a rash. They can appear anywhere on the genitals—on the penis or labia, inside the vagina, on the scrotum or between the genitals and rectum.

SYMPTOM RELIEF

Blood and tissue tests, cultures and prescription medications are the only way to diagnose and treat genital
sores. But there are steps you can take to help in proper
treatment. Here's what the experts suggest.

Don't play doctor. Self-medicating a genital sore by raid-
ing the medicine cabinet of friends or family is one of the
worst things you can do, according to Mary Ellen
Brademas, M.D., chief of dermatology at St. Vincent
Hospital in New York City.

"Don't think, 'My sister has some pills that might cure
this,' " she says. Antibiotics and other drugs interfere with
the blood and tissue tests you'll have to have before the
doctor can diagnose the sore.

Time wounds the healing process. The longer you delay

trip to a doctor, the more difficult it will be to identify and
eat the sore, Dr. Brademas says. So make an appointment
ght away.

Be safe, not sorry. The best way to guard against geni-
al sores is to have only one uninfected, monogamous sex
artner, Kay says. Other safer sex methods include limit-
ig your number of partners and making sure you know
heir histories of sexual diseases.

Erect a good barrier. Some sexually transmittable dis-
ases can still be transmitted from partner to partner even
vhen sores are not visible, Kay says. If there's the slightest
oubt about the possibility of healthy sex, always make
ure a latex condom is used. "But a condom's only effec-
ve on the area it covers," Kay says. Sores anywhere else on
ie genitals, the mouth or the rest of the body are still con-
igious.

GLAND SWELLING

WHEN TO SEE YOUR DOCTOR

Your swollen glands persist for more than two weeks
after an infection has passed.
You have swollen glands all over your body.
You have swollen glands and have not had a recent
cold or sinus, ear or upper respiratory infection.
You have a large, hard gland that doesn't move easily.
Along with swollen neck glands, you have fever, trouble swallowing, a chronic sore throat or trouble breathing, particularly if you smoke or drink alcohol.
One of your swollen neck glands is getting larger than
the others.

What Your Symptom Is Telling You

Your swollen glands may feel a little like Frankenstein neck bolts at the moment, but they're actually staging grounds for an army of good guys.

Scattered throughout your body are more than 500 lymph glands. They are gathering places for white blood cells—the cells that your body's immune system uses to fight infection. The glands swell when the white blood cells mount a defense against invading bacteria. The glands are also part of the drainage system that your body uses to carry away the debris that accumulates as it fights infection. The lymph glands drain into larger lymph nodes that are clustered in several areas of the body, including the armpit, groin and jaw. These nodes sometimes swell in response to an infection at a distant site—for example, an infected foot might produce a swollen lymph gland in the groin area.

A normal lymph node is a soft, rubbery, movable mass that is less than 1/4 inch in diameter. When glands swell, they become large, hard and tender.

The glands in the neck are most likely to swell—a common response to a cold or upper respiratory infection. Why the neck? Over 30 percent of your body's lymph glands lie above the collarbone in the neck and throat, says Frederick Godley, M.D., an otolaryngologist with the Harvard Community Health Plan in Providence, Rhode Island.

Swollen neck glands may also indicate either a viral sore throat or a bacterial infection, such as strep throat. Infections of the sinuses, ear or skin can also cause your neck glands to swell. And a dental problem can bring on the swelling, as can an infection resulting from a cat scratch. More serious, though less likely, causes of swollen neck glands are illnesses like mononucleosis, tuberculosis, syphilis and some types of cancer, such as Hodgkins' disease.

SYMPTOM RELIEF

Since swollen glands are most likely caused by an infection, the key to getting rid of them is to treat the underlying infection. Here's what you can do.

Try heat. While treating the infection, you can ease the pain in your swollen glands by applying a warm washcloth or heating pad for 15 minutes three or four times a day, Dr. Godley suggests.

Stamp out strep. It's important to treat strep throat because, left untreated, it could lead to rheumatic fever, a condition that can damage the heart, says Nelson Gantz, M.D., chairman of the Department of Medicine and chief of the Infectious Diseases Division at the Polyclinic Medical Center in Harrisburg, Pennsylvania, and clinical professor of medicine at the Pennsylvania State University College of Medicine in Hershey. That's why, if your swollen glands are accompanied by a persistent sore throat, you'll need to see your doctor. Your doctor will use a throat swab to take sample cells from your throat for a culture. If you do have strep, your doctor will prescribe a course of antibiotics to cure the infection, says Dr. Gantz.

Investigate other infections. Skin infections in the scalp, temple or face as well as sinus and ear infections, can cause your glands to swell, says Randy Oppenheimer, M.D., an otolaryngologist in Encinitas, California. Your doctor will treat these and any other infections with prescription antibiotics, he says.

Expect some tests. If the cause of your swollen glands isn't easy to determine, your doctor may ask you to return for several visits or further tests. In addition to blood tests or x-rays in certain cases, your doctor may sample some of the tissue within the lymph node using a technique called needle aspiration, says Dr. Godley. "In most cases, this is a short and simple in-office procedure," he says. After your skin is numbed with a local anesthetic, a needle is passed into the gland and some of the cells are withdrawn for examination.

Take a closer look at the lymph node. Your doctor may use x-rays to help diagnose the cause of your swollen glands. Or a single lymph node may be surgically removed after needle aspiration. In the unlikely event that you have a malignancy of the lymph system, Dr. Godley says, you would be treated with cancer-fighting drugs.

GROIN BULGE

WHEN TO SEE YOUR DOCTOR

- Any bulge should be brought to the attention of your doctor.

WHAT YOUR SYMPTOM IS TELLING YOU

Unlike a solid lump, a bulge is soft and usually retracts when you push or lie down on it. If you have a bulge, it's probably in your groin or on your upper thigh, and it's probably a hernia.

A hernia happens when there's a weakening of the muscles and connective tissue in the abdominal wall that keeps the intestines in place. The intestines pop through the wall, and that protuberance is the hernia.

Hernias are fairly common. Men are the more likely victims because they have a weak area in the groin muscle where it's intersected by the tube that carries sperm. Heavy lifting and straining during bowel movements increase your chances of getting a hernia. Laughing or coughing can trigger one, too.

Hernias are seldom life threatening, but they can lead to complications. If the intestine actually gets stuck in the opening, you can develop an intestinal blockage or even gangrene, says John C. Rogers, M.D., M.P.H., vice chairman of the Department of Family Medicine at Baylor College of Medicine in Houston.

Symptom Relief

Treatment for hernia is straightforward. Here's some information to help you choose your options wisely.

Forget the truss. A truss is an elastic or canvas pad that keeps the bulge from protruding. But trusses are bulky, and if the hernia enlarges, a truss can choke off blood supply to it and complicate treatment.

Consider surgery. Most doctors recommend surgery. "Wearing a truss is just a stopgap. The only certain way to cure a hernia is surgery," says Glen Hollinger, M.D., an internist at the Hospital of the Good Samaritan in Los Angeles.

In many cases, the surgery can be done as an outpatient procedure in less than an hour, and you can go home soon afterward. You can return to work and resume most normal activities within two to four days.

"Generally, hernia surgery is fairly minor and it prevents serious complications. So, in my opinion, it's well worth doing," says Dr. Rogers.

GUM PROBLEMS

WHEN TO SEE YOUR DOCTOR

- Your gums bleed and there is also swelling, puffiness, soreness or persistent bad breath.
- Sores develop under your dentures.

What Your Symptom Is Telling You

We're not talking about a stick of spearmint that loses its taste too fast. We're talking about problems with the foundation of your smile, the coral-colored tissue that anchors your teeth. We're talking, of course, about your gums. Love them—or leave your teeth behind.

The most common gum problem is bleeding, and it's a sign of inflamed gums, or what dentists call gingivitis. But gingivitis is just the overture for another and more serious "-itis": periodontitis. Once your gum problem has advanced this far, you can lose your teeth.

Gingivitis is caused by the buildup around the teeth and gums of *plaque,* a gunky, bacteria-filled concoction of food and saliva. As anybody who has ever been face-to-mask with a dental hygienist knows, not brushing and flossing regularly is the main reason for your choppers becoming a plaque warehouse. But other factors play a role in gum problems.

For one thing, this symptom is sexist. Women are much more susceptible to gingivitis than men, according to JoAnne Allen, D.D.S., a dentist in private practice in Albuquerque. During menstrual periods, women's gums generally are more swollen, tender and puffy, Dr. Allen says. Their gums also bleed more easily then. "That doesn't predispose women to gum disease, but it could make it worse if other factors like poor hygiene are present."

Also, she says, almost all women who become pregnant get a temporary gingivitis with swelling and bleeding that gets worse as the baby comes to term.

In fact, that baby might inherit the tendency for its mother's—or father's—gum problems. "Gum problems can be hereditary," says Paul A. Stephens, D.D.S., a dentist in private practice in Gary, Indiana, and president of the Academy of General Dentistry. "Some people just naturally get only a little bit of plaque on their teeth. Others seem to accumulate a lot very rapidly."

Certain medications can cause gums to bleed or swell, says Eric Z. Shapira, D.D.S., a trustee on the national board of the Academy of General Dentistry and a dentist in private practice in Half Moon Bay, California. Medications that can cause problems include oral contraceptives, antidepressants, decongestants, antihistamines, nasal sprays and medications for high blood pressure and heart disease.

And gum problems are more common among people with diabetes and leukemia and those who have dry mouths, who smoke or are under a lot of stress.

Those last two categories—smokers and the stressed— are especially susceptible to trench mouth, a disease common among the soldiers of World War I that is now known as necrotizing ulcerative gingivitis. (You have to add poor hygiene to that mix to be at risk.) People with this type of gingivitis have painful ulcers on their gums, bleeding and breath that goes beyond bad to hellish.

Dentures Can Cause Gum Woes

If dentures aren't properly fitted, or if the jawbone is so deteriorated that it can't hold dentures firmly in place, a person can get ulcerations on their gums. The sores aren't necessarily painful, says Samuel B. Low, D.D.S., assistant dean and director of postgraduate periodontics at the University of Florida's College of Dentistry in Gainesville. But that doesn't mean they should be ignored.

"It's a form of pressure atrophy, just like what happens to your arm when you're wearing a cast for a long time," he says. The surface of the gums becomes loose, and the bone beneath the gums can dissolve.

SYMPTOM RELIEF

Bleeding and sore gums are the same as most health problems: If you catch them before they get too bad, they're easy to reverse. "Gingivitis is absolutely reversible in the earlier stages," says Dr. Allen. To put bleeding gums in reverse, put your hands on floss and a toothbrush. But make sure to hold that toothbrush the right way.

Put a new angle on your brushing. The best way to get rid of plaque nestling at the intersection of your teeth and gums is to use a soft-bristle toothbrush held at a 45-degree angle to your teeth and moved gently in a sawing or circular motion. This motion is also effective for getting plaque off the teeth themselves.

Decide on daily. Ideally, you should brush after every

meal, says Bruce Pihlstrom, D.D.S., professor and director of the Minnesota Clinical Dental Research Center at the University of Minnesota in Minneapolis. If you can't do that, make sure to brush at least once a day.

For flossing, make a C and earn an A. The key to proper flossing is to hook the thread (whether it's waxed or unwaxed doesn't make a difference, say dentists) into the shape of a C around each tooth. Make sure you go slightly below the gum line, moving the floss back and forth and up and down until the teeth on both sides of the thread feel and sound squeaky clean, says Dr. Pihlstrom.

If you draw a little blood the first few times you floss, don't be too concerned: "Flossing causes a little bit of irritation on an area inflamed with gingivitis," he says.

Don't be a stranger to your dentist. "Most people should get a cleaning every six months, while others may want to see their dentist more often," says Dr. Pihlstrom. Those who might want to think about seeing the dentist more frequently include all those who were described at the beginning of this chapter as being more prone to gum disease, such as smokers and people with diabetes, people taking medications that can cause gum problems and people with a family history of gum disease.

Pregnant women, because they're more prone to gum problems, should see their dentist for a cleaning at least three times during their pregnancy.

There'll be a reason to frown if you don't see the dentist regularly. You'll have to remove your smile every night before going to bed. "People who wait longer than six months between visits tend to lose their teeth eventually," says Dr. Allen.

When Gingivitis Becomes Severe

Brushing, flossing and a routine biyearly visit with the hygienist won't make much difference if your gingivitis is severe or has advanced to periodontal disease. At that point, your dentist or hygienist has to get out his equipment to remove the plaque, which is now a concretelike substance called tartar or calculus that has hardened deep inside the pocketlike spaces between your teeth and deteriorating gums.

Let your dentist chip away. The dentist will chip and scrape away the calculus and plaque down to the surface of the roots of your teeth, a process called scaling and planing. It may require a local anesthetic, says Dr. Pihlstrom, and you'll probably need two or three appointments before the job is completed.

See a specialist. If the deterioration is severe, the dentist may refer you to a periodontist, a specialist in mouth, gum and bone disease. "A periodontist can give you a lot of options," says Dr. Pihlstrom. Among them are bone grafts, repair and rebuilding of deep gum pockets and restoration of the gum line.

Tips for False Teeth

Even if you've lost your real teeth and now sport dentures or a partial, you still should be good to your gums. Here's how.

Keep brushing. Dentures aren't called false *teeth* for nothing. You have to brush them, which helps prevent gum problems. You'll also want to brush your gums. And never leave your dentures in overnight—your gums need a break.

Get a new pair. A pair of dentures doesn't last a lifetime. "It's a big mistake to think that the first set is enough," says Dr. Low. That's because once you've lost your real teeth, the jawbone can erode, robbing your dentures of their snug fit.

"They get loose and cause irritation, but people tend not to do anything about it," he says. Your dentist should check your fit once a year, and chances are you'll need a new pair about every five years.

H

HAIR CHANGES

WHAT YOUR SYMPTOM IS TELLING YOU

Hair turned white from fright virtually overnight? Well, your head could look like the end of a cotton swab because of all the frightful stress you've been under—that new marriage, those bills, this job!

But most of those white hairs have been with you all along. The transformation came when stress literally spooked some of the *dark* hairs from your head—causing them to fall out, says Allan Kayne, M.D., who is in private practice at the Virginia Mason Medical Center and a clinical assistant professor of medicine at the University of Washington in Seattle. Fortunately, the majority of people experiencing this will see their hair regrow eventually, he says.

While suddenly going white is certainly dramatic, it's by no means the only change your hair can undergo. Fortunately, most hair changes are part of a natural process. Hair naturally begins to slowly turn gray for many during their thirties and forties.

Other hair changes may be caused by chemicals. Swimming in heavily chlorinated pools harmlessly turns blonde to green. Well water and iron in water work their own special magic, sometimes transforming entire towns into redheads, says David Cannell, Ph.D., corporate vice president of technology for Redken in Los Angeles.

Limp, lifeless hair, although sometimes a tip-off to nutritional deficiency, is more often caused by hair that already has a very small diameter and is coated with oil. "Fine hair usually doesn't have much body to begin with," says Dr. Cannell. "So when it gets coated with oil, it tends to get weighted down and flatten out."

Lack of protein, although not generally a problem for well-fed Americans, can force hair into a resting phase, leading to hair loss.

And then there are hair changes like split ends and dryness that are most commonly caused by grooming goofs, like overuse of blow dryers, hot rollers and chemical dyes.

SYMPTOM RELIEF

Before hair changes turn your coiffure into a disaster du jour, try these hair-care tips.

Feed your hair. Yo-yo dieters take note: Starvation dieting can create skinny hair. In fact, in impoverished countries, hair loss from protein deficiency is common, says Dr. Cannell. "If you're just getting a tiny amount of protein in your diet, hair becomes superfluous, and so you see a thinning, a withering and a decrease in the hair fiber as the follicle becomes atrophied," he says. "Generally, however, the average Western diet is quite sufficient in terms of vitamins, minerals and protein for hair growth."

Deal with stress. Don't scare the color out of your hair with too much stress. Manage stress by taking walks, using a relaxation technique, talking to friends or going on mini-vacations—before the situation is out of control (and you're out of dark hair).

Beauty Parlor Tricks

Creative hair care can also keep hair changes to a minimum. Try these tips.

Block pool chlorine with conditioner. Before diving in, work some creamy conditioner through your hair. "Putting a little in your hair before swimming will put a barrier between your hair and the chemicals in the water," says Dr. Cannell. And that means your blond hair is less likely to turn green, he says.

Try a special shampoo. Use a shampoo once a week that helps remove hair-product buildup from hair, says Dr. Cannell. Many hair-care products these days contain ingredients that can build up and cause unwanted hair-color changes, he explains. "Regular shampoos generally do not have very good mineral-removing capability," he says. There are products on the market that are applied to the hair and then left on for five to ten minutes for the sole purpose of removing buildup, he says.

Wash out excess oil. If your hair has gone limp, don't lament: You may not be shampooing enough, says Dr. Cannell. "Shampooing tends to make the hair fuller and fluffier. There are also plenty of body-building hair conditioners with protein that add substance to the hair and make it feel like there's more of it."

End split ends. Having hair trimmed regularly and keeping hair from getting too hot—with proper hair dryer handling—can prevent split ends, says Ron Renee, president of Aestheticians International Association in Dallas. Also important: using the correct daily shampoo and conditioner. For best results, both should have a pH (or acid) level between 4.5 and 5.5. You can check the pH level of your shampoo by ordering nitrozine paper test strips from your pharmacist, says Renee. Wetting the strip with your shampoo or conditioner will make it change color, indicating the pH level, he says.

HAIRINESS

WHEN TO SEE YOUR DOCTOR

- You experience a sudden increase of dark, coarse hair on your face, neck or body.
- You are also experiencing missed periods or a deepening voice.

WHAT YOUR SYMPTOM IS TELLING YOU

A young man is delighted when the peach fuzz on his upper lip transforms into a dark mustache. When this happens to a woman, the reaction is just the opposite.

Of course, some women (and men, too) simply have more body hair than others, especially if their ancestors came from Italy, Greece or one of the other Mediterranean countries. But if you're a woman and you suddenly sprout dark hairs where there was once only downy hair, it may mean that you have some kind of hormonal imbalance.

An imbalance can occur quite naturally, according to Lois Jovanovic-Peterson, M.D., endocrinologist with the Sansum Medical Research Foundation in Santa Barbara and coauthor of *Hormones: The Woman's Answer Book*. "When women reach menopause, they may notice that the hairs on their face, neck or abdomen are becoming darker and thicker," she says.

At menopause, the ovaries decrease their production of the hormone estrogen, which normally blocks the effects of testosterone, Dr. Jovanovic-Peterson explains. Testosterone is the hormone responsible for the changes that men go through at puberty, including the appearance of facial hair. Although testosterone is known as the male hormone, women also produce some. When estrogen levels start to decrease in a woman, her naturally occurring testosterone can begin to click in. The most common reaction: hair on the upper lip.

Besides menopause, other factors can influence testosterone levels and trigger hairiness. Younger women who crash diet can throw off their hormone balance to the point where ovulation ceases and testosterone production is increased. These women, too, may sprout a fuzzy upper lip or coarse hair elsewhere on their bodies, says Dr. Jovanovic-Peterson.

In addition, medications such as steroids and drugs to control high blood pressure may boost testosterone levels.

Besides hairiness, there are usually several other clues that should alert you to a hormonal problem that requires medical attention, says Dr. Jovanovic-Peterson. "Missed periods, bulkier muscles if you haven't increased your level of exercise or a deeper voice are all signs that should send you straight to the doctor," she says.

SYMPTOM RELIEF

Even if you've started to sprout unwanted hair, it is possible to have that smooth-body look again. Here's how.

Check your medications. If you're taking steroids or medication to control your blood pressure, ask your doctor whether some alterations in your medications might be appropriate.

Talk to your doctor about spironolactone. If you're still menstruating, your doctor can prescribe this drug, which prevents new hair growth by countering the excess testosterone, says Leslie I. Rose, M.D., director of the Division of Endocrinology at Hahnemann Hospital in Philadelphia.

Go on the Pill. Oral contraceptives are another option, according to Julianne Imperato-McGinley, M.D., associate professor of medicine at Cornell University Medical Center in New York City. The Pill suppresses the amount of testosterone released from the ovaries, limiting new hair growth, she says.

Take hormone replacement therapy. If you're past menopause, ask your doctor about hormone replacement therapy (HRT). HRT corrects the estrogen/testosterone imbalance and will stop unwanted hair growth, according to Lila Nachtigall, M.D., associate professor of obstetrics and gynecology at New York University School of Medicine in New York City.

Pluck it out. Medications and hormones will squelch new hair growth, but you will need to remove unwanted hair that is already there. If you only have a few stray hairs on your chin, nipples or eyebrows, you can tweeze them out. This method may backfire, however. "Plucking can irritate the base of the hair follicle and may stimulate hair regrowth," says Dr. Rose.

Lighten it up. Women have used bleach to lighten fuzzy upper lips for years. You should always test a bit of commercial hair bleach on a small area of your arm before using it on your upper lip hair, just to make sure it won't irritate your skin, says Fredric Haberman, M.D., clinical instructor of dermatology at Albert Einstein College of

Medicine in New York City and author of *The Doctor's Beauty Hotline*. And don't use bleach on your eyebrows.

Shave against the grain. Shaving does not make the hair grow back quicker or coarser, according to Dr. Haberman. Still, some women are hesitant to shave their faces for fear of a thicker stubble, he says. For close, smooth results wherever you shave—face, arms or legs—lather up with soap, baby oil or shaving cream to pre-soften the hairs. Then, using a sharp blade, shave "against the grain" (opposite from the direction of hair growth), rinse and apply moisturizer.

Strip it off. For defuzzing arms, legs, bikini areas or toes, wax stripping is smoother and longer-lasting than shaving and may produce softer and finer hair with repeat waxings, says Dr. Haberman. As hot wax hardens, it traps hairs that can be pulled out as the wax is stripped off. Cold wax involves wax bonded to strips of paper and is best for smaller, downier areas. To learn the painless way to wax, go to a salon for your initial waxing and pick up pointers, suggests Dr. Haberman.

Burn it off. You can use a chemical depilatory cream to remove hair anywhere on the body, except around nipples or eyes. Regrowth is less bristly, but the chemicals can be irritating, says Dr. Haberman. Try a test patch first. If your skin does not turn red, apply the cream and wipe away the hairs with a soft cloth. Afterward, wrap your skin in a cold washcloth to reduce stinging.

Zap it. "Electrolysis is the only way to permanently remove the unwanted hair you already have," says Dr. Jovanovic-Peterson. A current is sent down a probe to destroy the hair follicle. You'll need several electrolysis sessions to get rid of all the unwanted hair. Unless you have a top-flight operator, electrolysis may cause scarring or undue pain. "Ask your dermatologist for the name of a certified operator with a good track record of lasting results, good hands and a good deal of patience," says Dr. Haberman.

HAIR LOSS

WHAT YOUR SYMPTOM IS TELLING YOU

First your barber starts charging you half-price for a trim. Then your wife develops an odd habit of licking her palms and matting your stray hairs into place. Next you find yourself sarcastically referring to perfectly coiffed entertainers and newscasters on the tube as Mr. Hairdo. It's time to face the nearly bare facts: You're probably one of 50 million Americans suffering from male or (women, take note) female pattern baldness—the most common forms of hair loss.

The best way to know for sure: Most people shed 50 to 150 hairs from their heads a day. If you're a man and you're losing twice that many off the top in a broad pattern—and the only thing that has grown back looks like it belongs on a peach—you're a likely candidate. Female pattern baldness, however, doesn't seem to be limited to one particular area, says Larry E. Millikan, M.D., chairman of the Department of Dermatology at the Tulane University Medical Center in New Orleans.

If you've developed one or more coin-shaped bald patches on your head, you may have developed alopecia areata—a mysterious condition thought to be caused by allergies to your own hair, says Ronald C. Savin, M.D., clinical professor of dermatology at the Yale University School of Medicine. The condition is often temporary.

Less mysterious: Temporary hair loss in women who have just had children. Hormones apparently slow natural hair loss during pregnancy but boost it afterward, says Dr. Savin. It resolves within ten months after giving birth.

Drugs and medical treatments—like anti-gout and anti-arthritis medications and antidepressants—and poor nutrition can also spell temporary distress for your tresses. Among the worst: radiation therapy or chemotherapy for cancer, says Robert Richards, M.D., of Toronto, a spokesperson for the American Academy of Dermatologists.

SYMPTOM RELIEF

If you're trying to hang on to your hair, consider these tips.

Feed your scalp. It won't turn a desert into a forest, but good nutrition—like quality protein and iron—*do* seem to play at least a minor role in preventing hair loss.

In fact, severe dieting (200 to 400 calories a day) can actually provoke substantial temporary hair loss, says Dr. Savin. Good, low-fat sources of protein are lean chicken, beef and beans. Get sufficient iron from lean beef and enriched cereals, or even a good supplement. Too much vitamin A can actually cause hair loss.

Tricks of the Hair Trade

If growing new hair isn't an option—and it usually isn't—the only other alternative is making the most of what you have.

Have a discussion with your hairdresser. Because female pattern baldness is characterized by thinning throughout the scalp, proper styling can help hide hair loss in women. Men may also benefit. "Appropriate hairstyles and grooming methods can make the hair look much thicker," says Joel Moore, artistic and educational director for Revlon in Savannah, Georgia.

Flip over wigs. Made with real human hair, many wigs and toupees feature two-sided tape that can get wet and still stay in place, says Moore. Before making your selection, consult an experienced cosmetologist.

Wear a weave. During a hair weave, hair is matched and braided to your existing hair in a process that keeps it snug and lifelike. The only drawback: As your hair grows, the weave becomes loose and you have to go back for tightening, says Moore.

Medical Approaches

If you're willing to consider a medical solution, consult your doctor about these treatments.

Regain your hair with Rogaine? While initial reports

trumpeted Rogaine's (minoxidil) success in treating male and female pattern baldness, some experts are now more skeptical. Studies show that about 40 percent of the men who use minoxidil, the active ingredient in the prescription hair-growth product Rogaine, will have modest, though cosmetically significant regrowth, says Dr. Savin, who also serves as a consultant for the company that manufactures the drug. In the remaining 60 percent, however, hair loss is merely slowed or stopped by using minoxidil. Women, on the other hand, fare much better: Nearly every woman who uses the drug regrows 12 to 15 percent of her lost hair.

For best results, follow the directions strictly, says Dr. Savin. And instead of using mousse or a styling gel, which can water down the dose, style with hairspray.

If you don't see results in ten months, minoxidil may not be for you. Two to six months after you stop using the drug, "nature catches up with you, and you lose the new hair that you grew," says Dr. Savin. A month's supply, about two ounces, costs between $55 and $70.

Shave some size off that scalp. During a procedure called scalp reduction, doctors actually remove part of the skin from the scalp and then pull the areas with hair closer together, giving the illusion of more hair, says Dr. Richards. Candidates for scalp reduction include those with more vigorous side hair growth.

Plant some old hairs in a new place. During a hair transplant, hair is surgically removed from an area with more prolific hair growth—like the back of the head—and placed in the bald area. Contrary to popular belief, the transplanted hair will not spread. If successful, the hair merely grows—and no one misses it from where it used to be. "In hair transplantation there's no change in the number of hairs. It's just a mechanical redistribution," says Dr. Richards.

Consider cortisone. For the coin-size bald patches caused by alopecia areata, many doctors inject cortisone directly into the bald area. Results are usually impressive, says Dr. Savin. Cortisone injections are also used to grow eyebrows and eyelashes for victims of alopecia universalis, the more serious form of alopecia, says Dr. Savin.

HALLUCINATIONS

- Any hallucinations that occur, other than when you're just waking up or falling asleep, should be brought to the attention of your physician.

WHAT YOUR SYMPTOM IS TELLING YOU

The stories about people who've seen Elvis in convenience stores don't faze you, but when your neighbor tells you she saw a 30-foot-tall vision of Tiny Tim walking down your street, you politely ask her to tiptoe back to her side of the tulips.

A hallucination can range from a simple flash of light or color to clear visions of people, animals or plants.

Generally, hallucinations are an important warning signal that a person may have a mental health problem. Seeing things could be a symptom of schizophrenia, acute depression or grief. Hallucinations also can have physical causes, such as alcohol and drug abuse, a side effect of medications, Alzheimer's disease, cataracts, glaucoma, migraines, extreme dehydration or fatigue, high fever, kidney failure or brain tumors.

SYMPTOM RELIEF

The only times that hallucinations occur normally are when you are falling asleep or just waking up," says Betsy Comstock, M.D., a professor of psychiatry at Baylor College of Medicine in Houston. "As you wake up, for example, you may see a suit in your closet and think a man is standing there. That's fairly common and you don't have to go to a doctor about that. But any other time you see something that isn't there, you should get to your doctor." While hallucinations are a symptom of many serious ailments, your doctor may suggest a simple remedy after he has completed a thorough medical examination. And there's one thing you can do to help your doctor determine what's wrong.

Check your medications. Most of us know that illegal drugs such as marijuana and LSD can cause hallucinations. But so can some prescription and over-the-counter drugs, including antihistamines, anticonvulsants, antidepressants, antibiotics, tranquilizers, steroids and pain and cardiovascular medications. Prepare a list of all the medications you are currently taking—including over-the-counter drugs—and ask your doctor if you should make any changes.

HANDS AND FEET, COLD

WHEN TO SEE YOUR DOCTOR

- The discomfort limits your activities.
- You also have persistent swollen discolored fingers or swollen joints.
- A sore develops on your fingers or toes.

WHAT YOUR SYMPTOM IS TELLING YOU

It can happen every time when you hold a chilled can of soda or step into an air-conditioned movie theater. Suddenly, your fingers turn icy, white and numb. And your feet are so sensitive that they feel frozen to the bone after doing the dishes while standing on cool kitchen tiles. But sometimes the temperature isn't the cause at all. For some people, emotional stress is enough to turn their fingers and toes to ice.

An estimated 2 to 6 percent of all Americans have hands and feet that are overly sensitive to chilly temperatures and stress. Doctors call the condition Raynaud's syndrome, after the French physician who discovered it. With Raynaud's, a dip in the temperature or a rise in stress levels causes the small blood vessels in the extremities to go into spasm, narrowing to the point that blood can barely circulate through them. Fingers and toes turn waxy white, then blue, and are numb and cool to the touch. Then, when the fingers and toes get warm, they flush deep red and tingle and throb as blood returns full force. This kind of episode can take anywhere from a few minutes to several hours.

Seventy-five percent of people with primary Raynaud's syndrome—the most common kind—are women under 40. It's unclear why. "My guess is there's a link to female hormones, which affect the blood vessels," says Fredrick Wigley, M.D., director of rheumatology at Johns Hopkins University School of Medicine in Baltimore. In any case, the color changes, numbness and tingling may be the only symptoms, and they may get worse or better. The problem usually improves dramatically by menopause.

Secondary Raynaud's—a less common but potentially more serious kind—usually targets women over 40 and men. Factors that act on the blood vessels may trigger the problem. These include smoking, high blood pressure medicines and diseases such as rheumatoid arthritis, lupus (an autoimmune disease) and atherosclerosis. Certain wrist-flexing, wear-and-tear activities such as typing or operating vibrating power drills may increase susceptibility to secondary Raynaud's.

People with this type typically have more intense episodes that gradually worsen each winter and can affect just one finger, hand or foot. Secondary Raynaud's can lead to skin sores or tissue damage.

SYMPTOM RELIEF

Here are some tips to keep your fingers and toes toasty.

Plunge your hands into warm water. If you're involved in an activity that involves cold—stuffing a turkey, for example—it helps to run your hands under warm water periodically. "This forces blood vessels to remain open," says Murray Hamlet, former director of the Army's Cold Research Division in Natick, Massachussetts.

Move your arms like a windmill. Swinging your arms briskly in 360-degree circles for a minute or two helps drive blood into the fingers and can relieve vessel spasm, according to Donald R. McIntyre, M.D., a dermatologist in private practice in Rutland, Vermont. "Just keep the elbow, fingers and wrist straight," he says.

Sip some hot cider. When the thermometer plunges, hot fruit juice can help stoke up your body's furnace because the sugar provides instant energy, says Dr. Hamlet. Hot coffee is a cold-weather no-no, however. Caffeine constricts the blood vessels, further reducing blood flow. "Alcoholic hot toddies are worse," adds John Abruzzo, M.D., professor of medicine and director of the Rheumatology and Osteoporosis Center at Thomas Jefferson University Hospital in Philadelphia. Alcohol dilates the blood vessels, which gives a sensation of warmth, he says. But the dilated vessels are actually throwing off heat. "You'll shiver more," says Dr. Abruzzo.

Have a fish feast. Fish oil may help ease primary Raynaud's symptoms by reducing the painful blood vessel spasms that cause a shutdown of blood flow to fingers and toes, according to researchers conducting a small preliminary study at Albany Medical College in New York. They observed that 5 out of 11 people who took fish-oil capsules daily for three months had symptoms stop completely. Ask your doctor about taking these capsules. In the meantime, a daily serving of sardines, salmon or tuna may keep your fingers from getting frosty, says Joel M. Kremer, M.D., professor of medicine and head of rheumatology at Albany Medical School.

Go for the loose and layered look. "Getting chilled can trigger Raynaud's syndrome because it diverts blood away from extremities," says Dr. Abruzzo. You can keep warm all over by wearing loose, layered clothing, which helps trap heat, he says. For the layer closest to your body, cotton blends are better than pure cotton or wool because they wick away chill-causing perspiration.

Cover your head when it's nippy. "You lose up to 55 percent of body heat from your head," says Dr. Hamlet. So wear a hat whenever the temperature outside dips even slightly.

Wear mittens, not gloves. Keeping the fingers together helps them generate warmth and will protect them better than gloves, says Dr. Hamlet. Insulated mittens are best, he adds.

Wear hot socks on frigid days. If you're going to be outdoors—sitting in a chilly stadium, for example—take along chemical warmers. These are small heating pouches, available in sporting goods stores, that can be placed in pockets, gloves, boots or shoes. Battery-powered "hot socks" are also a good idea.

Buy a steering wheel cover. Gripping a cold, vibrating steering wheel drains the blood from your hands and can set you up for cold fingers.

Use oven mitts to handle frozen food. And don't be embarrassed to put on mittens to rummage around in your home freezer. You can also protect your fingers from the cold by using an insulated drinking glass or wrapping a napkin around your glass, says Dr. Hamlet.

Place mats over cold tiles. Consider using a mat with built-in heating coils in any tiled or bare-floored area where you stand for prolonged periods, says Dr. Abruzzo.

Bump up the bedroom temperature. Metabolism slows during sleep, so it's important to keep your body temperature high, says Dr. Abruzzo. Wearing socks and even mittens to bed will add extra warmth on cold nights.

Retrain your arteries. This technique, developed by Dr. Hamlet, really works. First, make sure the room where you're practicing is at a temperature that is comfortable for you—not too hot and not too cold. Sit for five minutes with your hands in an insulated container filled with hot tap water. Then wrap your hands in a towel and move to a chilly area—the porch or basement, for example. Now, unwrap your hands and dunk them into a second hot-water container for ten minutes. Then go back indoors for another two- to five-minute dip. Repeat this routine 3 to 6 times every other day for a total of 50 times. "Our studies showed that after the immersion procedure, hands remained seven degrees warmer when exposed to cool air," says Dr. Hamlet. The results can last two years or longer, he adds.

HEADACHES

WHEN TO SEE YOUR DOCTOR

- You've never had headaches before, but now you're getting them.
- Your headache persists for more than 72 hours or prevents you from doing normal activities.
- The headache feels like a sudden "explosion" in your head.
- You are also experiencing vision problems, difficulty talking, problems with coordination, weakness in your arms and legs or difficulty thinking clearly.
- You also have a fever or stiff neck.
- You get a headache whenever you exert yourself.
- You're also vomiting but don't feel nauseated.
- Your headaches are becoming more frequent and severe.

WHAT YOUR SYMPTOM IS TELLING YOU

Sometimes it seems like nothing feels worse than a nasty headache. It throbs, it bangs, it squeezes. It can feel as if it's twisting your head inside out and wringing all the energy from your body.

"Headaches are incredibly widespread," says George H. Sands, M.D., a neurologist and headache specialist at Mount Sinai Medical Center in New York City. Over 90 percent of Americans have at least one headache in their lifetime. In fact, nearly 60 percent of all men and over 75 percent of all women probably had at least one headache within the past month.

Nine out of every ten headaches are muscle contraction headaches, also known as tension headaches, says Egilius Spierings, M.D., Ph.D., director of the Headache Section at Brigham and Women's Hospital in Boston. Often triggered by stress and fatigue, these headaches are caused by sustained contraction of the head and neck muscles. Tension headaches usually strike in the late afternoon and can feel like a tight band is wrapped around your head.

The notorious migraine occurs when blood vessels in the scalp dilate. It often begins early in the morning with intense pain on one side of the head or behind the eyes. The pain can last for several hours or linger for up to three days. Some people who have migraines experience auras—flashes of light or zigzag lines—15 to 30 minutes before the headache occurs. Migraines also can cause nausea, vomiting and sensitivity to light. Migraines afflict less than 7 percent of Americans, but between 65 and 75 percent of the people who have migraines are women.

"Headache pain in women may be connected to the menstrual cycle," says Sid Gilman, M.D., professor and chair of the Department of Neurology at the University of Michigan Medical Center in Ann Arbor. "Migraine headaches are much less common after menopause."

Men, however, are more likely to get cluster headaches, an extreme burning or gnawing type of head pain in or around one eye that afflicts less than 1 in 100 Americans. Considered one of the most painful types of headaches, cluster attacks may last up to two hours once or twice a day for a month and then not occur at all for six months or several years, Dr. Spierings says.

Headaches also can be a sign of a cold, flu, high blood pressure, brain hemorrhage, stroke, brain tumor, meningitis, Lyme disease, tapeworm, glaucoma, abscessed tooth or caffeine withdrawal. They can also be side effects of certain drugs.

Symptom Relief

Fortunately, less than 5 headaches in 100 are a sign of a serious underlying illness, Dr. Spierings says. For the majority of us, headaches are a painful but routine part of life. You can, however, bring them under control. Here's how.

Get some sleep. Many tension headaches are relieved by getting some good sound sleep, says Donald Farrell, M.D., a professor of neurology at the University of Washington School of Medicine in Seattle. But sleeping can also *cause* a headache, says Dr. Spierings, if you get too little or too much. That's why it's important to set a regular bedtime and get up at the same time each morning.

Stop the nightly grind. "Some people are so tense during sleep that they will grind their teeth and wake up with headaches in the morning," Dr. Farrell says. (To put an end to tooth grinding, see page 651.)

Fuel your body. Skipping meals can cause headaches just as easily as missing sleep. "We're not sure why, but it may be that when your body runs low on fuel, it activates the part of the nervous system that increases tightness of the muscles throughout your body," Dr. Spierings says.

Play diet detective. "It's a good idea for people who get frequent headaches to consider the possibility that the foods they ate two to three hours earlier had something to do with their headache," Dr. Gilman says. The common offenders are foods that contain tyramine, an amino acid known to trigger headaches in many people. Foods or beverages containing tyramine or other headache-producing substances include most alcoholic beverages, aged cheeses, cured meats, pickles, chocolate, citrus fruits, pizza and anything containing monosodium glutamate (MSG). "If you suspect that foods are causing your headaches, try eliminating them one by one from your diet and see what happens," Dr. Spierings says.

Pass on red. The next time you're offered red wine, think twice. Red wine contains many chemicals that can dilate blood vessels and cause headaches, Dr. Spierings says.

No more third cups. Don't drink excessive amounts of

coffee. "If you drink three or more cups of coffee every day in the office and you sleep in late on Saturday, you could wake up with a headache because of caffeine withdrawal," Dr. Sands says. To prevent that, doctors suggest that you drink no more than one or two eight-ounce cups of coffee a day.

Stamp out the butts. "Smoking is bad for everyone, and it will make certain headaches worse," Dr. Sands says. "If you smoke, quit."

Make your own shade. "Some people will get a headache if they go to the beach and sit facing the glare of the water," Dr. Sands says. "I suggest these people wear good sunglasses and a wide-brimmed hat."

Get moving. "Exercise is a surprisingly effective treatment for headaches," Dr. Gilman says. "It seems odd, but there are people who will play a vigorous game of racquetball and find that their headaches go away." Exercise relieves stress and can trigger production of natural painkillers called endorphins, Dr. Sands says. Just walking 30 minutes a day three times a week may be enough to prevent headaches and enhance your health in other ways. If your headache is accompanied by a fever, you should seek medical advice and postpone exercise until you recover.

Get warm. "One important home remedy is using a heating pad on the neck and shoulders for 15 to 20 minutes daily. It's a very good way to gradually reduce the frequency of your tension headaches," Dr. Spierings says. The heating pad helps soothe tight muscles and prevents them from squeezing off circulation. In a pinch, you can try taking a warm shower or hot bath, but neither is as effective as a heating pad, he says.

Learn to relax. "Stress management such as biofeedback and yoga can be very valuable for people who suffer from recurrent tension headaches," Dr. Farrell says. (Biofeedback involves using an electronic device to learn how to control biological functions over which you don't normally have conscious control.) Ask your doctor to recommend someone who can teach you one of these relaxation techniques.

Imagine there is no headache. Guided imagery is a very effective way to rid yourself of headaches, says Dennis

Gersten, M.D., a psychiatrist in San Diego and publisher of *Atlantis: The Imagery Newsletter*. To try it, sit or lie in a comfortable position and close your eyes. Imagine you are lying on a beach with the sun comfortably warming you. The waves gently pour over you. Each time the waves roll back out to sea, they pull more and more tension out of your body.

After you're relaxed, Dr. Gersten suggests trying this imagery: Focus your attention on your headache. Imagine the pain has a certain size, shape and color. What does it feel like? Is it smooth or rough? Does it stay in one place in your head or does it move around? Allow the headache to turn to liquid. Allow the pain to roll down into your neck, then down into one shoulder, into your hand and finally your fingertips. Then allow the liquid to pour out of your fingertips and watch it as it flows out of the room or space you are in.

The Drug Alternatives

If natural remedies don't work for you, there are plenty of prescription and over-the-counter medications that may relieve your headache pain. Here's a sampling.

Reach for an aspirin. "Most people can find excellent relief from their headaches if they take two aspirin or acetaminophen," Dr. Gilman says. "Aspirin decreases inflammation, and both aspirin and acetaminophen are good pain relievers."

Don't forget the java. If you have a moderate to severe headache, try taking your aspirin with a strong cup of coffee, Dr. Spierings suggests. The caffeine in the coffee will speed absorption of the aspirin.

Take an antihistamine. Over-the-counter antihistamines that don't also contain pain medication (Benadryl 25, Dramamine, Chlor-Trimeton) may subdue your tension headache if you take one or two tablets every four hours, says Dr. Spierings. You can take up to 300 milligrams per day, but don't exceed the daily limit given on the package label, he says.

"These antihistamines can cause muscle relaxation if

taken repeatedly," Dr. Spierings says. "They're effective and they get you away from pain medications. They may make you drowsy at first, but the more you take them, the more effective they will become against your headaches and the less drowsy you will be."

Take a breath of big O. Oxygen is an effective weapon against cluster headaches and may also benefit people who get migraines, Dr. Sands says. Doctors aren't sure how oxygen relieves pain, but it does decrease blood flow to the brain and has a positive effect on the brain cells. Ask your doctor if breathing 100 percent oxygen from a tank might help you. If appropriate, your doctor can prescribe oxygen and direct you to a supplier.

Is it time for a prescription? For severe cluster or migraine headaches, you may need a prescription drug such as ergotamine, dihydroergotamine or sumatriptan. Ask your doctor if a prescription medication is right for you.

Be wary of painkillers. "There's nothing worse for a headache than using painkillers regularly," Dr. Spierings says. "Any pain medication, whether it is prescription or over-the-counter, should not be used more than twice a week for headaches, because regular use of these medications actually lowers your pain threshold and will increase the frequency of your headaches." If you're overdoing the painkillers, see your doctor, who can help you design a program to get rid of your headaches.

HEALING PROBLEMS

WHEN TO SEE YOUR DOCTOR

- A wound is inflamed, discolored or producing pus.
- A wound increases in size and severity.
- A cut or gash does not heal within four weeks.
- You have slow-healing leg sores and swollen ankles.

WHAT YOUR SYMPTOM IS TELLING YOU

Dad cut himself shaving the other day, and the gash is still red and sensitive. Mom had some minor surgery a while back, and the scar looks sore and infected. Little Johnny fell off his bike last month, and that skinned knee still hasn't gotten better. And Grandpa has developed these sores on his legs that just don't want to go away.

Not your typical family. And not your typical wound behavior. Usually the body is ready, willing and able to fix itself when it needs repair. But when healing proceeds at a snail's pace, you have to suspect that the body is encountering some obstacles.

In normal healing, a wound goes through three phases. Phase one: White blood cells and blood platelets rush to the wound to fight infection and begin repair. In phase two, these platelets release proteins called growth factors that stimulate the production of new tissue. In the final stage, the new tissue is accepted by the body and matures. At any stage, however, a lot of things can go wrong.

"There are six key elements to wound healing," says David Knighton, M.D., director of the Institute for Reparative Medicine in St. Louis Park, Minnesota. "Healing relies on good blood flow. Proper nutrition is essential. The effects of certain medications or diseases that inhibit tissue repair must be controlled or minimized. The wound itself must be clean and free from foreign bodies. It must be free from infection. And the wound must be safe from trauma and aggravation. A problem with just one of these elements will stall the healing process. The process will collapse and you're stuck with a nonhealing wound."

Of those healing elements, perhaps the most important is adequate blood flow. Why? Because the blood brings oxygen to the wound. "Oxygen enables the body's white blood cells to kill the infectious bacteria in the wound," says John M. Rabkin, M.D., assistant professor of surgery at the Oregon Health Sciences University in Portland. "It also plays a vital role in depositing collagen—an important protein needed to build new tissue."

Other factors also come into play. One is age: Older skin

just doesn't heal as fast as a youngster's. Swollen skin doesn't heal as well, nor does skin that has been treated with radiation. Scabs, while they protect the wound from the outside world, actually slow down the growth of new skin tissue. Finally, wounds that are kept moist heal much quicker than those that are dry.

Slow-healing wounds and sores are hallmarks of many diseases. Both diabetes and circulatory disease of the veins and arteries, for example, can cause severe ulceration in the lower legs. These conditions also cause poor circulation, which further inhibits healing. Other illnesses as well as the treatments prescribed for them can leave a person "immuno-suppressed"—that is, they impede the immune system from doing it's healing work. Sickle cell disease, anemia, hemophilia and any other disease that impairs the blood-clotting process or the formation of blood cells and platelets are prime examples. So are tuberculosis, cancer and AIDS.

SYMPTOM RELIEF

Contrary to the old adage, time doesn't heal all wounds. The immune system heals wounds. You can give a cut, burn or sore all the time in the world, but if it isn't provided with a proper healing environment, you're in for a long recovery. Here's how you can speed up the process.

Keep wounds clean. Top priority! Wash all wounds thoroughly with warm water and a gentle soap once per day, more often only if the wound gets dirty again. Try to remove any dirt or foreign objects you see in the wound, and if you can't, ask a doctor to do the job, says James Brand, M.D., assistant professor of family medicine at the University of Oklahoma Health Sciences Center in Oklahoma City.

Keep air out. Use bandages to keep moisture in and dirt and bacteria out, suggests Guy F. Webster, M.D., Ph.D., assistant professor of dermatology and director of the Center for Cutaneous Pharmacology at Thomas Jefferson University in Philadelphia. Adhesive bandages and taped gauze pads are usually just as effective as fancy surgical dressings. You can even use plastic wrap under the bandage to keep it extra airtight, says Dr. Webster. Just make sure the wound is clean, the bandage is secure and you change the bandage frequently, he says.

Baby your wound. Your wound won't heal if you pick at it or subject it to rough scrubbing, burns, chemicals, abrasives, bumps or bangs. Treat it gently, advises Dr. Knighton.

Apply heat. The direct application of heat—through a heating pad, a hot-water bottle, warm clothing or a warm bath—will stimulate blood flow to the wound site, according to Dr. Rabkin. Don't scald yourself; a few degrees above your body temperature will do the job. You can apply the heat 15 to 20 minutes at a time, several times a day.

Stock up on these healing nutrients. Certain vitamins, minerals and other nutrients are instrumental in the healing process. Among them: Vitamins C, A and E; zinc; magnesium; manganese and protein. Balanced meals and a daily multivitamin supplement are usually sufficient to get what you need, says Dr. Knighton. If you need more, a physician can recommend a good vitamin supplement program to meet your needs.

Fight infection with antibiotics. If your wound is producing pus, it's probably infected and you'll require oral antibiotics, says Dr. Rabkin. You can also apply a topical antibiotic ointment like Neosporin, Polysporin or Bacitracin (available at pharmacies). They'll help the infection a little, but the big thing they do is hold in moisture and prevent additional bacteria from getting in the wound.

Double-check your Rx. Many medications can slow down your immune system's effectiveness, says Dr. Rabkin. Ask your doctor if you should discontinue any of your medications or switch to something else.

Get plenty of exercise. Exercise will improve your blood flow, says Dr. Knighton. While working out, however, it's important not to traumatize the area you're trying to heal. That's why many people who have wounds on their legs are instructed to focus their workouts on the upper body.

Stop smoking. Smoking will reduce the amount of oxygen the blood can deliver to a wound, says Dr. Brand. The nicotine in the smoke is also a toxic substance that may interfere with the cells' ability to repair tissue.

Don't go in the pool. Think a dip in the pool is good for a wound or cut? Wrong, says Dr. Knighton. The chlorine will destroy new skin tissue. Reserve your swimming for fresh water or the ocean.

Avoid these healing hinderers. "The less stuff you put on a wound, the happier it is," says Dr. Webster. Repeated usage of antiseptics like hydrogen peroxide and iodine will kill new tissue along with bad bacteria, he explains. If you do use them, only use them during your initial cleaning. And if the wound hurts, don't apply an anesthetic. It will just aggravate the wound. You can take an aspirin or some other painkiller if you need to.

Keep an eye on scabs. Scabs should be removed, especially if pus is accumulating underneath. But don't rip them off! Soak smaller scabs in warm water several times a day and keep them bandaged. They'll soften up and fall off on their own. See a doctor to remove larger scabs.

Ask about growth factors for chronic wounds. Doctors can now help nonhealing wounds from diabetes and impaired circulation with growth-factor solutions. The solutions are prepared from the patient's own blood and applied directly to the wound to promote the growth of new cells and tissue, says Dr. Knighton.

HEARING LOSS

WHEN TO SEE YOUR DOCTOR

- Any hearing loss should be brought to the attention of your physician.

WHAT YOUR SYMPTOM IS TELLING YOU

When it comes to predicting someone's age, you may be better off checking their hearing instead of counting their gray hairs. That's because by age 60, nearly everyone suffers from some hearing loss, and after age 70, they continue to lose hearing steadily.

But there's at least one factor that ensures hearing loss long *before* age-related problems set in. And that's continued exposure to loud noise.

"Noise damage is caused by both the intensity of the sound and the duration of the exposure," says Charles P. Kimmelman, M.D., professor of otolaryngology at Manhattan Eye, Ear and Throat Hospital. "But because the effect of noise damage is cumulative, hearing loss from noise *adds* to the hearing loss you'll get from aging."

In fact, repeated exposure to high-decibel noise—like jet engines, gunshots or sternum-thumping rap music—actually deadens the sensitive nerve endings in your eardrums that help you hear, he says.

Not surprisingly, a ruptured eardrum can also cause temporary hearing loss, says Clough Shelton, M.D., an associate clinical professor of otolaryngology at the University of California, Los Angeles, and a member of the House Ear Institute at the University of Southern California. A number of things can rupture the eardrum, including severe ear infections and sports that cause pressure changes in the ear—scuba diving, parachuting and lifting heavy weights.

Certain diseases can also cause hearing loss. Among them are rheumatoid arthritis, syphilis, Menière's disease and otosclerosis. Menière's disease is a somewhat rare ailment that attacks the inner ear, causing dizziness and tinnitus (ringing in the ear). Otosclerosis, which affects mostly young adults and twice as many women as men, is a disease that causes the growth of calcium in the inner ear. People who have otosclerosis may feel as if one ear is plugged or they're listening to the world from inside a barrel.

Some particularly powerful prescription antibiotics, called aminoglycosides, may bring about hearing loss in some people.

Not all hearing loss is irreversible. In fact, in some cases, the cure is delightfully simple. Sometimes a sudden hearing loss in children is traced to something stuck in the ear. That something can be as simple as a wad of gum or paper.

Other hearing loss culprits include swimmer's ear, earwax buildup and otitis media—a common childhood inflammation of the middle ear, resulting in an accumulation of fluid behind the eardrum.

SYMPTOM RELIEF

Because a wide range of health problems can cause hearing loss, it's a good idea to see your doctor for diagnosis and appropriate treatment. For example, a course of antibiotics may clear up an infection causing the problem. Here are a few other possibilities.

Get a test. If you have even the faintest suspicion that a child may be hard of hearing, make an appointment with a pediatrician. Early detection and correction can actually prevent learning disabilities in children, says David Marty, M.D., a Jefferson, Missouri, otolaryngologist and author of *The Ear Book*. "Maybe a child's not doing well in school, or a child who's doing well in school starts bringing home failing grades—that's not necessarily the sign of a behavioral disorder," says Dr. Marty. It could simply mean that the child is not hearing what the teacher is saying, he explains. Treating the hearing loss may improve the child's academic performance as well.

Tune in to a hearing aid. When normal conversation is difficult to understand, it may be time to consider using a hearing aid, says Dr. Kimmelman. But the real question is how much you're willing to pay. "They come in all types, from compacts to limousines—generally from a few hundred dollars to about $2,000," he says. Even the least expensive hearing aid will do a fair job of amplifying sound. But by spending a little more you get better construction, higher fidelity and in some cases, the ability to remove background noise, says Dr. Kimmelman. By law, you don't need to see a doctor to buy a hearing aid, but it still may be a good idea. "The right way to do it is to see an ear specialist who can review the history of the problem and make sure that a proper diagnosis has been reached so that there are no serious medical problems underlying the complaint," say Dr. Kimmelman.

Get an electronic boost. If you're having a hard time hearing your television or radio, you might consider a set of earphones, says Dr. Kimmelman.

Consider surgery. If you have otosclerosis, an operation called a stapedectomy may be an option, says Dr. Marty. "The doctor will remove a small bone in the inner ear and generally replace it with a stainless steel wire prosthesis or some kind of plastic tube prosthesis that allows you to hear," he says.

Protect your ears. Wearing earplugs when you're working in the yard or participating in hobbies that create noise may seem inconvenient—but so is going deaf. Earplugs can be effective at protecting your ears if you frequently use a gas-powered leaf blower or a chainsaw or ride a snowmobile. These activities are all potentially damaging to your ears, says Jack Vernon, Ph.D., professor of otolaryngology and director of the Oregon Hearing Research Center at the Oregon Health Sciences Center in Portland.

But it might be best to avoid some activities—like loud concerts—altogether. The average rock concert generates 140 decibels of noise, nearly as much as a jet engine. "People who go to these events will regret it when they're older, because they're getting excessive exposure and damage already," says Dr. Kimmelman.

Get the wax out . . . carefully. Resist the urge to go after a plug of earwax with a cotton swab. You run the risk of puncturing an eardrum. (For tips on safe earwax removal, see Earwax Buildup on page 178.)

HEARING VOICES

WHEN TO SEE YOUR DOCTOR

- See your doctor any time you hear imaginary voices.

WHAT YOUR SYMPTOM IS TELLING YOU

We all talk to ourselves. If you drop a plate of food in your lap at a holiday gathering, you might think to yourself, "Boy, what a jerk I am." But you know you have a medical problem if a mysterious voice in your head suddenly replies, "Yes, you are."

"Hearing voices can be a serious symptom of psychosis or neurological impairment. It shouldn't be taken lightly," says Paul Fink, M.D., chairman of psychiatry at Albert Einstein Medical Center in Philadelphia.

Some doctors suspect that imaginary voices are actually a person's own inner thoughts, which for some reason develop a distinct pattern that the person identifies as a separate voice or voices. "When people with serious mental illnesses hear voices, they believe that the voices are real. They'll say, 'There's a voice telling me I should kill myself,' or 'There's a man telling me to kill my mother,'" Dr. Fink says. "They don't think it's a hallucination, and they feel like they have to do what the voice says."

More often than not, hearing voices is a symptom of schizophrenia, a serious mental illness that usually appears in early adulthood. But it also could be a sign of mania, Alzheimer's disease, depression or drug and alcohol abuse. On the other hand, it could be something as simple as a defective hearing aid or a side effect of medication.

And some people, particularly when they're profoundly depressed or just falling asleep, can hear voices calling their name. Doctors don't know what causes this phenomenon, but they believe that it is harmless.

"It has happened to me just once in my adult life," says Betsy Comstock, M.D., a professor of psychiatry at Baylor College of Medicine in Houston. "I was just walking down the street doing some shopping when I thought I heard my mother calling to me—and no one ever spoke my name like my mother did. A lot of people have that experience, but we don't think it's any cause for alarm."

Symptom Relief

If you hear imaginary voices regularly, you should see a physician as soon as possible, Dr. Fink says. After a thorough medical examination, your doctor may determine that you need to see a psychiatrist, who may want to prescribe antipsychotic or antidepressant medication. On the other hand, your doctor might be able to help you tame the voices in your head with a couple of simple remedies.

Evaluate your nonpsychiatric drugs. Hearing voices can be a side effect of certain medications, including anticonvulsants. Make a list of all the medications you are currently taking—prescription and over-the-counter—and ask your doctor if any of these drugs alone or in combination could be causing your problem.

Tune out. Although it's extremely rare, doctors have found that a few people who wear hearing aids and who have reported hearing voices actually are picking up transmissions from nearby radio stations through their hearing aids. If you wear a hearing aid and believe you are hearing voices, ask your audiologist to check your hearing aid to make sure it is working properly.

HEARTBEAT IRREGULARITIES

WHEN TO SEE YOUR DOCTOR

- You experience skipped beats, extra beats, flip-flops or pounding of the heart several times a week or more.
- Your heart fluctuates wildly from less than 50 beats to more than 100 beats per minute.
- See your doctor immediately if your heartbeat takes off chaotically at rates well above 100 beats per minute when you're not even exerting yourself.

What Your Symptom Is Telling You

As any musician can tell you, every band or orchestra needs a good rhythm section to lay down a solid beat and keep good time. If any of the players are out of tempo or rhythm, the entire band can rush ahead, lag behind or just plain fall apart mid-tune.

You can think of the heart as a little five-piece combo: two upper chambers (the atria) pump incoming blood over to two lower chambers (the ventricles), which pump it back out to the lungs and body. Instead of a drummer, a built-in pacemaker called the sinus node keeps the upper and lower chambers moving and grooving by sending out tiny electrical signals. But if something should disrupt those impulses, the heart's rhythms become inconsistent. If it's abnormally slow—below 60 beats per minute—doctors call it *bradycardia*. And if it's abnormally fast—over 100 beats per minute—they call it *tachycardia*.

Cardiologists call these disturbances in normal heart rhythms *arrhythmias,* and they can originate anywhere in the electrical pathway from the sinus node to the atria to the ventricles. Sometimes these disturbances are brief, sometimes sustained. Some can be alarming; others pass unnoticed.

"Many arrhythmias arise from external factors such as tobacco, stimulants, illegal drugs and certain medications," says Mark E. Josephson, M.D., professor of medicine at Harvard Medical School and director of Harvard-Thorndike Electrophysiology Institute and Arrhythmia Services at Beth Israel Hospital in Boston. "Some are associated with serious underlying conditions such as thyroid disease, anemia, coronary heart disease or heart failure. But a great many are simply normal occurrences in healthy hearts while sleeping, exercising or undergoing stress or emotion."

When a drummer misses a beat or two or the band plays a bit too loudly, you may not notice or even care. The same is true with heart palpitations—a sensation that the heart is pounding, skipping a beat or throwing in extra beats.

"Palpitations are just electrical misfires, often anxiety-

or stress-related, that everyone experiences from time to time, and unless they occur with great frequency, they are often harmless and insignificant," says Lou-Anne Beauregard, M.D., assistant professor of medicine at Cooper Hospital/University Medical Center in Camden, New Jersey.

Physicians are more concerned with other arrhythmias, such as those that originate in the upper portions of the heart. A "sick" or malfunctioning sinus node can produce bradycardias, tachycardias or alternate between the two. An atrium can take off in brief but regular discharges of 200 beats per minute—a condition known as paroxysmal supra-ventricular tachycardias (PSVT). Or it can go into fibrillation—an even faster, disorganized firing from multiple sites in the atrium. This broad class of tachycardias (rapid heart rhythms), which arise from the upper chamber of the heart, are known as supra-ventricular arrhythmias.

"Supra-ventricular arrhythmias are common, treatable and usually benign," says Jeremy Ruskin, M.D., director of the Cardiac Arrhythmia Service at Massachusetts General Hospital in Boston. Occasionally, people with serious heart disease experience supra-ventricular arrhythmias, which can (rarely) degenerate into life-threatening arrhythmias, he says. These life-threatening arrhythmias are those occurring in the ventricles. Ventricular tachycardias can flutter and flap at speeds well over 200 beats per minute and are almost always indicative of underlying heart disease. If the ventricle should fibrillate, the beats become so chaotic that the heart loses all effectiveness and shuts down. Ventricular fibrillation is the leading cause of sudden death in America.

SYMPTOM RELIEF

Keep in mind that the normal heartbeat range is 60 to 100 beats per minute, with some dips into the 40s and 50s being common for well-conditioned athletes. And any-time you find your heart doing the cha-cha when it should be playing a waltz, it's wise to see a doctor to confirm that there's no serious problem. Here are a few things to be aware of.

Find a distraction. Don't obsess over palpitations; find something to get them off your mind. You're more likely to notice and become anxious over them when you're alone and doing nothing, according to Dr. Beauregard. "People lying awake in bed often have an enhanced awareness, which increases as they absorb themselves in their own heartbeats," she says. Read a book; watch TV. Any new focus will do.

Check your medicine cabinet. The wrong dosage of medication can make your pulse rise or fall suddenly. So can certain over-the-counter products like antihistamines and asthma relievers. But if you are taking heart medication, the change in pulse may well be the desired result. Check with a doctor to see if you should halt, change or maintain your medication.

Cut back on your caffeine. Too many cups of coffee in the morning may lead to palpitations or tachycardias in the afternoon. Limit your intake of all caffeine beverages: coffee, tea and colas.

Practice good clean living. Tobacco and alcohol may not stunt your growth, but they can cause some crazy tachycardias and should be avoided, says Dr. Josephson. And stay away from illegal drugs. "Cocaine and marijuana users are frequent visitors to the emergency room with cases of erratic heartbeats," he adds.

Ask about anti-arrhythmic drugs. Your doctor can tell you whether you need drugs for bothersome heart palpitations. Commonly prescribed medications for managing atrial and/or ventricular tachycardias include quinidine, procainamide, digitalis drugs and beta blockers.

Hire a new drummer. The most effective means of controlling irregular heartbeat is by surgically implanting an artificial pacemaker, which takes over for the sinus node. These devices may be used as permanent or temporary measures to correct the rhythm.

HEARTBURN

WHEN TO SEE YOUR DOCTOR

- You persistently suffer from heartburn.
- If you're suffering from sudden, severe chest pain, treat it as a medical emergency and get help immediately.

WHAT YOUR SYMPTOM IS TELLING YOU

For all its fiery bluster, heartburn often amounts to nothing more than a false alarm. That's because most heartburn is just a couple of spoonfuls of stomach acid seeping back into your esophagus.

Of course, heartburn isn't a big concern as long it *is* heartburn—and not a heart attack.

"I can't tell you how many people show up in a hospital emergency room thinking they are having heartburn when they're really having a heart attack," says Jorge Herrera, M.D., assistant professor of medicine at the University of South Alabama College of Medicine in Mobile and member of the American Gastroenterological Association and the American College of Gastroenterology. "If it seems like you're having chest pain or pain unlike any heartburn you've ever experienced before, it *could* be a heart attack, especially if you're experiencing other symptoms, like shortness of breath, pain in your left arm or sweating."

But more often than not your pain isn't because your heart is starving for oxygen. It's because your esophagus (the food tube that leads to the stomach) is being painted with acid. How did that acid get there? There's a little "door" between your esophagus and your stomach. That door is called the lower esophageal sphincter (LES), and it opens to let food in and shuts to keep it there. Sometimes the LES swings back open and acid escapes.

A lot of different factors can reopen the door. There are

foods that don't agree with you (citrus, peppermint, chocolate and fatty and spicy foods top the list). Or just eating too much food of any kind. (In fact, overweight people are more prone to heartburn than thinner people, probably because they overeat). Caffeine, smoking and alcohol are common causes. Certain medications can cause distress when taken with food. And some, like aspirin, are simply hard on the stomach. Even wearing too tight a belt can force stomach acid upward. Heartburn is also a common complaint among pregnant women.

If your heartburn is persistent and you can't connect it with anything you're putting into your mouth, it could be the symptom of an ulcer. Or it could be the result of a hiatal hernia, which is actually a small portion of the stomach that has slipped through an opening in the diaphragm, says Andrew H. Soll, M.D., a professor of medicine and director of the affiliated training program for gastroenterology at the University of California at Los Angeles and chief of gastroenterology at Veterans Administration Hospital.

SYMPTOM RELIEF

If you have any hint that what you're experiencing is something other than heartburn, seek medical help right away. Also, if taking an over-the-counter antacid doesn't calm the fire within 15 minutes, you should make an appointment with your doctor for a checkup.

You should also see a doctor if your heartburn is chronic or your stomach is so sensitive that anything you eat makes you feel ill. He will evaluate you for a possible ulcer or hiatal hernia. Both can be treated with drugs, although sometimes surgery is necessary. (For more information on ulcers, see page 586.)

But if it's obvious that you've had heartburn, and you're having it again, here's what you can do.

Take an antacid. Most antacids contain chemicals that quickly absorb excess stomach acid, vanquishing a case of heartburn in no time, says Dr. Herrera.

Grab a glass of moo. Relief is as close as your refrigerator. Drinking three to four ounces of skim milk temporarily neutralizes stomach acid, says Dr. Herrera. If you're out of milk, try a glass of water. It might temporarily wash the acid out of your esophagus, he says.

Monitor your medicine. A number of medications can kick your stomach's acid production into high gear, says Dr. Soll. These include aspirin, other nonsteroidal anti-inflammatory painkillers (NSAIDs), certain heart and blood pressure medications and asthma medications. "It's unlikely that the drug alone will give you heartburn," says Dr. Herrera. "But if you are already suffering from occasional heartburn, your drugs may push you into frequent bouts."

If you suffer recurring heartburn, make a list of all prescription and over-the-counter medications you are currently taking and show it to your doctor. Your doctor may be able to suggest some alternatives.

Kick those butts. Lighting up increases stomach acid production and weakens the muscle at the end of the esophagus that is supposed to prevent stomach acid from creeping in, says Dr. Herrera.

Round up the usual suspects. Need another reason to avoid fat and alcohol? Working independently or together, the members of this double health threat can weaken the muscles that open and close your stomach, says Wendell Clarkston, M.D., assistant professor and director of the Fellowship Training Program in Gastroenterology and Hepatology at the Saint Louis University School of Medicine. "If you want to really suffer, have a double cheese pizza, a couple of beers and a few peppermints," he says.

Lose some weight. Pressure from excess weight can push stomach acid where it doesn't belong, says Dr. Soll.

Sit up straight. When you lie down within a few hours after eating a meal, stomach acid has a way of creeping into your esophagus and attacking sensitive nerve endings there, causing pain, says Dr. Clarkston.

Prop yourself up. Eating just before bed is never a good idea, but if you can't help it, you can avoid an upset stomach if you prop the head of your bed up about six inches with a couple of bricks or wooden blocks. Gravity will help prevent stomach acid from working its way into your esophagus, says Dr. Clarkston. This is a particularly helpful technique for women in the late stages of pregnancy.

Using an extra pillow will *not* work, by the way. It will make you bend at the middle and increase pressure on your LES.

Loosen up. Because skin-tight clothes and severely cinched belts can also push acid from the stomach into the esophagus, you should steer clear of tight-fitting outfits, says Dr. Clarkston.

HICCUPS

WHEN TO SEE YOUR DOCTOR

- Hiccups persist for more than one hour.
- You've been having bouts of hiccups several times a day or several days a week.
- You also have chest pain, heartburn or difficulty swallowing.

WHAT YOUR SYMPTOM IS TELLING YOU

Boo!

Still have them, eh? Ah well, the old sneak-up-from-behind-and-scare-the-ever-lovin'-bejeebers-out-of-them trick never was a sure-fire remedy for the hiccups anyway.

And what is? For all the advances of medicine over the years and decades, science still has not found a sure cure for those annoying little spasms that temporarily make you sound like the town drunk.

A normal hiccup is just an audible tic. The phrenic nerve that excites the muscles of the diaphragm, for reasons unknown, lapses into uncontrollable spasms, says Ravinder K. Mittal, M.D., an associate professor of medicine in the

Department of Internal Medicine at the University of Virginia in Charlottesville.

The esophagus also can be provoked into involuntary contractions, according to John Renner M.D., president of Consumer Health Information Research Institute in Kansas City, Missouri. An improper swallow or food stuck in your esophagus triggers a nerve spasm in the esophagus near where it meets the stomach.

Hiccups come and go innocently enough, but sometimes when they persist, they indicate a more serious medical problem, according to Monte Bobele, Ph.D., associate professor in the counseling psychology department of Our Lady of the Lake University in San Antonio. People recovering from gastric or back surgery often gasp their way through extended bouts of hiccups. Others get post-surgery hiccups in reaction to an anesthetic.

Developing kidney failure may bring on continual or recurring hiccups, Dr. Mittal says, as could a growing abscess or tumor in or near the chest, diaphragm or esophagus.

And some people develop hiccups for psychological reasons, Dr. Bobele says. In a reaction similar to the paralysis some soldiers suffer when they're afraid of combat, these people subconsciously give themselves hiccups as a way to avoid something disagreeable.

SYMPTOM RELIEF

To cure hiccups you need to stop the spasm in the diaphragm or esophagus. You can do this by either distracting the person's attention from the affliction or making him or her gasp. That's usually all it takes.

"If hiccups don't go away, you're trying too hard to make them go away," Dr. Bobele says. "You're focusing on your chest and actually tightening your diaphragm. But tensing up and trying to suppress that next expected hiccup only worsens it." Here's how to do it right.

Swallow something bitter. Ingesting something with an overwhelming taste might jar you out of your spasm, Dr. Mittal says. Try sucking on a lemon or swallowing a teaspoon of vinegar.

Heed a gag order. Put your finger down your throat as if you're forcing yourself to throw up, Dr. Mittal says, although don't go so far as to actually vomit. A little gagging might be enough to disrupt the rhythm of your hiccups.

Drown them. Steadily drinking a large glass of water with regular, evenly paced swallows could disrupt the hiccups' rhythm, Dr. Renner says. It also will help wash away any food at the bottom of your throat that might be irritating the nerve down there.

Drink upside down. "Bottoms up" takes on a whole new meaning with this hiccup cure. Bend at the waist over a sink, Dr. Bobele says, and drink water from the side of the glass farthest from your body.

Attempt some scare fare. Startling the hiccup victim—by suddenly popping a bag or shouting boo provides a momentary jolt that can interrupt the spasm, Dr. Bobele says.

Leave 'em hanging by a thread. A popular cure for infant hiccups among Hispanics in southern Texas calls for placing a red thread or strip of red cloth in the middle of baby's forehead, near the bridge of the nose. "Maybe for the baby, crossing his eyes or diverting his attention is all that's needed to stop the hiccups," Dr. Bobele says.

Sweeten it. Sprinkle some sugar on the back of your tongue and swallow, Dr. Bobele says. Or mix a teaspoonful into a shot of bitters and gulp it down.

Pull on it. Open your mouth wide the next time you're under a hiccup attack, grasp your tongue, give it a gentle yank and hold on to it for several seconds. That's the cure that was preferred by President Kennedy's personal physician, Dr. Bobele says. (Attempting to pronounce "Ich bin ein hiccupper" with tongue in hand is optional.)

Put money on it. Finally, Dr. Bobele's favorite remedy for the average hiccup, which he says has yet to fail: The next time someone starts to hiccup, take out a $5 bill, place it on the table and bet the hiccupper that he or she can't hiccup again in the next minute. Without fail, the person can't release another real hiccup.

"Once you stop trying to make them go away, you bring a whole other set of muscles into play, and the spasms stop," Dr. Bobele says. "It works all the time. I haven't lost money yet."

Go for tests. If your hiccups are irritatingly frequent or the spells exceptionally long, your doctor probably will take x-rays after giving you some barium liquid to drink to highlight any obstruction in your esophagus, Dr. Renner says. To quell severely persistent hiccups not caused by some obstruction, your doctor may prescribe a medication depending on where he thinks the problem lies.

HIP PAIN

WHEN TO SEE YOUR DOCTOR

- After an injury, even a minor one, your hip pain persists or grows worse.
- The pain is interrupting your sleep or interfering with your work or home activities.
- You also have open sores on your feet, or leg pain.

WHAT YOUR SYMPTOM IS TELLING YOU

When you say hip and your doctor says hip, you may be talking about two different places. To most people, hip pain can refer to pain in the side of the upper thigh or the side of the upper buttock—the area right around the curvy part in women. But to a doctor, hip pain means pain felt in the groin—where the hip joint itself lies.

Hip pain can be tricky to decipher for other reasons. You can feel pain deep in the hip joint itself. You can feel pain in the tissues around the joint—in a bursa, for example. (The bursae are fluid-filled sacs that cushion the bony part of the hip close to the surface. If a hip's bursae become inflamed, you have bursitis.) There are tendons around the hip, too, tying it to the legs and the back. And these can also become inflamed (often after an injury), a condition called tendinitis. And the pain in your hip doesn't have to start there. You might have "referred" pain—you *feel* it in your hip, but the source is somewhere else, like your back. The cause of hip pain can even be outside your body: a too-soft mattress or ill-fitting shoes.

Arthritis is a common cause of hip pain. Usually, it's osteoarthritis—the "wear-and-tear" kind that affectsalmost everyone to some degree as they get older. Osteoarthritis in your hip is particularly likely to be a problem if you've ever suffered a fractured hip or pelvis. It's possible, too (though less common), that rheumatoid arthritis is making its presence known in your hip. This is the potentially disabling type that usually strikes when you're young.

Occasionally, a structural defect is at the root of hip pain. A curved spine or one leg that is slightly shorter than the other can cause your hip to hurt.

While carrying extra weight is not exactly a structural defect, your hip doesn't know that. Extra pounds can contribute to hip pain no matter what the cause.

SYMPTOM RELIEF

Hip pain is a hindrance and a hassle—no doubt about it. Fortunately, there are many ways to relieve it.

Use heat to soothe. Moist heat is your first ally against hip pain, because moisture helps the heat penetrate further, says William Loomis, D.O., a Spokane, Washington, osteopathic physician and president of the American Association of Orthopedic Medicine. Soak a towel in hot water, wring it out and place it over your hip for 20 minutes three or four times a day, he suggests. You might want to place a dry towel on top of the wet one to help hold in the heat. Or you can use a moist heating pad.

Take it easy. You should cut back on exercise (but not totally eliminate it) for a few weeks when the pain is at its worst, says Robin Dore, M.D., a rheumatologist in private practice in Anaheim, California. Give yourself a chance to heal. Perform only stretching, not weight-bearing exercises.

Smooth on a deep-heating ointment. Both the ointment itself and the soothing rub will ease tight hip muscles. Try Ben-Gay, Flex-all 454 or Eucalyptamint, available at most pharmacies. Never use menthol-containing ointments with a heating pad, however, as serious burns may result.

Make that a massage. Whether it's your own hands or a spouse's, massage is a masterful healer for hip pain, says Dr. Loomis. "Massage focuses on surrounding tissues, where so much of the pain originates, rather than the joint," he says. "Since there are so many kinds out there, from Swedish to Shiatsu, you should experiment to find out which gives you the most relief."

Ask about medicines. If over-the-counter standards like aspirin and acetaminophen haven't eased your pain, your doctor may prescribe stronger medicines. Your doctor may also recommend cortisone injections or tablets, Dr. Loomis says. "It's great for quick reduction of inflammation within the first few days after an injury."

Sleep in comfort. Avoid lying on the painful hip, suggests Dr. Dore. And for softer support, use a foam egg crate mattress over your regular mattress.

Walk in the right shoes. Buy *running* shoes for walking—not walking or aerobic or cross-training shoes. Running shoes are extra light and specially designed to increase stability of the foot, says Bill Arnold, M.D., rheumatologist and chairman of the Department of Medicine at Lutheran General Hospital in Park Ridge, Illinois.

Customize your cane. If you need a cane or walker for extra steadiness, be sure it's the right size, suggests Earl Marmar, M.D., an orthopedic surgeon at Einstein Medical Center, director of the Einstein/Moss Joint Replacement Center and assistant clinical professor of orthopedic surgery at Temple University in Philadelphia. "If Grandpa's cane from Ireland is the wrong size for you, it will increase your hip pain," he says. Ask your doctor to refer you to a medical supply store where you can be properly measured.

Lose some weight. It's easy to overlook as a cause, but excess body weight can greatly increase hip pain, says Dr. Marmar. "Every time you take a step, two to three times your body weight goes through the hip in terms of the pressure exerted on the joint," he explains. "Each pound lost represents two to three pounds less pressure on your hip."

Pinpoint your pain. If you do go to your doctor for hip pain, be prepared to talk about *exactly* where it hurts and when. Tell your doctor what kind of pain you're experiencing—whether it's dull or sharp, whether it comes or goes, whether it hurts more when you're moving or still, and what kinds of movements seem to make it worse.

Don't get testy. If your doctor suspects arthritis, you may need to undergo several diagnostic tests, as there are over 100 types of arthritis, says Dr. Marmar. Be prepared for a bone scan or perhaps MRI (magnetic resonance imaging). Your doctor may also prescribe anti-inflammatory medicines and refer you to a physical therapist for exercises and heat and ultrasound treatments.

Examine your architecture. If a curved spine or slightly shorter leg has altered your gait, you may be unaware of it. Here's a home test from Sidney Block, M.D., a rheumatologist in private practice in Bangor, Maine: Stand undressed with your back to a mirror and a hand mirror angled over your shoulder so you can see yourself from the rear. Or ask a family member to look at you from the rear. If the height of your knees seems unequal, if your pelvis seems tilted downward in one direction or if your back looks curved, you may have discovered the problem.

Fortunately, your gait is correctable—usually quite easily. You may need a prescription shoe lift or just an over-the-counter lift inside one shoe, Dr. Block says. If the difficulty is severe, your doctor will refer you to an orthopedist or othotist (a physical therapist who specializes in braces, special shoes and other appliances).

Go for repairs. Usually, a hip fracture will require surgical repair, says Dr. Marmar. One procedure preserves your natural bone and implants a pin in the hip to strengthen it. For a more serious fracture, or even severe arthritis, a surgeon may remove the affected joint and replace the hip entirely with a prosthesis.

An infection in the hip may require surgery as well as intravenous antibiotics, Dr. Marmar says.

And in the unlikely event that a tumor has caused your

hip pain, after the biopsy you will be treated with some
combination of radiation, chemotherapy and surgery.

See also Joint Inflammation; Joint Pain

HIVES

WHEN TO SEE YOUR DOCTOR

- Your face, eyes or throat begins to swell.
- You have frequent or persistent hives.
- Your symptom lasts for more than one day and is
  accompanied by a fever or other ill feeling.
- Your hives turn to blisters.

WHAT YOUR SYMPTOM IS TELLING YOU

Who named this obnoxious type of rash? It must have
been someone who felt as if a colony of bees had
swarmed under their skin.

You know you have hives if you otherwise feel well but
your skin seems to be having a raucous party that moves
from one place to another. Hives are bumpy, red, itchy
patches that go away in less than a day (more likely hours).
But the bumps, called wheals, often reappear elsewhere,
explains Glenn Kline, M.D., allergist and assistant clinical
professor of pediatrics at the University of Texas at
Houston. They're raised because histamine, a chemical in
the body, squeezes fluid out of blood vessels and it collects
under the skin.

Hives can be acute (a one-shot deal) or chronic (they last
for weeks on end or sometimes needle a person for years),
Dr. Kline explains. Anyone can get hives, but they often run
in families and are likely to prickle allergy-prone people
who have hay fever, dust mite allergies and eczema.

Acute hives often are allergic reactions to things you eat or touch. Artificial flavorings, colorings and preservatives, for example, are a common cause of hives, says Ivor Caro, M.D., a dermatologist and associate professor of medicine at the University of Washington School of Medicine in Seattle. Hives caused by bee stings are also acute; they usually go away in a few hours.

Some people's hands erupt in hives when they handle certain foods—tomatoes and some meats, for example. Remarkably, they often can *eat* those foods with no problem, says Arthur Daily, M.D., associate clinical professor of dermatology at Brown University in Providence, Rhode Island.

Occasionally, hives are even caused by "nerves" or stressful situations. "For example, during finals, I see a lot of students with hives," says Dr. Kline.

Other major causes: Viruses and certain diseases, such as lupus; medications, such as antibiotics and aspirin; sunlight; heat; cold; pressure (as in the pressure of a chairback when you sit, or a tight waistband); exercise and sweating. But virtually *anything* can cause hives.

SYMPTOM RELIEF

Often the cause of acute hives is very clear: You eat strawberries and soon you look like one. Chronic hives are usually more mysterious. Their causes are rarely uncovered, even by expert investigators, says Dr. Daily. Fortunately, both kinds of hives respond to a variety of treatments.

Be cool. When hives begin to blossom, you often can save your body from becoming a bouquet of red lumps by taking a cool shower, says Dr. Daily. That's a *cool* shower. Hot water stimulates histamine release and can turn you into a giant, walking wheal.

Have hives, will travel (to a pharmacy). Hives and histamines go hand in hand, so it makes sense to lull those red bumps into submission with oral *anti*histamines, such as Benadryl or Chlor-Trimeton. But if you don't want to be lulled to sleep as well, see a dermatologist for a prescription antihistamine that won't make you sleepy, such as Hismanal and Seldane. Only use prescription antihistamines if your hives are chronic, says Dr. Kline.

Or perhaps you *want* to sleep through your symptoms. In that case, Dr. Kline says to take the common drowsiness-causing antihistamines before going to bed, which will both help you sleep and probably take care of tomorrow's hives.

For stress-caused hives, Dr. Caro often prescribes Doxepin, a combination antihistamine and antidepressant medication. "It's often a tremendous benefit both to treat the hives and to help people relax," he says.

Taste no evil, touch no evil. If you break out in hives after eating specific foods or using various products, stay away from them. If the troublemaker is unknown, do a little hive hunting: Avoid diet drinks and foods with lots of additives. Avoid dusty places (and dust mites). And stop putting chemicals that you might be allergic to on your skin. Possible culprits include makeup, cologne, shampoo and soaps. Reintroduce them one at a time and see if they cause hives.

Use care with clothes. Avoid hive-raising chemicals in fabrics by washing new clothes before you wear them. Also, use mild, unscented detergents, and stop using softener sheets in the dryer, says Dr. Caro.

HOARSENESS

WHEN TO SEE YOUR DOCTOR

- Your hoarseness persists longer than a week.
- You are hoarse even though you have not had a cold, an allergy problem or a recent injury to your voice.
- You also have a lump or bump in your neck, persistent pain while talking or a greenish discharge from your nose.

WHAT YOUR SYMPTOM IS TELLING YOU

Your vocal cords—two small strips of muscle behind your Adam's apple—move apart as you breathe and vibrate back and forth as you speak. When your voice is hoarse, it means something is keeping the vocal cords from coming fully together or interfering with the way they vibrate.

That something is usually swelling—from hours of happy howling at your son's football game (he won but you lost your voice), talking over loud background noise, yelling at your kids or even singing out of your natural range.

People who use (or abuse) their voices a great deal can develop tiny nodules on their vocal cords that produce hoarseness. These nodules are so common that doctors often name the condition after the professionals they treat. Singers', speakers', ministers' and teachers' nodules have been joined by one doctor's favorite— aerobic dance in- structors' nodules. And in children, they're appropriately named screamers' nodules.

Of course, abusing or simply overusing your vocal cords is not the only thing that can cause hoarseness. A sinus infection or an upper respiratory infection such as a cold may swell the vocal cords, causing common laryngitis. And any condition that causes coughing or repeated throat clearing can also lead to hoarseness.

Another common cause of hoarseness is nighttime acid reflux—excess stomach acid that seeps up the esophagus into your throat while you sleep. What's tricky about this type of reflux is that you may not know you have it. One clue is unusually pungent morning breath. So if you have unexplained hoarseness *and* very bad morning breath, nighttime reflux may be the problem.

Allergies can be an indirect cause of hoarseness, since they cause the coughing, mouth breathing and postnasal drip that can inflame vocal cords. And substances that you may not be allergic to, like cigarette smoke and chemical fumes, can also irritate the vocal cords and cause hoarse- ness.

And all that cigarette smoke can cause hoarseness another way: By producing a tumor or growth on the vocal cords, a problem that hits smokers more than anyone else.

And no matter what the cause of your hoarseness, dry air makes it worse.

SYMPTOM RELIEF

You don't have to be banished from the choir forever. There are many ways to treat hoarseness and get your instrument back in tune.

Rest your voice. Total silence is the most healing gift you can give your worn-out voice, says Howard Levine, M.D., director of the Mount Sinai Nasal Sinus Center in Cleveland. At the least, avoid the extremes—whispering and shouting. "Whispering puts tremendous stress on the vocal cords," Dr. Levine says. "If you *must* speak, you're better off using a soft voice."

Humidify, inside and out. "Inhaling the steam from a good old hot shower is one of the best treatments," says Glenn Bunting, a senior speech pathologist at the Massachusetts Eye and Ear Infirmary in Boston. Or try a steam inhaler. "It's like getting a facial," he says. You also might consider using a humidifier in your bedroom to offset the damage from dry indoor heat, he adds.

You need to get enough water *inside* your body, too. He suggests this guideline for healthy water intake: Increase your water consumption until your urine is clear. If you're taking vitamins like beta-carotene or medications that change the color of your urine, then simply consume 10 to 12 eight-ounce glasses of water daily.

Invite a chicken to lunch. If your hoarseness is from a cold, try chicken soup. "There's a good scientific basis for chicken soup," says Dr. Levine. The heat creates humidity, and the garlic is a good mucus thinner. If chicken soup isn't your favorite dish, he suggests taking a garlic supplement. Follow the manufacturer's suggestions for the recommended amount.

Thin secretions. Robitussin syrup is good for thinning

out mucus, says Dr. Levine. But avoid antihistamines, which have a drying effect. A decongestant can also help reduce the flow of mucus, he says, but if you have a heart condition, check with your doctor before taking them. Certain oral decongestants may increase blood pressure.

Avoid aspirin. If your cold has produced a lot of inflammation, aspirin can cause more bruising of the vocal cords, says Dr. Levine, which can make your hoarseness worse. Choose a nonaspirin pain reliever instead.

Control your cough. Use a cough suppressant and expectorant to prevent coughing from further damaging your vocal cords, says C. Thomas Yarington, M.D., clinical professor of otolaryngology at the University of Washington in Seattle.

Don't gargle. Contrary to popular belief, gargling with mouthwash actually makes hoarseness worse, says David Alessi, M.D., an otolaryngologist in Los Angeles. Most mouthwashes contain alcohol, which irritates mucous membranes and dehydrates vocal cords. The gargled liquid doesn't actually get anywhere near the vocal cords, and the action of gargling itself is harmful. It will bang your vocal cords together and increase swelling.

Skip that drink. The alcohol in your cocktail has the same drying effect as the alcohol in a mouthwash, Dr. Alessi adds. If you're hoarse, soothe your throat with a nonalcoholic beverage instead.

Pass on the caffeine. "Stay away from caffeine—in coffee, sodas or chocolate," says Bunting. Caffeine is a drying agent, which won't help those inflamed vocal cords.

When You Need Medical Help

If vocal nodules are severe, or if a growth is discovered, your doctor can help.

Ask for voice therapy. If your vocal nodules don't clear up with voice rest and hoarseness-prevention techniques, your doctor may refer you to a speech pathologist for retraining your voice, says Dr. Levine. Surgery may be considered for severe cases.

Treat a tumor. If your doctor suspects a tumor is causing your hoarseness, don't let fear get in the way of help, says

Dr. Levine. Most vocal cord tumors are small, and if they're found in an early stage, they can usually be cured while preserving your voice.

Preventing Future Problems

Once you've cleared up your hoarseness, here's how to keep that frog on his lily pad.

Warm up. Anyone who uses their voice a great deal is a vocal athlete, says Bonnie Raphael, Ph.D., a vocal coach for the American Repertory Theatre in Cambridge, Massachusetts. And just like any other athlete, they need a warm-up. Try this one before your next speech or concert practice.

Gently stretch your neck muscles by moving your head around slowly while breathing easily and allowing your jaw to hang loosely. Roll your shoulders in a number of different directions, then shake them loosely. Sip some water. Move your tongue around a little both inside your mouth and out. Yawn a few times and hum a bit of a song while feeling the sound vibrations on your gently closed lips. Do the same routine after you've used your voice, and you'll help forestall hoarseness.

Avoid irritants. Cigarette smoke, chemical fumes and wood dust all can produce hoarseness, says Dr. Alessi. Avoid exposure to cigarette smoke—your own and other people's. And wear a filter mask in the workshop to protect your throat and vocal cords from wood dust and fumes, he suggests.

Stop clearing your throat. Clearing your throat is a common habit that can be hard to eradicate, says Bunting. To avoid the hoarseness that can result, try swallowing instead, he suggests. Take a slow, extended swallow as though you are actually swallowing a bite of food. It will alleviate the sensation that something is in your throat, he says. (For more tips on eliminating throat clearing, see page 626.)

Let your voice travel lightly. If you travel in airplanes a lot, your voice will encounter two enemies—very dry air and the necessity of talking above the background noise of the engines. Bunting suggests adding a steamy shower to your pre-airport routine and drinking a lot of water during the flight.

Get up close and personal. If you have to communicate in a noisy environment, "try to do it close up and in the other person's range of listening," says Bunting. "The best position is face-to-face, so they can read your lips."

HOT FLASHES

WHEN TO SEE YOUR DOCTOR

- Your hot flashes are so severe or frequent that they result in fatigue, depression or mood swings, or they interrupt your sleep.

WHAT YOUR SYMPTOM IS TELLING YOU

Many women ease gently into menopause, experiencing only minor symptoms. Their hot flashes may call for no more than a little discreet fanning now and then. For other women, though, these episodes may seem more like close encounters with a blast furnace.

Whether your own hot flashes are experienced as delicate flushes or the engulfing flames, rest assured they're normal. Hot flashes are the body's reaction to a decreased supply of the hormone estrogen, which occurs naturally as women approach menopause.

Not all women experience hot flashes, but more than half do. In some, estrogen production decreases gradually, producing few hot flashes. But for others, the ovaries stop estrogen production abruptly. Or estrogen production may stop and start a couple of times before it ceases altogether. "For these women, hot flashes can be a real roller-coaster ride," says Brian Walsh, M.D., who is an assistant professor of obstetrics/gynecology and reproductive biology at Harvard Medical School and director of the Menopause Unit at Brigham and Women's Hospital in Boston.

If you're suffering from hot flashes, you'll recognize this description from Veronica Ravnikar, M.D., professor of obstetrics and gynecology and director of the Reproductive Endocrine and Infertility Unit at the University of Massachusetts Medical Center in Boston.

"First, you may get an aura—a feeling that something strange is coming on. Then, your internal core temperature drops abruptly. In response, your skin sweats to give off heat and balance itself with the drop in internal temperature.

"You may have one hot flash after another. Most occur at night, and when you do wake up, it will be a bolt upright awakening. Then you get hot and sweaty. Finally, you get so chilled you feel like you need a down comforter to get warm. Sleep is constantly interrupted."

SYMPTOM RELIEF

There's plenty you can do to turn down the heat on those hot flashes.

Solve it with soy. There's a startling difference in the rate of hot flashes and menopausal symptoms between cultures. One study showed that over 50 percent of U.S. and Western European women reported menopausal symptoms, while in Japan it was only 9 or 10 percent.

A joint study done by American, Finnish and Japanese researchers singles out soy products as a possible treatment for menopausal symptoms, says Barry Goldin, Ph.D., a biochemist and associate professor of community health at the Tufts University School of Medicine in Boston. Japanese women eat much more soy than Western women do, he says, and soy foods contain a natural estrogenic compound that may serve as a hot flash reliever.

Try adding soybeans, tofu, miso and other soy products to your diet, Dr. Goldin suggests. An added benefit is that these foods are low-fat.

Get help for bad habits. Doctors have noticed that smokers and heavy drinkers have more difficulty with hot flashes than those who don't, says Dr. Ravnikar. Talk with your doctor about support for beating these bad habits.

Cut back on coffee. Drinking more than a few cups of coffee a day can also turn on hot flashes, says Dr. Ravnikar. "Don't drink excess amounts of coffee," she advises. Any sort of chemical stimulant like caffeine can slightly raise blood pressure and heart rate—and trigger a hot flash.

Breathe them away. A recent study has shown that women given training in slow, deep-breathing exercises were able to reduce their hot flashes by 50 percent. Women participating in the study received eight one-hour treatment sessions every other week. Ask your doctor to refer you to an expert in deep-breathing relaxation techniques. (Many experienced yoga instructors can provide this kind of training.)

Try commonsense cool-downs. Anything that will make you feel cooler and more comfortable is an appropriate response to hot flashes, says June Lavalleur, M.D., director of the division of general gynecology at the University of Minnesota Hospital and Clinic in Minneapolis.

"Wear cotton clothing, which leaves you feeling cooler since it won't stick to your skin," she suggests.

Other relievers? Take a small fan to work to flip on when a hot flash hits, and dress in layers so you can easily shed or add clothing, says Lane Mercer, M.D., chief of gynecology at Northwestern University Medical School in Chicago.

Ease hot flashes with estrogen. If your hot flashes persist, you may want to discuss hormone replacement therapy (HRT) with your doctor. While HRT is not appropriate for everyone, there is no question that it relieves the misery of hot flashes.

"Estrogen comes in pills, transdermal skin patches, vaginal creams and in pellets that can be surgically implanted under the skin of the abdomen," says Dr. Lavalleur.

For women who need medical relief but can't take estrogen because of a current or past breast cancer, the prescription blood pressure medication clonidine may also bring relief, says Dr. Lavalleur.

See also Flushing

HYPERACTIVITY

WHEN TO SEE YOUR DOCTOR

- Your child's overactive and inattentive behavior interferes with his education and constantly aggravates the people with whom he comes in contact.

WHAT YOUR SYMPTOM IS TELLING YOU

Living with a hyperactive child can be like trying to lasso a hummingbird with a thread.

"Often, by the time the parents come to see a doctor about this problem, they have reached the end of their rope," says Paul Horton, M.D., a psychiatrist in Meriden, Connecticut. "They can't stand the child's behavior."

There's a long list of things that can cause hyperactivity in a child, including hearing or vision problems, thyroid disease, learning disabilities, boredom, depression, anxiety, lead poisoning, sexual abuse, mental illness and the side effects of medications. But if your child is hyperactive, the most likely cause is something known as attention-deficit hyperactivity disorder (ADHD). This is a disorder that makes it difficult for a child to concentrate, sit quietly or follow directions. Researchers estimate that it may affect as many as 5 percent of the nation's children.

Boys are up to five times more likely to have ADHD as girls. The disorder may be noticeable even before a child starts walking and can continue into adulthood, says Stephen Sulkes, M.D., associate professor of pediatrics at the University of Rochester Medical Center in New York.

No one is sure what causes ADHD, but some researchers suspect that a portion of the brain called the frontal cortex, which works with other brain regions to control movement and attention, isn't working properly, says Marty Teicher, M.D., Ph.D., a psychiatrist at the Harvard Medical School in Cambridge, Massachusetts.

Symptom Relief

If you suspect that your child is hyperactive, make an appointment with a pediatrician. You may find that something as simple as a new pair of glasses or switching medications will restore peace to the family. But if the diagnosis is ADHD, there's plenty of help available.

"The long-term prognosis for a child with ADHD is good if he receives proper treatment," says Larry Waldman, Ph.D., a psychologist in Phoenix and author of *Who's Raising Whom: A Parent's Guide to Effective Child Discipline.* "They can do fairly well in school and many tend to do very well as adults."

Consider drugs carefully. Your doctor may recommend a combination of drug treatments, including antidepressants and stimulants such as Ritalin. (Certain medications that act as stimulants in adults may improve a child's attentional focus and result in less active behavior.)

However, all of these drugs have side effects. Some are mild, like reduced appetite and insomnia. But in rare cases the side effects can cause facial tics, heart disease or liver damage, Dr. Horton says. Be sure that your doctor explains *all* of the risks of the medication to you. It also may be wise to get a second opinion from another pediatrician or child psychiatrist before allowing your child to take these powerful medications, says William Womack, M.D., associate professor of child psychiatry at the University of Washington School of Medicine in Seattle.

Once your child is on a drug, you should see improvement in his behavior within one to three weeks, depending on the medication. If you notice any side effects or perceive no improvement within that time, insist that the medication be changed or discontinued.

Reward good behavior. A star or point system that allows the child to earn credits for good behavior or completing a task is an effective way to motivate a child with ADHD, Dr. Waldman says. The child can exchange the credits for rewards such as an extra hour of television or a pizza. However, make sure that the tasks are within the child's capabilities and that the rewards are fairly immediate. "If a child doesn't get his reward for three weeks, it's going to be hard for him to remember why he was trying to be good instead of wild," says Ann Saunders, M.D., an assistant professor of psychiatry at Baylor College of Medicine in Houston.

Walk away from trouble. Children with ADHD often have temper tantrums. A simple way to lick this problem is just to walk away when your child has a tantrum, Dr. Waldman says. If the child follows you into another room, lock yourself in the bathroom or your bedroom so that the child can't get to you. Once your child realizes he no longer has an audience for his outburst, the tantrums might end. "It also gives the child the message that he is responsible for calming himself down, and you know that he can really do it," Dr. Saunders says.

Criticize caringly. Even when your child doesn't do a task well or behaves less than perfectly, try to find a way to praise him. "If it takes 30 minutes and several reminders for your child to put on his shoes avoid saying, 'Look how much time you wasted putting your shoes on!' " Dr. Saunders says. "Instead, try saying, 'All right, you finally got your shoes on. I knew you could do it, but let's see if you can do it a little faster next time.' Even if you feel as if the effort was 200 percent yours, don't forget to acknowledge that he accomplished the task."

Slow down, you're going too fast. Many children who have ADHD have no concept of time or speed. "If you ask one of these kids to walk across a room fast, and then walk back slow, you can hardly tell the difference," Dr. Saunders says. Relaxation exercises such as deep breathing or yoga may help. (Your doctor may be able to refer you to someone who teaches yoga to children.) Games like Simon Says, which make the child listen carefully and do a task at the proper time, can teach him how to slow down and pay attention.

Divide and conquer. Children with ADHD have extremely short attention spans and have difficulty following complex directions. That's why it's important to break tasks down into very small bits. If your child has 25 math problems, ask him to do 5 at a time throughout the evening until the homework is completed, suggests Dr. Womack. In addition, when you give your child instructions, keep them short and simple. "If your directions are longer than one sentence, that's too long for these kids."

I

INCONTINENCE

WHEN TO SEE YOUR DOCTOR

- You urinate when you shouldn't, because you have no sensation that your bladder is full.
- Self-help methods don't keep you dry.

WHAT YOUR SYMPTOM IS TELLING YOU

The problem is certainly common enough. Some 30 percent of all women have some inability to restrict their urine. Many have borne children or are past menopause, but age and pregnancy history aren't always a factor, according to Margaret M. Baumann, M.D., associate chief of staff for geriatrics and extended care at the Veterans Administration West Side Medical Center in Chicago. Men are less likely to experience incontinence, but they, too, can be troubled by the problem, especially after a prostate operation.

Incontinence falls into three main categories, although people can leak through because of a combination of causes. First, there's *stress incontinence*, in which you urinate accidentally when you laugh, cough, sneeze or exert yourself. This happens either when the bladder neck shifts position out of reach of the internal muscles that put pressure on it or when those muscles themselves fail to work effectively, because of age, surgery or childbirth.

In *urge incontinence*, the bladder develops a "mind of its own," contracting and emptying whenever full despite an individual's conscious efforts to resist. Stroke, Alzheimer's disease, years of very forcefully urinating to compensate for bladder stones or an enlarged prostate and aging can all cause this kind of incontinence.

"I tell my patients with urge incontinence that their bladder's now acting like a baby's bladder," explains Joseph M. Montella, M.D., an assistant professor and director of the Division of Urogynecology in the Department of Obstetrics and Gynecology at Jefferson Medical College of Thomas Jefferson University in Philadelphia. "It fills to a certain capacity, they feel the urge to go, the bladder contracts on its own, but they cannot control it."

And in *overflow incontinence*, you completely lose the sensation that you have to go. Medications or advancing neurologic disease can deaden the nerves responsible for alerting you to the need, Dr. Montella explains. But you also can develop overflow incontinence from habit—years and years of continually suppressing the urge. "It happens to shift workers, truck drivers, teachers and doctors," he says. Then when they do go, they don't empty completely because the bladder has lost strength. And a half-full bladder takes a lot less time to top off again.

In figuring out why you can't control your urine, doctors look to DIAPPERS—a handy acronym that stands for delirium (neurological problems from aging or stroke); infection (such as cystitis or a sexually transmitted disease); atrophic vaginitis (a deterioration of muscles from hormone deficiency); psychological problems (severe depression); pharmacological causes (prescription drugs such as diuretics, beta blockers, antidepressants and sleeping pills); excess urine (simply drinking a lot of liquids or suffering from a disease like diabetes); restricted mobility (which prevents you from getting to the bathroom before you go) and stool impaction (severe, chronic constipation also affects how you hold your urine). Any of those factors, alone or in combination, should be considered first in trying to help you go only when you want to.

Such common sense causes all too often are overlooked, says Dr. Baumann. "I can't tell you how many doctors don't check for a urinary tract infection," she says. "Drugs, infections, vaginitis—it's amazing what's overlooked."

SYMPTOM RELIEF

Incontinence can be supremely humiliating—for you to discuss with your doctor. "People are embarrassed about it," Dr. Montella says. "Plus, a lot of doctors are not comfortable with the subject because they don't know what to do about it if there's no identifiable source. It's a real gray area." And then there are those commercials for adult diapers. While they have alerted people that the problem exists, he says, he feels they may convey the idea that the only solution is to wear diapers.

Quite the contrary. Incontinence is not a natural part of aging or a woman's fate. Nor is surgery or diapers the only recourse. If you learn what to do and get the right kind of help, you'll almost always be improved, if not cured," says L. Lewis Wall, M.D., Ph.D., an assistant professor of gynecology and obstetrics at Emory University School of Medicine in Atlanta.

It's appropriate to see the doctor for diagnosing and treating this symptom. However, here are several things to consider.

Measure your output. Stopping the flow could be as easy as drinking less liquid. And if it's not, doctors will want at least a 24-hour record of how much and how often you're urinating. You can use a two-liter soda bottle to measure your output. A large volume of urine, say four or five liters, isn't necessarily causing your incontinence, Dr. Baumann says, "but it could be contributing to it."

Look in your medicine cabinet. A whole host of drugs can cause you to urinate more or to relax your pelvic muscles enough to make you lose control over your urination, says Dr. Baumann. These include diuretics, calcium channel blockers, antidepressants, sedatives, certain blood pressure medications and some antihistamines. This is a very likely cause of incontinence in elderly people, she says.

Banishing incontinence may be as easy as taking your water pills for high blood pressure in the morning instead of before you go to bed, says Dr. Baumann. Ask your doctor if any of your prescription or over-the-counter medications could be responsible and whether it's possible to make substitutions. "Usually there are alternatives to medications that contribute to incontinence," Dr. Baumann says.

Muscle up your reflexes. Time-honored Kegel exercises are the mainstay for coping with many kinds of incontinence, Dr. Montella says. If performed properly and diligently, "Kegeling" can bring relief or a cure to between 70 and 90 percent of the people with stress incontinence.

The first time you "Kegel," you can locate the muscles that you're going to be working with by deliberately stopping the flow of urine while you're going to the bathroom. Or insert a finger into your vagina or rectum and try to squeeze it without tensing your abdomen, thighs or buttocks.

This could be difficult to do, especially if the muscles are weak. "Many people can't do Kegel exercises correctly from verbal or written directions," Dr. Baumann says. So if you can't feel the muscles, ask your doctor to refer you to someone who is able to teach you these movements.

A common Kegels prescription is to contract (or squeeze) the muscles ten times in a row for ten seconds and do this three times a day. You'll need between 8 and 12 weeks of concerted effort before you'll see results.

Don't practice when you're actually going to the bathroom, though. "It's a really bad habit to perform Kegels while your bladder's contracting to urinate," Dr. Montella warns. "If it doesn't send urine back up into the kidneys, it can decrease your bladder's capacity by exercising that muscle instead and making it thicker." That could *contribute* to your continence problem.

And make sure to relax fully between contractions. "Physiologically, a muscle that doesn't relax can't contract effectively the next time," Dr. Baumann says.

Take an antihistamine. Minor stress incontinence might be helped simply by taking over-the-counter drugs like Sudafed, Actifed and Contac, Dr. Montella says. Those and other cold preparations contract smooth muscles, like the urethra, that can't be voluntarily controlled. But the effect lasts only a few hours and ends when you stop taking the medication. "They may not help stress incontinence caused by a misplaced bladder neck," he says, "and you shouldn't do this for a long time without a doctor's okay. You can set yourself up for some problems and side effects with long-term use."

Go by the clock. Retraining the bladder to go when you want to, not when it wants to, often can effectively cure (or at least manage) urge and overflow incontinence. You can both expand bladder capacity and force it to empty regularly. First, keep a 24-hour log of when you urinate, how much you urinate and how long you last between going to the bathroom or incontinence accidents. Maybe it'll be an hour, maybe several hours. "You'll see lots of variations," Dr. Baumann says, "so you take the minimum time between episodes and work from there."

For a week or two, whether you really need to or not, go to the bathroom according to your schedule of the minimum time you can last until you leak. "At the very least, if you go by this, you shouldn't run into any problems," Dr. Baumann says.

But, especially as you strengthen your pelvic muscles through Kegels, you can try to expand the periods between urination, starting out with just an extra five or ten minutes every week or two with a goal of being able to hold it in for three to four hours. "If you leak a little, it's okay," Dr. Montella says. Stick to your slowly expanding schedule. "The idea is to hold it and try to suppress that contraction. You're telling your bladder, 'You won't empty until I say so.'"

Approach surgery with caution. Except for stress incontinence caused by a misplaced bladder neck, surgery is a last resort for incontinence problems, according to Dr. Montella. Operations to sever the nerves to the bladder or expand its capacity with a piece of intestine are things "you don't really want to do unless you have to," he says.

Use a siphon. If timed bladder training doesn't help you with overflow incontinence, you might consider self-catheterization, in which you insert a tiny tube through your urethra and into your bladder to drain out the urine. "It's uncomfortable and requires a little coordination," Dr. Montella says, "but people can learn how to do it in ten minutes, and only under a doctor's care."

Call on an expert. Your family doctor may be able to help you deal with your incontinence, but it might be a better idea to try to locate a urologist, gynecologist or urogynecologist in your area who specializes in keeping people dry. Ask your doctor for a referral or contact a medical school in your area for information.

INSOMNIA

WHEN TO SEE YOUR DOCTOR

- You've been having a problem falling asleep almost nightly for more than a few weeks.
- You dread going to bed because you're anxious over your ability to fall asleep.
- You're dead tired during the day and can't concentrate or function adequately.
- You're relying on alcohol or drugs to fall asleep.

WHAT YOUR SYMPTOM IS TELLING YOU

Everyone suffers through an occasional sleepless night. Lying wide awake night after night is another matter. Insomnia is almost always a sign of another problem—either a medical condition or an emotional tumult.

Chronically painful conditions such as arthritis can keep the sandman from your door, as can something as fleeting as an itchy bout of poison ivy. A fight with your spouse can leave you punching the pillow all night, while trouble at work turns into tussling with the covers.

Also, a change in your regular routine can alter your natural biological rhythm enough to cause a problem. Going on dayturn from the night shift can get in the way of a good night's sleep, for example, as can jet lag following a coast-to-coast flight.

Insomnia often starts with a few wide-eyed nights caused by, say, an injury or a minor emotional disturbance, according to Edward Stepanski, Ph.D., a clinical psychologist and director of the insomnia clinic at the Sleep Disorders and Research Center at Henry Ford Hospital in Detroit. Those few sleepless nights create habits that can lead to a long-term problem—you take a nap during the day or a nip at night. You watch TV in bed or raid the fridge at 2:00 a.m. Before you know it, you're doing these things on a regular basis and you've developed what's known as behavioral insomnia.

"All of the things most people do to supposedly improve their sleep will actually worsen it," says Dr. Stepanski. "The original problem goes away, but the insomnia remains. They've developed terrible sleep habits that wouldn't allow anyone to sleep, plus now they're watching the clock and they're very fearful as bedtime approaches." By then, the natural rhythms of the chronic insomniac are so out of whack it's like they're doing the watusi while the band plays that old country waltz.

SYMPTOM RELIEF

If you slept well before, you will sleep again, experts say. But don't expect miracles from a one-night experiment with good sleep habits. "Your sleep probably took a long time to get as bad as it is," Dr. Stepanski says. "It will gradually get better. It isn't going to happen instantly the very first night."

Can't sleep? Then don't go to bed. "If there's one recommendation I would make for insomnia, it's to delay bedtime by an hour, maybe two hours," Dr. Stepanski says. One of the worst practices people follow is to go to bed when they're not really tired. "They don't even feel sleepy, but they think it's time they should go to bed," he says. And few events can tighten the tension like lying in the dark, listening to the bathroom faucet drip and wondering why you can't sleep.

Once you snuggle under the covers, if you don't fall asleep within 20 minutes, get up, leave the bedroom and muddle through something mundane. "Don't sweat it. Go ahead and watch the late show and ride it out," Dr. Stepanski advises.

Practice good sleep habits. Sleep experts like to rattle off a list of what they call sleep hygiene tips: Don't use the bedroom for anything but sleep or sex; get up at the same time every morning regardless of when you retire; don't take naps; exercise in the late afternoon or early evening; don't go to bed hungry. Most people trying to banish insomnia go down the list, trying each item for a day or two, then discarding it and returning to the old habit.

"They end up concluding that none of these things works, but you really have to try them all simultaneously and give them a chance," Dr. Stepanski says. "Instant sleep won't come the very first night you skip an evening cup of coffee or go to bed at 1:00 a.m. rather than midnight."

Warm up with water. A hot bath, whirlpool or Jacuzzi before retiring can relax muscles and warm you up for a sound sleep, says Suzan Jaffe, Ph.D., clinical director of the Sleep Program at Hollywood Medical Center in Florida.

Relax to the max. Gentle, quiet talk or a muscle-kneading massage can soothe the tension beast that scares off the sandman. So can yoga or relaxation training.

See the light. Bright light therapy can help you reset your natural sleep rhythm, especially if jet lag or time-shifting at work has induced the insomnia, Dr. Stepanski says. Try taking a half-hour walk in the early-morning sun. "It sends a message to the body to activate for the day," he says, "and you'll be more prepared to sleep at night."

Don't raid the fridge; don't light a butt. If you wake up in the middle of the night, never smoke a cigarette or go to the kitchen for something to eat. "I can take the best sleepers in the world and wake them up five nights in a row for a sandwich or a cigarette," says Dr. Stepanski. "On the sixth night and thereafter, they'll wake up on their own. Both should be absolutely forbidden in between bedtime and waking time."

Drugs are tough pills to swallow. Sleep physicians are extremely reluctant to prescribe sedatives, Dr. Jaffe says, except in the event of an obvious trauma, such as the death of a spouse, and even then only for a very temporary period. Improper withdrawal from sleeping pills can cause the insomnia the prescription was designed to treat, she says.

What about the occasional use of over-the-counter sleeping pills? "Don't routinely take them," Dr. Jaffe advises. "We don't know the long-term effects of them. But they're absolutely not benign. They contain ingredients that can cause addiction."

INTERCOURSE PAIN

WHEN TO SEE YOUR DOCTOR

- You have recurrent pain with intercourse.
- The pain is preventing you or your partner from enjoying sex.
- The pain is deep within your pelvis and is severe.
- The pain is accompanied by vaginal itching, discharge or dryness.
- You are also experiencing burning with urination.

WHAT YOUR SYMPTOM IS TELLING YOU

Not tonight, dear." You never thought you'd find yourself saying it quite so often. And it's not a headache that's lessening your libido these days. It's that sex is hurting—and you're not sure why.

Often something as simple as an unaccustomed sexual position will bring on pain. If it's only a twinge with a new position, don't worry—just mention it to your doctor at your next checkup, says Roger Smith, M.D., a professor of obstetrics and gynecology at the Medical College of Georgia Hospital and Clinics in Augusta.

Sometimes simple body mechanics can cause pain during intercourse—dryness or perhaps a small (or tense) vaginal opening. And emotional causes are important, too—if sex has become too rushed and stressed to savor, that may contribute to lack of lubrication and pain.

If the pain you feel is mostly on insertion, the most common causes are an inflammation or infection of the vulva or outer vaginal lips. If it hurts more when the penis is thrusting deeply, then a vaginal infection may be the problem.

A bladder or urinary tract infection is also a possible cause of painful intercourse.

SYMPTOM RELIEF

Pain with intercourse is not dangerous to your health, says Dr. Smith. But that's no reason to put up with it. Here's how to help bring pleasure back to lovemaking.

Re-position your positions. "You don't need a trapeze bar in the bedroom," Dr. Smith says. Even a slight change in position may help. "The best positions are where the woman controls the thrusting, whether she's on top or you're lying side to side," he says. "Find positions that are comfortable for you both, both mechanically and psychologically. If you can't find a pain-free position, tell your doctor which positions hurt most and which least. This information will help your doctor find out where to look for the problem."

Relax, don't rush. "If your vaginal muscles are tightening up and preventing intercourse, focus on gentle foreplay," Dr. Smith suggests. Often your sensitive body will respond clearly to emotions—like fear of pregnancy or pain or reluctance to have sex. Don't allow yourself to be rushed, and if your concerns persist, talk to your doctor about them. "Making love doesn't have to include sexual intercourse," Dr. Smith reminds us. "You can be tender and loose, and do things like brush each other's hair for an hour."

Quench the dryness. As you approach menopause, thinning and drying vaginal tissues are a common problem—with several solutions. If you feel dry only occasionally, try a water-based lubricant like K-Y Jelly or Surgilube. For continuing moisture, try one of the newer products like Replens, which brings fluid steadily into your vaginal tissues, suggests David Eschenbach, M.D., professor and chief of the Division of Gynecology at the University of Washington School of Medicine in Seattle. If the problem's chronic, you may want to discuss estrogen replacement therapy with your doctor.

Prevent bladder infections. If burning sensations occur during intercourse *and* urination, it's very possible that you have a urinary tract infection. Once your doctor has examined you, diagnosed a urinary infection and prescribed appropriate treatment, the most important part—preventing repeat infections—is up to you. "Urinate at regular intervals of no less than every three to four hours," says Jack Lapides, M.D., a urologist in Ann Arbor, Michigan. Otherwise, your bladder may stretch, retain urine, become inflamed and be invaded by bacteria.

Heal the herpes. If the herpes virus is at the root of your pain, you should avoid having sex until the outbreak is past. Although herpes needs long-term treatment, it can be urged into remission and even cured, says R. Don Gambrell, Jr., M.D., clinical professor of endocrinology and obstetrics and gynecology at the Medical College of Georgia Hospital and Clinics in Augusta. Your most important cautions during those painful episodes are to "avoid sex during outbreaks and use condoms at all times," he says. (For more information on dealing with vaginal infections, see Vaginal Itching on page 689.)

See also Vaginal Dryness

IRRITABILITY

WHEN TO SEE YOUR DOCTOR

- Your irritability persists more than a week and is adversely affecting your job performance and relationships with your family, friends and co-workers.
- You also feel under constant pressure at home or at work.
- You also have persistent headaches.

WHAT YOUR SYMPTOM IS TELLING YOU

That thick skin you used to have has suddenly worn thin. Gentle teasing from your spouse sparks a rage. A minor traffic snarl provokes a fury. A co-worker's well-intentioned criticism sets you off on a tirade that people in the office whisper about for days. The odd thing is you don't know why you're feeling so out of control.

"Occasional irritability is a normal part of being human," says Paul Horton, M.D., a psychiatrist in Meriden, Connecticut. "Adolescents, for example, go through periods of irritability. One moment they're surly and ten minutes later, they're fine. Parents shouldn't be overly concerned about that because adolescents are like tropical weather—they change from moment to moment.

"But irritability also can go hand in hand with almost any illness. Very often, people who are falling ill will become irritable but don't know why."

Irritability can be a sign of flu, a cold, premenstrual syndrome, fatigue, depression, anxiety, drug or alcohol abuse, stress, diabetes, schizophrenia, Alzheimer's disease, thyroid disease, stroke or brain tumor. It can also be a side effect of certain medications.

SYMPTOM RELIEF

Because so very many things can produce irritability, repeated or persistent bouts should be brought to the attention of your doctor. If you just wake up on the wrong side of the bed, however, or when you feel on edge, try these suggestions.

Identify the cause. If you sense you're more irritable than usual, take a moment to think about what might be causing it. "Identifying a cause can help you realize that your irritability is temporary, and you just need to be more patient and extra careful with people around you for a while. It can help you restrain yourself from doing or saying something you'll regret later," says Betsy Comstock, M.D., a professor of psychiatry at Baylor College of Medicine in Houston. Just knowing that premenstrual syndrome makes you irritable for two days a month every month, for example, can help you keep yourself in check.

Don't hide it. Instead of trying to hide your feelings, warn people around you that you feel grumpy. "People get into trouble when they don't acknowledge their feelings to others. If you don't tell people you're irritable, they'll be absolutely perplexed by your behavior," says Roland D. Maiuro, Ph.D., director of the Anger and Domestic Violence Program at Harborview Medical Center in Seattle. "If I have one of those days, I'll say, 'I just wanted to let you know that I'm not doing to well today. So if I seem irritable, please forgive me.' That can help people understand where you're coming from and defuse the situation."

Take the pause that refreshes. Try doing a task that will distract you from whatever is irritating you. "There's an old saying, 'Busy hands avoid mischief.' Some people just need to keep their hands busy," Dr. Comstock says. "Take a walk, do the laundry, write a letter, water the lawn. You need to do something that's going to reduce your stress and absorb some time—it should take 15 minutes to an hour, depending on how much cooling-off time you need—so that you don't react impulsively."

Do a systems check. Before you confront someone, make sure your thoughts and actions are under control, Dr. Maiuro suggests. Are you thinking in words that exaggerate, such as "always," "should," "ought" or "never"? Are you focusing on what you think of the person rather than solving the problem? Are you having thoughts of revenge or getting back at this person? Are you unable to sit still? Are you speaking loudly and pounding your fist on a table? Do you feel muscle tension in your back or neck? "If you're having any thoughts or feelings like that, then you're probably not ready to deal with the situation," Dr. Maiuro says. "If you confront someone at that point, you're likely to distort or complicate the problem rather than solve it."

Set a time. If someone does irritate you and you sense you'll explode if you start talking about the problem at that moment, try to negotiate a time when you think you can discuss the situation with the other person calmly, Dr. Maiuro says.

Think positive. If you find you're having negative thoughts like, "This is going to be a horrible day," try replacing that thought with positive thoughts, says Dennis Gersten, M.D., a San Diego psychiatrist and publisher of *Atlantis: The Imagery Newsletter*. "If you wake up in a bad mood, then close your eyes for a moment and visualize the day going smoothly and successfully," he says. "Use positive self-talk like 'I wonder what kinds of challenges today will offer me?' 'I wonder what I will learn today?' Repeating positive mood words such as 'connect,' 'go for it' and 'succeed' over and over again in your mind also may help your irritability fade."

J

JAUNDICE

WHEN TO SEE YOUR DOCTOR

- Your skin and the whites of your eyes turn yellow.

WHAT YOUR SYMPTOM IS TELLING YOU

Whoa! What's that you see in the bathroom mirror? A slight yellow/green tinge to the whites of your eyes and your skin? It's a sunny day and the shade is up. You look a little closer. The color change is definitely there...and it's definitely upsetting.

There are a couple of things that can give the *skin* a yellowish tinge—eating too many carrots for example. But only true jaundice turns the skin and the whites of the eyes yellow and even makes urine a dark tea or coffee color, according to William B. Ruderman, M.D., chairperson of the Department of Gastroenterology at the Cleveland Clinic–Florida in Fort Lauderdale.

Actually, this color change can be good news if you act on it. That's because jaundice is your body's way of alerting you to a liver infection or blockage of your bile duct. Normally, your gallbladder sends a continual supply of dark-colored bile through a bile duct to your liver to help you digest fats. Sometimes a gallstone (a hardened piece of cholesterol) or a growth blocks the bile duct, forcing bile into your bloodstream. Then bile's dark color starts to show up in the skin and eyes.

"It's as if a dye that's supposed to be going into your gut begins traveling through your system," says Samuel Labow, M.D., president of the American Society of Colon and Rectal Surgeons and a private practitioner in Great Neck,

New York. "And it shows up by coloring your skin, eyes and urine." You may also experience abdominal pain, he says.

Hepatitis, which causes painful liver inflammation, can also cause jaundice, says Dr. Labow.

SYMPTOM RELIEF

While jaundice itself doesn't directly threaten your health, it is a sign of something that needs medical attention.

Expect medications or tests. If your doctor suspects hepatitis, you may be placed on a low-fat, high-carbohydrate diet for the duration of the disease. If liver infection is not in the picture, your doctor will perform a number of diagnostic tests to find out what is blocking the flow of bile from the liver. Gallstones or a tumor have to be removed surgically.

JAW CLICKING

WHEN TO SEE YOUR DOCTOR

- Pain or discomfort accompanies a popping noise when you open or close your jaw.
- You also grind your teeth.

WHAT YOUR SYMPTOM IS TELLING YOU

The muscles that control your jaws usually work in harmony, allowing you to open and close your mouth smoothly—and silently. "But if the muscles are tired or overworked, or if you're chewing on a tough steak, they won't pull together evenly," says Van B. Haywood, D.M.D., an associate professor in the Department of

Operative Dentistry at the University of North Carolina School of Dentistry in Chapel Hill. One muscle pulls one way, another pulls in an opposite direction or doesn't move at all—and your jaw clicks.

Jaw clicking is very common, dentists say. The only reason it's so annoyingly noticeable is that it's right next to your ear.

Sometimes jaw clicking comes along with other symptoms—such as headaches, neck pain, stiffness or difficulty opening and closing the mouth. More serious problems with the jaw joint are known as temporomandibular joint disorder (TMD). Problems with this joint can develop when its supporting muscles and ligaments are overly stretched and out of alignment, according to Eric Z. Shapira, D.D.S., a trustee on the national board of the Academy of General Dentistry and a dentist in private practice in Half Moon Bay, California. And if the bony portions of the joint don't align properly, bone will grind against bone.

Bruxism, the nightly clenching and grinding of the teeth, increases the potential for additional problems, Dr. Shapira says. Not only is it one of the most common dental problems, but nine out of ten people whose jaws click also gnash their teeth, which can cause the jaw to deteriorate.

SYMPTOM RELIEF

Jaw clicking is an irritant, primarily because it's so audible. But unless you also have facial pain or unless the jawbones and muscles are deteriorating, doctors can't do much about it.

"You can't fix it any more than you can fix a knee that goes out," Dr. Haywood says. "It just gets dislodged, and then it goes back into place."

Here's how to silence some of that racket.

Ban the Bazooka. Don't ever chew gum, Dr. Haywood says. That puts a continuous strain on your jaw joint and muscles.

Avoid steak. You should never chew tough meat or vegetables. And stay away from triple-decker sandwiches. "If you have jaw clicking or popping, that stresses your joints tremendously," says Dr. Haywood.

Watch for wear. Tell your dentist about your jaw clicking and ask him to look for signs of bruxism-caused erosion on the chewing surfaces of your teeth, Dr. Shapira says. (For hints and tips on dealing with teeth grinding, see page 652.)

See also Jaw Problems

JAW PROBLEMS

WHEN TO SEE YOUR DOCTOR

- Your jaw hurts, especially when you talk, yawn or chew.
- You can't open your mouth more than two inches.
- You also feel pain in your neck, shoulders or ears.

WHAT YOUR SYMPTOM IS TELLING YOU

The jawbone's connected to the head bone—that much we know for sure. We also know that the joint we laypeople call the jaw is referred to by doctors as the temporomandibular joint. When it isn't working right, doctors say you have temporomandibular joint disorder (TMD or TMJ). From there, though, certainty fades amid assorted and often contradictory claims about the most common causes of jaw problems.

TMD "is the most vague area in dentistry," says Van B. Haywood, D.M.D., an associate professor in the Department of Operative Dentistry at the University of North Carolina School of Dentistry in Chapel Hill. "Causes and effects can be very confusing."

One manifestation of TMD is pain in the face or head.

TMD may create an audible click when you open and close your mouth. (If you have that clicking though, it doesn't necessarily mean you have TMD.) The joint can become inflamed and swollen. The damaged joint could lock your jaw open or closed. The muscles and ligaments could lose their elasticity, and you might develop a receding chin. The injury also can cause headaches, toothaches and ringing in the ears.

The jaw muscles and ligaments can hurt on their own, but they can also send pain to muscles in other places, such as your neck and shoulder, says Brendan C. Stack, Sr., D.D.S., an orthodontist and president of the National Capital Center for Craniofacial Pain in Vienna, Virginia, and past president of the American Academy of Head, Neck, Facial Pain and TMJ Orthopedics.

The possible culprits of TMD are many. It could be arthritis, which can just as easily affect your jaw joint as any other joint in the body.

Improper alignment of teeth could also tax the joint. Sometimes a whack to the jaw area can set TMD in motion. Teeth grinding and tight facial muscles brought on by stress can exacerbate the problem.

Finally, sinus infections and toothaches can put pressure on the muscles in your face, making you *think* you have TMD when you actually don't, Dr. Stack says.

SYMPTOM RELIEF

Because there's so much guesswork involved in getting to the source of your jaw problem, many things might work alone or together to ease your discomfort. Before you take your problem to the experts, here are a few things you should know and try.

Save the knife for last. Don't be tempted or persuaded to seek a fast surgical solution to your jaw problem, Dr. Haywood says. "First we identify bad habits or stresses that could contribute to the problem," he says, "then we look at things structurally and functionally. Surgery to realign the jaw or teeth is a last resort. You may be able to treat the pain by taking a common analgesic like aspirin."

Don't take it on your chin. If you have jaw pain, the best sleeping position is on your back or on your side, Dr. Haywood says. Sleeping on your stomach pushes the head to one side and places a lot of pressure on the jaw.

Press for less stress. A lot of people manifest stress by tightening muscles in their face and neck. Try to consciously relax these muscles as you go about your daily business. Keep your mouth closed but your teeth slightly apart. "If you walk with your fists clenched up, you're going to get a charley horse in your arm," says Dr. Haywood. "That's what happens when you go around with your teeth clenched."

Guard your mouth. An orthodontist or dentist practiced in treating TMD can devise a special mouthguard to realign your jaw, decompress your jaw joint and get your face muscle to relax, says Dr. Stack. The guard clasps onto your teeth in the back of your mouth, hidden from view.

Find an expert. Members of the American Academy of Head, Neck, Facial Pain and TMJ Orthopedics are specialists in the whole murky area of jaw problems, Dr. Stack says. You can obtain a referral to an expert in your area by calling their national office in Fort Worth, Texas.

JOINT CRACKING

WHEN TO SEE YOUR DOCTOR

- The cracking sounds start after you've experienced a fall or a blow to the joint.

WHAT YOUR SYMPTOM IS TELLING YOU

Nothing. Well, that's not entirely true, but unless you've been injured, cracking joints are no cause for concern.

There may be *reasons* why your joints snap, crackle and pop like a bowl of Rice Krispies, but it's not necessarily a sign of anything wrong.

The most common cause is a tendon rubbing against another tendon or ligament, says Robin Dore, M.D., a rheumatologist in private practice in Anaheim, California. When you're young and still growing, ligaments, tendons and bone may grow at different rates, so your adolescent child may sound like a tiny percussion section now and then. As you get older and the cartilage around your joints thins, the ligaments and tendons snap at you because they are rubbing against each other, Dr. Dore says.

If you're double-jointed, you have a slightly more interesting reason for the cracking: Your ligaments and tendons are longer and more elastic than normal, so the joints move farther than they should and crack more often. Most people normally outgrow being double-jointed by their mid- to late twenties, however, Dr. Dore says.

Other than the rub of a ligament or tendon, the only other known cause of cracking is a nitrogen bubble that suddenly depressurizes in the tissues of your joint as you move. It's like a teeny-weeny case of the bends inside a joint, says Kent Pomeroy, M.D., a physiatrist in Scottsdale, Arizona.

SYMPTOM RELIEF

If an injured joint starts making music, your doctor will probably want to x-ray it to rule out the possibility of fracture. Otherwise, there's nothing that needs to be relieved. Relax—you just have noisy joints.

JOINT INFLAMMATION

WHEN TO SEE YOUR DOCTOR

- Your joint is hot, red, swollen and extremely painful, and you don't know the cause.
- The inflammation doesn't respond to over-the-counter pain relievers like aspirin or ibuprofen.

WHAT YOUR SYMPTOM IS TELLING YOU

One of your joints feels like it has a little electric heater in it and someone left the setting on high. It's hot, it's red and it burns.

Obviously, there's no heater—but there probably is arthritis, the most likely cause of joint inflammation. The most common type of arthritis is osteoarthritis, which produces tiny growths called spurs on the bony part of the joint. Those spurs dig into surrounding muscles, tendons and ligaments, causing irritation and inflammation.

Gout is another form of arthritis, and its searing attacks of pinpoint inflammation—frequently confined to the big toe—can last up to a week. The inflammation comes from crystals of uric acid that lodge in the joint like slivers of glass. You get gout because your body can't metabolize a protein called purine, and the excess forms uric acid. In some cases gout is inherited; in others, it's a side effect of medication.

A third (and much less common) type of arthritis that causes inflamed joints is rheumatoid arthritis. This is actually what scientists call an autoimmune disease, in which the immune system treats the body like an infection and attacks it. In this case, the body part that is attacked is the joints. Lupus is another autoimmune disease that can cause joint inflammation.

But a *real* infection can also inflame the joints. For example, Lyme disease—a bacterial infection spread by the bite of the deer tick—can inflame one or many joints. (It frequently picks the knee.)

Two less likely causes of joint inflammation are a kind of rheumatism called *polymyalgia rheumatica* and a form of arthritis called *ankylosing spondylitis*.

And, of course, if someone kicks you in the knee (or you injure any joint) it's going to get inflamed. (Even an *old* injury can act up, causing inflammation.)

SYMPTOM RELIEF

Half the battle in healing an inflamed joint is detecting the cause. Inflammations caused by an injury are usually obvious—you fell on your elbow or banged your knee and it flared up.

Beyond that, diagnosis is murky and medical, and you should see your doctor so he can figure out what's wrong. He may use a needle to draw a fluid sample out of the inflamed joint. The fluid might contain bleeding from a recent injury, bacteria from an infection, uric acid crystals or serum, a substance that shows the inflammation is from an old injury that's acting up.

Help for Arthritis Inflammation

Arthritis is a serious medical problem, and you should work with your doctor to create a total program of coping strategies and pain control. Here are a few helpful suggestions.

Put your joints under wrap. A wrap or splint using an elastic bandage will help keep a painfully inflamed joint stable, says Robin Dore, M.D., a rheumatologist in private practice in Anaheim, California. Get your doctor to show you how to put on the wrap or splint, and ask him how long you should use it without removing it.

Let those dishes sit. "If you have rheumatoid arthritis, save your dinner dishes for the next morning," suggests Bill Arnold, M.D., a rheumatologist and chairman of the Department of Medicine at Lutheran General Hospital in Park Ridge, Illinois. "Many people with painful hands love to do dishes in the morning, because the warm water feels so good." (For more tips on dealing with stiff, painful, inflamed finger joints, see Finger Deformity on page 222.)

Be precise with your prescription. Rheumatoid arthritis generally responds well to a combination of methotrexate (a powerful drug that helps slow the destruction of the joint) and nonsteroidal anti-inflammatory (NSAID) medicines, says Robert Thoburn, M.D., clinical associate professor of rheumatology at the University of Florida in Gainesville. "NSAIDs have a high potential for stomach ulceration, however, so be sure to follow your prescription exactly." If you're disabled by the pain, your doctor may prescribe a steroid medication, which brings quick relief until the methotrexate begins to work.

Banishing Gout Pain

There are several things you can do to ease the painful inflammation of an acute attack of gout.

Wait out a bout. Elevate the affected joint and rest it as much as possible, says Edward Lally, M.D., chief of rheumatology at Brown University and Roger Williams General Hospital in Providence, Rhode Island. Attacks of gout usually last no longer than four to seven days.

Wash out the acid. "Drink lots of water to wash the uric acid out of your system and help prevent uric acid kidney stones," says Dr. Dore.

Use medicines short-term. The pharmaceutical weapons of choice for battling gout are anti-inflammatory drugs, says Dr. Lally. They're usually prescribed for short-term use—the length of a typical attack. To treat the pain as well as the inflammation, doctors sometimes prescribe Indocin, Naprosyn or Voltaren. The most often used medication is colchicine, which is usually very effective. If the attack is particularly severe, your doctor may prescribe injections or tablets of steroid anti-inflammatories, such as cortisone.

Review your other medications. Medications that you're taking for other problems can spark an attack of gout, says Dr. Lally. Some diuretics, for example, can cause your body to retain uric acid. Ask your doctor to check your prescriptions and over-the-counter drugs to see if they need to be changed.

Avoid purines. In many cases, gout can be controlled by medications. However, it may be helpful for those with high uric acid levels to avoid purine-rich foods, such as organ meats, gravies and some seafoods like anchovies, sardines and herring. These are only some of the culprits that can trigger an attack. For further purine protection, ask your doctor about a medicine called allopurinol, which lowers uric acid levels.

Treating Other Types of Inflammation

Lyme disease is cured with intravenous antibiotic therapy, says Leonard Sigal, M.D., chief of rheumatology at the University of Medicine and Dentistry of New Jersey Robert Wood Johnson Medical School in New Brunswick. You can receive the three- to four-week treatment at home.

Polymyalgia is curable with steroid medicines. You may have to take them for three to five years, but they do the job, says Herbert Kaplan, M.D., a rheumatologist at the Denver Arthritis Clinic.

The more serious joint-inflaming conditions, such as rheumatoid arthritis, ankylosing spondylitis and lupus, require ongoing medical treatment. Your doctor will prescribe specific medications and appropriate exercises, says Dr. Dore.

See also Joint Pain; Joint Stiffness; Joint Swelling

JOINT PAIN

WHEN TO SEE YOUR DOCTOR

- Your joint pain is severe or unexplained.
- The pain lasts more than one week.
- The joint is hot, red or swollen as well as painful.
- You get no relief from the use of aspirin, ice packs or heat.
- You have recently injured the joint, particularly with a sharp blow.

What Your Symptom Is Telling You

Your joints usually serve you effortlessly—they glide like
the parts of a miraculous machine through all the
movements of your day. Then, one of these vital parts starts
to hurt. What's going on?

It could be any one of a hundred things, says Robert
Thoburn, M.D., a clinical associate professor of rheumatology at the University of Florida in Gainesville. But
though joint pain has many possible causes, the major con-
tenders are arthritis, rheumatism or an injury.

There are over 100 types of arthritis, including gout and
rheumatoid arthritis. But the type that most commonly
causes joint pain is osteoarthritis, sometimes called the
wear-and-tear disease.

Osteoarthritis is the result of a series of small injuries that
occur over a long period of time. Years of hard work and
overuse (like constant typing or incessant use of one motion
in a sport, such as a golf swing or tennis serve) cause tiny
fractures in the joint's cartilage and underlying bone, and
the joint begins to deteriorate. (Oddly enough, *underuse*
through lack of exercise can also cause the problem.)

Rheumatism is the medical term for inflammations of
the muscles, tendons, ligaments and bursae (tiny, pillowing
sacs) that surround the bony part of the joint. This kind of
pain—better known as bursitis or tendinitis—also results
from the wear and tear of aging, or from overuse.

A single injury to a joint—such as a sharp blow or
strain—can also cause joint pain, as can a torn cartilage or
ligament. And sometimes the pain you feel may actually
originate somewhere else. A healthy knee might hurt
because of arthritis in the hip, for example. Or inflammation in the wrist from carpal tunnel syndrome might cause
pain in the shoulder.

Arthritis can snake like ivy through your family tree.
Can you bend your hand down and touch your thumb to
your wrist like Uncle Edward? If you can, you may have
inherited unusually mobile joints. While they come in
handy in yoga class, hypermobile joints tend to wear out
and become arthritic earlier because your extra-stretchy lig-

aments and tendons have trouble holding the joints stable.

Other causes of joint pain may include a viral or bacterial infection, a hormonal or nervous system problem or—rarely—certain types of cancer.

SYMPTOM RELIEF

The most important approach to joint pain is to work with your doctor for the right diagnosis, ruling out any serious medical problems or infections, says Bill Arnold, M.D., a rheumatologist and chairman of the Department of Medicine at Lutheran General Hospital in Park Ridge, Illinois.

If your pain results from osteoarthritis, the most common cause of joint pain, your doctor will prescribe specific medications, injections or exercise.

If your doctor says you have gout or rheumatoid arthritis, you will be treated for inflammation (heat and swelling) in the joints as well as pain.

But no matter what the cause of your pain, there's a lot you can do on your own to relieve it.

Turn up the heat. "The more chronic your pain, the better heat is," says Dr. Arnold. "Heat helps to relax muscles around the joint." Moist heat is particularly effective, he says. Take a wet towel, put it in the dryer but remove it while the towel is still wet and hot. Then place it against the joint, putting a dry towel on top to keep the heat in. Or you can use a moist heating pad, wrapping it around the painful joint for 20 to 30 minutes.

Ice it. If you are suffering from a recent injury or from pain that has recently appeared, use cold instead of heat, says Dr. Arnold. "The sooner you put ice on, the better off you are. That's why baseball pitchers slap it on in the dugout," he says. Here's Dr. Arnold's recommendation for an ice pack: "Buy a one-to-five-pound bag of frozen peas or kernel corn and wrap it around the painful joint. You've got yourself an ice wrap. And then you can eat it for dinner." You can leave the ice pack on for 20 minutes at a time.

Rest what hurts. If you have pain in just one joint or area, like the knee or neck, use a brace or support to rest it, says Dr. Arnold. If many of your joints are involved, plan for 15 minutes of rest for every hour that you're awake. For ten hours of activity, you'll need one to two hours of rest. "Just put your feet up and relax," he says. (See specific joint pain entries for more information on dealing with pain.)

Mix your OTCs. Over-the-counter or nonprescription painkillers will ease arthritis pain, says Dr. Arnold. But be aware that steady use of anti-inflammatory drugs like aspirin and ibuprofen can increase your risk of an ulcer. Dr. Arnold suggests this solution: Say you find that if you take four aspirin tablets daily, your joint pain is relieved. Instead of taking four aspirin daily, take two aspirin and two acetaminophen tablets. This will reduce the quantity of anti-inflammatory medicines entering (and irritating) your stomach. Acetaminophen will not help with inflammation, but it is an effective painkiller that is easy for the stomach to tolerate, explains Dr. Arnold.

Explore your range of motion. For problems of the soft tissue around the joint, like bursitis and tendinitis, staying limber and flexible will prevent those tissues from tightening up and hurting even more, says physical therapist Kathleen Haralson of Washington University School of Medicine in St. Louis.

Each joint has its own natural range of movement, she explains, and each individual has to find the fine line between overuse and keeping it limber. "Listen to your body," she says. "Don't overstretch, just try to exercise in your normal range of motion several times a day, depending on how painful it is." For example, if you have a painful shoulder, raise your arm over your head until it hurts just a little bit. "You need to move the painful body part as far as you can, but do not force it," she says. "This is what a physical therapist would do with you."

Get your whole body moving. People have less pain in their joints when they exercise regularly at low to moderate intensity, says Haralson. Her top pick is swimming or walking in water. "Getting into hip-deep water and fast-walking to your capacity is wonderful," she says. Stationary bicycles, treadmills and low-impact aerobic dance are also good choices.

If your condition keeps you chairbound, you can still get a good workout, Haralson says. Sit in a chair, put on some moderate- to fast-paced music and march with your arms until you work up a good sweat, she suggests.

Get a little assistance. "For people with arthritis or rheumatism, there's a device out there that can make your life a little less painful, especially for dressing, hygiene and kitchen activities," says Haralson. "These devices include zipper pulls, buttoners, long-handled shoehorns, long-handled combs, elastic shoelaces or Velcro fasteners." She also suggests using something to get your weight off the painful joint, like a cane, crutch or walker.

Try the antidepressants for anti-pain. Your doctor may prescribe tricyclic analgesics, also known as tricylic antidepressants, for musculoskeletal pain. These medicines may be very helpful for the insomnia and fatigue that often accompany rheumatism, says Sidney Block, M.D., a rheumatologist in private practice in Bangor, Maine. They're prescribed in smaller doses than those used for depression, and they are not addicting. "They relieve pain, help promote a good sleep pattern and can be used for long-term pain problems," says Dr. Block.

Get physical with a therapist. Ask your doctor about a prescription for physical therapy, suggests William Loomis, D.O., an osteopathic physician in Spokane, Washington, who also serves as president of the American Association of Orthopedic Medicine. Physical therapists treat the muscles and underlying ligaments around the joint by improving the joint's blood supply, which promotes healing. They can help you with range-of-motion exercises and also apply healing techniques such as ultrasound waves, which go deeper into the injured tissues than any at-home, self-help techniques, says Dr. Loomis.

See also Joint Inflammation; Joint Swelling

JOINT STIFFNESS

WHEN TO SEE YOUR DOCTOR

- Your joint stiffness lasts more than six weeks.
- The stiffness follows a blow to the joint.
- The stiffness in your joints is worse in the morning and improves as the day does on.

WHAT YOUR SYMPTOM IS TELLING YOU

Whether you think of them as simple hinges or ball-and-socket wonders, your joints allow you all the marvels of motion. Then a joint stiffens up—and to bend for the newspaper, reach for a rose, twist in your chair, hold a cup or even head out on that health-promoting walk becomes an uncomfortable challenge.

Most of the time, joint stiffness is related to the normal changes of aging and is not a symptom that arthritis may be just down the road. The ligaments and tendons that help joints function may become overstretched from years of use, leaving the joints less stable and more prone to wear and tear. And as a person ages, the lubricating membrane that normally allows each joint to slide and glide through its motion may become dried and contracted, constricting the joint's movement.

If a joint has been hurting you, then becomes stiff and "rickety"-feeling, your body may actually be making its own splint to protect the joint from further injury. Muscles surrounding the joint go into spasm to prevent the joint from moving, and those spasms contribute to stiffness.

You may notice the stiffness most when you first get out of bed in the morning, and feel it loosening up during the day. You may have swelling along with stiffness, though swelling is more likely when the stiffness results from an injury.

If you've been bedridden or stuck in a cast or have spent

the winter on the couch watching sit-coms, your joints may feel frozen and stiff simply because of lack of exercise.

A long-since-forgotten injury may cause a joint to stiffen up years later. A new injury or episode of overuse (is it your bowling arm?) can bring on stiffness.

Rarely, some neurological or muscular disorders may be part of the problem, though these conditions will usually be signaled by other, more noticeable symptoms.

SYMPTOM RELIEF

If the stiffness in your joints is severe or persistent, you'll want to see your doctor for a clear diagnosis. But no matter what the cause, here are some basic comforts that will help stiffness loosen its hold.

Relax with moist heat. Take a wet towel, put it in the dryer, but remove it while the towel is still wet and hot, says Bill Arnold, M.D., a rheumatologist and chairman of the Department of Medicine at Lutheran General Hospital in Park Ridge, Illinois. To relieve those muscles, just wrap the moist hot towel around the affected joint and leave it on for 20 minutes or so. You might want to place an additional dry towel on top to hold the heat in. Or, you can use a moist heating pad.

Get a head start on stiffness. If you've been feeling stiff for a while, and know that it's worse in the early morning, head off the stiffness with over-the-counter anti-inflammatory medication, Dr. Arnold suggests. "You can wake yourself around 5:00 a.m. and take Advil or Nuprin with a glass of milk, and by the time you get going at 8:00, you'll feel better," he says. "Or try taking two tablets the night before, and you may find that they will last you until the morning."

These medicines will help reduce pain in the joints as well, Dr. Arnold says. Steady use of anti-inflammatory drugs can lead to stomach problems, and taking them with milk will soften this effect.

Keep it moving. You can resist stiffness with gentle range-of-motion exercises to help your joint stay flexible

and limber, says Kathleen Haralson, a physical therapist a
Washington University School of Medicine in St. Louis.

A slight variation in range of motion from person to per
son is perfectly normal, Haralson says. People wit
extremely mobile joints have a large range of motion, an
bodybuilders may have less.

"Whatever is normal for you, you don't want to lose,
she says. "Don't overstretch, but gently move the joint a
far as you can several times a day," she suggests.

Regular exercise for your whole body is a good practic
to keep all your joints toned and limber. Work yourself u
to a brisk 20-minute walk at least three times a week.

See also Joint Inflammation; Joint Pain; Joint Swelling

JOINT SWELLING

WHEN TO SEE YOUR DOCTOR

- The swelling lasts more than seven days.
- Your joint is red and hot as well as swollen.
- You also have fever or chills.
- You have already been diagnosed with arthritis, but thi
  swelling is new or a different type than you've had before
- If the joint has been punctured, see your doctor *imme-
  diately*.

WHAT YOUR SYMPTOM IS TELLING YOU

Have you been pushing yourself lately? Maybe you sur
vived a stint of aerobic housecleaning—only to notic
a newly swollen elbow or wrist. Or perhaps you twisted
knee during that heroic lunge to catch a fly ball at the com
pany picnic.

Rather than its usual firm, sturdy feel, the joint no

feels puffy and soft. A newly injured joint swells because of a small amount of internal bleeding, which stretches the skin and surrounding tissues.

Other things besides brand-new injuries can cause joint swelling, however. An old injury can flare up with swelling from fluids that have collected in the joint. (In some people, a previously injured joint even acts like a barometer, swelling in response to changes in the weather.)

Arthritis is another common cause of swelling in the joints. When you have a swollen (and sometimes painful) joint anywhere in your body for more than six weeks, it's probably arthritis. (You can also develop arthritis with no visible swelling.)

When a joint is not just swollen but also red or hot to the touch, it is inflamed. Bacteria, a virus or fungus—all of which can enter through a break in the skin—may be attacking the joint, causing infection. Even without infection, however, arthritis or injury can inflame a joint.

SYMPTOM RELIEF

When you injure a joint, keep this in mind: If pain begins to lessen and you feel strength starting to return to the joint within 24 hours, you're already beginning to mend. In the meantime, here are several ways you can help your swollen joint return to normal size.

Cool it. The first weapon against swelling is ice, says Robin Dore, M.D., a rheumatologist in private practice in Anaheim, California. "Cover the ice with a plastic baggie or towel and apply it 15 to 20 minutes, three times a day," she suggests.

Stabilize it. You can immobilize a swollen finger joint with a taped-on Popsicle stick, Dr. Dore says. "Put one tip of the stick at the tip of the finger, the other in the palm of your hand, and wrap adhesive tape around the finger," she explains.

For a swollen toe, use the adjoining toe as the splint. Simply wrap the tape around the swollen toe and a toe next to it, says Dr. Dore.

One caution about splinting comes from Sidney Block, M.D., a rheumatologist in private practice in Bangor, Maine. "A day or two is as long as you should splint without checking with your doctor," he says. If you splint for too long you could end up with an extremely stiff joint called a flexion contracture.

When Arthritis Causes the Swelling

If you have arthritis, you don't need to report each episode of swelling to your doctor, says Dr. Block. Unless the pain or swelling is unusual or particularly severe or accompanied by fever, just mention it at your next visit. Between visits, here's how to deal with the swelling.

Warm it up. If you have a history of arthritic swelling, hot packs are more effective than cold, Dr. Block says. Reserve ice for injuries.

Reach your range. Gentle range-of-motion exercises help keep your joints functioning. Move the joint gently in every direction as far as it will go. Keep the joint moving but don't overdo it. And be sure to have your doctor's okay before you begin.

Range-of-motion exercises stimulate the muscles to pump the debris produced by inflammation out of the joint and into the body's lymph system, which carries it away, says William Loomis, D.O., an osteopathic physician in Spokane, Washington and president of the American Association of Orthopedic Medicine.

Ask about soundwaves. If swelling is persistent, your doctor may refer you to a physical therapist for a soothing ultrasound treatment, Dr. Loomis says. Ultrasound waves penetrate painlessly into the swollen tissues around the joint, improve the joint's blood supply and promote healing.

Treat Infections Carefully

If an infection is causing the swelling, your doctor will treat you with a course of appropriate antibiotics. Here's what to keep in mind for home treatment.

Avoid ice. Use moist heat instead of an ice pack on an infected joint, says Dr. Dore. Ice will cause blood vessels to contract and actually keep the infection in place. Heat will open up the blood vessels so white blood cells—the body's immune defense against infection—can reach the area. Some infections may even drain through the surface of the skin when moist heat is applied, she says. Wrap the joint for 20 minutes in a towel that has been dipped in hot water and wrung out.

See also Joint Inflammation; Joint Pain; Joint Stiffness

K

KNEE LOCKING

WHEN TO SEE YOUR DOCTOR

- Your knee freezes in either a bent or extended position.
- You are unable to fully extend or flex your knee.

WHAT YOUR SYMPTOM IS TELLING YOU

You're kneeling or squatting on the floor and suddenly you can't stand up. Or perhaps you're walking or playing sports and one leg becomes frozen in position. Or you try to rise out of your seat...but you can't.

It's almost as if a vise has clamped onto your knee and is preventing it from moving. Well... almost. Something very real is probably preventing your knee from moving.

"In normal situations, the knee is a smoothly operating mechanism, like a door hinge swinging open and shut," explains Edward J. Resnick, M.D., professor of orthopedic surgery at Temple University Hospital in Philadelphia. "But if you put a jam in the door or an object in the hinge, that smooth movement may be obstructed or frozen in position."

This is what orthopedists call a *true* locking of the knee: something that physically prevents the knee from fully straightening out or bending and holds the knee rigidly in place. It's often painful, and since it can occur while climbing stairs, sitting on the ground, or being in some other vulnerable position, it can be quite frightening.

Usually, the locking is caused by a torn piece of cartilage, or possibly a loose bone fragment resulting from a bone disorder called osteochondritis dissecans. "The cartilage fragment or bone chip moves freely in the knee cavity until it gets trapped between two joint surfaces, impeding your ability to straighten the knee," says David W. Lhowe, M.D., orthopedic surgeon at Massachusetts General Hospital in Boston and professor of orthopedic surgery at Harvard Medical School.

Sometimes the obstruction is from a misalignment of the bones and muscles around the knee. "Weakness of the muscles on the inside of the thigh or tightness of the outer muscle can throw off the alignment of the kneecap," says Lyle Micheli, M.D., director of the Sports Medicine Division at Boston Children's Hospital and associate clinical professor of orthopedic surgery at Harvard Medical School. "The kneecap comes out of groove with the thigh bone, derails and gets stuck, not allowing you to bend or extend. When the muscle returns to normal, the kneecap gets back on track and movement proceeds normally."

True locking is fairly rare. But many times, say following an injury, a person will experience an inability to move the knee. That can *feel* like a locking of the knee, but in reality there's nothing physically interfering with the movement of that knee. Doctors call this a pseudo-lock.

"A pseudo-lock is simply a reaction to pain. The pain mechanism won't allow the joint to extend or flex fully," says Phillip J. Marone, M.D., director of the Jefferson Sports Medicine Center at Thomas Jefferson University Hospital in Philadelphia and team physician for the Philadelphia Phillies professional baseball team. Sometimes the pain that creates a pseudo-lock is brought on by a twist or a bump to the knee. Or it could just as easily be a bad case of stiffness from sitting too long.

SYMPTOM RELIEF

Although a locked knee may simply unlock with a little rest, don't assume you've been cured. Serious knee damage can occur if your lock was brought on by a loose piece of bone or cartilage. Any restriction of knee movement should be treated by a doctor. The problem may have to be corrected surgically.

See also Knee Pain

KNEE PAIN

WHEN TO SEE YOUR DOCTOR

- Your pain makes it hard for you to walk.
- The knee feels loose or unable to support your weight.
- You also have severe swelling, redness or discoloration that doesn't diminish after 24 hours.
- Unexplained pain lasts for more than three days.
- Pain following an injury doesn't diminish within five days.

WHAT YOUR SYMPTOM IS TELLING YOU

Those #*&!%@ knees! You push them just a little too far and the next thing you know, you feel like you've double-crossed the Godfather!

As one of about 50 million Americans with knee problems, you've just joined the Painful Knee Club. Our knees have always been vulnerable to an assortment of bumps, bangs and bruises. But as we have become an older and more active society, our hapless knees now bear more burdens and face more wear and tear than ever before. Hence the club's ever increasing membership.

A fall, twist or bang on the knee can obviously qualify you for membership. So can an old injury that never healed properly and now acts up in response to changes in the barometer. But most recurrent or unexplained knee pain comes from overuse.

The knee is held together by tough ligaments that connect, protect and stabilize the joint; cartilage that cushions the bones; and tendons that join muscles to bone. But even these resilient tissues have their limits. Too much bending and twisting, too much running or too much jumping can cause them to rupture or become inflamed.

Damage to these tissues also takes its toll on the sensitive surfaces of the knees' bones. "The tissues in the knees work like the shock absorbers in a car," says M. Solomonow,

Ph.D., director of the bioengineering section at the Louisiana State Medical Center in New Orleans. "If you make a lot of sudden stops or subject these components to stresses they weren't designed to handle, they wear out. In a car you'll hear the sound of metal on metal; in a knee you'll feel the pain of bone rubbing on bone."

Many overuse pains are lumped under the umbrella term chondromalacia patellae—a fancy way of saying pain in, around and under the kneecap.

But not all overuse pains belong in this category. Suppose you have an active teen in your house complaining of pain just south of the kneecap. It could be Osgood-Schlatter disease, commonly called growing pains—a condition arising from excess stress on the tendons of the lower leg bone. Combine lots of physical activity with the rapid muscle and bone growth of puberty, and you get one miserable kid with a painful, bony enlargement or bump on the upper part of his lower leg, just in front of and below the kneecap.

When the knee is subjected to misuse as well as overuse, it can develop a condition called synovitis. Your mother may have called it water on the knee, because the achy joint now bears a striking resemblance to a water balloon. Synovitis is from a bang or twist that causes certain tissues in the knee to fill with blood or other fluids.

Another knee condition related to overuse is sometimes called housemaid's knee. It's really a form of bursitis—irritation to the front of the knee causes a bursal sac in front of the kneecap to fill up with fluid. Its most common cause: prolonged kneeling on hard surfaces.

The knee is also a potential site for a painful condition called osteochondritis dissecans—a necrosis, or death, of a segment of bone or cartilage. Its cause is unknown. Eventually, the dead cartilage or bone chip can break off and produce even more pain as well as a locked knee.

In some instances, nasty knee pain can actually originate elsewhere in the body, such as the toe, foot, spine or hip. Fallen arches or weak ankles can cause your foot to overpronate (rotate too far inward), putting too much force on the knee. And if you have poor posture or an improper gait, it can focus pain directly to your knees.

The knee is also a favorite target for arthritis in its many forms. Osteoarthritis results from the breakdown of cartilage and other joint tissues after years of wear and tear. Rheumatoid arthritis is characterized by a progressive development of pain and swelling in joints and their connecting tissues, which can be coupled with other symptoms like fatigue, weight loss and low-grade fever. And gout is a metabolic condition in which severe arthritis develops when uric acid is deposited in joints and other tissues.

In addition, the knee is also a potential site for tumors and cysts as well as painful bacterial infections.

SYMPTOM RELIEF

The key to silencing most angry knees is not to subject them to the kind of activities that ticked them off in the first place. Repeated abuse is a sure-fire means of provoking a ferocious response.

Treat painful knees with kindness and they'll behave. Let these tips show you how.

Use RICE on injuries. Whether from an acute trauma like a sprain or simple overuse, injuries respond best to RICE: an acronym for rest, ice, compression and elevation. "Rest is the key component," says Edward J. Resnick, M.D., professor of orthopedic surgery at Temple University Hospital in Philadelphia. "Then after a period of limited activity, doctors like to see a gradual resumption of activity and exercise."

Supplement several days of rest with applications of ice: 15 minutes at a time, several times a day to reduce swelling. Compress the knee by wrapping it snugly, but not too tightly, in an elastic bandage to limit movement. And elevate the knee with pillows to drain fluids from the joint.

Take an analgesic. Aspirin and ibuprofen are powerful pain and inflammation fighters that will help sore, swollen knees. Acetaminophen will help pain, but won't do anything for swelling.

Warm your wobbly knees. Cold is fine for injuries after they first occur, but most lingering pain responds best to moist warmth, says Dr. Resnick. He recommends a warm, moist towel, a hot-water bottle, a moist heating pad, a warm bath or a whirlpool.

Drop a few pounds. "If you're overweight, losing weight is a good way to reduce some of the painful forces acting on your knees with each step," says David W. Lhowe, M.D., orthopedic surgeon at Massachusetts General Hospital in Boston and professor of orthopedic surgery at Harvard Medical School. "Contact forces on joint surfaces in the knee can range up to eight times body weight. Lose 10 pounds, and you'll reduce those forces by 80 pounds, which is a lot."

Support your arches. A simple over-the-counter arch support in your shoe can prevent overpronation, says Peter Francis, Ph.D., professor of physical education at San Diego State University. People who pronate severely may require a professionally fitted arch device.

Cushion your knees. If you must spend periods of time on your knees, take some of the stress off your kneecaps by wearing cushioned knee pads. And take frequent rest breaks so that the stress isn't applied constantly.

Avoid squatting. Squatting and deep knee bends put enormous stress on the knee and can cause cartilage tears or possible rupture of the quadriceps tendon. Repetitive squatting can also produce prolonged episodes of knee pain in certain individuals, says Dr. Lhowe.

Find alternatives to running. Nonpounding activities like biking, walking and swimming can provide the same benefits as running, but are much kinder to your knees, says Dr. Francis. If you must run, increase your warm-up time, cut back your mileage, run on softer surfaces and always wear quality running shoes.

Send your knees to the gym. "Poor muscle tone is often the real culprit underlying most chronic knee problems," says Phillip J. Marone, M.D., director of the Jefferson Sports Medicine Center at Thomas Jefferson University Hospital in Philadelphia. "That's why in 80 percent of all cases, painful knees will respond to a sensible exercise program focusing on building flexibility and strength, particularly in the quadriceps and hamstrings [the large muscles at the front and backs of the thighs]."

See also Joint Inflammation; Joint Pain; Joint Swelling

L

LEG PAIN

WHEN TO SEE YOUR DOCTOR

- The pain lasts more than three days.
- You also experience numbness, coldness or weakness in your legs.
- Pain occurs in *both* the upper and lower leg.
- You notice bluish skin coloration, ulceration or tender lumps below the skin.
- You sustain an injury that produces swelling or discoloration or you suspect bone damage from the injury.
- You have an overuse injury that does not improve after three weeks.

WHAT YOUR SYMPTOM IS TELLING YOU

Several years ago, Secretariat—perhaps the greatest thoroughbred in racing history—suffered a leg injury. Even though his career was long since over and he had been put out to stud, the pain was such that the legendary Triple Crown winner had to be destroyed.

It's a thoroughly sad story. But look on the bright side—you're not a horse!

As with Secretariat, injuries are always the first suspect when leg pain arises. Something like a broken bone is usually pretty obvious, because it's caused by a sudden trauma, like a fall. Ditto for a muscle tear or strain. But an overuse injury comes on gradually. This category includes the malady every athlete knows all too well—shin splints.

"Shin splints is a catchall term for any sharp overuse pain in the bones and tissues of the lower leg," says Lyle Micheli, M.D., director of the Sports Medicine Division at

Boston Children's Hospital and associate clinical professor of orthopedic surgery at Harvard Medical School. In reality, shin splints are things like stress fractures, tendinitis or compartment syndrome—an irritation of the tissue that surrounds the shin muscles. And shin splints have many causes, including hard running surfaces, inadequate footwear, not warming up or overzealous exercise.

The legs are also hot spots for various types of painful diseases of the veins or arteries. Thrombophlebitis—an inflammation and clotting of the veins—creates a feeling of heaviness, along with a throbbing or burning sensation below the skin. In its "superficial" form, this disease produces tender skin redness and is not cause for concern. But deep vein thrombophlebitis (DVT) can produce sore, oozing skin ulcers. And a DVT clot that breaks away could be fatal if it lodges in the lungs.

In addition, insufficient blood flow from atherosclerosis (hardening of the arteries) can lead to what doctors call intermittent claudication. A person who has this condition experiences a dull cramping sensation that comes on with exercise (when the muscles require more oxygen-rich blood) and goes away with rest. Intermittent claudication, which is fairly common, usually shows up in the calves but sometimes appears in the upper leg as well. In rare cases, blood flow problems can be caused by a limb-threatening aneurysm (ballooning) in an artery behind the knee.

It's also possible for leg pains to originate somewhere other than in the leg, particularly in the spine. This is called referred pain. "Any abnormality in a disk or the spinal canal—a tumor, an infection—can refer pain to the legs with little or no pain in the back," says Steven Mandel, M.D., clinical professor of neurology at Jefferson Medical College and an attending physician at Thomas Jefferson University Hospital in Philadelphia.

Sciatica is a common type of referred pain. The sciatic nerve runs from the spine down the leg. Just sitting on a hard stool or wearing a tight work belt can pinch the nerve upstairs and produce a stabbing pain farther down the leg.

Also, the leg itself can experience entrapments—constrictions of nerves that produce burning, tingling, numbness or weakness. This kind of pain often shows up in people who sit, squat, stand or kneel for long periods.

Finally, the cause of pain can be in the bone itself. Osteomyelitis, for example, is an infectious bone disorder that can be acutely painful.

SYMPTOM RELIEF

An aching leg can make you feel like a plow horse bound for the glue factory. Here are some tips to get your gimpy gams back in racing form.

Be attentive to your symptoms. Try to identify what makes your pain worse and what may make it better. Pay particular attention to the kinds of activities that affect the intensity or duration of your pain, advises Michael F. Nolan, Ph.D., physical therapist and associate professor of anatomy and neurology at the University of South Florida College of Medicine in Tampa. If constant or repetitive leg motion is part of your job, consider taking frequent rest breaks.

Chill out with ice. Several days of ice-pack applications is perfect for relieving pain from an injury, says Dr. Micheli. Wrap ice cubes in a towel and apply them to the painful area for 15 minutes at a time, whenever you need relief. Just make sure the pain is from an injury. Ice can aggravate the pain associated with vascular disease, says Robert Ginsburg, M.D., director of the Cardiovascular Intervention Unit at the University of Colorado Health Science Center in Denver.

Try compression. An elastic bandage will relieve pain and swelling from a quad or hamstring pull, says Dr. Micheli. (The quadriceps and hamstrings are muscles at the front and back of the thighs.) For relief from painful thrombophlebitis, compression support stockings do a fine job, says Dr. Ginsburg. These are prescription stockings designed for vascular pain relief. Knee-high support hose from a department store can actually constrict blood flow and increase pain, he says.

Get a leg up. Elevating an injured leg drains the fluids that cause painful swelling, says Dr. Micheli. It can also provide fast relief for the dull, aching heaviness of thrombophlebitis.

Warm away vascular pain. A warm, not hot, heating pad, blanket or other warming device provides fast, soothing relief for thrombophlebitis, says Dr. Ginsburg. Don't use heat on the first three days following an injury, however. It could make swelling worse.

Preventing Leg Pain

If leg pain plagues you on a regular basis, there are several things you might want to try to keep it at bay.

Be heart smart. "The same lifestyle changes that can prevent a heart attack can reduce vascular leg pain," says Dr. Ginsburg. "Give up smoking, stop eating fatty, cholesterol-laden foods and shed some pounds. A regular exercise program, especially a walking program, will re-establish quality blood flow throughout the leg."

Find exercise alternatives. People who have shin splints should cut back on the activity that brought on the pain (usually running) and find less stressful alternatives, like biking or swimming, advises Gary M. Gordon, D.P.M., director of the Running and Walking Clinic at the University of Pennsylvania Sports Medicine Center in Philadelphia.

Work your abs. Sit-ups and other stomach-strengthening exercises can relieve strain in the lower back, thus reducing referred leg pain, says Dr. Nolan.

Empty your pockets. Sitting on your wallet can bring on sciatica, says Dr. Mandel. Wearing tight belts and tight pants can also irritate nerves. So pick your pockets and trade in your designer jeans for a pair of comfortable chinos.

Use padding. Cushioned seats or knee pads can lessen the severity of hard surfaces and prevent sciatica and nerve compression, says Dr. Mandel.

See also Calf Pain

LIBIDO LOSS

WHAT YOUR SYMPTOM IS TELLING YOU

The last time you were hot in bed was when the air conditioner broke. And the only thing that gets turned on once the lights go out is the alarm clock buzzer.

Maybe your spouse pesters you to do the mattress dance more than you want to. You may even oblige, but you don't really want to and don't really enjoy it. Is something wrong with you?

Sex therapists don't like to play a numbers game when talking about frequency of intercourse and what's considered normal. They're more concerned with determining what's right for a couple to maintain a healthy relationship.

"If you're in a relationship and you make love one or two times a month or less, that might be considered low," says Shirley Zussman, Ed.D, a certified sex and marital therapist in New York City and director of the Association for Male Sexual Dysfunction. "But who's to say what level of desire is more desirable?"

Low libido becomes a problem that should be addressed only when it is perceived as a problem, sex therapists say. "It's usually only in the framework of a relationship that it becomes an issue," Dr. Zussman says. "It's when there is a discrepancy in desire between the person and the partner, or when people feel there's something wrong with them because they have a low level of desire."

Everyone experiences peaks and valleys in sexual desire, an ebb and flow in libido that could be caused by any of a variety of factors, from a bad childhood to a bad day to a bad illness, from too much stress to too little time. Occasionally, a hormonal imbalance or prescription drug will sap sex drive. And, of course, there's a difference between sexual drive and sexual function. You may be able to become aroused and experience orgasm yet have little or no interest in doing so. (That's why seeking professional advice from your doctor or a qualified sex therapist is not a bad idea if your problem persists.)

If your lowered libido persists and you perceive that you have a problem, what can you do about it?

SYMPTOM RELIEF

Libido is an appetite, Dr. Zussman says. And it often can be difficult to help someone acquire a taste for something—or to acknowledge to themselves that they really do have a craving for something delightful. "You can present tempting foods like a luscious dessert," she says, "but that won't necessarily help someone who doesn't feel like eating or who denies the pleasure of eating sweets."

Here's what sex therapists might suggest to cultivate a sexy sweet tooth and put a lilt in your libido.

Sample from the sexual spice rack. For many couples, sex becomes as exciting as doing the dishes because they do the same thing all the time. Reading a sex manual and trying new positions or new techniques may add a renewed dash of zest to making love, Dr. Zussman says.

Don't forget to touch. People with low libidos often are reluctant to express any sort of affection toward their mates, according to Jo Marie Kessler, registered nurse practitioner, certified sex therapist and educator in private practice in San Diego. They may believe their gestures amount to teasing or will spark a debate over making love, but the loss of touch makes their partners feel unwanted and unloved.

"I always encourage them to maintain or resume expressions of affection—a kiss on the cheek or lips, casual touches on the arm or shoulder, a brush of their hair," she says. "Both partners need to demonstrate that they care, but with the understanding that the display of affection is not a signal for sex."

Read something risqué. You don't have to don sunglasses and a trench coat and creep into an adult bookstore, Kessler says, "but you could read some romance novels, love poems or erotic literature to try to nurture or enhance your own sensuality."

Spend an hour in the shower. Don't treat bath time as just a three-minute clean-up before you dash out the door to work. "Avail yourself of all the sensual experiences in the shower or tub," Kessler says. Feel the pleasure of the water as it dances on your skin. Lather yourself gently and sen-

sually, perhaps with a loofah sponge rather than a wash
cloth. Use bath salts and lightly scented candles.

Let your fingers do the talking. Take the time and plea
sure to know your own body and your partner's withou
any pressure to have intercourse and orgasm, Kessler says
"Focus on the leisurely exploration of each other's bodies
and share the joy and intimacy of that alone." Touch eac
other, feel and caress each other's genitals, notice the sen
sations of your two bodies as they move about. Tell eac
other what feels good.

Don't hesitate to help yourself. Sexual self-gratificatio
is not dirty or wrong, Kessler says. In fact, a person wit
low libido can use masturbation to learn what feels good t
his or her body, so that sex provides positive feedbac
instead of negative feedback. Practice first in private, sh
suggests, where you won't be so self-conscious, then broac
the topic of mutual masturbation with your mate.

Mind over Sexual Matters

In conjunction with sensual enhancement techniques, se
therapists also suggest other kinds of strategies to lift lo
libido. "You can deal with the immediate problem wit
techniques, but that might not help forever or to save
relationship," Dr. Zussman says.

Here are a few more approaches.

Dig yourself out of the dumps. Depression can produc
some very physical symptoms and is one of the most com
mon causes of inhibited sexual drive, Dr. Zussman says
"When you're depressed, you have an interest in practicall
nothing. Certainly your libido will be decreased, too. It jus
flies out the window." (See Depression on page 144.)

Look in your medicine chest. A number of prescriptio
and over-the-counter drugs, especially certain types of psy
chiatric and antidepressant medications and some hig
blood pressure pills, could dampen libido for both men an
women, says Richard C. Reznichek, M.D., a certified se
therapist, assistant clinical professor of urology at UCL
and urologist in Torrance, California. Some drugs also inter
fere with your ability to be aroused. If you're using medica
tions that you think are responsible for decreasing your se

drive, don't stop taking them, Dr. Reznichek advises. Speak first with your doctor and ask for alternative drugs.

Ask for help. From your spouse, that is. At least at first. He or she may, after all, have been the first to note the low libido. Whether it's exploring each other's sensuality, experimenting with new positions or trying to get in the mood more often, explain to your spouse that you may feel awkward, self-conscious and a bit stressed in attempting to change, but that you want to do it for the sake of the relationship, Dr. Zussman says. "Evoke their cooperation. Tell them that you'll need their help and understanding."

Talk to yourself...or perhaps to a friend. Ask yourself why your sex drive jackknifed into a ditch, Dr. Zussman says. Has it always been that way? What was happening in your life or relationship when it veered? Mull it over in your head, then talk to your partner, a friend or a family member who knows you well, Dr. Zussman advises. They may help spark some insight.

Take time to address your stress. He works. She works. He's tired at the end of the day. She comes home late several evenings a week. The kids have homework that needs to be checked. The ambition to excel professionally, the demands of raising children, the need to maintain social connections—all those stressors put the brakes on sex drive, Dr. Zussman says. "That can put you in a state of apathy when it comes to sex," she adds.

None of those everyday, everyweek worries leaves much time, ambition or emotional energy for making love, Dr. Zussman says. She suggests that a couple may need to give sex a higher priority in their relationship. "Try making a date with your partner. Not just to make love, but to talk with each other, hold each other and share your feelings and concerns with each other. That may help to restore your sexual interest."

Help for Those Hormones

It's also entirely possible that your libido is being K.O.'d by a hormone imbalance in the body. Here's what you should consider.

Deal openly with menopause. Some women may notice a declining interest in sex during menopause, Kessler says. It's a common side effect while the body is attempting to adjust. Estrogen replacement therapy can help return your libido to normal, she says. "Once the unpleasant symptoms of menopause have stopped, the drive returns and could even be enhanced." If you are going through menopause, ask your doctor about hormone replacement therapy.

Wait out the pregnant pause. Hormonal changes during pregnancy, especially the last trimester, and lactation often can dampen the drive for sex, according to Kessler. "Hormones are present in different levels at these times," she says. "Loss of libido immediately after childbirth and during lactation is nature's way of spacing children."

Test your testosterone. If you're a man who seemingly has no psychological reason for a lack of desire, you may want to ask a doctor to perform a blood test that will gauge your body's level of testosterone, according to Dr. Reznichek.

Low levels of the male hormone aren't a common cause of sapping your sexuality, but it always must be suspected, Dr. Reznichek says. Depending on the cause, a physician could prescribe either testosterone injections or a medication that counteracts other hormones that are suppressing naturally occurring testosterone, he says.

LIGHT-HEADEDNESS

WHEN TO SEE YOUR DOCTOR

- You've felt light-headed for more than two consecutive days.
- The light-headedness recurs frequently.
- You have fainted.
- You have chest pain.

What Your Symptom Is Telling You

Your head suddenly feels as weightless as one of those satellites you've seen astronauts toss around like a balloon in space. You grab onto a wall to steady yourself as the world around you begins to dim and your legs start to buckle. For a moment, you feel faint, but then manage to recover.

Feeling light-headed or faint is a common complaint, doctors say. In many cases, it means that your brain is momentarily getting less oxygen than it needs to remain fully alert. This can happen for many reasons—from an emotional surprise such as a marriage proposal to an emotional shock such as learning a loved one has died.

Light-headedness can be the first sign of a health problem, such as anemia, low blood pressure or low blood sugar. It also can be a sign of more serious conditions such as diabetes, internal bleeding, heart disease or stroke.

"There is some common sense involved. If you have a moment of light-headedness when you're about to give a speech, the chances are that you have stage fright and aren't having a cerebral hemorrhage," says Robert Slater, M.D., an assistant professor of clinical neurology at the University of Pennsylvania School of Medicine in Philadelphia.

Symptom Relief

For the most part, light-headedness is a problem that can be easily relieved. Here's how.

Drink plenty of fluids. If you become dehydrated, your blood pressure will drop and you might feel light-headed. Drinking at least six eight-ounce glasses of water every day will help prevent this problem.

Don't forget to eat regularly. Skipping meals can result in low blood sugar, a common cause of light-headedness, says Dennis O'Leary, Ph.D., director of the Balance Center at the University of Southern California University Hospital in Los Angeles.

Indulge your sweet tooth. If you suspect your light-headedness is caused by low blood sugar, then try eating a piece of candy or chocolate or drinking a glass of orange juice with a teaspoon of sugar added. That may be all you need to do to relieve the problem, says Ronald Amedee, M.D., associate professor of head and neck surgery at Tulane University Medical Center in New Orleans.

Cool off. Hot, humid days can drain the body of fluids and make you feel light-headed. "My advice in that situation is to get into an air-conditioned room and drink at least a couple of glasses of water, and you'll probably feel a lot better very quickly," Dr. Amedee says.

Reel in your drugs. Some drugs, particularly those used to treat high blood pressure, can cause light-headedness, Dr. Amedee says. Ask your doctor to review your medications with you.

Bow your head. If you feel light-headed, lie down or lower your head between your legs. That will increase blood flow to your brain and heart and reduce your chances of fainting, doctors say.

Brown-bag it. Often, hyperventilation causes light-headedness because overbreathing decreases the amount of oxygen and increases levels of carbon dioxide in your body. If you are hyperventilating, try holding your breath for several seconds or place a paper bag over your nose and mouth and take slow, deep breaths until the light-headedness is gone.

See also Fainting

LIGHT SENSITIVITY

WHEN TO SEE YOUR DOCTOR

- Your eyes suddenly become sensitive to bright light and the discomfort lasts more than an hour.
- You also have pain or pressure in your eyes or see colored halos around lights.
- Your eyes are becoming increasingly sensitive or the sensitivity is interfering with daily activities.

WHAT YOUR SYMPTOM IS TELLING YOU

It's normal to experience momentary discomfort as your eyes adjust to light. When you emerge from a darkened theater into the afternoon sun, for example, that sudden glare is sure to make you squint. But what if ordinary daylight makes you wince and shield your eyes like a criminal caught in a prison yard's floodlights?

In most cases, sensitivity is no cause for alarm. A cold, a sinus infection, even a speck of dirt can stimulate the nerves leading from the eyes to your brain, sending eye-pain messages that make you wince in ordinary daylight.

Certain antibiotics, antihistamines and other medications can also make your eyes temporarily more sensitive to light. So can an eye infection.

If bright, sunny days, or harshly lit rooms *always* make you squint, it may simply mean that you have sun-sensitive eyes, just as some people have sun-sensitive skin, according to Jason Slakter, M.D., attending surgeon in the Department of Ophthalmology at the Manhattan Eye, Ear and Throat Hospital. Or, if you've adopted the prudent habit of wearing sunglasses to shield your eyes from damaging ultraviolet rays, the downside is that now your eyes may be less tolerant to bright light. "This sort of sensitivity isn't harmful," says Dr. Slakter.

Bright light intolerance can also be a by-product of the aging process, adds Dr. Slakter. By age 40, he says, it's common for people to become more sensitive to glare from light bouncing off a car's polished hood, for example, or from light reflected off of a lake or snowy bank. This glare sensitivity occurs as the eyes' aging lenses become thicker or more opaque, thus scattering and magnifying light.

Another, less common disorder, called macular degeneration, damages the light sensor cells that normally help the eye adapt to bright light. The most common form of the disease is more prevalent among older people. A sensitivity to light can also be one of the early warning signs of glaucoma, although you most likely will also experience trouble with your vision and have pain.

Symptom Relief

Any problem that comes on suddenly should be brought to the attention of your doctor as soon as possible. If it turns out to be glaucoma, the sooner you can begin treatment, the better your chances are for saving your eyes. (To find out more about glaucoma, see Eye Pain on page 195.) If you're having a problem adjusting quickly from bright light to dim light while driving, for example, it could be an early warning sign of macular degeneration. Unfortunately, few treatments exist for the most common form of this disease, which may lead to tunnel vision in reverse—or the inability to see straight ahead.

If your problem is nothing more than oversensitive eyes, here's what you can do to help cut the glare.

Buy the best sunblockers. If you have sun-sensitive eyes, you need sunglasses with three main features, says Dr. Slakter. For starters, the tag on your sunglasses should indicate that the lenses screen out at least 90 percent or more of harmful ultraviolet-alpha and beta (UVA and UVB) radiation. Besides helping you see comfortably in harsh light, they may also ward off cataract formation and macular degeneration down the road, adds Mitchell H. Friedlaender, M.D., director of corneal services in the Division of Ophthalmology at the Scripps Clinic and Research Foundation in La Jolla, California, and coauthor of *20/20: A Total Guide to Improving Your Vision and Preventing Eye Disease*.

The lenses should also be polarized to eliminate the glare from reflected sunlight. "You'd be surprised what a difference polarized lenses make when you're fishing on a sun-dappled lake or skiing down a sunlit snow slope," says Bruce Rosenthal, O.D., chief of low vision services at the State University of New York, College of Optometry in Manhattan.

The third feature—a metallic, mirrored coating—further reduces the amount of light that reaches the eyes by reflecting it away. ("To those around you, the lenses look like mirrors," says Dr. Friedlaender.)

Shield your eyes when you're on medication. Light sen-

itivity can be a temporary side effect of a number of common medications such as antihistamines, antibiotics or
blood pressure medication, according to Dr. Friedlaender. If
you're taking one of these medicines and notice that you're
squinting in bright light more than usual, make sure you
wear sunglasses outdoors. You may also need a second pair
of glasses with a lighter, tinted lens to wear in harsh, indoor
light, he adds.

See also Eye Pain

LIMPING

WHEN TO SEE YOUR DOCTOR

You have a limp from an injury or a pain in your body
that does not go away after five days.
- Any unexplained limp, especially in children, should be
seen by a doctor.
- See your doctor immediately if the limp comes on suddenly and is accompanied by muscle weakness on one
side of the body, numbness, fever or radiating pain.

WHAT YOUR SYMPTOM IS TELLING YOU

A limp is okay if you're Gabby Hayes or Walter
Brennan—they made careers out of hobbling and wob-
bling across the silver screen. Unfortunately, Hollywood
doesn't have much of a demand for comical cowboys these
days. Besides, most of us would probably prefer to carry
ourselves with the grace of Fred Astaire or Ginger Rogers.

Maintaining a smooth, even gait is much more complex
than putting one foot in front of the other. It requires a variety of systems and body parts exerting forces and moving in
precise harmony. "Any kind of neural, muscular or skele-
tal abnormality can disrupt this harmony and produce an

imbalance in the way we walk," says Howard Hillstrom,
Ph.D., director of the Gait Study Center at the Pennsylvania College of Podiatric Medicine in Philadelphia.

A commonly seen abnormality is a difference in the
lengths of one's legs. "A limp will frequently develop
because one leg is measurably shorter than the other," says
Howard Dananberg, D.P.M., podiatrist and director of The
Walking Clinic in Bedford, New Hampshire. But in some
people, there is only an *apparent* discrepancy in limb
length. This can happen if you experience contraction or
spasms of the muscles that run on one side of your body
from your shoulder to your pelvis. "Although the legs are
really the same length, one side is so tight, the leg functions
as if it were shorter," says Dr. Dananberg.

Legs that are too big because of excess weight can also
produce problems. Being overweight can produce collapsed
arches, turned-in knees, poor posture and can worsen any
underlying imbalance. Large thighs can also force you to
adopt unusual walking patterns.

Now, suppose that all your body parts are the right
size—only they're not quite in the right place. "Any part of
your body that's out of alignment can produce an imbalance, just like a bad tire can do to your car," says Peter
Francis, Ph.D., professor of physical education at San
Diego State University. One such alignment problem is
excessive pronation—inward rolling of the foot—usually
from fallen arches. Another cause of imbalance might be a
kneecap that "derails" from its normal track of movement.

Sometimes all your parts are where they should be, only
they're not doing what they should do. An example of this
is functional hallux limitus—a locking of the big toe. This
locking can block your ability to extend your thigh, causing
you to drag your leg and flex your waist awkwardly.
Stiffness in the joints of the leg or a muscle weakness that
affects the motion of one or more joints might also cause a
leg to drag.

If any of the bones, muscles or nerves in a leg or foot are
injured, you may limp to minimize the pain. You may even
be in pain and not even be aware of it! Suppose you're a
frequent jogger, a "weekend warrior" or a former high

school football star. The wear and tear of overuse, aging joints or old injuries that did not heal properly may start producing a little pain. Before you even notice it, your body starts limping as a defense mechanism.

Sciatica, a pinching of the sciatic nerve, which runs from the spine through the leg, can also bring on some horrendous hobbling.

Some limps are created purely by habit. For instance, carrying books, a briefcase or a heavy pocketbook on the same side everyday can throw your body off kilter. If you do a great deal of standing on the job, you may tend to unconsciously shift your weight to one leg, even when walking.

The worst-case scenario is that a limp could be the first sign of a bacterial infection in the leg or foot. It can be the initial sign of multiple sclerosis. A limp can even indicate a neurological problem such as nerve damage, neuromuscular disease, a lesion on the spine or a brain tumor. Fortunately such problems are rare.

SYMPTOM RELIEF

Correcting a limp can be tricky business. Most people don't have the patience or the awareness of their movements to re-train their gaits on their own, says Dr. Hillstrom. If you try to treat the effect and not the cause, the problem can get worse. And with so many possible causes, it really requires a physical therapist, podiatrist, orthopedist or walking specialist to find the right one. In the meantime any of the following tips can help put that spring back into your step.

Get a lift. You can easily correct leg length discrepancies, toe lock, fallen arches, pronation and other problems with the use of a prescription, custom-fitted heel lift or arch support, says Dr. Dananberg. "A store-bought device can provide some short-term relief for a minor limp, but it could be detrimental for the limp that has been getting progressively worse." Try an over-the-counter product for two weeks. If it doesn't produce results, see a specialist.

Shift your load. If you overuse one half of your body, start using the other half of your body more, says Dr. Francis. Get in the habit of carrying things on the *other* arm or try a back-pack. If you stand a lot, shift your weight to your other leg or try to place your weight evenly on both legs.

Trade in your chair. Sitting all day in an uncomfortable or unbalanced chair can produce stiffness of joints, numbness of legs and pain from the neck down. Dr. Hillstrom recommends using a chair that has good back support, adjustable height to prevent neck arching or foot dangling and a soft but sturdy cushion on the seat.

Check your shoe size. "Most people don't realize that their foot size can change with time," says Dr. Dananberg. Cramming your tootsies into a tight or poorly fitted shoe can lead to limping, so make sure that you have the proper fit. Also look for flexibility of the soles across the balls of the feet, a raised arch and a slightly raised heel.

Lose a few pounds. Getting rid of excess weight can help ease up many conditions that lead to limping, says Dr. Francis.

Walk on flat surfaces. Walking is an excellent exercise for improving posture . . . as long as you're level. If you limp, you should try to avoid hills, inclines and uneven terrain that can make you lean to the side or cause foot pronation, says Dr. Dananberg.

Swing your arms. A natural, healthy walk involves legs *and* arms. When your right leg is forward, your left arm swings forward; when your left leg is forward, so swings your right arm. If you have difficulty doing this, it may be a sign of stiffness or weakness in the shoulders, says Dr. Francis. This should be checked by a physician who will recommend appropriate strengthening and flexibility exercises.

Pedal with one foot. If you have an obvious imbalance in leg strength or lack flexibility in a joint, you may benefit by focusing strength-building or range-of-motion exercises on that body part, says Dr. Francis. An excellent strength-builder is to pedal on a stationary bike with one leg. Devote more riding time to the weaker leg until it becomes equal in strength to the other. Stop if you feel pain or if the limp worsens.

LIP CHAPPING

WHEN TO SEE YOUR DOCTOR

- Your chapped lips develop severe cracks and fissures.

WHAT YOUR SYMPTOM IS TELLING YOU

If your rough, peeling chapped lips could talk (on their own, that is), they'd beg for two things: moisture and something to seal the moisture in. But how do lips *lose* their moisture? If you have a common habit—lip-licking—you have a sure setup for chapping. Here's how it happens.

In dry air—a centrally heated house in winter, for example—moisture evaporates from your lips. Unconsciously, you notice that dry feeling and lick your lips to wet them again. Then, when this wetness evaporates, it robs your lips of even more moisture, so you feel the urge to lick again. A sunburn on the lips can also tempt you to lick and cause them to chap.

Another common cause of chapped lips is an allergic reaction to dyes in lipstick.

Some people have chapping mostly in the corners of their mouths, and the cause may be the shape of their lips. If your lips turn down at the corners when your face is relaxed, saliva may collect in the corners and cause the outside edges of your lips to chap.

SYMPTOM RELIEF

Chapped lips can be irritating and unsightly. The good news? You can almost always cure them yourself.

Soak to hydrate. To give your sore, chapped lips the ultimate treatment, use daily cool salt water compresses, suggests Caroline Koblenzer, M.D., a clinical associate professor of dermatology at the University of Pennsylvania in Philadelphia.

"Use one teaspoon salt to one pint water. Soak a wash-cloth in the solution and lay it over your lips. Keep it cool and moist for a while, then pat dry," she says. You might try doing this just before going to bed. Do it daily for one week.

Seal in the moisture. Right after the compress, apply a thick coat of an emollient ointment like Vaseline or a lip balm containing waxes or lanolin to hold the moisture in, says Alan R. Shalita, M.D., professor and chairman of dermatology at the State University of New York Health Science Center at Brooklyn.

Step up to cortisone. If a week of compresses and emollients don't do the trick, you can add over-the-counter 1 percent hydrocortisone ointment to your regimen, says Tor Shwayder, M.D., a pediatric dermatologist at Henry Ford Hospital in Detroit. Use the hydrocortisone under your emollient ointment, he suggests. Try this for two weeks.

Don't lick the problem. It's tough to stop licking your lips because the behavior is mostly unconscious, like blinking. But stopping *is* the first step in healing, says Dr. Shwayder. And he says the first step in stopping is just knowing that lip-licking is causing the problem.

Change lipstick. If you suspect that an allergy to an ingredient in your lipstick is causing your lips to chap, Dr. Koblenzer offers this easy home allergy test: "Put a little dab under an adhesive dressing on your inner arm and leave it there for 48 hours," she says. "If you're truly allergic to something in the lipstick, you'll have an itchy reaction."

Your other lipstick options? Either avoid using it altogether or opt for a hypoallergenic brand, she suggests.

Don't get burned. The delicate skin on your lips is easily damaged and chapped by sunburn, says Dr. Shalita. While you're developing the lip ointment habit, be sure to choose a lip balm that contains sunscreen, he suggests.

LIP DISCOLORATION

WHEN TO SEE YOUR DOCTOR

- If your lips suddenly turn blue and you also have a rapid heartbeat, you're sweating or coughing and you have difficulty breathing, see a doctor immediately.
- If your child has blue lips and/or nails and a harsh cough, fever or difficulty breathing, see a doctor immediately.

WHAT YOUR SYMPTOM IS TELLING YOU

If your lips are blue, your body is sad—it isn't getting enough oxygen.

When you are exposed to intense cold, your body directs the flow of blood away from the skin to its core in an effort to provide adequate blood to keep vital organs like the heart, brain and kidneys warm and to conserve the body's heat. This reduces the oxygen supply to the tiny blood vessels near the skin's surface. Seen through the skin of your lips, this oxygen-poor blood looks inky blue.

Blue-tinged lips can also be a sign that your blood has become oxygen-deprived from breathing toxic fumes or from smoking.

If your lips are blue and your skin is pale, you may have iron-deficiency anemia. Iron is a vital component of hemoglobin, the substance that gives blood its red color. Besides nutritional deficiency, other causes of low iron levels include heavy menstrual periods or ulcers—any health problem that results in the regular loss of blood.

In children, blue lips plus a barking cough can indicate a severe form of croup, a common respiratory condition.

Lips that *suddenly* turn from red to blue—along with a rapid pulse and difficulty breathing—are your body's way of saying that your heart or lungs are in trouble. You may have a severe heart problem, or your lungs may not be getting enough oxygen because of pneumonia, bronchitis, asthma or emphysema. A blood clot in the lungs could also do this. Get to the emergency room.

SYMPTOM RELIEF

If your lips turn blue without an obvious cause, see your doctor. He'll probably test you for circulatory problems or anemia. If your lips turn blue because you're sensitive to the cold, here's what to do.

Swaddle yourself from head to toe. Wrap up in a giant towel or blanket that covers your head. "The warmer you can get your entire body, the quicker you'll raise your core temperature and blood can flow back to your lips as well as fingers and toes," says John Abruzzo, M.D., professor of medicine and director of the Rheumatology and Osteoporosis Center at Thomas Jefferson University Hospital in Philadelphia. Drinking steamy liquids can help the process by dilating blood vessels and promoting better blood flow. But pass up coffee, says Dr. Abruzzo. Caffeine narrows the vessels. (For more tips on warming your extremities, see page 276.)

Do some jumping jacks. Aerobic movement involving nonstop motion of your arms and legs gets blood moving and delivers oxygen to the tissues. "It will quickly bring a rosy flush to your skin and lips," says Dr. Abruzzo.

Nix the nicotine. Cigarette smoke chokes off oxygen and also narrows blood vessels, says Dr. Abruzzo.

LOWER BACK PAIN

WHEN TO SEE YOUR DOCTOR

- Your pain lasts more than 72 hours.
- Your pain is so severe that it interferes with your work.
- Your pain seems to radiate to your legs, feet or toes.

WHAT YOUR SYMPTOM IS TELLING YOU

There's no doubt about it: Lower back pain can be a real pain in the you-know-where—interrupting your work, keeping you from your hobbies, forcing you to hobble around the house.

Complain if you want—just don't buy the myth that you have to put up with it. While a tiny group of back pain sufferers (less than 1 percent) *do* end up needing surgery, your pain is probably nothing more than your body serving notice that you've been overdoing it. You've pushed your back ligaments, muscles and joints to do too much, and now they're rebelling.

"If you ask someone what caused their problem, they usually tell you they did too much. They exercised too much or they worked too hard or they lifted too much or they slipped...something of that nature," says David Imrie, M.D., coauthor of *The Back Power Program* and medical director of Medifit of America in Teaneck, New Jersey. "The problem, I believe, is that we are generally involved in too *little* physical activity, so when we do too much, we get into trouble.

"Most back pain comes from muscle weakness, muscle tightness and joint problems—things you can't see on an x-ray," he says.

Another cause of lower back pain is a slipped or injured disk—the jellylike cushion that works as a shock absorber between the vertebrae of the spine. How can you tell if you've slipped a disk? Severe pain may radiate from your back into one of your legs.

SYMPTOM RELIEF

Before you try any self-help treatments, you can determine whether you need to see a doctor immediately by taking this test: While lying on a firm bed or mattress, straighten one leg and raise it 90 degrees. If you have pain radiating down your leg, seek medical help as soon as possible.

If your lower back is merely whimpering for help, try these treatments for fast relief.

Hit the floor. For this remedy from Brent V. Lovejoy, D.O., a member of the board of trustees of the American Osteopathic College of Preventive Medicine and director of the Rocky Mountain Medical Group in Denver, you'll need some floor space, a pillow and a small ice pack (a bag of ice wrapped in a towel or cloth will do.) Lie on your back on the floor and put a pillow under your knees—that raises them slightly, taking some of the pressure off your lower back. Now place the ice under the painful area for about 20 minutes. If lying on the ice is too uncomfortable, dispense with it. Just lying in this position will provide some relief, says Dr. Lovejoy.

Be cool. Ask your spouse or a friend to rub the painful area with ice for at least 20 minutes every couple of hours. Continue ice treatment until three days after the injury. In addition to numbing the pain and relaxing muscle spasms, ice also reduces swelling, says Hubert Rosomoff, M.D., D.Med.Sc., medical director of the University of Miami Comprehensive Pain and Rehabilitation Center in Miami Beach.

Some like it hot. You may also benefit from moist heat applied to your achy back. Try using either a hot-water bottle or a towel that has been soaked in hot water. The warmth increases the flow of blood and oxygen to the injured area, which speeds healing, says Dr. Lovejoy. Because heat can promote swelling, don't use it until 72 hours after the injury, he says.

S-t-r-e-t-c-h. Once your homemade anesthetic (ice) has kicked in, gently stretch your back. The best technique in an emergency, according to Vert Mooney, M.D., professor of orthopedic surgery at the University of California, San Diego, Medical Center and director of the Spine and Joint Conditioning Center: Lie on your stomach, then bend your arms, placing your hands flat on the floor directly under your shoulders. Slowly raise your torso onto your elbows for ten seconds, lower your body and repeat. This movement forces nutrients and oxygen into the disks of the lower spine and forces out waste products like lactic acid, helping ease muscle spasms, says Dr. Mooney.

Hit the hay. For severe lower back pain, bed rest is of some value, but the amount must be limited. In fact, for every three hours that you're down, doctors say you should be on your feet for between 20 minutes and an hour. "We know the detrimental effects of staying on your back," says Dr. Lovejoy. "You lose calcium from your bones and your muscles begin to weaken."

Hit the streets. Some people seem to improve by taking a short walk, says Dr. Lovejoy. The reason: Unlike sitting, walking *reduces* the amount of stress on your lower back.

Kill the painkillers—if you can. Prescription pain relievers *will* help the most severe cases of back pain. But try limiting their use to two to three days after an injury, recommends Dr. Lovejoy. These powerful, addicting narcotics merely treat the pain—not the cause. "I rarely allow my patients to use them," he says.

Ask for an NSAID. Nonsteroidal anti-inflammatory drugs are available over-the-counter. These medications help reduce the swelling often associated with muscle and other soft-tissue injuries, says Dr. Lovejoy. Aspirin is one form of NSAID, but you may also consider taking ibuprofen, which is thought to be a more powerful NSAID, says Dr. Lovejoy.

Try a chiropractor. Either a chiropractor or an osteopath is capable of manipulating your spine to help alleviate back pain. Both use x-rays and detailed patient histories to make their diagnosis, says Dr. Lovejoy. Osteopaths are licensed to prescribe drugs, but chiropractors are not. "About 50 to 60 percent of all back problems can be seen once or twice for manipulation and be resolved," he says.

Take TENS. If your back pain just keeps on coming back, you might want to ask your doctor about transcutaneous electrical nerve stimulation (TENS), a small but powerful emergency back pain treatment. Electricity from a compact device courses through electrodes taped to your back, stimulating the lower back muscles and ending spasms. Although not a muscle strengthener, TENS units may also be used after surgery to help reduce pain, says Dr. Lovejoy.

Beating Back Pain at Work

You undoubtedly feel safe sitting at your desk in that air-conditioned office. But did you know you're just as likely to develop lower back pain as someone who works outdoors? In one study, researchers discovered that women who worked in offices had the same kind of degenerative back changes—like loss of water from their spinal disks—as meter maids, says Annie Pivarski, a back-care consultant and personal trainer in San Francisco who helped rehabilitate the back of San Francisco '49ers quarterback Joe Montana following back surgery in 1986. To keep from beating up your back at work, try these tips.

Be a clock watcher. It's not enough to merely shift your weight in your seat. You have to *move*. Stand up at least once an hour and stretch, says Pivarski. Here's one good stretch from Dr. Lovejoy: Stand erect and place your hands on your lower back. Bend backward slightly by lifting your chest up and out. Hold, then relax and repeat. Now slowly increase your stretch by tilting your head back and leaning backward as far as comfortable. Hold the position for just a moment. Now slowly raise your head, then your body so you are standing erect again. Repeat.

Divide and conquer. Structure your work routine so that you alternate between standing and sitting, says Pivarski. "Anything that would allow you to change your position can help remedy this overuse syndrome," she says.

Pull up the right chair. Even so-called ergonomic (user-friendly) chairs can have a devastating effect on your back if they're not right for *you*. If possible, get a chair that has an adjustable, contoured seat so that your hips are slightly higher than your knees. If the chair is too low, you'll feel pressure on your tailbone; too high and you'll feel pressure on your lower thighs.

If the chair has armrests, they should be adjustable so that your arms can rest freely at your sides. Armrests that are too long prevent you from you moving close enough to your desk, causing you to lean forward in your seat. Leaning forward causes more load on the lower back than just about anything else that people do," says Pivarski.

Kneeling chairs can also help reduce strain on the lower back depending on the tasks at hand, she says. (Kneeling chairs are definitely not the answer for people who also have knee problems, she adds.)

Go on a roll. Whether it's a specially designed foam roll or simply a small pillow placed at the small of your back when you sit down, lumbar supports help retain the natural curve of your spine while you're seated, says Pivarski.

Do a computer chin-up. If your computer screen is too low, you run the risk of leaning forward while typing and straining your back and neck, Pivarski says. Leaning backward isn't good either. A good guide: Make sure that the center of your screen is at chin level. A couple of old phone books placed under your monitor may be all you need to push your screen up to the proper level.

Driving Dos and Don'ts

Another place where your lower back can get into trouble is the front seat of your car. Frequent driving doesn't have to put you on the road to back pain. Consider these tips.

Sit pretty. Instead of diving behind the wheel when you get into your car, back in and sit gently, then turn and swing your legs inside. "Most people don't get in and out of their cars properly," says Dr. Rosomoff.

Resist low riding. Ever notice the people who sit so low and far back in their cars that they can barely see over the steering wheel? They may look cool, but they're begging for lower back problems, says Pivarski. "What often happens is that in stretching out your legs, you pull your back away from the back of the seat and you start to slump. That's bad news for your lower back," she says. Adjust your seat so you're sitting slightly reclined when you drive.

Prop yourself up. Available at most drug and medical supply stores, a low-back support is also helpful when riding in or driving a car, especially if yours has bucket seats, says Pivarski. Avoid the wooden bead kind, she warns, as they can cause problems during an accident.

Give yourself an hour. It may sound impractical, but doctors suggest that after sitting in a car for an hour, you should take time to stop, get out of your car and stretch your back. Failing that, you can also shift your rear end from side to side, wiggle your feet and tighten your stomach muscles to help give your back a break.

Home Back Savers

Instituting these back-saving steps at home will go a long way toward relieving repeated episodes of lower back pain.

Sleep sweetly. From now on, before going to sleep, place one pillow under your head and two pillows under your knees, says Dr. Lovejoy. Alternatively, you can lie on your side with your head on top of a pillow and a pillow under your feet and lower legs, he says. These positions will ensure a good night's sleep for you and take pressure off your lower back. Also, a firm mattress is better for your back than one that sags, he says.

Easy does it. Bounding out of bed may be the stuff of business legends, but it's actually a good way to beat up your back. Why? While you were sleeping, the disks in your spine were filling up with water, making them plump and causing some stiffness in surrounding muscles. To protect against sudden moves that can cause microtears in the spinal disks, simply roll onto your side and push yourself up with your arms. Finally, swing your feet onto the floor, says Pivarski.

Be sink smart. Bending over the sink to brush your teeth or shave can also strain your lower back. Instead of merely leaning into the effort, open the cabinet door below the sink and rest your foot inside. Then brace yourself with one hand, says Pivarski. You can also put your foot on a small stool or box. Switch feet every few minutes.

Get a leg up. Instead of sinking into your favorite easy chair, reduce the strain on your back by keeping one knee higher than the level of your hips. One technique: Rest one foot on a stool in front of you, says Dr. Lovejoy.

Stretching: The Right Moves

Because a flexible back is usually a pain-free back, most doctors recommend that your treatment include stretching. Dr. Lovejoy suggests including these stretches in your low back protection plan.

Knee to chest. Lie on your back and bring both knees to your chest. Hold the position for a slow count of 20. Then return your feet to the floor and relax. You can also perform this stretch with one leg at a time.

Cat stretch. Get down on your hands and knees. First relax, letting your back sink down and sag. Now arch up and stretch like an angry cat for ten seconds. Repeat ten times.

Lateral trunk stretch. Lie on your back with your knees bent and your feet flat on the floor. Now cross your right leg over the left. Let both knees drop slowly to the right toward the floor. Take the stretch only as far as is comfortable for you and then hold the position for ten seconds. Switch legs and repeat.

Building a Better Back

After you've stretched, you can increase your strength and protect against lower back pain with this following series of doctor-recommended exercises. Not convinced they're important? A study of Los Angeles firefighters found that those who exercised regularly with weights had half as many back injuries as their less-active colleagues, says Dr. Lovejoy.

Abdominal curl. Lie on your back with your knees bent and your feet flat on the floor. Now slowly lift your head and shoulders off the floor, keeping your eyes fixed on the ceiling. Hold this position for a two count, then slowly lower your head and shoulders back down. Repeat 20 times.

Opposite arm and leg lifts. Lie on your stomach with your arms stretched out in front of you. Now lift your right arm and left leg several inches off the floor and hold for a count of ten. Rest and repeat, using the opposite arm and leg. If you recently suffered back pain, do the exercise only one or two times. As your strength increases, consider strapping on one-pound ankle weights and holding a can of soup in each hand, says Jennifer Stone, head athletic trainer at the U.S. Olympic Training Center in Colorado Springs.

Get aerobic. Some of the best exercises for your lower back don't seem like back work at all. Any aerobic activity, like walking or swimming, challenges most of the body's muscles, including the ones in your lower back, says Dr. Lovejoy. Perform your favorite aerobic exercise three times a week for at least 20 minutes, he says.

LUMPS

WHEN TO SEE YOUR DOCTOR

- Any lump or any change in a lump that has been already diagnosed should be brought to the attention of your doctor.

WHAT YOUR SYMPTOM IS TELLING YOU

No, you probably don't have cancer. But another c-word—caution—is *strongly* advised if you have a lump.

"Most lumps you feel under your skin aren't cancerous and are probably harmless. But it's up to your physician to make that judgment," says Glen Hollinger, M.D., an internist at the Hospital of the Good Samaritan in Los Angeles.

A lump is most commonly a cyst, abscess, benign tumor or lipoma—a harmless round, fatty growth that has the consistency of modeling clay. Lumps can occur in almost every part of the body, but usually are found in the breasts, arms, legs and back.

SYMPTOM RELIEF

In most cases, finding a lump isn't a cause for panic," Dr. Hollinger says. "But I urge you to let your doctor know about it as soon as possible," says Dr. Hollinger. Here are a few things you should be aware of.

Let it be. Lipoma, the most common kind of lump, probably doesn't need treatment. "It's a meaningless lump and really not worth worrying about unless it gets infected, which usually doesn't happen," says John C. Rogers, M.D., M.P.H., vice chairman of the Department of Family Medicine at Baylor College of Medicine in Houston. A woman who has a lipoma near the bra line may find it very uncomfortable, however, and may decide to have the lump removed. The procedure can be done in a single visit to the doctor's office.

Get an abscess drained. If the lump is a cyst or an abscess, your doctor will probably recommend having it drained, which is another simple office procedure. The doctor makes a small incision, allows the fluid to drain from the lump, covers the area with a surgical bandage and you're done.

Know your body. Regular self-examination is the best way to insure early detection of breast and testicular lumps, Dr. Hollinger says. Women should examine their breasts five to seven days after the end of their periods or on the same day each month if they have gone through menopause. Men should examine their testicles for lumps at least once a month. If you don't know how to do a proper breast or testicular exam, ask your doctor to show you.

Get treatment. The reason to have a doctor check any new lump—or any lump that changes color or size—is to find out whether it shows signs of being cancerous. If it is, the earlier you get treatment, the greater your chances of recovery. Treatment will depend on several factors, including the type of cancer, its size and location and the likelihood of it spreading to other parts of your body.

See also Breast Lumps

M

MALAISE

WHEN TO SEE YOUR DOCTOR

- A feeling of the blahs persists for more than five days.
- Your abdomen hurts or you've noticed changes in your bowel movements.
- Urination is painful or difficult, or you have a discharge from your vagina or penis.

WHAT YOUR SYMPTOM IS TELLING YOU

An indefinite feeling of lack of health often indicative of the onset of an illness"—that's what Webster has to say about this symptom, which means that it could be a sign of *any* and *every* disease.

But let's investigate a little more thoroughly. Whenever you have malaise, other, more revealing symptoms will undoubtedly provide a better indication of what's troubling you, according to Clayton W. Kersting, M.D., a family physician in Newport, Washington. "Malaise means 'a vague feeling of uncomfortableness.' Doctors hate the word 'vague,' so we have to go from head to toe asking questions for a more specific cause of the problem."

At the least, a bout of the blahs might be all in your head, the result of too much stress or work and not enough play time, Dr. Kersting says. If you're constantly sad and lack motivation, you may be depressed. Or perhaps you're not eating well and not getting enough nutrients. Maybe you're not sleeping enough.

Infections and viral illnesses often produce a listless feeling, says Anne Simons, M.D., an assistant professor of family and community medicine at the University of California in San Francisco and coauthor of *Before You Call the Doctor.* And you don't have to be visibly ill. "A hidden infection like chronic sinusitis or a tooth infection may not be immediately obvious, but it'll make you feel sick," she says.

Anemia could be behind your blahs, especially if you also feel weak or light-headed. Women who have heavy menstrual periods and the elderly are especially susceptible, Dr. Simons says.

An underactive thyroid can cause malaise, Dr. Kersting says. If you have an underactive thyroid, you'll probably also feel weak, sleep more than usual, gain some weight, miss some periods and feel cold.

Heart and lung problems may be responsible if you feel chest pains or can't breathe sufficiently. Intestinal abnormalities—from stomach viruses to tumors—will disrupt your bowel movement in addition to making you feel bad. Urinary tract infections, pelvic inflammatory disease and prostate malfunctions interfere with urination and produce a burning sensation when you do urinate.

SYMPTOM RELIEF

So now not only are you tired of being down in the dumps and singing the blues, you're overwhelmed by the possible causes. Pick yourself up with some of these malaise erasers.

Give yourself a break. You may just need to inject some fun in your life. "When was the last time you had a vacation or did something nice for your spouse and kids?" Dr. Kersting asks. "Go to the movies, then set your priorities for the more enjoyable things."

Stock your refrigerator. Concentrate on eating more nutritious foods. And pick up a daily multivitamin and mineral supplement. "A healthy diet is important to feeling healthy," Dr. Kersting says.

Put some metal into your mettle. An iron supplement may bolster your spirits if you're suffering from a deficiency, Dr. Simons says. Vitamin B12 supplements may help your blood if you're elderly. "Anemia caused by iron or B12 deficiency may be a sign of a more serious problem, like internal bleeding, an ulcer or cancer. Be sure to ask your doctor if these supplements are appropriate for you," she says.

Move your body. Exercise makes you feel better physically and emotionally, Dr. Kersting says, so start a workout program. Select an activity you like to do so you'll stay with it. "If you don't like bicycling, don't buy a stationary bicycle," says Dr. Kersting.

Take your temperature. Fever is an indication of an infection somewhere in the body, Dr. Simons points out. If you have an infection, antibiotics probably will help.

Have a look under the hood. Schedule a checkup and physical with your doctor, making sure you go from head to toe mentioning any other symptoms that are bothersome.

Don't worry. Never ignore even a hazy notion of not feeling well, but at the same time, never frighten yourself by assuming the worst. "I think a lot of the times if people get a vague symptom, they worry it's cancer or something serious," Dr. Simons says. "In fact, it's rare that those things cause only malaise."

MENSTRUAL CRAMPS

WHEN TO SEE YOUR DOCTOR

- Your cramps are so severe that you cannot attend school or work or keep up your usual activities.
- Your cramps are accompanied by nausea, headaches, diarrhea and vomiting.
- You also bleed very heavily or pass clots for more than one day.
- You have severe cramps and you take birth control pills.
- Your painful cramps began suddenly in adulthood.
- Your cramps are not relieved by taking aspirin or ibuprofen.
- You've just begun to menstruate, and your first or second period causes very severe cramps.

WHAT YOUR SYMPTOM IS TELLING YOU

Menstrual cramping is one of the few symptoms on a schedule. Cramps arrive with the same relentless regularity as the mortgage payment or the utility bills...and are about as welcome.

Ever wonder why something as natural as a woman's monthly cycle should be accompanied by varying degrees of discomfort? Well, so have medical researchers. They've found that a woman's body produces hormones known as prostaglandins to help the uterus contract and shed its lining. The uterus has to contract to create the menstrual flow, and many women experience the contractions as cramps.

Fortunately, most of the time menstrual cramps are relatively mild. More than 50 percent of women experience some sort of cramping, usually starting one to three years after they begin their periods, says Susan Coupey, M.D., a researcher studying common menstrual disorders at Montefiore Medical Center in the Bronx.

How painful your cramps are will depend on how much prostaglandin your body produces, says John Jennings, M.D., a gynecologist at Bowman Gray School of Medicine of Wake Forest University in Winston-Salem, North Carolina. But if you have persistent, really excruciating cramps, there may be other factors at work as well. You may have an overgrown uterine lining—a condition called endometriosis. Endometriosis often makes cramps hurt worse, Dr. Jennings says.

Or if you cramp during a period that's much heavier than usual, your uterus might be squeezing out blood clots caused by fibroids, says Charles Debrovner, M.D., professor of obstetrics and gynecology at New York University School of Medicine in New York City and a gynecologist at New York University Hospital. Fibroids are benign muscle tumors in the uterine wall. And sometimes a woman may experience cramping that signals the loss of an undiagnosed pregnancy.

SYMPTOM RELIEF

If your monthly period is accompanied by cramps, who cares if they're common—they *hurt*! Though you can't help having cramps, there are many things you can do to ease the ache.

Swim away from the pain. Not only does exercise release endorphins—your body's own natural painkillers—but it can take your mind off the cramps. "Of all the things you can do if you have bad cramps, swimming is the least traumatic and most helpful," says Marcia Storch, M.D., director of the women's unit of New York University Student Health Services in New York City and co-author of *How to Relieve Cramps and Other Menstrual Problems.*

Relax your muscles for relief. If you feel too cramped up and uncomfortable to even consider swimming, try this gentle exercise from Dr. Storch. It will help relax the muscles that cause the cramps.

Lie on your back on the floor or a bed with your knees bent, your feet flat on the floor or bed and your arms at your sides, palms down. Lightly bounce your belly up and down for a couple of minutes, keeping the muscles loose. While you are bouncing, take short, quick panting breaths. Bounce and breathe for ten breaths. Do this series five times. Rest between series. (Quick, shallow breathing can make you dizzy.) Next, place a big, heavy, soft-covered book (a big-city phone book is fine) across your abdomen. Slowly breathe in through your nose, filling your abdomen and chest with air and pushing the book up. Hold for a count of five. On six, begin exhaling slowly through your mouth, and let the book drop slowly. Contract your stomach muscles and hold for a count of five. Continue deep relaxed breathing for a couple more minutes.

The book creates pressure that can help relieve abdominal spasms, says Dr. Storch.

Put heat where it hurts. Heat feels very good on a crampy abdomen, says Dr. Jennings. Using a hot-water bottle or heating pad increases blood flow and circulation to your uterus and may help lessen the impact of the naturally occurring chemicals that cause the cramps, he says.

Try relaxing in a warm bath or placing a heating pad or hot-water bottle on the abdomen for 15 minutes. You might want to try gently massaging over-the-counter deep-heating creams or oils into the abdomen. (Warning: Never use these creams and a heating pad at the same time. Combining the two can cause severe burns.)

You can also warm your tummy by sipping hot liquids—clear soups, broth or a nice cup of herbal tea.

Chill out your cramps. Some women find that applying cold instead of heat eases cramps. Try putting an ice pack on your abdomen for 15 to 20 minutes, says Dr. Debrovner. The cold constricts blood vessels, which can bring relief, he explains.

Check out calcium. "Does your diet consist mainly of low-calcium foods like fruits and vegetables? Then make a special point of seeking out low-fat yogurt and low-fat milk," recommends James G. Penland, Ph.D., a psychologist with the U.S. Department of Agriculture's (USDA) Human Nutrition Research Center in Grand Forks, North Dakota.

At least four different studies have shown that calcium offers strong relief from menstrual cramps. Yet, on average, American women tend to consume only about 600 milligrams of calcium daily. (The Recommended Dietary Allowance is 800 milligrams.)

In one USDA research project, Dr. Penland found that women who consumed 1,300 or more daily milligrams of calcium reported a reduction in menstrual cramps. Not only did they report less pain, but also less water retention, improved moods and better concentration.

"One cup of low-fat yogurt will give you about 400 milligrams of calcium, and there are about 300 milligrams in a cup of low-fat milk," Dr. Penland says.

Keep active. Don't give up your normal routines, says Dr. Jennings. If you get up and move around, it can take your mind off the cramps and divert you from the pain.

Coddle yourself a little. Anxiety can increase pain by over 30 percent, says Dr. Storch. So experiencing anything you associate with comfort and ease may help the pain. She suggests tea, hot milk or even chocolate if these are strongly associated with comfort.

Inhibit cramps with ibuprofen. Though the naturally occurring hormone prostaglandin is a normal partner in the menstruation process, some women are extremely sensitive to it, says Dr. Debrovner. Ibuprofen drugs, such as Advil, are among the most effective prostaglandin inhibitors, he says.

Timing is critical to head off the pain of cramps, however. The earlier you take the medicine, the better it works, he says.

"Take it with food at the very first twinge or the very first sign of flow," he suggests. "Usually, ibuprofen for the first day or two of your period is all that's needed."

Love away the pain. Cramps are often accompanied by uncomfortable sensations of pelvic congestion and heaviness caused by dilated blood vessels. Having an orgasm sometimes helps ease the discomfort, says Dr. Debrovner, because the uterine contractions you experience during orgasm also contract the dilated blood vessels that cause that congested feeling.

When Professionals Can Help

If despite your efforts at home treatment, cramps continue to create discomfort every month, consider discussing the problem with your doctor. There are several treatments that might help.

Try the Anaprox antidote. Of all the prescription drugs that calm cramps, Anaprox is the drug of choice for most women, says Dr. Storch, because it's more rapidly absorbed into your system.

"And if you anticipate the cramps, you'll end up taking less medicine," she says. Do you know your period will arrive tomorrow and that heavy cramps are par for the course? "Take an Anaprox before going to bed," she suggests.

Check out biofeedback. If you'd prefer a nondrug cure for cramps, ask your doctor for a referral to a clinical psychologist or psychiatrist in your community who offers biofeedback training.

In biofeedback, you use a monitor that tells you when your muscles are tense and when they're relaxed. Gradually, you learn to identify and "create" relaxed muscles.

A study supervised by Jack May, Ph.D., a psychologist at Florida State University in Tallahassee, showed that women who received biofeedback training reported a very significant reduction of menstrual pain and discomfort.

"Ask for training for a few days at mid-cycle, to learn the techniques for reducing menstrual cramps," Dr. May suggests. "Then when your cycle begins, you can use the biofeedback for cramps control."

See also Pelvic Pain

MENSTRUAL FLOW, HEAVY

WHEN TO SEE YOUR DOCTOR

- Your periods are so heavy that they interfere with your lifestyle or regular activities.
- You are passing clots and never have before.
- You feel weak or dizzy during your period.
- Your heavy periods are not preceded by your *usual* premenstrual symptoms, such as breast tenderness, abdominal bloating or food cravings.
- You are also experiencing bleeding between periods.
- Your periods are also more than 45 to 50 days apart.

WHAT YOUR SYMPTOM IS TELLING YOU

What does "heavy" mean? Well, what is heavy to you might feel normal to Judy down the block. But doctors say that needing to change your pad or tampon more than once an hour is a reasonable measure of heavy.

Overzealous dieting or exercising may cause unusually

heavy periods, says Charles Debrovner, M.D., professor of obstetrics and gynecology at New York University School of Medicine in New York City and a gynecologist at New York University Hospital.

Other possible causes of heavy bleeding include infections, clotting problems and polyps or fibroids (benign growths in the uterus).

SYMPTOM RELIEF

If heavy periods are not the norm for you, see your doctor for diagnosis and treatment. But these tips may help in the meantime.

Lighten up. Scaling back on your busy schedule may help lessen the flow, says Dr. Debrovner.

See it out with C. One simple remedy for a very heavy flow is to take higher doses of vitamin C, says Dr. Debrovner. Vitamin C firms up the walls of tiny blood vessels in the uterus called capillaries and helps decrease monthly blood flow, he explains. He recommends a dose of between 1,000 and 2,000 milligrams daily, beginning a few days before your period and continuing until it ends. (Get the go-ahead from your doctor before taking any supplements.)

Pump up your nutrients. "Make sure your diet includes plenty of B vitamins and iron," says Wulf Utian, M.D., Ph.D., chairman of the Department of Reproductive Biology at Case Western Reserve University in Cleveland. Vitamin B12 and folate are important nutrients for building healthy blood volume and blood quality. "Iron is needed for hemoglobin, another important blood component," he says. The level of B vitamins and iron in a typical daily multiple vitamin should be sufficient.

Help from Your Doctor

When uterine growths or undetermined causes result in heavy periods, your doctor can help with medication, or in some cases, surgery.

Reach for anti-inflammatories. Prescription-strength

nonsteroidal anti-inflammatory drugs (NSAIDs) may often correct the problem when no specific cause has been found, says Susan Haas, M.D., a reproductive endocrinologist and assistant professor of obstetrics, gynecology and reproductive biology at Harvard Medical School. Your doctor is most likely to prescribe mefenamic acid, which you take up to three times daily during your period, she says. Although ibuprofen is an over-the-counter drug of the same type as Ponstel, Dr. Haas notes, it has not been proven as a treatment for heavy menstrual bleeding.

Avert anemia. In some women, extremely heavy periods may cause several days of mild anemia, says Dr. Utian. In this instance, your doctor may prescribe birth control pills to regularize and lessen the flow. Why the pill for heavy periods? During the first half of the menstrual cycle, the ovaries produce only estrogen, which causes the uterine lining to grow very thick and bleed more when it is shed during a period. When birth control pills containing both estrogen and progesterone are taken, the lining grows less thick, producing less bleeding.

Have the growths removed. If you are diagnosed with polyps or fibroids, your doctor may recommend surgery to remove them. Depending on the size and location of the growths, either abdominal surgery or a newer procedure called *hysteroscopy* may be needed. During hysteroscopy, a fiber-optic device with tiny surgical instruments attached is passed through the cervix to remove the growths, says Dr. Haas. Seventy-five percent of women who have this procedure are permanently helped, Dr. Haas says.

Another procedure, called *endometrial ablation*, coagulates the entire uterine lining. Fifty to 80 percent of women with heavy bleeding experience no bleeding at all after this procedure, says Dr. Haas.

Before either of these surgeries, your doctor will prescribe drugs called GnRH agonists for a few months to shrink any growths and cause your periods to stop, Dr. Haas says. "They are used as a short-term fix to allow your body to build blood cells back up before surgery," she says.

MENSTRUAL FLOW IRREGULARITY

WHEN TO SEE YOUR DOCTOR

- You also bleed in between periods or after intercourse.
- You also bleed heavily or for more than ten days.
- Your periods are more than a week off schedule or you miss more than an occasional period.
- Your irregular periods are accompanied by fever.
- You also experience severe cramps, and they are not relieved by ibuprofen or aspirin.

WHAT YOUR SYMPTOM IS TELLING YOU

Ever watch the easy blur of rubber balls that a good juggler can produce? Then consider what many women try to keep aloft all at once: jobs, relationships, family responsibilities . . . never mind time to relax. Imagine those whirling balls, and it's easy to see how your own juggling act can become high-performance stress. And it's stress that is the major cause of menstrual irregularity, according to Lane Mercer, M.D., chief of gynecology at Northwestern University Medical School in Chicago.

Whether the stress is a major life event like a divorce or a daily struggle like deadlines, your body says to itself: This is probably not a very good time to reproduce. But your "body language" in this case is *chemical:* It stops producing progesterone, the hormone that triggers ovulation and menstrual bleeding.

Of course, stress isn't the only cause of irregular periods. In pre-teens and teens, the mechanisms that control ovulation and menstruation aren't mature, and missed periods are common, says Dr. Mercer. As women move into their twenties, menstrual cycles usually become regular.

Menstrual irregularity also is common in the midforties

as you approach menopause. Although you still menstruate, you may find yourself going 30 or more days without a period.

The stress of gaining or losing a lot of weight can also play tricks on your hormones and change your menstrual calendar, Dr. Mercer says. Other dietary factors, such as vegetarianism, can also play a role.

There can be medical causes for irregular periods as well, including infection, uterine polyps or fibroids, cancer and structural abnormalities of the uterus.

SYMPTOM RELIEF

Though the cause of irregularity is usually common and harmless, if it persists more than a few months, you should see your doctor to determine treatment. Here's a look at the options your doctor may suggest.

Rule out the infection connection. If your irregular periods are accompanied by pain or fever, you may have an infection, says R. Don Gambrell, Jr., M.D., clinical professor of endocrinology and obstetrics and gynecology at the Medical College of Georgia Hospital and Clinics in Augusta and author of the *Estrogen Replacement Therapy User Guide*. Your doctor will probably treat an infection with antibiotics, he says.

Reset the cycle. If you are between the ages of 20 and 40 and your irregularity persists longer than three months, your doctor may have you take a progesterone medication called Provera for about three months, says Dr. Mercer. This drug will mimic the progesterone you normally get from ovulation. After that, he says, your body will often correct itself.

Check out the vegetarian variation. Research has shown that vegetarian women have four times more irregular or absent periods than nonvegetarian women. The researchers believe the high amounts of fiber in the typical vegetarian diet cause estrogen levels to drop, making menstrual irregularity more likely, says Tom Lloyd, M.D., a reproductive endocrinologist at the Milton S. Hershey Medical Center in Hershey, Pennsylvania.

"If you're vegetarian, ask your family physician or gynecologist to check your circulating estrogen levels," advises Dr. Lloyd. If your levels are low, your doctor may prescribe a dietary change or supplemental estrogen in the form of tablets or a patch, he says.

Factor out fibroids and polyps. If fibroids—fleshy growths in the uterus—are interfering with your cycle, your doctor will first treat any hormonal abnormality, says Dr. Gambrell. Often fibroid surgery is not necessary, he says.

If the problem is caused by polyps—grapelike growths in the uterus—they can usually be removed very simply in the doctor's office, he says.

Doctors can treat fibroids or structural abnormalities of the uterus that are causing stubborn bleeding problems with surgical remedies, including endometrial ablation, a procedure in which the lining of the uterus is cauterized, says Dr. Mercer. In severe cases, your doctor might recommend a hysterectomy, the removal of the uterus.

MENSTRUAL SPOTTING

WHEN TO SEE YOUR DOCTOR

- Spotting happens at the time you normally expect your menstrual period, and you could possibly be pregnant.
- Unexplained spotting persists for more than three months.
- Your spotting is accompanied by fever or pelvic pain.

WHAT YOUR SYMPTOM IS TELLING YOU

About 5 percent of women will experience spotting—a light staining of blood—regularly with ovulation. The key to this harmless kind of spotting doctors say, is that it happens almost every month near the middle of your menstrual cycle. Often this spotting is accompanied by mild pain on the right or left side of the abdomen. (However, in some women, *lack* of ovulation, which causes the uterine lining to grow thicker and then shed small areas of tissue at different times, may also be a cause of spotting.)

If you are experiencing spotting that does not seem related to ovulation, there can be a variety of causes, including infections of the vagina, bladder, cervix or edometrium (uterine lining). Other possible causes include polyps, little fleshy growths in the uterus; cervical dysplasia, abnormal cells in the cervix; cancer; pregnancy complications; the wrong birth control pills or hormonal imbalances.

SYMPTOM RELIEF

Your doctor will have to diagnose and prescribe treatment for unexplained spotting. Here's what to expect.

Clarify the cause. Your doctor will perform a careful physical exam, examining the outer areas, the vaginal lining and cervix, says Wulf Utian, M.D., Ph.D., chairman of the Department of Reproductive Biology at Case Western Reserve University in Cleveland. If necessary, he may take small tissue samples for closer examination under the microscope.

Harmonize the hormones. You may need to keep a temperature chart to determine whether or not you are ovulating, says Susan Haas, M.D., a reproductive endocrinologist and assistant professor of obstetrics, gynecology and reproductive biology at Harvard Medical School. If lack of ovulation turns out to be the cause of your spotting, your doctor will probably prescribe hormones, either in the form of birth control pills or progesterone.

Although birth control pills are a frequent treatment for this type of spotting, Dr. Haas says, for some women they may also be the cause. In that case, your doctor will adjust your birth control prescription.

Treat any infections. If an infection of the vagina or bladder is the cause of your spotting, your doctor will prescribe a course of antibiotics to clear it up, says Brian Walsh, M.D., assistant professor of obstetrics/gynecology and reproductive biology at Harvard Medical School and director of the Menopause Unit at Brigham and Women's Hospital in Boston.

Safeguard the cervix. Occasionally the cervix (the narrow opening to the womb) produces abnormal cells. This condition, known as dysplasia, can cause spotting and is usually easy to treat. Your doctor can use a laser to vaporize the abnormal cells, says Dr. Walsh. Dysplasia is very common, he adds, and two-thirds of the time represents no threat to your health. Dysplasia can be a precursor of cancer, though, so careful monitoring and treatment are vital, he says.

If you have been diagnosed with dysplasia, you can help protect the cervix by shielding it with a condom or diaphragm during intercourse.

MIDBACK PAIN

WHEN TO SEE YOUR DOCTOR

- Your pain lasts for more than three days.
- You are experiencing extremely severe or shooting pains.
- You also have numbness in your midback.
- You have heart disease.

WHAT YOUR SYMPTOM IS TELLING YOU

What is it with "mid"? You could be having a midlife crisis or midriff bulge. (Or, worse, both at once!) But maybe the worst "mid" of all is midback pain. It *hurts*.

The most common cause of midback pain is strained ligaments and muscles. They're strained because they're chronically weak or because you've lifted something the wrong way. A less common cause is arthritis of the spine. Another possibility is scoliosis, a disease that alters the natural curve of the spine.

Because the gallbladder is close to the back, gallstones can also cause midback pain. So can heart disease, aneurysm (ballooning of an artery), pneumonia, peptic ulcers and kidney infections. Finally, there's a cause of midback pain that every mother remembers: pregnancy.

SYMPTOM RELIEF

If your pain is severe or lasts more than three days, see your doctor. Problems like ligament tears, ulcers, kidney infections and gallstones require medical treatment.

Most of the time you can relieve midback pain on your own. Here's how.

Turn on shower power. For some folks with midback muscle pain, relief is only a hot shower away, according to Karl B. Fields, M.D., associate professor of family practice and director of the Sports Medicine Fellowship at Moses Cone Memorial Hospital in Greensboro, North Carolina. The heat from a shower increases blood flow to the area, which helps speed healing, he says. For severe pain, take at least two showers a day.

Try a mild water workout. You definitely won't work up a sweat with this routine: While water from your warm shower begins to soothe you, re-establish movement in your midback by gently twisting and bending for a few minutes. But *don't* move more than two to three inches from side to side and front to back, says Dr. Fields.

Go soak. Soaking in a whirlpool or tub in very warm water (104°F) for 20 minutes or so raises your internal temperature, causing painful muscle spasms to relax, says Dr. Fields.

Have a ball. This massage technique works best on mid- and lower back pain, says Patrice Morency, licensed massage therapist and sports injury management specialist in Portland, Oregon, who works with Olympic hopefuls. Take two tennis balls, put them in a sock, and tie the end of the sock. Lie down on the sock, making sure a ball is on either side of the spine. Then gently roll your back up and down, allowing the tennis balls to massage your back until you get relief, she says.

Chill and twist. After wrapping an ice pack on the painful area with an elastic bandage, gently rotate your trunk from left to right. Repeat this movement several times a day, says Vert Mooney, M.D., professor of orthopedic surgery at the University of California, San Diego, Medical Center and director of the Spine and Joint Conditioning Center. "It's going to hurt a *little* at first," he says, "but you need to make sure that you get some movement each day. Complete rest is the wrong thing to do." Too much time in bed allows muscles to weaken, he says. Do not do this exercise if it seems to make the pain worse.

Muscling Away Midback Pain

Once the pain has subsided, it's time to start thinking about making your midback pain-proof. One of the best ways: strengthening your abdominals, says Dr. Fields. "If you don't maintain good abdominal strength, you get fatigued, and when you're fatigued, you're much more likely to get muscular injury," he says. Try these techniques.

Pelvic tilt. Stand up straight with your back against a wall. Slowly tilt your pelvis up, pressing the small of your back into the wall and hold for three to four seconds. Repeat ten times. "We're trying to tilt the pelvis into a more anatomically correct posture," says Dr. Fields.

Trunk twist. With your arms held out from your sides (or resting on your hips) and your hips held stationary, carefully turn your trunk, upper body and head from side to side 20 times.

Curl-ups. Lie on your back on the floor with your hands by your sides and your knees bent. Slowly curl your upper body, lifting your shoulders two to three inches off the floor. Lower and repeat. "It would help everyone to do 20 to 30 of these a day," says Dr. Fields.

MOLES

WHEN TO SEE YOUR DOCTOR

- You have a mole that changes in size, shape or color.
- You have a mole that burns, bleeds, itches or stings.
- You develop a new mole that grows rapidly.

WHAT YOUR SYMPTOM IS TELLING YOU

Moles can be as perplexing as ice hockey, cribbage, Star Trek conventions, politics and most television shows.

"Nobody has really figured out why people have moles. They make no sense and don't appear to serve any purpose," says Kevin Welch, M.D., assistant professor of dermatology at the University of Arizona Health Sciences Center in Tucson.

In most cases, moles are like harmless hitchhikers, taking a free ride on your back, arms, legs or face. They can last 10 to 40 years, then fade away.

Only about 1 in 100 people are born with moles. Usually, they develop at the age of five or six, says Marc Bauder, M.D., a family practice physician in Sun City West, Arizona.

"The average person is not born with moles nor does a person who lives an average lifetime die with moles," Dr. Welch says. "They tend to come and go as you age, so by the time you're 70 or 80, you have very few of them."

But while doctors know little about the origin of moles, they do know that any dramatic change in a mole could be a warning sign of skin cancer—both the malignant (melanoma) and benign (basal cell carcinoma) varieties. They also know that prolonged sun exposure increases the chances that a mole will become cancerous.

"Your risk of skin cancer isn't really determined by how many or how large your moles are," Dr. Bauder says. "It has more to do with your cumulative sun exposure during your lifetime. Excessive sunlight can either produce a new skin cancer out of existing normal-looking cells or cause a mole to go bad and turn into a cancer."

SYMPTOM RELIEF

There really isn't any way you can prevent getting a mole," Dr. Bauder says. "But if you notice any change in a mole, see your doctor as soon as possible."

Early detection of skin cancer is vital, particularly if it is melanoma. "Of all skin conditions, melanoma is the leading cause of death. So it's very important to be diagnosed early, while the melanoma can be cured," says Martin A. Weinstock, M.D., Ph.D., chief of dermatology at the Veterans Affairs Medical Center in Providence, Rhode Island.

Here's what you need to know about moles.

Take a hard look. Each month, do a head-to-toe examination of your skin. Look for any changes in size, color, shape or appearance of any mole, Dr. Bauder says. Use a hand mirror to check areas that are hard to see, like the back of the legs. If you're unsure how to do a self-exam, ask your doctor to show you.

Let your doctor do it, too. Your doctor should inspect your skin at least once a year, says Robert J. Friedman, M.D., clinical assistant professor of dermatology at New York University School of Medicine in New York City. If you have a family history of skin cancer (melanoma) and you have many moles, have your skin checked twice a year.

It pays to be suspicious. A change in a mole doesn't automatically mean skin cancer. Often, it is just a result of some minor bump or bruise. Still, it would be wise to get any suspicious-looking mole checked out. Most likely, your doctor will simply shave off the mole and send it to a lab for a biopsy. Even if it is cancerous, removal of the mole may be the only treatment you'll need.

Create a barrier. Wearing a sunscreen with a sun protection factor (SPF) of at least 15 will protect your skin—and your moles—from most of the sun's harmful rays, Dr.

Welch says. If you have lots of moles on your legs, using sunscreen may be especially important. In a study of 341 nurses, researchers found that people with 12 or more moles on their lower legs had 4.2 times greater risk of developing melanoma than those who had no moles on their legs.

See also Birthmark Changes

MOOD SWINGS

WHEN TO SEE YOUR DOCTOR

- Your mood swings are unpredictable or seem disproportionate to the situation.
- Your moods feel uncontrollable.
- You sometimes have periods of intense elation followed by severe depression.
- Your sleep patterns are disrupted.

WHAT YOUR SYMPTOM IS TELLING YOU

A person with a mood problem is like a human roller coaster. One minute he's up, the next minute he's down. And he never seems to be able to get off the ride. His mood swings are intense, sudden and out of control.

SYMPTOM RELIEF

Chronic and severe mood swings—like chronic depression or panic attacks—are a psychological disorder, a health problem every bit as real as a physical ailment. (In fact, sometimes they're the *result* of a physical problem, like a premenstrual syndrome.) And just like a physical problem, they can be treated.

Ask yourself if it's PMS. A woman's turbulent moods might be caused by premenstrual syndrome, which is a hormone-sparked collection of emotional upsets and physical discomforts that for some women begins mid-cycle. There are many recommendations for dealing with the mood swings of PMS. Some nutritionists say calcium and vitamins B, C and E work well. Other experts suggest regular exercise, like walking. In some cases, medication may work. If you think your mood swings are caused by PMS, talk it over with your doctor.

Try a salt that lowers the pressure. If your doctor determines that you have a mood disorder—even a mild one—he'll probably prescribe the drug lithium. "Lithium carbonate can decrease mood alterations in the majority of people with mood problems," says Paul Wender, M.D., distinguished professor of psychiatry at the University of Utah School of Medicine in Salt Lake City.

Lithium treatment has to be customized so that you always have an adequate level of the medicine in your blood, he explains. For that reason, your doctor will start you on a somewhat high dose, reducing it gradually. In the beginning, you may have some side effects, including fatigue, mild nausea, frequent urination and very mild hand tremors. They'll diminish or disappear once the right dose has been determined.

And don't worry about addiction. Dr. Wender explains that lithium is not addicting and is safe for long-term use.

Reach out to resource organizations. Help is just a postcard away. Contact the Depression Awareness, Recognition and Treatment (D/ART) Program for free information. Write to: D/ART, National Institute of Mental Health, Parklawn Building, 15C-05, 5600 Fishers Lane, Rockville, MD 20857.

See also Depression; Personality Change

MOUTH BURNING

WHEN TO SEE YOUR DOCTOR

- The burning sensation is accompanied by a sore on or discoloration of the tongue, cheeks or gums.
- Burning seems to be located near, below or above dentures or a partial or on the tongue.
- The burning sensation continues for more than a week.

WHAT YOUR SYMPTOM IS TELLING YOU

Bite into a jalapeño pepper and you'll get an idea of what it's like to have a burning mouth—or at least one of the variations. Someimes it doesn't feel like fire at all. Some people say it feels like a hot knife is being jabbed into their mouths. Others say it feels like their mouths, tongues or gum tissue is shrinking and withering up like wet rawhide left to dry out in the desert sun. Still others describe it as an abrasive, sandpaper feeling.

Whatever it feels like, you know it if you have it, and you're probably frustrated because none of the doctors you've seen knows what to do about it. And if you're like many people who have this irritating sensation, you *have* seen several doctors for it.

"People who come to me with burning mouth usually have a long, complex pattern of seeing doctors, dentists, nutritionists and psychiatrists for this," says Louis M. Abbey, D.M.D., professor of oral pathology at Virginia Commonwealth University/Medical College of Virginia School of Dentistry in Richmond. "When no physical cause is found, they're often told it's all in their heads or they're branded neurotic. And some of them actually do border on being neurotic because of the pain and stress of not finding a reason or cure for the burning."

For all but about 5 percent of the people with burning mouth, no cause can be found, Dr. Abbey says. And most are women at or past the age of menopause and otherwise in good physical, mental and dental shape. "The places of burning in their mouths vary, and there's often no demonstrable lesion you can see," says Dr. Abbey. "But I'm convinced most of them have a real complaint."

An oral infection like candidiasis is one real complaint that can cause burning mouth, according to R. Gregg Settle, Ph.D., research associate in the department of otolaryngology/head and neck surgery at the University of Pennsylvania School of Medicine in Philadelphia. So are conditions like uncontrolled diabetes, food sensitivities, nutrient deficiencies and a lack of saliva. Improperly fitting dentures or an allergy to the denture material also may produce a burning mouth.

SYMPTOM RELIEF

Many doctors may examine an individual for only one probable cause of burning mouth, Dr. Settle says. "Any attempt to look at one treatment to the exclusion of others is unlikely to succeed," he says. "I suspect burning mouth is caused by a lot of different things that converge into that final symptom." Sometimes therapy focusing on a sole cause is successful; sometimes not. In the meantime, here are some things you can do to put out the fire.

Get wet. Extreme dryness in the mouth may feel like a burning, according to Michael W. Dodds, Ph.D., who holds a bachelor of dental surgery and is an assistant professor in the Department of Community Dentistry at the University of Texas Health Science Center in San Antonio. Certain medications, illness, aging and radiation therapy can sap the salivary glands of their punch. (See Mouth Dryness below for remedies to wet your whistle.)

Ask about hormones. Many women with burning mouth are near menopause or actually going through it. For this reason, a number of doctors have experimented with estrogen replacement therapy to relieve the symptom. The results have been mixed, Dr. Settle says. Ask your doctor whether this therapy is appropriate for you.

Diet may do it. A food sensitivity or allergy may ignite your mouth, Dr. Abbey says. "You have to look at your whole diet—new or unusual foods, new medications, new drinks, a new toothpaste, new chewing gum." If you've recently started eating a new food or using a new product, try eliminating it and see if that helps, he advises.

Put out the flames with B vitamins. A deficiency of virtually any of the B vitamins or iron-deficiency anemia could be causing the burning," Dr. Abbey says. (This is uncommon in America.) Try taking a daily multivitamin supplement and see if it helps.

MOUTH DRYNESS

WHEN TO SEE YOUR DOCTOR

- You have to drink fluids frequently to alleviate thirst and the dry feeling in your mouth.
- Dryness interferes with eating or speaking.

WHAT YOUR SYMPTOM IS TELLING YOU

If you have dry mouth—doctors call it xerostomia—your salivary glands seem as unproductive as a dead creek bed. Dry mouth is no minor inconvenience, says Michael W. Dodds, Ph.D., who has a bachelor of dental surgery degree and is an assistant professor in the Department of Community Dentistry at the University of Texas Health Science Center in San Antonio. "With a chronically arid mouth, it becomes quite difficult to speak, chew, swallow and taste," he says. "All of these things make life pretty unpleasant, in general."

Saliva is also essential in preventing tooth decay and gum disease. "A dry mouth accelerates tooth decay dramatically, in just a period of months," Dr. Dodds says.

Normally, the antibacterial, high-alkaline saliva neutralizes erosive acids from plaque that eat at your teeth. High concentrations of calcium and phosphate in your spittle also repair the very early stages of tooth deterioration.

"If you don't get that washing and flushing," says Eric Z. Shapira, D.D.S., a trustee on the national board of the Academy of General Dentistry and a dentist in private practice in Half Moon Bay, California, "it'll lead to a plaque buildup. And if your hygiene isn't what it should be, you'll end up with gingivitis or worse." (Gingivitis is the first stage of a gum disease that, left untreated, can lead to tooth loss.)

The primary cause of dry mouth is the use of medications, Dr. Dodds says. In fact, xerostomia is a common side effect of some 400 drugs, including antihistamines, decongestants and antidepressants. Many diuretics and medications to counteract high blood pressure and muscle spasms also can dry out the mouth. Even over-the-counter antihistamines and decongestants will suck the saliva from your mouth, Dr. Shapira adds.

Having a stuffy nose can also cause a dry mouth. "People who breathe through their mouths because of allergies or adenoids or whatever also experience dry mouth," Dr. Shapira says. A number of vitamin deficiencies—particularly of riboflavin or vitamin A—can dry out the mouth as well.

Saliva production may slow as you are, leading to complaints of a dusty mouth. Diabetics who can't control their blood sugar often are thirsty because of diminished salivary secretion, caused by frequent urination. People with Sjögren's syndrome, a disease akin to rheumatoid arthritis that affects mostly women past menopause, also have dry mouth. And radiation therapy for head or neck cancer can destroy salivary glands if they're not protected.

SYMPTOM RELIEF

Most treatments for dry mouth require a lot of chewing, Dr. Dodds says. "The more you chew, the more saliva you produce," he explains. "Chewing stimulates the salivary glands, much like exercising a muscle. If you don't use them, they kind of wither away." But those remedies assume you have functioning salivary glands. If the glands don't work, chewing won't help.

Crunch a cube. Chewing on crushed ice not only moistens your mouth, says Timothy Durham, D.D.S., director of adult general dentistry at the University of Nebraska Medical Center in Omaha. It also demands the jaw action necessary to turn on the salivary glands.

Buy gum! Chewing sugar-free gum is an anywhere, anytime way to stimulate saliva. "The combination of jaw action and the sweetness of the gum acts to increase saliva flow," Dr. Dodds says. "But I have to emphasize sugar-free, because sugared gums promote tooth decay."

In studies he has conducted, Dr. Dodds found that people's saliva flow increases considerably if they chew gum for ten minutes every hour. "For some people it may not have to be that long," he says, "but others may have to keep chewing all the time."

Button your lip—and tongue and teeth. If you don't care to chew gum, try sucking on a large fruit pit, Dr. Dodds suggests. "The presence of something in the mouth just seems to help people produce more saliva," he says. Conventional hard candies and breath mints produce the same result. Just make sure they're sugar-free.

Take many sips. Drink as much water as you want and swish it around your mouth and through your teeth, says Dr. Durham.

Don't drink your meals. Liquid diets are becoming an increasingly common cause of dry mouth, Dr. Dodds says. Contrary to what you might think, a meal in a milk shake "will retard production of saliva because you're chewing less frequently," he says. "Those on a liquid meal-substitute diet may possibly notice the output of saliva decreases over the course of a couple of weeks."

Fill up on fiber. Diets high in fiber and bulk also seem to stimulate your salivary glands, Dr. Dodds says. The reason for the action, he says, seems to go back to the chewing—high-fiber foods often require more gnawing and gnashing.

Moisten with a multiple. Vitamin deficiencies could be robbing the moisture from your mouth, Dr. Shapira says. A lack of riboflavin or vitamin A can cause a dry mouth, as can pernicious anemia from a vitamin B12 deficiency. Try a daily multiple vitamin supplement.

Fake it. For comfort and lubrication, a doctor can prescribe artificial saliva for people who have chronically dry mouths and little or no salivary gland action, Dr. Dodds says. The gel contains the same enzymes and minerals as real saliva but lingers in your mouth only a short time, so you have to use it frequently.

MOUTH SORES

WHEN TO SEE YOUR DOCTOR

- See your doctor anytime you develop an unexplained sore or discolored spot anywhere in your mouth—painful or not.

WHAT YOUR SYMPTOM IS TELLING YOU

Almost anything that goes wrong in your body can cause a mouth sore.

"Ninety-eight percent of diseases can be diagnosed by lesions in the mouth," says Eric Z. Shapira, D.D.S., a trustee on the national board of the Academy of General Dentistry and a dentist in private practice in Half Moon Bay, California. "Even chickenpox and the measles include mouth sores as a symptom."

If you notice a white substance like thick curds coating your mouth, tissues or tongue, you may have a yeast infection called oral candidiasis. This is especially likely if the coating has been there awhile and you have a yeasty taste in your mouth, according to Louis M. Abbey, D.M.D., a pro-

fessor of oral pathology at Virginia Commonwealth
University/Medical College of Virginia School of Dentistry
in Richmond. A few candida strains may create red sores
instead.

In addition to diseases, there are a few other fairly common causes for mouth sores. Denture wearers often get
ulcers on their gums and elsewhere in their mouths, says Dr.
Shapira. A poor fit or inadequate cleaning is almost always
to blame, and the sores, which are usually painless, can
linger for a long time.

Vitamin B deficiencies (especially of riboflavin) can
cause small sores at the corners of your lips, according to
Dr. Shapira.

Aspirin can also cause problems. That little white pill
can be a life-saver to ease aches and pains when you swallow it, but it can wreak havoc in your mouth if you place
it on an aching tooth.

"People come to me with these huge ulcerations in their
mouths, and I'll ask what happened," Dr. Shapira says.
"They say, 'I had this toothache, so I put an aspirin on it.'
Well, aspirin happens to be an acid. It burns and irritates
the tissue."

Long-time use of chewing tobacco or snuff can turn
your gums, cheeks or the insides of your lips a whitish
color, according to Paul A. Stephens, D.D.S., a dentist in
private practice in Gary, Indiana and president of the
Academy of General Dentistry. The discoloration, called
leukoplakia, can be a precursor of cancer. Smoking can
cause a similar discoloration.

And, of course, mouth sores can be from minor problems like biting your cheek or tongue or developing a
canker sore.

SYMPTOM RELIEF

What doesn't hurt you now ultimately could hurt you
later on if you don't have a dentist or doctor examine it, Dr. Shapira says. A painless mouth sore could be a
precursor of oral cancer. "Get it checked out," he cautions.

Eschew the chew. The leukoplakia caused by chewing

tobacco should go away, Dr. Stephens says, if you pull the plug and give up your chaw. So should the discoloration from smoke—if you snuff out the habit for good. If the whitish stains remain after you've sworn off tobacco, see your doctor.

Get that prescription filled. To get rid of a candida infection, doctors may prescribe nystatin or other drugs, Dr. Abbey says. Be sure to follow your physician's instructions on how to take the medication, or ask your pharmacist if you're unsure.

Make a beeline to the vitamin section. A balanced multivitamin supplement that contains both vitamin C and the B vitamins can help ward off mouth sores, says Dr. Shapira. Ask your doctor if this daily supplement is appropriate for you.

Swallow aspirin—don't suck on it. Aspirin works best in your bloodstream, not when it's applied topically, says Dr. Shapira.

Make sure your dentures fit. Because poorly positioned false teeth can cause mouth sores, have your dentist check the fit at least once a year, says Dr. Shapira. If you gain or lose weight, your dentures may no longer fit properly, because your mouth tissue can expand or shrink.

See also Canker Sores; Cold Sores

MUSCLE CONTROL LOSS

WHEN TO SEE YOUR DOCTOR

- Any loss of muscle control requires medical attention.

WHAT YOUR SYMPTOM IS TELLING YOU

Ever try to follow directions from someone who is shouting "Turn right!" while urgently pointing to the left? In your confusion, you can easily miss the turn altogether and keep going straight ahead. In essence, the same sort of confusion happens inside your brain when illness causes you to lose control of your muscles.

Losing control of your muscles means that a communications breakdown is happening in your nervous system, says John Byer, M.D., an associate professor of neurology at the University of Missouri—Columbia School of Medicine. Somewhere in the complex network of nerves that travels from the brain through the spinal cord to the muscles, the message that you want to move your arm, leg or other body part is getting garbled or isn't being translated properly.

Loss of muscle control has a multitude of causes, including extreme exhaustion, drug and alcohol abuse, head injury, multiple sclerosis, muscular dystrophy, Parkinson's disease, stroke and catalepsy (a rare form of muscle weakness that affects some people when they experience strong emotions, such as intense anger or joy).

SYMPTOM RELIEF

Loss of muscle control is almost always serious. Any loss of muscle control, even if it lasts for less than ten minutes, should be brought to the attention of your physician, because early diagnosis and treatment may improve your chances of recovery and prevent further damage to your nerves, muscles and brain. With the exception of exhaustion (see Fatigue on page 216), conditions that cause loss of muscle control involve a comprehensive program of medical treatment that must come from a physician.

MUSCLE CRAMPS

WHEN TO SEE YOUR DOCTOR

- Your muscles frequently cramp during and after exertion or at rest.
- You have cramps that "lock" and don't release for minutes at a time.
- A cramp recurs several times in a single day.

WHAT YOUR SYMPTOM IS TELLING YOU

Muscle cramps are an "equal opportunity" pain: They don't discriminate between the star athlete and someone who barely moves. You may be competing in a long-distance bike race, taking leisurely laps in the pool or sleeping soundly in bed. Suddenly, a muscle seizes up and grips you in pain.

A cramp is caused by anything that interferes with the muscle's natural ability to contract and relax. Take a foot spasm, for example. When feet are flexed for propulsion while swimming or when tight bedsheets force your toes downward, the muscle tendons become overstretched and the nerves extending through your foot and into your calf can become hyperexcitable. When this happens, the nerve signals become confused, according to Robert Nirschl, M.D., assistant professor of orthopedic surgery at Georgetown University School of Medicine in Washington, D.C. The result: a painful cramp. "Your muscles may get the message to contract, but not to relax," he explains.

Profuse perspiration can also cause a muscle cramp. Heavy sweating drains your body of important minerals: potassium, sodium, magnesium and calcium. These minerals, called electrolytes, carry electrical charges to the nerves that control a muscle's impulse to contract and relax. Lack of fluids can upset the delicate balance of electrolytes, causing nerve signals to misfire.

If you've actually injured a muscle from overuse, a cramp may go into a continuous contraction, or spasm. While "cramp" and "spasm" are often used interchangeably, a spasm generally means the muscle fibers have "locked up" to protect the injured muscle.

People who have conditions that interfere with blood circulation or muscle metabolism can experience repeated cramps. These conditions include diabetes, rheumatoid arthritis and thyroid disease.

SYMPTOM RELIEF

Here's how to ease out of the grip of a muscle cramp, no matter what the cause.

Stretch and squeeze. Stretch a cramped leg muscle with one hand and alternately squeeze and release the muscle with the other hand. "This mechanical kneading restores blood flow and generally helps relax the spasm and tightness in seconds," says Dr. Nirschl.

Point your toes back toward your chin. This is a quick way to halt a leg cramp while swimming, according to Harry Daniell, M.D., clinical professor in the Department of Medicine at the University of California, Davis, School of Medicine.

Cool it. If stretching doesn't release a cramp and the muscle's in painful spasm, an ice massage will numb the area, according to Irene von Estorff, M.D., assistant professor of rehabilitation medicine at the New York Hospital–Cornell Medical College in New York City. Rub the ice over the cramped muscle for three to five minutes. Make sure to keep the ice moving so you don't harm skin tissue.

Pinch your upper lip. Oddly enough, pinching the area above the upper lip with your finger and thumb can make a leg cramp vanish, according to Dr. Nirschl. He's not sure why this works, but there are two possible reasons: The upper lip may be a pressure point that helps relax the muscle. Or, he says, it simply may be that the pain of the pinch distracts you from the pain of the cramp until it releases on its own.

Quench your thirst pronto. "If you're exerting yourself, dripping with sweat and suddenly feel a cramp in your thigh, take a few swigs of water or whatever fluid is handy," says Robert Wortmann, M.D., chairman of the Department of Medicine at East Carolina University School of Medicine in Greenville, North Carolina. If you follow swigging with stretching, the cramp should vanish quickly.

Keep on sipping. "To prevent cramping during a sweaty workout, take three or four normal swallows of water every ten minutes," says Owen Anderson, Ph.D., editor of *Running Research News*.

Pass up the salt. Whatever you do, avoid taking salt tablets or very salty liquids such as soft drinks when you're perspiring. "Salt actually draws fluid out of muscles and into the stomach," says Dr. Nirschl.

Pack a sports drink on a hot day. If you're going to be sweating profusely during a long hike, you may need to replace potassium and other electrolytes that plain water can't provide. "Sipping electrolyte sports drinks such as Gatorade at regular intervals may be a good idea," says Dr. Nirschl. These replacement drinks also contain glucose, which helps electrolytes get absorbed quicker than plain water.

Do wall push-ups before bedtime. "In a study with 44 people, we found that calf-stretching exercises, performed three times per day for a week, helped cure nocturnal leg cramps," says Dr. Daniell. To perform the calf stretch, he says, stand facing a wall about two feet away. Place your hands on the wall and slowly lean forward, keeping your heels in contact with the floor. Hold the position for ten seconds and relax for five seconds. Do this two more times.

Serve yourself a quinine nightcap. "This age-old remedy seems to work for nocturnal leg cramps," says Dr. Daniell. Possibly, quinine make nerves less excitable. In any case, taking quinine and vitamin E tablets (like Q-vel) or 12 ounces of plain tonic water each night probably won't hurt, and it may help. But talk to your doctor first.

See also Muscle Pain; Muscle Spasms

MUSCLE PAIN

WHEN TO SEE YOUR DOCTOR

- You also have tender areas in the neck, shoulders, chest, hip, back and buttocks.
- You also have a fever.

WHAT YOUR SYMPTOM IS TELLING YOU

Last Saturday you spent the morning painting the kitchen ceiling. Then in the afternoon you played touch football with your nephews. You probably would have been okay—if only you hadn't decided to clean the garage on Sunday.

All that activity felt great while you were doing it. But by Monday morning, your muscles let you know—in no uncertain terms—that they didn't like the way they were being treated. Unfortunately, they only have one way of communicating this sort of thing: pain.

Think about it. They can hardly drop you a note that says, *"Stop what you've been doing and let us rest a while!"* But pain delivers that message very effectively.

When you take a look at what's going on inside the muscle itself, it's easy to understand why overuse hurts so much. Once they're pushed beyond what they're used to doing, muscle fibers start to tear. Muscles that are *severely* overworked may develop hundreds of tiny tears.

Overuse is not the only cause of muscle pain. If your muscles hurt all the time—particularly those in your shoulders, neck and hips—you could have what doctors call fibromyalgia. This simply means "pain in the fibrous muscle tissue." Fibromyalgia can hurt so bad that it keeps you from getting a good night's sleep and leaves you tired throughout the day.

Some doctors believe fibromyalgia is triggered by muscle stress, injury or illness. Others believe a sedentary lifestyle and the muscle tension it causes plays a major role. "Muscles are made to move," says Paul Davidson, M.D., associate clinical professor of medicine at the University of California School of Medicine in San Francisco and author of *Chronic Muscle Pain Syndrome*. When they're held immobile—while you're sitting at a desk all day, for instance—muscles tense up. They can actually tense up to the point of pain. This triggers a vicious cycle: The achiness interferes with deep sleep, so you wake up tired, stiff and sore. Movement becomes difficult, so your muscles remain tense and achy.

You may have fibromyalgia if pressing on tender points in your neck, shoulders, chest, back and buttocks makes you jump with pain, says Dr. Davidson. Suspect fibromyalgia if you've also had all-over achiness longer than three months, especially if you are in your late forties or older.

In addition, general muscle soreness can be from a flu-like virus or a reaction to a diuretic or blood pressure medication. If the pain worsens, it could indicate a thyroid condition or arthritis.

SYMPTOM RELIEF

Whether your muscle pain is recent or long-standing, here's how to deal with it.

Put your muscles on RICE. Even athletes follow the RICE rule (rest, ice, compression and elevation), especially following the first day of practice, according to Robert Nirschl, M.D., assistant professor of orthopedic surgery at Georgetown University School of Medicine in Washington, D.C. When muscle pain from overuse strikes, rest your sore muscles for at least 48 hours so they can begin to repair. During rest time, apply ice—"the most effective anti-inflammatory agent around," says Dr. Nirschl. Ice works to constrict blood vessels, dull the pain and also relax muscle fibers that have locked into spasm. Wrap some ice cubes in a thin cloth and apply the pack to the sore area for 20 minutes at a time.

If the sore muscles are in your arms or legs, you can also control swelling by compressing the affected area with a not-too-tight elastic bandage. Then, elevate the limb above the heart. Lie down and prop it up on some pillows.

Get help from your medicine cabinet. Taking aspirin or ibuprofen should reduce pain within a half-hour or so, says Dr. Nirschl. If it doesn't make a dent in your pain, see your doctor for a review of the problem.

Melt the pain away. If your muscles aren't swollen, you can't beat a warm bath for soothing lingering soreness or stiffness, says Dr. Davidson. Warmth improves circulation to damaged muscles and also carts off lactic acid, muscle waste products that build up in overused muscles and contribute to pain. "If you can't slip into a bath, use a heating pad on the painful muscle for 15 minutes," says Dr. Davidson. For longstanding achiness, a steam bath or sauna seems to penetrate deeper, he adds.

Get stroked. "There's a reason why animals lick their wounds," says Carol Warfield, M.D., assistant professor of anesthesia at Harvard Medical School and director of the Pain Management Center at Boston's Beth Israel Hospital. "The massaging action may provide pain reduction," she says. In people, massaging an aching muscle could increase the body's output of natural painkillers, combat stiffness and help restore movement. For the best results, warm the area, then gently massage it. Stop rubbing if it makes the pain worse.

Balm the soreness. Those tingly, icy-hot sports liniments containing menthol, such as Ben-Gay, may cause warming just below the skin, according to Christopher MacGrew, M.D., assistant professor in the Department of Family Practice at the University of New Mexico Medical Center in Albuquerque. "Just don't use these creams under heating pads or elastic wraps," he says. "This can damage the tissues." Using the two together can also cause severe burns.

Fight Off Fibromyalgia

Skip some rope. Or go for a brisk walk. Or take your bike out for a spin. Studies show that regular aerobic exercise helps reduce tenderness and promotes sound sleep. Continual movement also increases oxygen to the muscles and may boost endorphins, the body's natural painkillers. The key is to adapt to exercise gradually, says Dr. Davidson. "If your muscles ache early in your exercise program—like aching calves when you first start walking—work through the pain gently. Slow down but don't stop. You won't harm any muscles by doing this," he says. Aim for a minimum of 30 minutes of exercise three times a week.

Take a seventh-inning stretch. Tender spots typically settle in the upper back and shoulders, often as a result from sitting in a fixed position doing desk work, says Dr. Davidson. You need to get up periodically, he says. Stretch your arms like you're reaching for the sky. Roll your head in circles. Remember to breathe deeply while you stretch, he adds. This also releases tension and brings oxygen to your muscles.

Practice good sleep habits. "People with fibromyalgia who often wake up with aches and pains each day are not getting healthy, deep sleep," says Robert Bennett, M.D., professor of medicine and chairman of the Division of Arthritis and Rheumatic Diseases at Oregon Health Sciences University in Portland. Without this restorative sleep, he says, they actually produce less of the growth hormone needed for muscle repair. Restful sleep can do a lot to promote healing, he says.

His advice? Keep the bedroom quiet, dark and about five degrees cooler than the rest of the house. Avoid alcohol, caffeine or heavy meals at supper. And don't exercise strenuously within six hours of bedtime. If these measures fail, your doctor can prescribe a low-dose antidepressant for better sleep. (For additional tips for getting a good night's sleep, see Insomnia on page 326.)

MUSCLE SPASMS

WHEN TO SEE YOUR DOCTOR

- Pain and stiffness don't ease up within the first three days.
- If a back or neck spasm is accompanied by tingling, numbness or weakness, see your doctor immediately.

WHAT YOUR SYMPTOM IS TELLING YOU

You swoop down to pick up a piece of paper off the floor. You cradle the phone with your chin while chatting. You hoist your groceries out of your trunk. Suddenly, you're ambushed by a tightness that painfully twists your body like a corkscrew.

When a muscle goes into spasm, all the fibers within the core of a muscle contract simultaneously. This most commonly occurs when you suddenly move or overextend a tensed-up muscle that hasn't been properly prepared for the movement.

Quickly bending over after sitting, for example, can overstretch your back muscles and injure the area. In response, the surrounding muscle fibers instantly tighten, forming a kind of protective splint that guards the back against further irritation. This triggers a back-stabbing cycle: Contracted fibers squeeze off blood flow to the muscle, creating irritation and more pain. The additional pain triggers even tighter contractions. You're caught in a painful vise without a chance of the muscle relaxing on its own.

Unlike an ordinary muscle cramp that also involves a sudden contraction, a spasm does not usually release with movement. If your back locks in spasm, you *can't* move.

The prime targets for spasms are the muscles in the neck and back, according to Irene von Estorff, M.D., assistant professor of rehabilitation medicine at the New York Hospital-Cornell Medical College in New York City. These areas are often tight, tense and more vulnerable to becoming overstressed by the least little thing, she says. A cool breeze, for example, might blow over neck muscles already tensed from working at a computer or playing tennis. These muscles suddenly clench against the chill. Now you have the classic "crick" and probably won't be able to turn your head to see out your car's side window.

A sudden spasm in your back or neck that's accompanied by numbness, tingling or weakness, could mean a ruptured disk or nerve injury.

SYMPTOM RELIEF

Spasms have a way of holding on stubbornly. To release that grip, try any of these techniques.

Get off your feet. "Lying down will take the strain off already stressed tissues," says Karlis Ullis, M.D., assistant clinical professor in sports medicine at the University of California, Los Angeles, UCLA School of Medicine. If the spasm is in your back, gently bring your knees up to your chin and hold them there for a minute or more (as long as there is no pain). "This should help release some of the shortened connective tissue and muscle fibers," says Dr. Ullis. (For other techniques that deal specifically with back pain, see Lower Back Pain on page 382, Midback Pain on page 406 and Upper Back Pain on page 662.)

Try a gentle ice massage. "Rubbing an ice cube directly over the sore area in slow circles can numb the area in about five minutes flat," says Dr. von Estorff. (If you can't reach the area yourself, ask a friend or family member to lend a hand.) What's more, at first the ice narrows the blood vessels, then they open up superwide. This allows a rush of healing blood to flow in, helping to release the clenched fibers. "Just be sure to keep the ice moving so you don't freeze and injure surface tissues," says Dr. von Estorff. Repeat the rub once an hour.

Swallow a pain reliever. Aspirin or another nonsteroidal anti-inflammatory such as ibuprofen are "the best pain relievers you can get without a prescription," says Robert

Nirschl, M.D., assistant professor of orthopedic surgery at Georgetown University School of Medicine in Washington, D.C. Acetaminophen may bring less effective relief because it's not an anti-inflammatory, he says.

Limber gently; don't jerk. After icing, moving slowly and gently will help restore normal circulation and ease fibers back into their customary patterns of contraction and relaxation, according to Dr. von Estorff. Don't stretch too aggressively, however. "Stretching could make the spasm worse," she says.

After icing your sore shoulder, for example, simply move it through its full range of motion. Do this by gently raising your shoulders up to your ears, rolling them forward, then back, and also moving your arm diagonally across your chest. "This actually reprograms the fibers in the shoulders, telling them where to go so they don't clench up again," says Dr. Ullis. (For other techniques dealing specifically with shoulder pain, see page 534.)

Get it warm. If the spasm still has you in its grip after three days, you can try treating the area with heat, says Dr. von Estorff. Once the acute pain and swelling subside, heat will nudge blood flow to the sore site, she explains. Simply wrap a hot, wet towel around the area, cover it with plastic wrap and then wrap it with a dry towel to seal in the heat. Apply these hot packs five times a day for no more than 20 minutes at a time.

Break up the knot. Once the pain and swelling have subsided somewhat, you may be left with a tough little knot of muscle that is still in spasm. Try pressing your thumb, finger or even the tip of a broomhandle directly into a stubborn spasm, says Dr. von Estorff. This may help move the built-up fluid, relax the muscle and separate fibers, she says. If direct pressure doesn't do the trick, you may need to see a doctor who specializes in musculoskeletal pain.

See also Muscle Cramps; Muscle Pain

MUSCLE WEAKNESS

WHEN TO SEE YOUR DOCTOR

- You have unexplained muscle weakness that persists beyond a day or two.
- If you're suddenly unable to lift your limbs, see your doctor immediately.

WHAT YOUR SYMPTOM IS TELLING YOU

The coffee pot feels like it weighs a ton. It takes two tries to heave-ho the trash. Even raising your arm to brush your hair takes effort.

It's no wonder your arms feel like someone pulled the plug on your power source. Yesterday, you pruned the shrubs in your front yard and hauled a half-dozen cartons of discarded junk from the basement. You didn't know it then, but your home maintenance marathon actually damaged your muscles.

Pushing out-of-shape muscles to the brink tears the proteins inside the muscle fibers, according to Priscilla Clarkson, Ph.D., professor of exercise science at the University of Massachusetts in Amherst. Normally, these proteins link up to make muscles flex. This allows you to lift, push and do countless other movements.

When proteins tear from overactivity, they can't link up properly. And you have less power to perform even simple movements. "Depending on the extent of damage, it can take up to five days for the proteins to repair and for muscles to regain strength," says Dr. Clarkson.

You don't have to be hauling heavy boxes for muscles to lose their steam. One of the hallmarks of the flu is weakness, often to the point where you can barely lift your head off the pillow. That's because the virus causes inflammation of the muscle fibers. This interferes with proper contraction, according to Irwin Siegel, M.D., associate professor of orthopedic surgery at the Rush Presbyterian-St. Luke's Medical Center in Chicago.

The longer you stay bedridden, however, the weaker you'll be. Just as overdoing it stresses the protein in muscles, "underdoing" it harms muscles in another way. Movement builds up the proteins needed for muscle contraction. If you're barely stirring, the proteins deteriorate. "After a week spent flat on your back with the flu, you'll be weak as a kitten for days afterward," says Dr. Siegel.

Fluid loss—from severe sweating, vomiting or diarrhea—can also cut off the power juice to muscles. When you lose fluid, you drain away salt and also trace amounts of potassium, magnesium and calcium. A delicate balance of these minerals—called electrolytes—allows electrical signals to travel through the nerves to the muscles. These signals from the brain tell the muscles when to flex. Losing fluid upsets the electrolyte balance, and the signals may get confused before contraction can occur.

But muscles can't live on fluid alone. They'll wimp out if they're starved of the nutrients they need to do their work—proteins and carbohydrates. Protein from food is converted into your body's muscle fiber protein. And carbohydrates, which is stored in the muscles as glycogen, or found in the blood as glucose (blood sugar) provide fuel for muscle activity.

Muscles that slowly become weaker for no apparent reason could indicate a disease or condition in the body. Possible disorders include: anemia, which shuts off oxygen to muscles; diabetes, which interferes with the body's use of blood sugar; a thyroid condition, which interferes with the body's use of protein; or a nerve injury, which interferes with the brain's signals to the muscles.

Muscle weakness that develops slowly and is accompanied by pain can indicate lupus (a severe disorder that causes the immune system to attack the body) or polymalgia rheumatica (a common source of muscle pain in middle-aged people). And sudden muscle weakness can indicate food poisoning or a medication overdose and requires immediate medical attention.

SYMPTOM RELIEF

To overcome temporary muscle weakness from overactivity, flu, fluid loss or poor diet, try these self-help measures.

Lighten up. When you overdo it, you need to let your muscles rest, but it's important to give them *some* activity while they heal, says Dr. Clarkson. Continuing to perform light chores allows your damaged muscles to repair themselves without sustaining further damage, she explains. Give yourself a few days before doing any heavy lifting, she adds. If you push it, you'll further damage the fibers, and it may take longer to regain your strength.

Get back to exercise slowly. If you've been inactive because of sickness for a few days, it will take double your downtime before your muscles build back up to full steam, according to Dr. Siegel. If, for example, you've been in bed with the flu for three days and missed your daily walk, give yourself six days to work back up to top speed.

Replace lost fluids with sport drinks. Carbohydrate-electrolyte products can help recharge muscles weakened from severe vomiting, diarrhea or profuse sweating. "As a bonus, they also contain glucose, which can refuel muscles and speed fluid from your stomach to your bloodstream," says Robert Hackman, Ph.D., professor of nutrition at the University of Oregon in Eugene.

Eat a balanced diet. "Don't expect to have a lot of muscle stamina if you're restricting yourself to diet soda and rice cakes," says Dr. Clarkson. Your daily diet should include protein, which is found in red meat, milk, cheese, eggs, chicken, fish, lentils and soybeans. You should also have generous helpings of complex carbohydrates, found in pasta, breads, fruits and vegetables. Your body breaks down these foods to glucose, for muscle power. These foods also provide a mix of vitamins and minerals that assist in the chemical reaction needed to fuel muscles. "Think of vitamins and minerals as 'oil' for the muscle engine," says Dr. Clarkson.

Help from the Doctor

If your muscles suddenly become weak for no apparent reason, view the situation as a potentially life-threatening emergency and go to the nearest hospital for treatment. And if your muscles have slowly become weaker for unexplained reasons, see your doctor to get a handle on what's happening. He'll probably order a blood test to rule out anemia or other conditions, a urine test to detect diabetes and an electromyagram (EMG) to test if the muscles are receiving electrical signals from the nerves.

N

NAIL CHANGES

WHEN TO SEE YOUR DOCTOR

- You notice long-lasting and unexplained changes in the color of your nail unrelated to an injury.

WHAT YOUR SYMPTOM IS TELLING YOU

A black or blue nail tells the world that you and your hammer will probably never appear on "This Old House." Reddish yellow nails demonstrate that you change your nail polish nearly as often as the channel on your TV set. Nails that split and break can be a sign that you're spending too much time with your hands in the sink. Nails that take on a convex, spoonlike appearance may mean respiratory deficiency or simply that you're not getting enough iron. Nibbled nails and hangnails can betray your anxiety level.

And then there are the nail changes that seem like they're out of your hands.

Grooved nails (called Beau's lines) are caused by trauma, an illness or an accident that actually damages the nail's matrix—the production center for the new nail.

Chalky or crumbly nails signal a close encounter of the fungal kind. And the skin condition psoriasis can cause tiny pits in fingernails.

"There is a whole host of conditions that manifest themselves through nail changes," says Mark Scioli, M.D., an orthopedic surgeon at the Center for Orthopedic Surgery in Lubbock, Texas. "The nail is really a picture of the health of the body."

Symptom Relief

O nce you've identified the source of your symptoms, try
these treatments for nicer nails.

Chalk Talk

Unfortunately, chalky, crumbly fingernails and toenails are
much worse than they're cracked up to be.

Tenacious bacteria and fungi sometimes attack a nail or
its matrix after it's been damaged. They can also be a problem in anyone with a propensity toward skin problems such
as psoriasis. Fungal infections often spread to other nails,
says Dr. Scioli.

Here are some steps toward fungus-free nails.

Take a test. Instead of relying on your doctor's observa-
tion, ask him to have your nail tested for the exact cause
of your problem, says Richard K. Scher, M.D., professor of
dermatology and nail specialist at Columbia Presbyterian
Medical Center in New York City. "Samples taken from the
nail can confirm what type of fungus is afflicting you," he
says.

Buy a counterpart for your clippers. Instead of using the
same clippers for cutting all nails, you can help prevent the
spread of fungus to other nails by purchasing an extra pair
and using the old one on just the infected nail. Clean both
pairs with alcohol after use, says Dr. Scher.

Take a little (or a lot) off the top. Armed with a pair of
the appropriate nail clippers—fingernail clippers for fingernails, toenail clippers for toenails—carefully trim as low as
possible, says Dr. Scher.

Attack with an antifungal. After the infected portion of
the nail has been removed, apply an ointment containing
fungus-fighting ingredients such as imidazoles, says Dr. Scher.

Use griseofulvin with caution. Because topical antifungal
cream is often ineffective against nail fungus, your doctor
may prescribe griseofulvin for a stubborn case. Taken
orally, this antibiotic slows the growth rate of the fungus
while helping the body fight it. But be patient: It usually
takes 4 to 6 months to clear fungus on the fingernails and
12 to 18 months for toenails. And be careful: Although it's

been on the market for over 30 years, extended use of the drug has been found to cause liver problems like jaundice in a very small of number of patients, says Martin L. Kabongo, M.D., Ph.D., dermatology coordinator for the family practice residency program at Bon Secours Hospital in Grosse Point, Michigan. If your doctor prescribes griseofulvin, make sure he also intends to monitor your white blood cell count for blood abnormalities after you start taking the drug.

Substitute those socks. If you sweat a lot, which creates a breeding ground for fungus and bacteria, change your socks more than once a day, says Dr. Scioli.

Pat on some powder. An over-the-counter antifungal foot medication like Tinactin or Lotrimin sprayed or sprinkled on your feet and in your shoes twice a day may also aid in the fungus-banishing effort, says Myles Schneider, D.P.M., an Annandale, Virginia, podiatrist and coauthor of *How to Doctor Your Feet without a Doctor.* (For more tips on fighting the fungus that causes itchy feet, see page 229.)

Strategies to Stop Splitting

Nails can split when moisture robbers like harsh chemicals and cold weather steal their strength. But protecting them is easy. Here's how.

Go soak. Soaking your nails for 15 minutes at bedtime in plain warm water can help prevent splitting, says Dr. Scher.

Take time to trim. Nails are less likely to split if trimmed after a soak, says Dr. Scher.

Lay on the lanolin. Smoothing a moisturizer with lanolin on nails after a soak helps seal in moisture and keeps the nail from drying, says Dr. Scher.

Glove yourself. Because repeated wetting and drying of hands helps weaken nails, wear rubber gloves with cotton lining when washing dishes, says Dr. Scioli.

Keep an eye on biotin. Large doses of this little-known B vitamin reportedly reduced the brittleness of nails in two-thirds of the patients participating in a Columbia University study, according to Dr. Scher. The study began after researchers in Switzerland discovered that biotin supplements helped prevent race horses' hooves from splitting. The connection: "Hooves and nails are basically made of the same thing—keratin," says Dr. Scher.

Although more work needs to be done, researchers believe biotin somehow helps strengthen the keratin in the nail, he says. Until research is done on people, however, he recommends that you be content with the biotin that you'll find in good multivitamin supplements.

Preventing Polish Problems

Prudent nail polish policies can pay off *before* you develop dry or yellowed nails, or cracked cuticles. Consider these tips.

Buff 'em up. Gently buffing the surface of the nail with an emery board after removing the polish will keep your nail color natural-looking, says Dr. Scher.

Lay on another layer. An extra layer of colorless base coat will protect the nail and prevent discoloration, says Dr. Scher.

Never on Sunday. To help prevent your nails from drying out if you wear polish, enjoy the color for six days and then allow your nails to go bare for a day. Another important anti-drying aid: Use a nail polish remover that contains acetate rather than acetone, he says.

Be alert to allergies. "If you have *any* allergies, check with your dermatologist or family physician before you embark on any artificial nail use," says Dr. Scioli. "If you have allergic reactions, I wouldn't advise using things like lacquers or adhesives. They can cause chronic cuticle problems."

NAUSEA

WHEN TO SEE YOUR DOCTOR

- Nausea persists for more than two days or frequently recurs.
- You're pregnant and nausea is so severe that you can't eat or drink.

WHAT YOUR SYMPTOM IS TELLING YOU

You're wedged in the back of a rickety bus that's bumping along a winding country road. The air's a stifling mix of stale perfume, diesel exhaust and somebody's lunch. In fact, you're perilously close to losing *your* lunch.

When you're queasy from a bus ride or a too-greasy burger from Bob's Bar and Grill, it's hard to believe that nausea is sometimes a *helpful* sensation. But it is.

"Nausea is nature's way of suppressing your appetite," says Ronald Hoffman, M.D., director of the Hoffman Center for Holistic Medicine in New York City. Whenever something irritates your digestive tract—whether it's a burger or bacteria—a signal is relayed to "vomiting central" in the brain. The brain tells your mouth to start salivating, your digestive tract to do the rumba, your windpipe to narrow and your appetite to shut down. You perceive all these bodily activities as a single symptom: nausea. "And that keeps you from putting anything else in your stomach and further irritating it," says Dr. Hoffman.

But nausea isn't always a digestive system defense mechanism. The balance center in the inner ear can also spark nausea. When you're rocking in a boat, for example, your brain receives a mixed message: Your eyes are steady on a book or deck chair, but the fluid in your inner ears is rocking with the boat movement. This sensory mismatch triggers the release of stress hormones that make your stomach muscles quiver. This stomach distress creates the wretched feeling—often followed by the equally wretched vomiting—that we know as seasickness.

Fortunately, there's Dramamine. But certain other drugs, such as anesthesia, chemotherapy medications and tricyclic antidepressants, can *cause* nausea.

Other causes include migraine headaches, emotional stress or unpleasant odors. And severe hormone shifts—most notoriously, during the first trimester of pregnancy—can trigger recurring nausea.

Persistent nausea can also indicate a serious digestive problem such as colitis, ulcers, gastroenteritis or gallstones. In those diseases, however, nausea is usually accompanied by pain and other symptoms. Nausea can also be one of the signs of a heart attack, some types of cancer and kidney or liver disorders.

Symptom Relief

If you have severe, persistent nausea, see your doctor. But for "normal," everyday queasiness there are a number of things you can do to make the experience a little less—well, nauseating.

Eat something. This is probably the *last* thing you want to do. It should be the first. "Eating something bland and starchy at the first twinge of nausea may help control irregular stomach rhythms," says Kenneth Koch, M.D., professor of medicine at the Hershey Medical Center at Pennsylvania State University. Crackers or toast are good choices, but skip the butter. Fatty foods are too hard on the stomach, says Dr. Koch, and can make nausea worse.

Drink something. Right, not another beer. Tea or water are best. You could also try a sugary drink like apple juice or a soft drink, because sugar can help regulate stomach rhythms, says Roger Gebhard, M.D., gastroenterologist at the Veterans Administration Medical Center and professor of medicine at the University of Minnesota in Minneapolis. But drink it in small quantities at room temperature and drink it flat, he adds. Cold drinks and carbonation will only irritate your stomach more. And whatever you do, don't drink milk. "Milk will actually become cottage cheese in a churning stomach," says Dr. Koch.

Take a spoonful of syrup. Emetrol is a sugary, over-the-counter antinausea drug that's very similar to cola syrup, a time-honored home remedy. Emetrol, however, doesn't have caffeine and has a little phosphoric acid added to settle the stomach, says Dr. Gebhard.

Remember to breathe. Anxiety, says Dr. Koch, can stimulate the stress hormones that trigger nausea. To reduce anxiety, take several slow, deep breaths, especially when you first feel woozy. Deep breathing can also soothe your stomach contractions.

Review your medications. Tricyclic antidepressants can cause nausea if the dosage is too high, says Dr. Hoffman. If you're taking this medication (or any prescription drug) and experience unexplained nausea, call your doctor and ask whether your medication could be causing the problem and whether it should be adjusted.

Just do it. If you're still feeling like you need to throw up, don't try to stifle it. It may be the best thing to do if something doesn't agree with you or you have the flu, says Dr. Koch.

How to Calm Motion Sickness

If cruising the ocean blue leaves you green around the gills, here's what you can do for smoother sailing.

Take your medication early. Over-the-counter motion sickness medication, such as Bonine and Dramamine, is most effective if you take it at least an hour before you set sail, says Dr. Koch. Your doctor can also prescribe a scopolamine patch before the trip. Worn behind the ear, it delivers antinausea medication to your bloodstream for four days. The downside to these medications is that they can make you drowsy.

Try ginger. Scientific studies show that the herb ginger can work nearly twice as long as Dramamine with none of the side effects. Take three or four 400-milligram ginger capsules 15 minutes before leaving and every four hours once you get underway, suggests researcher Daniel

Mowrey, Ph.D., director of the American Phytotherapy Research Laboratory in Salt Lake City.

Come up on deck. Enclosed spaces aggravate motion sickness. And once on deck, you should stand near the center of the ship, where there is less pitching motion, says R. J. Oenbrink, D.O., a physician in private practice in Tequesta, Florida, who often works on ships.

Keep your eyes on the level. On a boat, keep your eyes on the horizon. In a car, focus on the distant terrain ahead of you. It's helpful to stabilize your vision even though your inner ears are registering a lot of motion, says Dr. Koch.

Press your wrist. The Chinese technique of acupressure helps short-circuit motion sickness in even the most weak-kneed sailors, says Dr. Koch. The spot is located exactly in the middle of your wrist, three finger-widths down from the wrinkle that separates your palm and your wrist. You can buy elastic acupressure wrist bands that exert constant pressure on the correct point. But, says Dr. Koch, acupressure seems to work better if you exert a strong rubbing pressure on the point.

Morning Sickness

Morning sickness (which can occur any time of day) usually appears during early pregnancy. Episodes generally disappear after the third month. If you have morning sickness, you'll want to discuss it with your doctor. Here are a few helpful recommendations.

Have a little breakfast right away. Eating crackers or another bland food before you get out of bed can help prevent nausea, says Jennifer Niebyl, M.D., professor and head of Obstetrics and Gynecology at the University of Iowa in Cedar Rapids. She also suggests eating several small meals throughout the day.

Sip ginger tea. Danish researchers discovered that powdered ginger root reduces nausea and vomiting, which was so severe it required hospitalization.

Many pregnant women benefit from this herb. To try it, dissolve a teaspoon of powdered ginger in a cup of hot water. Drink the tea every four hours as needed.

Be aware of B6. Dr. Niebyl conducted a study in which women who took 25 milligrams of vitamin B6 three times daily for three days reduced severe nausea. Women who took a placebo—a fake, look-alike pill—had no benefit. But B6 only worked for *severe* cases. "The nutrient had no effect on mild nausea," says Dr. Niebyl. Ask your doctor whether B6 supplements are right for you. (Pregnant women should check with their doctors before taking any over-the-counter medications or nutritional supplements.)

Rehydrate with fruit juice. If nausea has advanced to the vomiting stage, you'll need to drink lots of fluids—especially carbohydrates like fruit juice—to guard against dehydration, says Dr. Niebyl. If you can't keep any food or drink down, see your doctor immediately.

NECK PAIN

WHEN TO SEE YOUR DOCTOR

- Your neck pain persists for more than three days or keeps coming back.
- You suffer from neck pain after a fall or accident.
- Pain radiates from your neck down your arms or legs.

WHAT YOUR SYMPTOM IS TELLING YOU

Follow your instincts and you may be on to something. But allow your body to follow your chin as you sit, stand or walk, and you're probably in for some neck pain.

If you go about with your shoulders slumped and your chin thrust ahead, your head is no longer balanced properly atop your neck. Instead, the ligaments and other soft tissues of your neck have to deal with as much as 18 pounds of improperly distributed weight—definitely the wrong way to use your head!

"We think the big problem with the neck and the rest of the spine is that the joints are held at an extreme position for a long period of time, and that abnormal stress and strain eventually leads to pain," says physical therapist Wayne Rath, co-director of Summit Physical Therapy and senior lecturer of the McKenzie Institute International (U.S. Headquarters) in Syracuse, New York, and clinical assistant professor in the Department of Physical Therapy at Thomas Jefferson University in Philadelphia.

Various structures in your neck can give rise to pain. A ruptured disk—one of the rubbery, doughnut-shaped cushions between your vertebrae—can cause difficulty. So can problems with the muscles, joints or ligaments in the neck. Any of these can be hurt during an injury. The most common, whiplash, usually happens when a car is rear-ended. It makes the neck snap violently back and forth. The gradual degeneration of any of the structures in the neck from aging or overuse can also cause neck pain.

SYMPTOM RELIEF

Perched above your back, your sore neck may seem like it's an island of pain unto itself. But in fact, your neck will respond to many of the same pain-relief treatments that work for your lower back. (For those feel-good techniques, see Lower Back Pain on page 382.) There are, however, several specific remedies that can help provide fast relief for neck pain.

Collar your pain. Some people report that cervical collars, available at medical supply stores and most drugstores, may provide temporary relief by keeping your neck immobile, says Philip Paul Tygiel, a physical therapist who serves as a consultant for the University of Arizona University Medical Center Back Pain Clinic in Tucson. But it's not a good idea to keep your neck immobile for too long a time, he says. Wearing a cervical collar for more than a couple of days can weaken your neck muscles, making you susceptible to further injury, he says. If your pain continues for more than three days, see your physical therapist or doctor.

Wait it out. "Research shows that roughly 80 to 90 percent of the people who suffer neck pain and choose to do nothing are over their pain within two to three days," says Rath.

Improve your posture. "Poor posture isn't just how you sit and stand. It's how you hold your body when you function—moving, sitting, standing, bending, lifting, playing golf, whatever. It's how you hold your body while you are active or inactive," says Rath. And poor sitting posture, he says, is the worst offender of all.

"Think of your neck as a golf tee and your head as a golf ball. What happens if the tee is inserted at a 30-degree angle? Take a look at how people hold their necks," he urges. "What keeps their head from rolling off? All the muscles and ligaments under that strain." To maintain good posture: Sit up straight and tall, raise your chest up, lower your chin slightly and pull your head back so that your ears are directly over your shoulders, not in front of them.

If you suffer repeated bouts of neck pain, ask your doctor to evaluate your posture and, if necessary, recommend someone who can give you training in how to improve your posture.

Control that cough. If you accentuate your coughs and sneezes with a wind-up and delivery that would make a pro baseball pitcher proud, be forewarned: You could injure your neck. Instead, cough or sneeze while maintaining good posture or even while tilting your head and neck slightly back, says Rath.

Hold the phone. Rather than propping the phone between your head and shoulder—which can strain the soft tissues in your neck and the muscles in your upper back— hold the phone in your hand. Or better yet, buy a headset or speaker phone, says Hubert Rosomoff, M.D., D.Med.Sc., medical director of the University of Miami Comprehensive Pain and Rehabilitation Center in Miami Beach. "When you're cradling the phone like that, you're altering your posture and changing your head and neck attitude in an abnormal way," he says. "Don't do it—it's a disaster."

Get hold of a copy holder. Instead of twisting your trunk and neck to read copy while typing at your computer, install a copy holder that's flush with the screen. "That's probably one of the best tools someone can have," says Annie Pivarski, a back-care consultant and personal trainer in San Francisco who helped rehabilitate the back of San Francisco '49ers quarterback Joe Montana following back surgery in 1986.

Check that pillow. The wrong pillow is a common cause of neck pain. But rather than taking someone else's advice, find one that keeps *you* pain-free. Those filled with barley hulls can be molded to provide neck support when you sleep. But any cervical pillow that provides support to the neck ligaments can be very helpful. Above all, avoid pillows that push your head forward.

Go on a roll. Available at most medical supply stores, a cervical roll is designed to slip under your neck while you're sleeping, reducing strain on neck joints, says Rath.

Neck Exercises Prevent Pain

Everyone knows that exercise strengthens muscles and increases flexibility. Even gently exercising your neck helps lubricate and speed nutrients to the area, says Tygiel. Here are a few neck exercises that are particularly helpful.

Head turns. Move your head up and down by slowly dropping your chin to your chest and then bringing your head slowly back up to a normal position. Repeat ten times. Next, slowly lean your head from the left side to the right side and then back to normal. Repeat this ten times. Now slowly turn your head from side to side and return to the normal position. Repeat this ten times also. Do all of these exercises in the "pain-free" range only. (Don't worry if you hear cracking noises.)

"Most people don't take the joints in their neck through normal motions every day, so this is good therapy," says Tygiel.

Press it. Place the palm of your hand against the back of your head and gently press while resisting with your head. Hold for a count of ten. Repeat with your palm on your forehead. Now place the palm of your right hand against the right side of your head and press, again resisting the movement with your head. Repeat on the left side. Do this set of exercises once a day.

Say no to the spin. Rolling your head around in a circle—as some people do to "loosen" their neck muscles—can actually cause more damage. Avoid it, says Tygiel.

See also Neck Stiffness; Upper Back Pain

NECK STIFFNESS

WHEN TO SEE YOUR DOCTOR

- You feel a grating sensation when you turn your head.
- You were in an accident that snapped your head back and forth, and your neck is still stiff after two days.
- If you also have swollen glands, fever, a headache or feel nauseated, see your doctor immediately.
- Your stiff neck is accompanied by tingling or sharp pain that shoots down to your fingers.

WHAT YOUR SYMPTOM IS TELLING YOU

You woke up with a stiff neck. Consider the experience a wake-up call for you to pay more attention to your sleeping habits.

Of course, car accidents, falls, arthritis and even a cold draft can cause a stiff neck. But it's far more likely that you fell asleep in a position that strained the joints of the neck, resulting in inflammation and stiffness.

"If you take any joint, put it at an odd angle and leave it that way, you'll have stiffness," says Tab Blackburn, a physical therapist and vice president of the Human Performance and Rehabilitation Centers in Columbus, Georgia.

Other possible causes for stiff neck—like influenza, polio and meningitis—are far more serious. These conditions, however, announce themselves with other unpleasant symptoms, including nausea, headache and swollen glands.

SYMPTOM RELIEF

It helps to have a stiff upper lip to survive a stiff neck. In addition, here's what you can do to help ease the pain.

Some like it hot. Applying heat directly to the neck for 20 to 30 minutes two or three times a day will often alleviate the discomfort, says Blackburn. If you don't have a heating pad, try this: Run hot water over a towel, wring it out, roll it up and wrap it around your neck. Another method: Take a long, hot shower and allow the water to strike the back of your neck, says Blackburn. Do not use heat if the stiffness is the result of an injury that happened in the past two days. Heat will only aggravate the injury, making the pain worse.

Make motion your lotion. Gentle stretching and movement can help restore flexibility to a stiff neck, says Blackburn. "If you can move the neck gently four or five times a day, it's literally like pouring lotion on it," he says. He recommends carefully turning the head from side to side. Look over your right shoulder for a count of five, then look over your left shoulder for a count of five. Repeat the movement three times.

Try a topical. Rubbing ointments on a stiff neck doesn't treat the cause of the problem, but it can help relieve pain, says Blackburn. Over-the-counter topical ointments like Icy Hot and Tiger Balm contain ingredients that make the area feel warm. Other ointments are made with salicylic acid, the pain-relieving ingredient in aspirin. (Those who are aspirin-sensitive should check with their doctors before using these ointments.) But no matter which kind you choose, nothing beats the therapeutic value of having someone rub on a topical ointment *for* you. "There's something about the laying on of hands that's soothing and relaxing," says Karl B. Fields, M.D., associate professor of family practice and director of the Sports Medicine Fellowship at Moses Cone Memorial Hospital in Greensboro, North Carolina.

Shut that bedroom window. A cold breeze blowing on you may force you to snuggle in an awkward position just to stay warm, resulting in a stiff neck, says Dr. Fields.

Get a proper pillow. Propping yourself up on two or three pillows may be comfortable, but your neck doesn't appreciate all that padding. A single soft feather pillow or one made with barley hulls is easily manipulated to provide gentle support for the neck—rather than pushing your head forward. Also helpful: orthopedic pillows. Most have their centers hollowed out so your neck is supported and your head lies flatter, says Blackburn. You can buy an orthopedic pillow at some pharmacies and medical supply stores.

Reserve the couch for sitting. Nothing beats a Sunday nap, but next time, steer clear of the couch. Couches usually don't provide enough room or support for sleeping, says Blackburn. If you can't bring yourself to go to bed for 20 minutes in the middle of the afternoon, try stretching out on the floor to catch those Zs.

See your doctor. If stiffness persists for more than two days and these gentle home remedies don't help, your doctor may be able to help you find relief. He might recommend wearing a neck brace or send you to a physical therapist for a massage or an ultrasound treatment.

See also Neck Pain

NIGHT BLINDNESS

WHEN TO SEE YOUR DOCTOR

- You're having sudden or increasing difficulty seeing in dim light.
- You're having difficulty driving at night or performing other activities because of glare.
- You're unable to see stars in the night sky that are visible to others.

WHAT YOUR SYMPTOM IS TELLING YOU

The movie's theme song has started, the theater is pitch black and you're groping to find an empty seat. You're relieved to find yourself a good spot right in the middle without having tromped on too many toes. In a matter of minutes, you can see all 20 rows in front of you (...and the creepy guy in the seat next to you!). That's how it should work. But if you still can't make out your popcorn bucket after five minutes or so, it means that your nighttime vision isn't all that it should be.

Poor night vision is fairly common, especially among people who are nearsighted, says George Sanborn, M.D., associate clinical professor of ophthalmology at the Virginia Commonwealth University/ Medical College of Virginia in Richmond.

Other possible causes include diabetes, cataracts, macular degeneration (an eye disease in which a part of the retina gradually falls apart) or an inherited eye disease called retinitis pigmentosa. In rare cases (rare in the United States, but common in the third-world countries) night blindness is caused by a severe vitamin A deficiency.

SYMPTOM RELIEF

Here are some tips to help you see in low light.

Cut the glare. Your optometrist or optician can put an

antireflective coating on your glasses that cuts glare and increases the light coming into your eye, according to Bruce Rosenthal, O.D., chief of low vision services at the State University of New York, College of Optometry in Manhattan.

Wear your specs. If you're mildly nearsighted and don't have to wear your glasses all the time, at least wear them after sundown, advises Dr. Sanborn.

Forget fluorescents. After age 60, many people find that they see better with the increased wattage of incandescent (yellow) lights rather than fluorescent lights, says Dr. Rosenthal.

Think bright. If your doctor diagnoses macular degeneration, you need all the light you can get, especially while reading, says Jason Slakter, M.D. attending surgeon in the Department of Ophthalmology at the Manhattan Eye, Ear and Throat Hospital. In the early stages of this disease, positioning an arc-type halogen reading lamp behind your shoulder is ideal for providing bright light where you need it.

Eat smart. There is evidence that the antioxidant nutrients can help control many conditions responsible for poor night vision, according to Mitchell H. Friedlaender, M.D., director of corneal services in the Division of Ophthalmology at the Scripps Clinic and Research Foundation in La Jolla, California and coauthor of *20/20: A Total Guide to Improving Your Vision and Preventing Eye Disease*. Antioxidants work by counteracting naturally occurring tissue damage to the eye, he explains.

The key nutrients are vitamins A, C and E; zinc and beta-carotene, which is converted to vitamin A in the body. If your diet consists mainly of whole grains, fruits and vegetables, you should be getting the nutrients you need. But it's a good idea to ensure your intake with a daily multivitamin and mineral supplement.

Don't get caught in the headlights. Driving after sundown can be a challenge, especially when a stream of headlights is headed your way. "As a rule, you want to keep oncoming headlights in your peripheral vision so they don't momentarily blind you," says Dr. Slakter.

Wear sunglasses before entering tunnels. In daylight,

putting on sunglasses about a mile before entering a dark tunnel helps your eyes get partially adapted to the dark, says Dr. Slakter. Once inside the tunnel, remove your sunglasses and you'll be able to see in the dim light.

NIGHTMARES

WHEN TO SEE YOUR DOCTOR

- Your bad dreams are so bothersome or frequent that they impede your ability to fall asleep or remain asleep.

WHAT YOUR SYMPTOM IS TELLING YOU

Plaid lizards with teeth the size of elephant tusks and eyes like yellow hurricanes gnaw at your ankles as you stand immobile in a desert of broken glass. Well, no problem—if you're asleep!

Everyone has an occasional nightmare. You awake with a frightened start and bolt up in bed, heart thumping, brow damp. You're scared. If you're a little kid, you're really scared. And as the terror trails off, you wonder why you dreamed what you dreamed and how you can prevent it from happening again. Most likely, it's nothing more than a sign that you're under a touch of stress. Or maybe your blood pressure pills are acting up.

Psychologists and sleep experts still debate whether dreams reflect emotional turbulence. "It depends on whom you talk to," says Mark Mahowald, M.D., director of the Minnesota Regional Sleep Disorders Center at Hennepin County Medical Center in Minneapolis. Some say dreams are random brain-wave activities that the sleeping brain tries to choreograph into a plot. Others see greater significance—ancient archetypes, repressed fears and desires, symbolic solutions. "My guess is that it's somewhere in between, but closer to the random side," Dr. Mahowald says. "Virtually all mammals dream. My cat dreams, but I'm not sure what he's resolving."

Nonetheless, people under stress are more likely to have nightmares. "Nightmares are like anxiety attacks while dreaming," says Paul Gouin, M.D., director of the Sleep Disorders Program at Ingham Medical Center in Lansing, Michigan. "It's not a sign of a serious medical condition, but you might wonder if your mind might be calling attention to something you've suppressed during the day."

SYMPTOM RELIEF

So the loathsome lizard may or may not mean much, after all. You just don't want it lurking about in your head when you're abed. What do you do about this reprehensible reptile?

Don't lose any sleep over it. Literally and figuratively. The nightmare is usually not the manifestation of an underlying psychiatric disturbance, Dr. Mahowald says.

Reassure children. "Just tell them that everything is okay and that it was just a bad dream," says Dr. Mahowald. Kids can have a difficult time distinguishing between waking reality and the bizarre stuff that bad dreams are made of, so it might be a good idea to check under the bed and in the closets, just to show them that waking up banishes the boogey man.

The bugaboo may be a drugaboo. If nightmares gnaw at your psyche, the beast may be in the bottle in your medicine cabinet. "A wide variety of medications can dramatically change the severity, content, quality and quantity of dreams," Dr. Mahowald says. "The first thing we do for people complaining of nightmares is to find out what, if any, medications they are taking." Several prescriptions for high blood pressure and almost all drugs for Parkinson's disease tend to increase dream activity and may prompt nightmares, he says. If you're on any of these medications and are having nightmares, discuss it with your doctor.

Medicine might muzzle the monster. Occasionally,

physicians will prescribe tricyclic antidepressants to squelch nightmares. But this is an option you might want to consider only if the nightmares are seriously disturbing your sleep. Sleep experts usually frown on the drugs because they limit the rapid eye movement (REM) part of sleep so that you don't dream at all. "It's like going after sparrows with a deer rifle," Dr. Gouin says.

Rewrite your nightmare. When dreams turn ghastly, why not rewrite the script, Dr. Mahowald asks. "If you're bothered by a dream or if the nightmare is recurrent, you can change the ending of it while you're awake." In dream rehearsal, you run through the plot of the nightmare repeatedly during the day, changing the horrific happenings into nicer notions. At night, your mind remembers the plot revisions and incorporates them into the dream.

Talk about the terror. Because nightmares could represent underlying, unresolved emotional conflict in your life, some form of therapy may help. "Find out what's behind it," Dr. Gouin advises. "Find a friend, a confidante, a psychotherapist you can talk it through with."

Another Terror in the Night

What about when you (or more likely, your child) lets loose with a blood-curdling shriek that pierces the night? Just another nightmare? Maybe not. Nightmares often are confused with sleep terrors, which are seemingly similar but completely different.

People with sleep terrors are not even dreaming, Dr. Mahowald says. Sleep terrors are akin to sleepwalking, because both occur in the deep stages of nondream sleep.

Unlike someone having nightmares, a person with sleep terrors never actually awakens. In fact, they're difficult to rouse. And once they are awake, they can't remember what scared them or even that they jolted up in bed with a cry that would daunt Dracula.

Ride it out, gently. Sleep terrors are just part of the maturation process in kids. "These things just happen," Dr. Mahowald says. "The best thing you can do is console the sleeping person and guide them back into a lying position."

If the behavior is potentially dangerous, extremely disruptive or bothersome to other family members, it may be treated with medication or behavioral therapy, says Dr. Mahowald.

NIGHT SWEATS

WHEN TO SEE YOUR DOCTOR

- You sweat at night despite a cool room temperature, especially if the episodes come and go with regularity.
- The sweating is accompanied by fever, fatigue, discomfort or pain in the body.
- You are also experiencing a sleep disorder, such as sleepwalking, nightmares, apnea or insomnia.

WHAT YOUR SYMPTOM IS TELLING YOU

You retire to your bedchamber, eagerly anticipating a cozy night's sleep. But instead of drifting off to a sea of tranquillity, you awake to find yourself in your own little Sea World...and you're playing the part of Shamu, the performing killer whale!

If you're suffering from night sweats, you know that this scenario is not exactly an exaggeration. One drenching episode can quickly make your bed look like the set of an Esther Williams movie, leaving you, your clothing and your linens completely soaked.

The good news is that these nocturnal water follies are extremely rare. They're usually one-shot deals with completely harmless origins: a warm room, too many blankets, a bad dream or something you ate. It's also completely natural for women going through menopause to experience night sweats. And if you're an excessive daytime sweater, your propensity for wetness can easily carry over into the night.

"Emotion and stress commonly cause sweating, and you can carry those feelings with you to bed," says Ernest Hartmann, M.D., director of the Sleep Disorders Center at Newton-Wellesley Hospital in Newton, Massachusetts. "Nightmares, sleepwalking and sleep apnea can also cause night sweats," he adds.

"Recurrent night sweats are usually the body's attempt to fight off the effects of a fever," says Hinda Greene, D.O., staff physician of internal medicine with Cleveland Clinic–Florida in Fort Lauderdale. "The best-case scenario is that the fever is brought on by a low-grade infection, a cold, the flu—one of the more common illnesses."

There are also several relatively serious conditions that can trigger night sweats. These include tuberculosis, hepatitis, immune system disorders, thyroid disorders, leukemia, strokes, bowel disease and heart disease.

SYMPTOM RELIEF

Repetitive night sweats are unusual and are not to be treated lightly. It may take a little detective work on the part of your physician to find the cause. Here's what your doctor might consider as well as a few soak stoppers you may want to try on your own.

Lower the room temperature. "The first and most logical assumption is that you are using too many covers and the room is kept too warm," says Philip R. Westbrook, M.D., director of the Sleep Disorders Center at Cedars-Sinai Medical Center in Los Angeles. "Most sleepers only really need a light blanket and a room temperature of 65°F for a comfortable sleep. If a fan or air conditioner will cool you down, by all means use it."

Get on the stick. "Excessive daytime sweaters may be prone to night sweats and may take the same preventive steps they would use in the daytime," says Dr. Westbrook. "This would include the use of an antiperspirant, rubbing alcohol or body powder before retiring."

Drink more water. "Any time you have sweating, you need to increase your water intake to replenish what is lost," says Dr. Greene. She recommends at least 12 glasses per day (4 more than the average person requires) at room temperature to cool down your core temperature without shocking the system. Drink one glass just before going to bed. Showering or sponging with cool (not cold) water can also lower core temperature to inhibit some sweating.

Ask about estrogen. "Over half of all menopausal women will experience night sweats because of the decline of estrogen," says Lila Wallis, M.D., clinical professor of medicine at Cornell University in Ithaca, New York. "For some relief, your doctor can prescribe estrogen and other hormone supplements and medications." If you're going through menopause, ask your doctor whether hormone replacement therapy is appropriate for you. (For more tips on dealing with hot flashes, see page 315.)

Take aspirin. Check your temperature. If you're harboring a lingering fever, taking aspirin or acetaminophen during the day or before bedtime can break that fever. But, says Dr. Greene, it will do so by causing you to sweat. The good news is that it may be the push that's needed to finally lick the underlying infection.

Forget about nighttime exercise. "Don't take part in heavy physical activity before going to bed," warns Dr. Wallis. "This will only increase your body's core temperature and can serve as a spark to ignite sweating later in the night." Stay away from hot tubs, showers and saunas at night, too.

Avoid midnight snacks. "You shouldn't have a completely full stomach at bedtime," says Dr. Westbrook. "A midnight snack will just lie in your stomach all night, making you uncomfortable and thus producing sweating. Spicy foods and hot beverages can also bring on some severe night sweating."

Say no to nightcaps. That late-night cocktail, coffee or cigarette can raise your pulse, blood pressure, body temperature and adrenaline levels, says Dr. Greene. It's an open invitation for a difficult, if not sweaty, night's sleep.

Keep a sleep log. If you are at a loss to explain what could be causing your night sweats, Dr. Hartmann suggests keeping a record of your sleep activity. Note anything relevant before you went to sleep, such as what you wore or the room temperature. When you wake, jot down anything you can remember during the night, how you feel and the condition of your bed. Also record your daytime activities, food consumption and stresses. Continue logging the information for a few weeks—you may see patterns emerging that can give your doctor a better indication of the cause.

NIPPLE DISCHARGE

WHEN TO SEE YOUR DOCTOR

- The discharge is clear and yellow, watery or bloody.
- One or both nipples discharge continuously.

WHAT YOUR SYMPTOM IS TELLING YOU

You notice it while pulling on your bra in the morning. Or when doing your monthly breast check. Suddenly you find a drop or two of milky fluid oozing from your nipple. Your hand freezes. Your mind floods with fear.

Is this a sign of something serious?

Not necessarily. In most cases, it's as normal to have a slight discharge ooze from your nipples as it is to have a trace of oil seep from your skin.

Like skin follicles, the ducts leading to the nipples naturally contain some fluid, according to Susan Love, M.D., director of the Breast Center at the University of California in Los Angeles and author of *Dr. Susan Love's Breast Book*. "The ducts of the nipples are pipelines; they're made to carry milk to the nipple," notes Dr. Love. "The fact that there's a little fluid in the pipes shouldn't be surprising." The discharge colors can range from gray, green or brown to white.

If you squeeze your nipples, you may produce more discharge, adds Norman L. Sadowsky, M.D., clinical professor of radiology at Tufts University School of Medicine and chief of the Faulkner-Sagoff Breast Center in Boston. "Squeezing and other forms of nipple pressure mimic a baby's suckling," says Dr. Sadowsky. Squeezing may stimulate the production of prolactin, the hormone responsible for making the breasts produce milk and other fluids.

In a nursing mother, nipple discharge can occur spontaneously even without direct stimulation of the breast. "A hungry baby's cry can bring on a blouse-drenching milk discharge in seconds flat," says Dr. Sadowsky.

But even a woman who isn't nursing will have discharge if her nipples are squeezed or stimulated long enough, studies show. When researchers attached a gentle breast pump suction to the nipples of a group of women, most had discharge, whether they were young, old, many years past the birth of their last child or had never been pregnant.

In fact, just about any kind of breast stimulation can produce a discharge from the nipples—a strong shower spray, a mammogram, an ill-fitting bra or clothes rubbing against the breasts during exercise.

You're also more likely to experience discharge when your hormone levels change. A woman's hormone levels can fluctuate when she goes on or off birth control pills, enters menopause or takes hormone replacement therapy. Besides hormones, a number of things can cause discharge from both nipples, including antidepressants and blood pressure medications.

If the secretion is thick, yellow, brown, green or puslike, you could have an infection within your breast. A clear, watery or bloody discharge could signal a tumor, which is more likely to be benign than malignant. "That's why it's important to keep alert to the consistency, color, persistence and location of the discharge," says Dr. Sadowsky.

SYMPTOM RELIEF

Here are a few tips to ease your mind and control discharge.

Get help. If you experience discharge that seems in any way abnormal, bring it to the attention of your doctor. If you have an infection, your doctor will prescribe an appropriate antibiotic.

Get a sports bra. If you are prone to discharge, make sure your clothes don't rub against your nipples, especially during exercise. "Going braless in this circumstance is not a good idea," says Dr. Sadowsky. "Your clothes will continually stimulate your breasts and may make the problem worse."

Wear leakproof pads. If you are nursing, you can avoid embarrassing breast milk leakage by wearing absorbent breast pads inside your bra, says Dr. Sadowsky.

NOSE, RUNNY

WHEN TO SEE YOUR DOCTOR

- The drainage from your nose is thick and colored.

WHAT YOUR SYMPTOM IS TELLING YOU

Your runny nose may feel like a leaky faucet, but it's actually a perfect piece of self-correcting plumbing.

Nasal drainage is your body's way of washing out the nose, says Robert Enberg, M.D., an allergist at Henry Ford Hospital in Detroit. The problem could be an allergen or a cold virus, and your body is simply trying to get rid of it by flushing your nose with a fluid composed of proteins, salt water and antibodies.

Colds obviously cause a lot of runny noses, but if your nose is runny most of the time, the odds are 50 to 80 percent that you have an allergy, says Dr. Enberg. Certain medications—such as the beta blockers that control heart disease and high blood pressure—also trigger a runny nose. So does a sinus infection.

A nasal condition called vasomotor rhinitis can sometimes produce persistent nasal congestion and postnasal drip, along with sneezing and an occasional runny nose. "With this problem, your nose will suddenly run like a faucet for a few minutes—often first thing in the morning—so you have to grab a tissue quickly," says Dr. Enberg.

A severe change in temperature can cause vasomotor rhinitis (it's common among skiers). Changes in humidity can also bring it on, as can stress, hormonal changes and fatigue.

SYMPTOM RELIEF

If your nose is running, here's how to make it walk—and even sit down.

Don't take a multiple medication if you don't need it. If a runny nose is your only symptom, take a nonprescription antihistamine, says Dr. Enberg; if your nose is stuffed up, try a decongestant. Cold medications often include a variety of drugs to deal with multiple symptoms. It's best to take only the medicine your symptom calls for, says Dr. Enberg.

Review your medications. Because several medications can actually *cause* your nose to run, you should list all medications you are currently taking—both prescription and over-the-counter—and go over the list with your doctor. A change may be in order.

Try a prescription spray. If over-the-counter antihistamines don't dry up the runniness, your doctor may suggest a steroid nasal spray, says Richard Mabry, M.D., clinical professor of otolaryngology at the Southwestern Medical Center in Dallas. For certain severe cases of vasomotor rhinitis, your doctor may want you to try a prescription spray called ipratropium.

Hang on to your exercise habit. If you have just a head cold, with no fever or coughing, moderate exercise like walking will actually boost your body's ability to fight off the cold, says David Nieman, Dr.P.H., professor of health sciences at Appalachian State University in Boone, North

Carolina. Dr. Neiman's research has also shown that exercise will reduce your risk of catching the next cold bug that goes around.

Soothe your sinuses. If a sinus infection is causing the drainage, Dr. Mabry recommends a nasal douche. "Dissolve 1/4 teaspoon salt in four ounces of water. Over the sink, pour some into your hand, sniff it up into your nose and then blow it out, one nostril at a time," he suggests. You can also buy bottled nasal saline spray at pharmacies. (For other hints on battling sinus problems, see page 540.)

Attacking the Allergies

If allergies are causing your runny nose, here are a few ways to deal with them.

Try an antihistamine. If your allergies are fairly mild, over-the-counter antihistamines may be all you need, says Dr. Mabry.

Ask for prescription relief. If antihistamines make you feel drowsy, ask your doctor to prescribe a nonsedating antihistamine. Another highly recommended prescription medicine for allergies is cromolyn. This drug stabilizes cells in your nose and helps them resist runniness when they come in contact with an allergen. "Cromolyn is one of the safest medicines in the world," Dr. Mabry says.

Steroid medications and allergy shots are the next levels of treatment for more severe allergies, he says.

Avoid the allergen. When you know a certain plant or food causes your allergic runny nose, avoid it whenever possible. Try eliminating suspicious foods one at a time from your diet and gradually reintroduce them to see which are the culprits, says Dr. Mabry.

Fill up on fluids. Drink plenty of liquids to replace what you're losing with a runny nose, and use a humidifier in your bedroom to keep your nasal membranes healthily moist, suggests Dr. Mabry. Clean out your humidifier daily with vinegar to deter molds or fungus.

Learn the bedroom basics. To allergy-proof your bedroom, use plastic covers over the mattress and box springs, clean curtains monthly and remove rugs and upholstered furniture. Use lint-free bedspreads, synthetic rather than feather pillows, and don't sleep with stuffed toys. Keep your closet uncluttered and the door closed to keep dust down.

Use allergy strategies all over the house. Vacuum rather than sweep to clean floors, use disposable bags in your vacuum cleaner and dust daily with a damp cloth.

Try pure products. Use hypo-allergenic and unscented cosmetics, cleaning aids and detergents to ease your allergy woes, says Dr. Mabry.

NOSE, STUFFY

WHEN TO SEE YOUR DOCTOR

- You have tried home remedies for five days with no relief.
- You are troubled by a stuffy nose at the same time every year.
- You also have a fever and facial pain.
- You're producing thick greenish or yellowish mucus.
- Your stuffy nose is interfering with your sleep or causing a snoring problem.

WHAT YOUR SYMPTOM IS TELLING YOU

You feel like your nose is stuffed with socks, and not only can you not smell anything, but you're starting to wonder if breathing is still an option.

When your nose is stuffed up, the membranes that line it are swollen—perhaps from a cold or other viral or bacterial infections or an allergy. A chronic sinus infection may also leave you feeling stuffy—as well as tired. And certain medications—both over-the-counter and prescription drugs—can trigger stuffiness.

Don't keep blowing, because it's also possible that your nose is blocked by something besides mucus. Although it's probably been years since you tried the jelly-bean-in-the-nostril trick to impress your friends, it is possible to have a structural blockage caused by a deviated nasal septum, a benign nasal polyp or some other growth.

SYMPTOM RELIEF

Take a deep breath (through your mouth, for now) and read on for relief.

Wait it out. If a cold or other viral infection is stuffing you up, there's a time limit on your suffering, says Robert Enberg, M.D., an allergist at Henry Ford Hospital in Detroit. These infections almost always go away in a week or two, he says.

Humidify when the air is dry. From October through May, you'll keep your nose in better health if you humidify the bedroom, says Richard Mabry, M.D., clinical professor of otolaryngology at Southwestern Medical Center in Dallas. An ultrasonic vaporizer is less likely to grow harmful molds than the cool-mist varieties, says Dr. Mabry, but regular cleaning is critical whichever model you choose. Use a diluted bleach solution of one tablespoon bleach to one quart water to clean your vaporizer weekly, he says.

Spray with saline. Nasal saline, a diluted salt water spray available without prescription, such as Ocean or Ayr, is balm to those dry, stuffy nasal passages, says Dr. Enberg. If you make up a new batch every day or two, you can also use do-it-yourself saline: 1/4 teaspoon salt in seven ounces of previously boiled water. You can use nasal saline as many times a day as you need for relief, he says.

Steam away the stuffies. A nasal steamer humidifies dry, stuffy noses, says Alexander Chester, M.D., clinical professor of medicine at Georgetown University School of Medicine in Washington, D.C. It's also effective to create your own steamer, he says. Boil a pot of water, drape a towel over your head and the pot, and inhale the steam through your nose for about 15 minutes three or four times a day, he suggests. Be sure to keep your face at least 18 inches from the water to avoid burning yourself.

Reach over-the-counter for relief. Over-the-counter cold remedies may ease your stuffy nose, says Dr. Mabry. Use oral decongestants to ease congestion. Use antihistamines only for "wet" symptoms, like sneezing, itchy eyes and runny nose that suggest allergies. Use a combination remedy if you feel you need both, but avoid multi-symptom medicines that pack cough suppressants, drying agents, antihistamines, decongestants and pain relievers into one formula, he says.

Don't exceed the limits. Do-it-yourself doctoring is okay for nasal congestion with clear mucus and those "wet" symptoms that suggest allergies, Dr. Mabry says. Limit your use of over-the-counter decongestant sprays to five days or less. If overused, they cause a rebound effect that will leave you even more stuffed up than before.

Check your medicines. A number of medications, including beta blockers, medications for high blood pressure and high-dose estrogen, can cause nasal stuffiness. Let your doctor know about all medications you're taking, and ask him if switching medications would be helpful.

Cut back on chocolate. Concentrated sweets, particularly chocolate, may trigger swelling in your nasal membranes, says Dr. Chester. So avoid those sweets until your stuffy nose has cleared.

Pile on the pepper. "Cook with red pepper," suggests Varro E. Tyler, Ph.D., professor of pharmacognosy at Purdue University in West Lafayette, Indiana. Capsaicin, the active ingredient in red pepper, causes the mucus lining of your nose to increase secretions. "It'll make your nose runny and help clear it out," Dr. Tyler says.

Take your nose for a walk. As long as it's just a head cold, and you have no fever or flu, moderate exercise is good for your stuffy nose, says David Nieman, Dr.P.H., professor of health sciences at Appalachian State University in Boone, North Carolina. And exercise can help prevent your next cold, too. Research has shown that the immune system is strengthened during exercise and for about four hours afterward, Dr. Nieman says.

Decongest with a warm bath. When you come in from the cold after your walk, climb into a nice hot bath, suggests Dr. Chester. It'll warm your entire body and increase circulation in your nose, with a decongesting effect, he says.

Be happy without happy hour. When your nose is congested, avoid beer, wine and cordials, says Dr. Chester. By-products from the fermentation process of these beverages, called tyramine and tannin, will swell your nose further and block your sinus ducts. Red wine is worse than white, but distilled spirits may be less of a problem, he adds.

Take your nose to tea. A Chinese herb called ephedra is a good nasal decongestant, says Dr. Tyler. You can often find it in teas in health food stores, but make sure you're getting *Ephedra sinica*, the Chinese or Indian variety. The American species of ephedra lacks the active ingredient you need. Dr. Tyler cautions that ephedra will also act as a mild stimulant and should be avoided if you have high blood pressure or heart problems. Drink two cups a day until you feel better.

What if It's an Allergy?

If your doctor says your chronic stuffy nose results from an allergy, these are the basic treatments.

Avoid the allergen. If you work outdoors, you can't avoid ragweed, but you can banish the kitty from the bedroom. Learn what you're allergic to, and learn to avoid it whenever possible, says Dr. Enberg.

Take your medicine. Your doctor may prescribe various medicines for your allergic stuffy nose. Antihistamines, decongestants, a prescription nasal spray called cromolyn sodium and nasal steroid sprays will all bring relief.

Give it a shot. If your allergy-caused nasal congestion is severe and chronic, your doctor may recommend allergy shots, which desensitize your body to the allergen.

Swear off the moo juice. About 10 percent of people with chronic stuffy nose may have a milk allergy, says Dr. Chester. Try avoiding milk products for two weeks to see if this clears the congestion.

Read up on allergies. Need basic information on allergies? A helpful booklet called *The Allergy Almanac* can be ordered for $1 from the Foundation for Allergy Care and Treatment, P.O. Box 13367, Silver Spring, MD 20911-1336. (Allow four to six weeks for delivery.)

Removing Obstructions

If an obstruction or blockage is what's making you feel stuffed up, your doctor can help. Here are some possible surgical procedures.

Remove nasal polyps. A benign fleshy growth called a polyp results when the membrane lining your sinuses extends down into your nose, says Dr. Mabry. In most cases, your doctor can remove nasal polyps right in the office.

Straighten out the septum. If you ever got whacked on the nose, you may have a stuffy nose because of a crooked or deviated septum—that piece of cartilage that divides your nostrils. A procedure called septoplasty corrects the crooked septum, Dr. Enberg says.

NOSEBLEED

WHEN TO SEE YOUR DOCTOR

- Your nose is bleeding in gushes and won't stop even after you have pinched it tightly closed for five minutes.
- You also have high blood pressure, diabetes or any blood-clotting problem.
- You are taking aspirin regularly.
- Your nosebleed began with blood going down the back of your throat rather than out of your nose.
- Your nosebleeds are recurrent.

WHAT YOUR SYMPTOM IS TELLING YOU

Most nosebleeds seem worse than they actually are. The amount of blood lost is normally less than a tablespoon, and only 5 to 10 percent of nosebleeds ever need a doctor's care.

Noses are susceptible to bleeding because of their fragile anatomy. The inside of your nose is lined with hundreds of tiny blood vessels just inside your nostrils, and they are very vulnerable to trauma.

What's traumatic to your nose? Well, for one thing, there's digital trauma. Say again? Okay—nose-picking. Even though you've no doubt matured beyond the vigorous nose hunts of childhood and now probe adultly with a tissue-wrapped finger, the result can still be the same. Even a cotton swab can irritate the lining of the nose.

Another nasal trauma is the cold, dry air of winter. In that kind of weather, a simple sneeze or vigorous nose-blowing can trigger a bleed in almost anyone.

Older people have more nosebleeds. Older women are particularly vulnerable, since menopause causes shrinking and drying of the body's tissues, including those lining the nose.

Another type of shrinking—rapid weight loss, whether it's from dieting or illness—can also cause nosebleeds.

And speaking of illness, there are a couple of conditions, such as allergies, that can cause or contribute to nosebleeds. That includes two *inside* the nose: nasal infections and a fluid-filled, benign growth called a nasal polyp. And although high blood pressure doesn't *cause* nosebleeds, it does make them worse.

Finally, a number of medications can cause the problem. Using steroid nasal sprays for a runny nose may make you more susceptible to nosebleeds. Other medications include birth control pills, aspirin, ibuprofen and anti-arthritis medications like Naprosyn, Tolectin and Motrin.

SYMPTOM RELIEF

There are several very effective methods for dealing with nosebleeds, even chronic ones. Here are four good ways to stop the bleeding *now*.

Squeeze and hold. Your first response: Squeeze your nostrils and hold them tightly together, says Sanford Archer, M.D., an assistant professor of otolaryngology at the University of Kentucky in Lexington. A nosebleed will usually clot on its own, says Dr. Archer, but adding pressure makes it stop more quickly and helps form a scab. And forget the oft-heard advice to hold your head back. That doesn't do any good and will just make you feel like choking.

Use a clothespin. Tired of pinching? An ordinary wooden spring-type clothespin will work as well as your fingers, says Jordan S. Josephson, M.D., an otolaryngologist in Brooklyn. Hold your nose, lean forward and apply the clothespin.

Try Neo-Synephrine. Moisten a piece of cotton with Neo-Synephrine, an over-the-counter decongestant spray available at pharmacies. Put the cotton in your nose and then pinch your nostrils together firmly for five minutes, suggests Alan Sogg, M.D., an ear, nose and throat specialist in Cleveland.

Stiffen your upper lip. Dr. Archer says there's a scientific basis for this folk cure: Put a little wad of cotton inside your upper lip against the gum. One of the major blood vessels supplying the interior of the nose goes right through the upper lip, he says, and the pressure from the cotton will help to suppress the bleeding.

Ice it. Along with any of these methods, an ice pack applied to the forehead and bridge of the nose will also help to stanch the bleeding. "It will cool things down and make clotting a little quicker," says Dr. Archer.

Preventing a Recurrence

One of the most annoying things about nosebleeds is that they can tend to repeat themselves. Here's how to prevent their return.

Let it be. While your nose is healing, no more digital trauma or even nose-blowing, says William H. Friedman, M.D., an otolaryngologist and director of the Park Central Institute in St. Louis. You may dislodge the scab and cause a fresh nosebleed.

Moisturize your nose. After a nosebleed, use a nonprescription nasal saline spray to keep your nasal membranes moist, says Dr. Archer. Use the spray as often as you'd like.

Petroleum jelly is another good moisturizer, says Dr. Archer. "Put a ball of it on the tip of your finger. Then scrape your finger against your nostrils so that the Vaseline goes into your nose. The trick is to do this without inserting your finger. Do this three or four times a day, and within five days the scab should be completely healed."

When applying moisturizers, be careful not to inhale a gob. Vaseline or any other petroleum-based moisturizer can cause a form of pneumonia if it gets inside your lungs, warns Susan R. Wynn, M.D., an allergist in private practice with Fort Worth Allergy and Asthma Associates in Texas.

Humidify the air. A humidifier or vaporizer is an excellent idea, both for your bedroom and your office, says Dr. Josephson. However, says Dr. Friedman, daily and thorough cleaning of those devices is critical so that there is no buildup of molds.

Drink plenty of water. Keep a healthy level of moisture in your nose (and throughout your body) by drinking at least six glasses of water a day, says Dr. Friedman.

Switch to acetaminophen. If you've been taking aspirin or other nonsteroidal anti-inflammatory medicines, ask your doctor whether you can use acetaminophen instead, suggests Dr. Sogg.

More Help from Your Doctor

If your nosebleeds are persistent, your doctor has several ways to help.

Pack it away. Your doctor can stop a serious nosebleed by packing your nose with surgical gauze and sponges. This must be performed by a specialist, Dr. Josephson says, as all packing carries a risk of toxic shock syndrome, a rare illness caused by poisonous bacteria entering the bloodstream.

Seal the blood vessels. An otolaryngologist can seal broken blood vessels in your nose by cauterizing (precise surgical burning), by applying silver nitrate or by tying off the blood vessels with tiny stitches.

Eliminate polyps. If your doctor finds that a nasal polyp is causing the bleeding, he'll have to determine what is causing the polyp, says Dr. Sogg. He may ask for a CT scan or x-ray of your sinuses. If infection is found, Dr. Sogg recommends a minimum of three weeks on antibiotics, with a steroid nasal spray or a course of oral steroids to reduce swelling. "If the infection is treated, the polyp may resolve completely, along with your nosebleeds," he says.

Ask for a blood checkup. "If you have repeated nosebleeds, get a blood count to rule out clotting problems," says Dr. Sogg.

NOSE DRYNESS

WHEN TO SEE YOUR DOCTOR

- The inside of your nose is so dry that the skin cracks and bleeds.
- Your eyes and mouth are also very dry.

WHAT YOUR SYMPTOM IS TELLING YOU

Who enacted Prohibition in your proboscis? It's dry up there!

That moisture-craving schnozzola may be uncomfortable, but it rarely is a sign of a disease, according to Susan R. Wynn, M.D., an allergist in private practice with Fort Worth Allergy and Asthma Associates in Texas. In fact, the cause may even be something that you can remedy quite easily. "The biggest reason for dry nose is a side effect of drugs, usually antihistamines taken to dry up a runny nose," says Dr. Wynn. "You've had one problem, but now you've tipped yourself too far over to the other side." Nasal sprays, some bronchodilators and drugs containing atropine (which might be found in eyedrops, pain relievers and heart medications) also could dry out your nose.

Climate is another common cause of the complaint, according to Elliot Middleton, Jr., M.D., professor of medicine and pediatrics at the State University of New York at Buffalo and allergist at Buffalo General Hospital. "When the heat's up and the humidity's down, nasal passages can dry out," he says.

A dry nose also is a symptom of two rather rare disorders, keratoconjunctivitis sicca, in which not only the nose but the mouth and eyes are chronically lacking in moisture, and Sjögren's syndrome, a disease related to rheumatoid arthritis that attacks mucus and salivary glands, Dr. Wynn says.

SYMPTOM RELIEF

If you can't repeal Prohibition entirely in your nose, at least you can become a bootlegger. Here's how.

Think drink. From water to juices, drink more fluids, Dr. Middleton says. "Good hydration is important," he says. "And it's better to hydrate your tissues from the inside rather than to apply something topically."

Check out your medications. If you're taking antihistamines or anything with atropine in it, ask your doctor if you can cut back the dosage or stop completely, Dr. Wynn advises. And you might have your doctor review any medications you're currently taking to determine whether any other changes are appropriate.

For a solution, try saline. Squirt a little oasis into your nasal desert with a saline spray, such as Ocean or Ayr. Use the spritz, which you can buy at any pharmacy, three or four times a day, or however often you need to add some moisture to your nasal passages, Dr. Wynn says.

Put a splash in the air. Use a humidifier to spray moisture into the air of your home by day and set up a vaporizer in your bedroom to run while you sleep, Dr. Wynn suggests.

Be careful with cream. Apply a moisturizing cream just inside your nostrils to soothe very dry or cracked skin, Dr. Wynn says, but be careful not to inhale a gob. Vaseline or any other petroleum-based moisturizer can cause a form of pneumonia if it gets inside your lungs, she warns.

NOSE REDNESS

WHEN TO SEE YOUR DOCTOR

- Your nose is persistently red.
- You also have acnelike bumps on your nose.

WHAT YOUR SYMPTOM IS TELLING YOU

When you're skiing down a snowy slope, a red nose is as natural as windblown hair. It gives you that "I'm-having-healthy-fun" look.

A red nose can send a very different message when it suddenly appears after you simply enter a chilly room, drink hot coffee or give a speech in front of a crowd.

A red nose that seems to come out of nowhere can be explained in three words, according to Jonathan K. Wilkin, M.D., director of the Division of Dermatology at the Ohio State University Hospitals in Columbus: "oversensitive blood vessels."

Smokers and people with thyroid conditions often have oversensitive blood vessels. In those people, simply entering an air-conditioned room can make their blood vessels clamp down as tight as a vise, he says. This diverts blood away from the skin's surface. When their body warms up, however, the blood vessels open superwide. This brings a rush of blood to the nose, turning it rosy red.

A red nose can also be triggered by emotional stress. Stress causes a surge of adrenaline, which overdilates the blood vessels. In people who are prone to this kind of reaction, public speaking, a breakneck schedule or a fiery argument are all likely to result in a red nose.

But if your nose turns red frequently or the redness persists, you may have rosacea—a common skin disorder in which the blood vessels in the nose become enlarged. Five percent of the population has rosacea, which usually becomes noticeable around age 30 to 40. In this condition, the blood vessels leak, causing a low-grade inflammation that makes the nose (and also the chin, cheeks and forehead) look like you spent too much time in the sun.

The redness can come and go but may gradually become permanent and more noticeable. It is sometimes accompanied by pus-filled pimples. In advanced stages, the nose can take on a lumpy, swollen W. C. Fields appearance, as a result of tissue buildup.

Rosacea's exact cause remains a mystery, says Dr. Wilkin. "We do know that it targets fair-skinned people, particularly those who blush more easily and frequently," he says. Women are more likely than men to have rosacea, which may point to a hormonal link. "Many women first notice a red nose at menopause, when estrogen levels fluctuate and hot flashes begin," says Dr. Wilkin.

Sudden redness on the nose and face can also be caused by wind, high humidity and vigorous exercise as well as medications used to treat high blood pressure.

Scrubbing your face too hard and skin-care products to which you are sensitive can make the redness worse. So can alcohol, spicy foods and spending too much time in the sun.

Symptom Relief

Here's how to tone down a ruby nose.

Turn the tap to tepid. "Hot showers, saunas and steam rooms can force your blood vessels to overly dilate and stay that way all day," according to Robert A. Weiss, M.D., assistant professor of dermatology at Johns Hopkins University School of Medicine in Baltimore.

Wash your face like it is fine silk. "Stay away from abrasive cleaners and washcloths," says Dr. Wilkin. Use only mild soap and water, and lather up with your fingertips. Blot dry and follow with a supergentle moisturizer, such as a baby lotion. Avoid products containing perfumes and alcohol.

Use leprechaun makeup. As eerie as it sounds, applying sheer green makeup to red skin produces a flesh tone that virtually erases the redness, according to Joseph Bark,

M.D., chairman of the Department of Dermatology at St. Joseph's Hospital in Lexington, Kentucky, and author of *Retin-A and Other Youth Miracles*. The green "color correcting" makeup by Estée Lauder and other brands are sold at department stores.

Blow on your soup. Any hot liquid should be tepid before you drink it to avoid triggering a vessel response, says Dr. Wilkin.

Lay off the jalapeños and tequila. Spicy foods and alcohol cause blood vessels to dilate, which can make a red nose worse, says Dr. Weiss.

Suck on ice. "Holding ice in your mouth tricks your body's thermostat and keeps blood vessels from overdilating in heated conditions such as entering a hot car or exercising," says Dr. Wilkin.

Spritz your face with cool water. This also helps keep a red nose at bay during a workout.

Dress like a masked bandit. A scarf pulled up over your nose on wintry days protects against overchilling and tripping off a vessel reaction, says Dr. Wilkin. A thin shield of petroleum jelly smeared on your nose works well, too, adds Dr. Bark.

Take a deep breath. Stress relaxation may help counter the adrenaline hormones that dilate the blood vessels, says Dr. Wilkin. Before a speech, for example, take several slow, deep breaths and imagine your body floating on a calm sea.

Don't treat bumps with pimple creams. If your red nose is accompanied by acnelike bumps, your doctor can prescribe an antibiotic such as tetracycline together with a topical gel. This two-pronged treatment interrupts the inflammatory response and helps control eruptions. If necessary, laser treatment can remove persistently dilated blood vessels and improve your complexion.

NUMBNESS

- Any unexplained numbness—especially if it is accompanied by symptoms affecting the head, vision or an entire side of your body—needs immediate medical attention.

WHAT YOUR SYMPTOM IS TELLING YOU

It usually isn't quite as scary as a Stephen King novel, but numbness can certainly be an unsettling experience.

In most cases, the tingling sensation you feel when your arm or leg goes numb is a harmless signal that you've momentarily pinched a nerve. Once you change position, the nerve revives in a few seconds.

Numbness is also more common as you get older. "It's more likely to occur as we age because the body just doesn't bounce back as well as you get older. So the same amount of pressure on a nerve is more likely to produce numbness in an older person than a younger person," says C. Conrad Carter, M.D., a clinical professor of neurology at the Oregon Health Sciences University in Portland.

Another cause of limb numbness is the hyperventilation some people experience when they're anxious or afraid. While numbness usually is a harmless symptom, doctors stress that any sudden, unexplained numbness could be a sign of a serious illness and should be checked out.

Among the more serious causes of numbness are poor blood circulation, rheumatoid arthritis, multiple sclerosis, diabetes and carpal tunnel syndrome—a compression of the nerves of the wrist, which causes numbness in the hand and fingers.

Numbness also can be a warning sign of an imminent stroke or transient ischemic attack (TIA), a mini-stroke that temporarily causes symptoms of a major stroke such as paralysis or blurred vision. Without proper medical treatment, a TIA can lead to a full-blown stroke that may cause permanent physical or mental impairment.

SYMPTOM RELIEF

It's important that you not belittle the symptoms you're having, even if they only last for a few minutes," cautions Gilbert Toffol, D.O., a neurologist in Phoenix. "If you have a sudden numbness or weakness in any part of your body, and there isn't a logical explanation for it, you should seek medical care immediately."

If, however, your numbness is a problem of limbs "falling asleep," here's what you can do to wake them up.

Move that body. Regular exercise such as walking, running and swimming increases blood circulation and may help reduce the numbness you feel when sitting, sleeping or standing too long. But be careful which exercise you choose to adopt. Sports such as bicycling that involve a lot of sitting can cause numbness in the groin and actually contribute to the problem, Dr. Carter says. You should check with your doctor about which exercise is appropriate for you, he advises.

Quit smoking. Smoking can impair blood circulation and increase the likelihood that you'll feel numb in your hands, arms, toes and legs.

Move the wallet. If you have numbness in a leg, it's a possibility that carrying a thick wallet or other objects in your back pockets is contributing to your problem. "Carrying a wallet in your back pocket can put pressure on the sciatic nerve that runs along the buttocks and continues down the back of the leg," says Paul Gross, M.D., a neurologist at the Lahey Clinic in Burlington, Massachusetts. The solution? Find another place to carry your valuables.

You deserve a break. If you do a lot of repetitive tasks such as typing, knitting, sawing or hammering, you can develop carpal tunnel syndrome. If you take a break every 30 to 60 minutes and gently rotate the wrist for a minute or two, you may prevent this problem, says Alexander Reeves, M.D., professor of neurology and anatomy at the Dartmouth Medical School in Lebanon, New Hampshire.

O

OVEREATING

WHEN TO SEE YOUR DOCTOR

- You never seem to have a feeling of fullness.
- To compensate for overeating, you take laxatives or force yourself to vomit.
- You seem to eat a lot, but you're losing weight.
- You're chronically depressed.

WHAT YOUR SYMPTOM IS TELLING YOU

When you're tired, you sleep. When you're happy, you smile. When you're hungry, you eat. When you're not hungry, you eat. When you're *awake,* you eat.

We often eat out of habit, not hunger. "A lot of people regularly open up a bag of chips when they watch TV," says G. Michael Steelman, M.D., vice president of the American Society of Bariatric Physicians, who is in private practice in Oklahoma City. "When I walk into a movie theater, no matter how full I am, I think of a bag of popcorn."

Sometimes, that habit can become an obsession.

People who binge or who have the eating disorder called bulimia lose all sense of dietary control and eat thousands of calories at one sitting. Then they throw up or take laxatives. The problem often occurs in people who have low self-esteem after chronic failure at dieting. "After a while, it becomes a pattern of addictive behavior that can't be stopped," says Katherine A. Halmi, M.D., director of the eating disorders program at the New York Hospital-Cornell Medical Center in White Plains.

People who *do* try to stop an addictive behavior—smoking—often find themselves overeating. One reason is habit:

They're used to doing something with their hands and mouth, so they eat. Or they could be battling the misery of nicotine withdrawal with the nurturing pleasure of food.

Using food for nurturance is why people with depression often eat a lot, according to Donald S. Robertson, M.D., medical director of Southwest Bariatric Nutrition Center in Scottsdale, Arizona, and coauthor of *The Snowbird Diet*.

Sometimes it's not the mind that causes overeating—it's the brain. People who have low levels of the brain chemical serotonin often crave carbohydrates. In rare cases, a person who has a tumor or an injury to the hypothalamus section of the brain has no sense of feeling full when they eat.

A glandular problem can also cause overeating. An overactive thyroid, for example, can throw the metabolism into high gear and increase hunger. And untreated diabetes—a disease of the pancreas gland—robs the body of fuel, so the body compensates by revving up the appetite.

Some medications stimulate the appetite, leading to overeating. Cortisone, often prescribed for inflammation, is "notorious for increasing appetite," says Dr. Steelman. Steroids, antibiotics, antidepressants and pain relievers can also be a problem.

SYMPTOM RELIEF

Somebody with a chronic case of the munchies is different from somebody who eats thousands of calories at one sitting and then forces themselves to vomit. If you find yourself eating out of habit rather than out of hunger, here are some tips for you. But if you think you have an eating *disorder*—a serious psychological problem with food—see your doctor. And see your doctor, too, if you've noticed an increase in appetite and food consumption, but you're not gaining weight; you may have a glandular disease.

Bulk up. Dietary fiber satisfies the appetite more quickly and can keep you feeling full for a while, Dr. Steelman says. You can add fiber to your diet by eating more whole grains, fruits and vegetables.

Work off your appetite. "Regular exercise is one of the best natural appetite suppressants," Dr. Steelman says. Intermittent exercise won't have the same effect, though, so don't expect a Sunday stroll to do the trick. By "regular," Dr. Steelman means five to seven times a week.

Learn new table manners. If you eat whenever you're watching TV or reading in your favorite chair, you have to break the association between that activity, the place you do it and food. "Pick out one area in the house that's the designated eating area," Dr. Steelman says. "Sit there only when it's time to eat. When you are finished, leave the area. If you isolate eating to one specific spot, you weaken the effect of environmental cues on your appetite."

Avoid diet pills. Over-the-counter diet pills do little to curb eating. "If there is any effect, after a while it wears off and you'll start taking more and more," Dr. Robertson explains. "You could get into serious trouble with blood pressure and heart rhythms."

Check your medications. If your appetite seems to be stimulated after taking medications, tell your doctor, who may be able to substitute a drug without that side effect.

P

PARALYSIS

WHEN TO SEE YOUR DOCTOR

- Any paralysis should be brought to the attention of your physician immediately.

WHAT YOUR SYMPTOM IS TELLING YOU

Except for a few times when your mother insisted that you sit still and not move a muscle, you've been in motion all of your life. You've walked, jumped, run, swum, danced, stood, clapped, winked and snuggled.

But imagine not being able to move at all. Paralysis is a sign that there is a disruption of communication somewhere between the brain and the muscles in the body. That problem could be located in the muscle, the nerves leading to the muscle, the spinal cord or the brain itself.

"There aren't many good things that cause paralysis," says John Byer, M.D., an associate professor of neurology at the University of Missouri–Columbia School of Medicine. "You could have a momentary paralysis because you've slept on your arm and compressed a nerve, but most of the other causes of paralysis are very serious."

Paralysis can be caused by muscular dystrophy, tumor, multiple sclerosis, head and spinal injuries, stroke and transient ischemic attack (TIA)—a mini-stroke that can temporarily paralyze one or more parts of your body for less than 15 minutes. TIAs, however brief, should not be ignored, because they can be an important warning sign of a major stroke that can cause permanent paralysis.

SYMPTOM RELIEF

Sudden complete paralysis is fairly unusual," says C. Conrad Carter, M.D., a clinical professor of neurology at the Oregon Health Sciences University in Portland. But if paralysis or weakness comes on suddenly in any part of the body, you should seek medical attention immediately, because any delay may reduce your chances of recovering at least some movement.

PELVIC PAIN

WHEN TO SEE YOUR DOCTOR

- You experience sharp, sudden pain in your pelvis.
- Pelvic pain lasts more than two days or is recurrent.
- You are also experiencing burning with urination, increased frequency of urination, nausea, vomiting or diarrhea.
- You are pregnant.
- You've had loss of appetite and are now experiencing pelvic pain.
- You had a sexually transmitted infection at any time in the past or have had multiple sexual partners.

WHAT YOUR SYMPTOM IS TELLING YOU

Unfortunately, some of the qualities that make a woman's uterus such an ideal breeding chamber for a growing fetus—warmth and moisture—also make it an ideal breeding ground for bacteria. And bacterial infections in the uterus can cause considerable pelvic pain.

Urinary tract infections (UTIs) can also cause pelvic pain in both men and women. Women are much more likely to suffer from UTIs, however. (In fact, while men *may* experience pelvic pain, the symptom is almost invariably a woman's complaint.)

Another major cause of pelvic pain is pelvic inflammatory disease (PID)—an inflammation of the fallopian tubes. Sexually transmitted disease is the most likely cause of PID, but other types of infection may also be to blame.

In some cases, your doctor may be able to pinpoint the cause of the pain as soon as you describe its nature and location. If PID is your problem, for example, you'll hurt on both sides of the pelvis. On the other hand, pain from a ruptured ovarian cyst comes on suddenly, more on one side than the other.

Endometriosis—a growth of the uterine lining outside of the uterus—causes chronic pelvic pain, painful periods and painful intercourse. Ectopic or tubal pregnancy also causes pelvic pain.

And if you have appendicitis, you'll probably lose your appetite first, then develop pain near the navel, then in the lower right area of your abdomen.

Not all pelvic pain is cause for concern, however. If you routinely have mild pain at the midpoint of your menstrual cycle, don't worry, says David Soper, M.D., a gynecologist at the Virginia Commonwealth University/Medical College of Virginia in Richmond. Some women experience this type of pain when they ovulate, and it's perfectly normal and harmless.

SYMPTOM RELIEF

Fortunately, there's help for all these pelvic problems. Here's a look at the most important way you can help yourself, and that is to see your doctor for a complete exam.

Clear up current infections first. If your doctor finds a UTI, he may prescribe an antibacterial medication, says Jack Lapides, M.D., a urologist in Ann Arbor, Michigan. You can go a long way toward preventing repeated UTIs by urinating more frequently. What's frequent? No less than every three hours during the day, and even once or twice at night if the problem's persistent, he says. Urinating right after sexual intercourse may also help head off infections.

Ask for an analgesic. If your pain is caused by a ruptured ovarian cyst, the only treatment you'll probably need is a prescription analgesic, says David Eschenbach, M.D., professor and chief of the Division of Gynecology at the University of Washington School of Medicine in Seattle. Rarely, excessive bleeding from a ruptured cyst requires surgery.

Your doctor may also prescribe pain medications like ibuprofen for pelvic pain from other causes, says Dr. Soper.

Get medical treatment for endometriosis. There are several ways to treat endometriosis, depending on the severity of the pain and the extent of the overgrowth. Simply taking birth control pills may end the pain of endometriosis. Alternately, there are prescription medications—GnRh agonists—that cause the overgrown tissue to shrink by shutting down the menstrual cycle and producing a temporary "chemical menopause." GnRh agonists, however, can only be taken for the short term—six months or so.

If medication doesn't end pain from endometriosis, your doctor may recommend a surgical procedure called laparoscopy. This procedure calls for inserting a fiber-optic viewing device equipped with a tiny laser through a belly-button incision, says Dr. Soper. The doctor can then vaporize the troublesome tissue. In some cases, hysterectomy—the removal of the uterus—is recommended. But this should only be done as a last resort—and after a second opinion is obtained.

Treating and Preventing PID

In one sense, you're lucky if your pelvic pain indicates pelvic inflammatory disease. For countless women, PID is "silent" or painless, and they may face increased risk of infertility or ectopic pregnancy without ever realizing that there's a problem. Though PID is not to be taken lightly. Treatment usually relieves acute pain, but 10 percent of women become infertile after PID.

PID is treated almost solely with antibiotics, says Dr. Eschenbach. PID usually calls for oral antibiotics, he says. More severe PID may require intravenous antibiotics in the hospital.

Heading Off Trouble

Preventing a recurrence of PID is largely in your control.
Here's how.

Waste the weed. "One thing you can do for yourself is to
quit smoking," says Polly Marchbanks, Ph.D., an epidemiologist and chief of the Centers for Disease Control and
Prevention (CDC) Epidemic Intelligence Service in Atlanta.

Surprised? Almost everyone knows that cigarette smoking increases cancer risk to lungs and throat. Fewer people
may realize that smoking can also cause cancer in the bladder, pancreas and cervix. Dr. Marchbanks and researchers
at the CDC have discovered a link between smoking and
PID as well.

Don't douche. Douching may cause PID by driving
infectious material up into the uterus or by disturbing normal vaginal bacteria, says Dr. Eschenbach. The vagina is
perfectly capable of cleaning itself through normal secretions.

Recognize your risks. Since sexually transmitted diseases
are a prime cause of PID, protection is paramount.
Researchers at the Center for Reproductive Health Policy
Research at the University of California in San Francisco
offer this reminder: Mutual monogamy is safest; acquiring
new partners increases your risk for PID.

Protect yourself. Both mechanical and chemical barriers
are highly effective in preventing PID. These include latex
condoms, diaphragms and spermicides.

Don't ignore infections. Prompt treatment for symptoms
suggesting vaginal infections is an important ally against
PID, the researchers say. And remember to abstain from sex
during treatment. If your doctor says your type of infection
can be sexually transmitted, be sure to refer your partner
for treatment as well.

See also Stomach Pain; Vaginal Itching

PENILE DISCHARGE

WHEN TO SEE YOUR DOCTOR

- Any unusual discharge needs to be discussed with your doctor.

WHAT YOUR SYMPTOM IS TELLING YOU

A variety of causes could produce a persistent drip from the penis, doctors say. But most likely, in this age of war on sexually transmitted diseases, you've just been handed a dishonorable discharge.

"The vast majority of penile discharges are the result of sexually transmitted diseases," says Michael Warren, M.D., chief of the Division of Urology at the University of Texas Medical Branch in Galveston. The discharge can be thick or thin and vary in hue from white to yellow, greenish or red.

The two most common disease suspects are gonorrhea and chlamydia, according to Michelle Topal, supervisor of the Centers for Disease Control and Prevention National Sexually Transmitted Disease Hotline in Research Park, North Carolina. Both have similar signs. Chlamydia produces a discharge around the head of the penis and perhaps some pain when urinating. Gonorrhea also inflicts some urinary burning or pain.

The leak may let loose as soon as 2 to 5 days after having sex with an infected partner, or it could take as long as 14 days, Topal says. A chlamydia infection shows itself as a discharge anywhere from one to four weeks after intercourse.

Another common cause is an infection or irritation of the urethra, a disease known as nonspecific urethritis, says Irwin Goldstein, M.D., a professor of urology at Boston University School of Medicine. An infection or inflammation of the prostate also may prompt a penile discharge. Both kinds of infections can be transferred to a sexual partner, he says.

SYMPTOM RELIEF

If you're experiencing penile discharge, you absolutely must see your doctor for diagnosis and treatment. There are, though, some facts you should know before and after your visit.

Take your medicine. Only antibiotics can dam the flow of a penile discharge, doctors say. Ceftriaxone and doxy-cycline are used for gonorrhea and chlamydia, while other antibiotics are prescribed for urethritis or prostate problems.

Keep it to yourself. Don't take the chance of infecting someone else if you have a discharge from your penis. "You can't risk passing it on," Dr. Warren says. That means no unprotected sex until the problem is diagnosed and treated.

Don't write your own prescription. You can't presume to treat your own infection by rummaging around in the medicine cabinet and swallowing the antibiotics left over from your spouse's dental surgery. "There's precious little you can do until you see the doctor, and you don't want to change the symptoms by taking something," Dr. Warren says.

Stay clean. You should always keep the penis clean by wiping away the discharge and washing with mild soap and warm water. "Just basic hygiene," Dr. Warren says. (Your doctor will want to see the discharge, so don't cleanse the area just before going to his office.)

Pick up the phone. Most cities have free telephone services for people who have questions about genital problems like penile discharge that they suspect are sexually transmitted, Topal says.

PENILE PAIN

WHEN TO SEE YOUR DOCTOR

- A painful erection or erection-like swelling unrelated to sexual thoughts or arousal persists for an hour or more.
- You suffer any injury to your penis.
- Your penis painfully curves when it becomes erect.

WHAT YOUR SYMPTOM IS TELLING YOU

Nature plays a cruel joke when the body's main source of pleasure becomes a focus of pain. Penile pain comes in several forms, most of which are apparent only when the penis is erect.

Prolonged penile swelling, called priapism, may start out as a normal erection, and it may look like one, but it actually isn't. "The penis is only *acting* like it's sexually aroused," says Irwin Goldstein, M.D., a professor of urology at Boston University School of Medicine. "What we're really looking at is a malfunction of the regulation of blood flow in and out of the penis." Priapism usually results from an injury or a medication. Some men with diabetes or sickle cell disease also are prone to priapism, according to Bruce H. Blank, M.D., a clinical associate professor of urology at Oregon Health Sciences University School of Medicine in Portland.

An injury can actually break an erect penis, causing pain and even priapism. "I've treated people who have had a toilet seat fall on their erections," Dr. Goldstein says. "I've seen people who've had a door slam on their penises while having sex in a car."

It's also possible to miss the vagina during intercourse, cracking the erection against the woman's pelvis or thigh. "It just breaks. It's as simple as that," says E. Douglas Whitehead, M.D., a urologist, co-director of the Association for Male Sexual Dysfunction in New York City

and an associate clinical professor of urology at Moun
Sinai School of Medicine of the City University o
New York.

"It sounds a little difficult to believe that that can hap
pen, but it can. The penis actually breaks. It snaps, and yo
hear it." The penis also may turn black and blue, he says.

Once the initial pain of the injury subsides, you ma
smile smugly at what seems to be your new-found stayin
power, but that grin will soon give way to a grimace. No
even orgasm and ejaculation, which normally cause a
erection to subside, will relieve a pseudo-erection. Bu
there's nothing fake about the pain. "It's like a rubber ban
wound around your finger, only worse," says Dr. Goldstein
"It's horribly sore. The pressure is so great."

That pressure comes from a laceration of an arter
inside the penis. Too much blood is flowing in and canno
flow out. The urethra, which carries urine from the bladde
also could be fractured, which can cause an infection.

The penis also can be harmed when not erect, and th
blow doesn't have to hurt a lot or fall on the external por
tion of the organ to cause arterial damage that may even
tually lead to impotence. "Blunt trauma anywhere from th
tip of the penis to the anus can injure an artery and induc
blockage," Dr. Goldstein says. "Most people fail to appre
ciate that there's just as much of the penile mechanism
inside the pelvis as there is outside of it."

Fractured arteries or erectile tissue that don't result i
priapism still might heal improperly or form scars. The scar
ring not only inhibits blood flow but also prevents uniform
expansion of the penis. "Normally, the soft tissue expand
in all directions," Dr. Goldstein says. "When a scar ha
formed, expansion can't occur there. It's like putting a piec
of duct tape on a balloon and trying to blow it up."

Infection or inflammation in the urethra can also form
scars, Dr. Whitehead says. And arterial hardening in th
penis is often seen in men with an arthritic-like shortenin
or stiffening of the hands called Dupuytren's contracture.

No matter the cause of this scarring, the result i
Peyronie's disease, a sometimes painful bend in the erec
penis. The curve, not noticeable when flaccid, could b

light, or it could be so dramatic that the mechanics of intercourse become impossible. "I've seen guys with 90-degree bends to their erections," Dr. Goldstein says. "I've had some with curves of 120 degrees or more."

SYMPTOM RELIEF

The biggest impediment to curing painful erections or swelling is not the problem itself but the hesitancy of men to seek help right away. In the absence of sexual arousal, "a prolonged erection is very dangerous, because it will destroy erectile tissue," according to Dr. Goldstein. "You'll have substantial erection problems if it's not treated in 4 hours. And the damage could be irreversible after 12 hours." For prolonged erections, "everybody's so embarrassed about having them that they delay and delay and delay, hoping that it'll go down," Dr. Goldstein says. "But the longer they delay, the more likely they'll get permanent tissue injury." Here's what to do.

Get to the emergency room. Swallow your pride and march yourself to the emergency room posthaste, urologists urge. "The chance of achieving long-term potency by having this medically managed immediately is virtually 100 percent," Dr. Goldstein says. "With no treatment, the chances of becoming impotent range from 25 to 75 percent."

Forget about self-treatment. Over the years, several home remedies for prolonged or painful erections have been suggested, some of them from authoritative medical journals, according to Dr. Goldstein. Cold showers, ice-water enemas, cold compresses—"none of that would be helpful," he says, "and the delay only increases the chances of permanent damage."

Pretend it's just a runny nose. If the prolonged erection is caused by drugs or the blood otherwise cannot drain out of the penis, a doctor probably will inject the penis with a medication that constricts the blood vessels. "The erect penis is like a runny, congested nose," Dr. Goldstein says. "The tissue is congested and swollen, and the treatment is like giving you a dose of Neo-Synephrine to constrict the tissue and allow blood to drain."

Don't let ice suffice. If the fracture is slight, with little bleeding and no urinary infection, doctors might send you home with ice packs and precautions to avoid intercourse until your penis has healed. Delighted as you are that you won't be having surgery, you may want to seek a second opinion, Dr. Blank says. "I've seen fewer incidences of impotence and deformity if you surgically treat the small fractures," he says.

Seek a less-invasive solution. When an artery is lacerated inside the penis, a doctor doesn't *always* have to operate. "We used to," Dr. Goldstein says, "but we found that's a little too invasive and injurious." Instead, a vascular radiologist often inserts a catheter into the artery and injects a blood clot to stop the bleeding. When the clot dissolves, the hole has healed.

If the urethra has been fractured, surgery may be required to divert the urine from pooling in the penis, according to Dr. Blank.

Check your medicines. Drugs also cause extended erections by interfering with normal blood flow, Dr. Goldstein says. Some antidepressants are common offenders, as are some drugs for head and back injuries. Improper use of drugs to help men achieve erections can also cause painfully prolonged erection. Make sure your doctor knows about all the over-the-counter and prescription medications you're currently taking.

Getting Things Straightened Out

Peyronie's may be painful, but it's not always necessary to operate to take the kink out of the erection, doctors say.

Wait it out. In about half the cases, the pain, if not the curvature, goes away in a year or two. "It doesn't always need to be treated," Dr. Whitehead says, "if there is only a slight curvature and little pain. If it interferes with sex or if there's a lot of pain, then it's something we look at." This is not a decision you can make on your own, however. You need to get the go-ahead from your doctor.

Ask about E. High doses of vitamin E have proved to be helpful in treating Peyronie's disease, Dr. Whitehead says.

Ultrasound may be the ultimate. Ultrasound therapy may put some pliability back into the scarred tissue, Dr. Whitehead says. Injections of anti-inflammatory drugs also may help.

Straightening the bend. If surgery is necessary, the physician will cut out the hardened tissue and replace it with more pliant skin, Dr. Blank says. In severe cases, a penile implant may be necessary. Ask your doctor about these options.

PERSONALITY CHANGE

WHEN TO SEE YOUR DOCTOR

- You suddenly have difficulty getting along with relatives, friends and co-workers.
- You feel socially withdrawn or isolated.
- You feel hopeless or helpless.

WHAT YOUR SYMPTOM IS TELLING YOU

You're normally a fun-loving, outgoing person, but you've suddenly become cranky, morose and humorless.

Your daughter jokes that she might ask an exorcist to rid you of this perplexing shift in personality. But you don't laugh because you actually think she might be right.

"When there is a sudden, noticeable change in how a person behaves, that's pretty ominous. That usually doesn't happen unless there is something major going wrong," says Betsy Comstock, M.D., a professor of psychiatry at Baylor College of Medicine in Houston.

Although our basic personalities are set by the time we're

30 years old, some gradual adjustments can occur throughout life, says John Moran, Ph.D., a Scottsdale, Arizona, psychologist. Men, for example, often become more nurturing as they age, while women tend to become more assertive, he says. But it may take years for those changes to occur. Sudden changes in personality that take place over a matter of days or weeks can be a serious symptom.

Among the many causes of sudden personality change are anxiety, depression, drug or alcohol abuse, premenstrual syndrome, Alzheimer's disease, stroke and brain tumor.

SYMPTOM RELIEF

The list of medical conditions that can cause a sudden personality change is quite long," Dr. Comstock says. "If this happens to you, it's important to get a complete physical and psychiatric evaluation as soon as possible." Your doctor will prescribe appropriate treatment.

See also Depression; Irritability; Mood Swings

PIMPLES

WHEN TO SEE YOUR DOCTOR

- Over-the-counter acne medicines aren't helping.
- Your pimples are forming scars after they heal.

WHAT YOUR SYMPTOM IS TELLING YOU

Remember when just one pimple was enough to ruin your week? Your family complained that you never came out of the bathroom. But it wasn't vanity that kept you glued to the mirror—it was desperation.

Acne usually begins in adolescence, when hormones

start to rage. Along with producing major bodily changes like the appearance of a beard or breasts, those hormones can also produce enough oil to keep J. R. Ewing in business for life. With the extra, thicker oil supply, the tiny ducts leading from the oil glands to the surface of the skin can become narrowed or clogged.

Sometimes, oil gets caught at a pore's opening, and when it hits the air, it oxidizes and turns dark, forming a blackhead. Those irritating dark spots are *not* from inadequate cleansing, dermatologists say. You could wash your face six times a day and still be prone to blackheads. When oil can't escape a plugged-up pore, a small white cyst, known as a whitehead, may form. Either a blackhead or a whitehead can become infected, producing the inflammation and redness of an acne pimple.

But the raging hormones of youth aren't the only cause of problem complexion. External oils on your skin—greasy cleansers, hair products or cosmetics, or even oils you encounter at work—may cause pimples. Stress plays a part, too. Some researchers say that chemicals released by the skin during stress can worsen inflammation.

Acne in adults is essentially the same as the plague of adolescents. Older skin tends to react a little differently, producing deeper lesions and fewer whiteheads and blackheads.

Another kind of acne is unique to adults. It's called rosacea or "the curse of the Celts." This is a skin condition common among rosy-cheeked people of Scotch-Irish descent. These people have a tendency to flush easily, and the increased blood flow to the skin overstimulates oil glands. Over time, this condition can produce acnelike pimples. (For information on how to deal with rosacea, see Nose Redness on page 474.)

SYMPTOM RELIEF

There's a lot you can do on your own to clear up pimples.

Use the right OTCs. Over-the-counter preparations can be a big help with acne, if you know which ones to use, dermatologists say. Oxy-5, Oxy-10 and Clearasil contain ben-

zoyl peroxide, which fights infection and promotes drying
says Ralph Coskey, M.D., a clinical professor of dermatol
ogy at Wayne State University School of Medicine in Detroit

Clearasil contains salicylic acid and sulfur to both cover
and dry up the pimple, says Tor Shwayder, M.D., a pedi
atric dermatologist at Henry Ford Hospital in Detroit.

Handle with care. Gentle cleaning is the watchword for
acne. Twice a day, cleanse your skin with an antibacteria
soap like Dial or Safeguard and an ordinary washcloth
says Stephen Webster, M.D., a dermatologist in Lacrosse
Wisconsin. "Don't use abrasive scrubs," says Dr. Coskey
"They can make acne worse."

Also avoid astringents, advises Thomas D. Griffin
M.D., a dermatologist at the Graduate Hospital in
Philadelphia. Astringents can be irritating, causing the
follicles to swell and leading to further breakouts.

Soak, but don't pick. Warm compresses can ease acne
inflammation, says Dr. Shwayder. Dip a washcloth in warm
water, wring it out and apply it to the affected area for 20
minutes twice a day. Avoid the temptation to pick at the
lesions, which can cause scarring.

Use nonclogging makeup. Use only cosmetics labeled
"noncomedogenic," which won't clog pores, advises Dr
Griffin.

Soothe your stress. Removing the sources of stress from
your life—along with daily relaxation techniques and exer
cise—will ease the stress that can aggravate acne, says
George Murphy, M.D., a dermatologist at the University
of Pennsylvania School of Medicine in Philadelphia.
"Studies show that stress may be part of your skin prob
lem," he advises.

Don't touch. Touching your face frequently only encour
ages inflammation, says Dr. Griffin. Try to become aware
of it and leave this nervous habit behind.

Help from the Doctor

Fortunately, even the worst case of acne can be temporary
Here's how your dermatologist can help.

Open the pores. A form of vitamin A called tretinoir

(Retin-A) has gotten a lot of press for its ability to reduce wrinkles. But the primary mission of Retin-A is to treat acne by peeling away the buildup of skin in clogged pores. Your doctor can prescribe Retin-A for as long as you're troubled with acne. At first your skin may be irritated, but your doctor can adjust the dose to the concentration that's right for you.

Another side effect of Retin-A is increased sensitivity to the sun, says Dr. Webster. If you're using Retin-A, apply a nongreasy sunscreen with an SPF (sun protection factor) of 30 *every time* you go outdoors, he says. "Check labels. You should look for a gel-type sunscreen that contains alcohol."

Kill bacteria. For persistent acne, dermatologists often prescribe benzoyl peroxide medicines to be applied to the skin. Benzoyl peroxide cuts down bacterial activity in the pores, and also produces a mild amount of peeling, says Dr. Webster.

Ask about antibiotics. Your doctor may also prescribe antibiotic creams or lotions to cut down on skin bacteria, says Dr. Webster. The normal bacteria in your skin break oil down into fatty acids, which may cause inflammation. For more severe lesions, your doctor may prescribe oral antibiotics, he says.

Peel pimples away. Fruit acids called alpha-hydroxy acids are effective new weapons in the acne-fighting arsenal, says Dr. Griffin. "A light chemical peel gives fairly quick control over acne," he says. "It may take two or three light peels, repeated monthly."

Your dermatologist will apply a diluted solution of glycolic acid in the office, he says. You will feel stinging and burning for about 30 minutes and experience some initial redness and swelling. If you have the peel done on a Friday, by Monday you'll have only mild flaking, which makeup can cover.

Zap them with zinc. Prescription zinc creams, sometimes mixed with an antibiotic such as erythromycin, may slow the inflammatory process and aid in healing, says Dr. Shwayder.

Approach Accutane with caution. Accutane is a powerful prescription drug for severe cystic acne that doesn't respond to any other treatment, says Dr. Coskey. But Accutane can cause birth defects and must be used with extreme caution in women of child-bearing age. If you're a woman using Accutane, your doctor will require that you use a reliable method of birth control and that you be tested regularly for pregnancy. Other side effects often associated with Accutane are extremely dry skin, nosebleeds, dry eyes, muscle aches and elevated triglycerides and cholesterol.

Accutane therapy lasts for 16 to 20 weeks, and is 80 percent effective for severe acne, says Dr. Coskey.

POST-MENOPAUSAL BLEEDING

WHEN TO SEE YOUR DOCTOR

- You have any bleeding at all after menopause—light or heavy.
- You are on hormone replacement therapy, and your bleeding is not on the cycle your doctor told you to expect.

WHAT YOUR SYMPTOM IS TELLING YOU

Although menopause has come out of the closet in recent years, there are still plenty of women around who remember when it was oh-so-delicately referred to as the change of life. Today women heading through menopause might be likely to counter that with, "So what else is new? Change *is* life!"

One of the changes menopause will bring to your body is the end of your monthly menstrual period. This doesn't mean, however, that your period suddenly stops. It's very common for women going through menopause to have irregular cycles for a number of years, says Brian Walsh,

M.D., assistant professor of obstetrics/gynecology and reproductive biology at Harvard Medical School and director of the Menopause Unit at Brigham and Women's Hospital in Boston.

Bleeding after menopause can have several causes. Lowered estrogen levels may cause thinning of the vaginal walls, which are then more likely to bleed, says Dr. Walsh. Growths in the uterus may cause bleeding, and some post-menopausal bleeding may even come from the bladder or rectum, he says.

You may be worried that your bleeding might be a sign of cancer. It's certainly possible, but uterine cancer has a dramatically high cure rate if detected early, says Dr. Walsh. Because this bleeding is such an early warning sign, an early cure is possible in 95 percent of cases.

SYMPTOM RELIEF

Fortunately, there is a wide variety of treatments and cures for bleeding after menopause. Polyps or fibroids within the uterus can be removed with microsurgical techniques, infections can be treated with antibiotics and estrogen can help vaginal tissues to heal, Dr. Walsh says.

Keep a calendar. If you are taking hormone replacement therapy, you should still keep a record of your cycle and see your doctor every six months to a year, says Veronica Ravnikar, M.D., professor of obstetrics and gynecology and director of the Reproductive Endocrine and Infertility Unit at the University of Massachusetts Medical Center in Boston. "Be sure to ask your doctor what bleeding to expect," she says.

Plan on protection. If your regular Pap smears indicate dysplasia, you can help protect yourself from further exposure to the virus that may be responsible for it by shielding the cervix with a diaphragm or using a condom during intercourse. Dysplasia is increased activity in the cells of the cervix that can lead to cancer if untreated. It can be cured with cryosurgery and possible cervical excision, followed by careful monitoring using Pap smears.

Stub out that cigarette. Giving up smoking will also hel
keep your cervix healthy. Several studies have shown a rela
tionship between cigarette smoking and cervical cancer.

POSTNASAL DRIP

WHEN TO SEE YOUR DOCTOR

- Your postnasal drip is thick, colored and lasts longer
  than a week.
- You also have a fever and facial pain or are coughing
  up mucus from your lungs.
- Your postnasal drip is chronic and you are also experiencing sore throat, repeated throat clearing or hoarseness

WHAT YOUR SYMPTOM IS TELLING YOU

Everybody has postnasal drainage all the time. Health
noses and sinuses make a quart of clear, thin mucu
every day. This continually flowing stream of mucus clean
humidifies and heats air before it's drawn down into you
lungs and, normally, you swallow the mucus without eve
being aware of it.

You only become aware of postnasal drip when th
mucus thickens. You may even produce *less* mucus than yo
do when it's clear and thin, but it feels like more. And tha
condition, of course, is what's often called postnasal drip.

The causes of postnasal drip?

The dry air from heating or air-conditioning systems o
stomach acid that irritates the back of your throa
Heartburn. Or air pollution—and not just the kind fror
cars and smokestacks. Indoor air pollution from cigarett
smoke can also bring it on.

Postnasal drip can also result from an allergy to molds
dust, dust mites, pollen or animal dander (the tiny particle
of skin that pets shed along with fur).

Chronic sinusitis—repeated sinus infections—is often accompanied by headache and (you guessed it) postnasal drip. In this case, you'll have to treat the sinusitis if you want to turn off the drip.

SYMPTOM RELIEF

Postnasal drip can be stubborn, but a variety of tactics can thin the flow.

Make moisture. Use nasal saline spray generously and as often as you like to thin secretions, suggests Robert Enberg, M.D., an allergist with Henry Ford Hospital in Detroit. "It's a mild decongestant, but acts essentially as a nasal moisturizer," he says. You can get nasal saline spray without a prescription at pharmacies. You can also put a humidifier in your bedroom to help keep secretions thin while you sleep, says Frederick Godley, M.D., an otolaryngologist with the Harvard Community Health Plan in Providence, Rhode Island.

Drink plenty of water. "For postnasal drip, stay well-hydrated with six to eight glasses of water every day," says Lee Smith, M.D., a physician in private practice in Princeton, West Virginia, and secretary of the American Academy of Otolaryngic Allergy.

Cut down on coffee. Water's a great liquid to take in, but caffeinated coffee is not, says Dr. Smith. Caffeine is a diuretic, which will dehydrate you and thicken that postnasal deluge. Enjoy a cup of decaf or herb tea, instead.

Skip the smoke...and the cocktail. "Stay away from any kind of smoke," Dr. Smith says. "If someone's smoking around you, ask them to do it elsewhere."

And the cocktail? Alcohol is another dehydrator to avoid while you have postnasal drip. If you *do* indulge, Dr. Smith recommends drinking three eight-ounce glasses of water before you go to bed, which will offset alcohol's drying effect.

Try mucus-thinning medications. Over-the-counter agents like Robitussin syrup, which contain guaifenesin, will thin postnasal mucus, says Richard Mabry, M.D., clinical professor of otolaryngology at Southwestern Medical Center in Dallas.

If the problem persists, your doctor can give you prescription medicines. Humibid is prescription-strength guaifenesin. Your doctor may also recommend guaifenesin in a prescription decongestant such as Entex LA, Guaifed and Deconsal, says Dr. Mabry.

Take allergy action. If your doctor thinks allergies are triggering your postnasal drip, then taking an antihistamine may be appropriate. (For other tips on allergy relief, see "Attacking the Allergies" on page 463.)

Check out your sinuses. If chronic sinus infection is causing that thick mucus flow, your doctor will prescribe antibiotics, decongestants and thinning agents, says Dr. Mabry. (For more ways to deal with sinus problems, see page 540.)

Clear the blockage. If simpler sinus remedies don't do the trick, your doctor may examine your nose and sinuses with a viewing instrument called an endoscope, to see whether a nasal polyp or deviated septum (that piece of cartilage that separates your nostrils) is the source of your sinus trouble. Some polyps will shrink with steroid treatment, says Dr. Enberg, and larger ones can be removed surgically with tiny instruments. Deviated septums can also be corrected surgically.

See also Sinus Problems

PULSE, SLOW

WHEN TO SEE YOUR DOCTOR

- Your pulse falls below 50 beats per minute and stays there, and you are not an athlete.
- You are also experiencing dizziness, weakness, fainting, fatigue or difficulty breathing.

What Your Symptom Is Telling You

If somebody called you "slow" it would be an insult. If they said the same thing about your *pulse*, it would be a word of praise. When it comes to your pulse rate, slow is generally healthier. Or at the very least, not unhealthy.

Although the normal range for an at-rest pulse is 60 to 100 beats per minute, heart rates below 60—known to doctors as bradycardias—are not all that abnormal or uncommon, according to Joseph P. Ornato, M.D., professor of internal medicine and cardiology at the Medical College of Virginia Hospital of Virginia Commonwealth University in Richmond.

"Often a slow pulse is a sign of completely normal physiology," says Dr. Ornato. "Well-conditioned athletes may have such strong hearts that their pulses are in the forties or even thirties. And in certain individuals, a slower-than-average heart rate, say in the fifties, may be what is normal for their body chemistry."

A slow pulse becomes a concern when it is accompanied by other symptoms. "A pulse becomes too slow when the heart's pumping ability is reduced," says James Willerson, M.D., professor of cardiology and chairman of internal medicine at the University of Texas Medical School at Houston. "When the heart rate is too slow, most people experience disturbing symptoms such as dizziness, fatigue and weakness before they complain about their heart rate."

The bradycardias that are most likely to produce these symptoms, and that most concern heart specialists, are those resulting from disturbances in the electrical impulses that regulate heart rhythm. These conditions, if left untreated, can cause the heart to slip into a state of cardiac arrest.

But a slow heartbeat can also be caused by conditions that are not related to the heart. You could experience a slow pulse following damage to the heart from a heart attack. If the thyroid gland is secreting too little hormone, heart rate can plummet. Hypothermia—a drop in body temperature—can also slow the pulse. Although unlikely in America, severe malnutrition can reduce the heart rate.

Many of the medications used to treat heart conditions—like beta blockers, calcium channel blockers and digitalis—do their jobs by reducing heart rate. So do tranquilizers and sedatives. Other drugs can also produce slow pulses as a side effect.

SYMPTOM RELIEF

If you otherwise feel fine and have no other symptoms, a pulse on the slow side probably doesn't mean a thing or need any treatment. Only a doctor can tell you if your pulse is indeed "too slow" and prescribe the proper treatment. Here are a few things you should know about.

Have your doctor check your medications. Make sure you're taking the proper medicine and the right dosage. And don't just decide on your own to stop taking your medication. In many cases, such as with certain heart medications, a slow pulse may be the effect your doctor is trying to induce.

Get up to speed with a pacemaker. "If a bradycardia is serious enough to produce other symptoms and interfere with the pumping function of the heart, the most effective treatment is the implantation of an artificial pacemaker," says Lou-Anne Beauregard, M.D., assistant professor of medicine at Cooper Hospital/University Medical Center in Camden, New Jersey. "This device keeps the heart rate going at a level where you can enjoy a normal, productive life."

PULSE, WEAK

WHEN TO SEE YOUR DOCTOR

- Your weak pulse is accompanied by other more serious and distressing symptoms, including fainting, dizziness, weakness, fatigue, sweating, breathlessness or weight gain.
- Besides feeling faint, your pulse is above 100 beats per minute or below 50 beats per minute.

WHAT YOUR SYMPTOM IS TELLING YOU

You eat right. You take care of yourself. You look good and feel good. But one day you take your pulse...and you don't like what you feel. Instead of thumping with the gusto you expect, your pulse is virtually nonexistent. Faint blips. Lifeless.

Now you panic. "What's happening?" you ask yourself. "The old ticker must be on its last legs. Or maybe I have some rare tropical disease! Or maybe aliens have sucked the life out of me and turned me into a zombie!! Or maybe..."

Or maybe you should just settle down and get a grip. Your best bet is to simply relax and forget about it. "Physicians place virtually no importance on the complaint of a weak pulse in the absence of any other symptoms," says James Willerson, M.D., professor of cardiology and chairman of internal medicine at the University of Texas Medical School at Houston. "It generally is not a sign of any disease, and usually it is just a perception in an untrained and frightened individual."

Many things may make your pulse seem weak. It may be harder to feel a pulse in a heavier person. Your pulse may be a little rapid because of nervousness. Your hands may be cold. Or you may be feeling for it in the wrong place.

What about those rare occasions when something out of the ordinary *is* going on? "It generally means that your blood pressure is low," says Dr. Willerson. "This is a normal occurrence in some people. Other times, it arises from a loss of blood or fluids, vomiting, dehydration, malnutrition or a medication overdose."

"Anything that diminishes the forward flow of blood, if it is severe enough, will produce a true weak pulse," says Joseph P. Ornato, M.D., professor of internal medicine and cardiology at the Medical College of Virginia Hospital of Virginia Commonwealth University in Richmond. "But most people would complain of more obvious symptoms long before a weak pulse: sweating, shortness of breath, dizziness and/or fainting."

Weak pulses, along with these other symptoms, may be seen with severe congestive heart failure: A heart, weakened

by disease, damage or infection, is unable to pump sufficient blood and oxygen to the rest of the body, causing a
backup of blood and fluids in the heart and lungs. In this
case, the pulse is likely to be very rapid as well as faint.

SYMPTOM RELIEF

Almost always, the perception that your pulse is weak is
nothing but a perception, and you don't have a thing to
be concerned about. But if you are showing other symptoms or remain distressed about it, keep these tips in mind.

Have your pressure checked. Your blood pressure may
be lower than the average, but whether you suffer from true
low blood pressure depends on a number of factors including your age, size and weight. A physician knows best if
your blood pressure is low enough to merit treatment.

Double-check your medications. Read labels for proper
dosages. Too much or not enough can lower your blood
pressure and can weaken your pulse. Ask your doctor if any
of your medications should be changed.

Ask your doctor about salt. Sometimes people with
chronically low blood pressures are advised to increase
their salt consumption or are given medications to aid their
salt retention. But most people with heart failure are told
the exact opposite. Your doctor knows what's best for you.

Limit your liquor. Alcohol quickly dilates blood vessels,
dropping blood pressure and causing your pulse to go from
hearty to hardly in no time.

See also Heartbeat Irregularities; Pulse, Slow; Pulse Racing

Pulse Racing

WHEN TO SEE YOUR DOCTOR

Your pulse rate frequently rises above 100 beats per
minute when you're not exerting yourself.
Your pulse doesn't return to its normal range per minute
within five minutes after ceasing vigorous exercise.
Seek emergency treatment if you're not exerting yourself or emotionally anxious or under stress, and your
pulse takes off chaotically at rates well above 100 beats
per minute.

WHAT YOUR SYMPTOM IS TELLING YOU

Hot-rod racers can "tach up" their engines by revving
them at super-high revolutions per minute. The human
heart can also tach up and rev at high rates—a condition
cardiologists call tachycardia. But unlike a Corvette or a
Porsche, the heart is built for comfort, not speed. And when
your heart puts the pedal to the metal, you can be in for a
harrowing ride.

Taken when at rest, a normal adult's pulse can be anywhere from 60 to 100 beats per minute. Anything over 100
is technically defined as a tachycardia. There are many
instances during which it is perfectly natural for the heart
to be racing out of this "normal" range, according to
Joseph P. Ornato, M.D., professor of internal medicine and
cardiology at the Medical College of Virginia Hospital of
Virginia Commonwealth University in Richmond.

"The heart will always beat faster when it has more
work to do and needs to pump more blood and oxygen to
the body," he says. "Exercise, emotion, nervousness, a large
meal are all common triggers. If you are overweight or out
of shape, the heart will need to work harder. And sometimes, a regular pulse slightly above the norm just may be
normal for certain individuals, depending on his or her specific body chemistry."

Illnesses or physiological changes in the body also put additional work demands on the heart. These include fever, high or low blood pressure, asthma, anemia, increases in thyroid hormone production and excess adrenaline. And frequently the heart will pound like a jackhammer in response to external stimulants like nicotine, caffeine, prescription and over-the-counter medications and illegal drugs. Severe lack of certain nutrients—notably potassium and the B vitamins—can also send your heart racing. In fact, fad weight-loss diets can get your mineral balance so out of whack that rapid pulse can become a problem.

Rapid pulses are commonly seen in people who have survived a heart attack or who suffer from congestive heart failure. "When the heart is damaged, one of the ways it has to increase its output is to increase its rate," says James Willerson, M.D., professor of cardiology and chairman of internal medicine at the University of Texas Medical School at Houston.

Sometimes a damaged or even a healthy heart can develop defects in its internal electrical system, causing it to send out rapid-fire signals. A frequently seen by-product of these electrical storms is paroxysmal supra-ventricular tachycardia (PSVT)—a sudden but brief acceleration of the heart at up to 200 beats per minute. Doctors view this type of electrical discharge as mostly bark and no bite. It's easily treatable and non-life-threatening.

Other times, the heart fires at super-high velocities, but in crazy, erratic rhythms. This is called atrial fibrillation. Former president George Bush suffered a much-publicized attack of this generally benign and easily treatable pulse rate acceleration while jogging in 1991.

Physicians are most concerned when these rapid rhythm disturbances occur in the lower chambers of the heart (the ventricles). They can fibrillate at rates of several hundred beats per minute, hindering or halting all heart activity. Ventricular rhythm disturbances can lead to sudden cardiac death.

Symptom Relief

It's always a good idea to have any tachycardia checked out by a doctor just to confirm that there is no serious heart problem. When your heart starts taching up, here's how you and your doctor can slam on the brakes.

Just say no. Avoid all the stimulating substances that can send your heart racing to beat the band: foods and beverages containing caffeine (coffee, teas, sodas), alcohol and illegal drugs, says Dr. Ornato. Smoking constricts arteries, making your heart work harder, and nicotine is a powerful stimulant. If you are taking medication, check the label for proper dosages, or ask your doctor if a change is needed.

Give some extra effort. You can stop some episodes of PSVT dead in their tracks by using one of several techniques called vagal maneuvers. If you're prone to tachycardia, review these maneuvers with your doctor to see if they are appropriate for you to try. They work by stimulating the heart's vagal nerves to induce a slower rate. They include:

- Pinching your nose and blowing.
- Coughing and gagging.
- Plunging your face in a bowl of ice water for several seconds.
- Squatting low, tensing up and straining your body as if you're trying to lay an egg.
- Contracting your abdominal muscles and "straining" like you are trying to move your bowels.

Work out and slim down. Losing weight reduces the heart's overall workload. And aerobic exercise improves your cardiovascular fitness by conditioning the heart, lungs and muscles to use oxygen more effectively, says Dr. Willerson. Exercise is also a great anxiety cure.

Avoid fad diets. High-protein powders and quick weight-loss products often have a disturbing side effect, says Mark E. Josephson, M.D., professor of medicine at Harvard Medical School and director of Harvard-Thorndike Electrophysiology Institute and Arrhythmia Services at Beth

Israel Hospital in Boston. They make your heart rate zoom, sometimes dangerously. Go on a doctor-supervised program instead.

Ask about slo-mo medications. Cardiologists treat recurring and persistent tachycardias with a variety of heart-slowing drugs, says Jeremy Ruskin, M.D., director of the Cardiac Arrythmia Service at Massachusetts General Hospital in Boston. These include beta blockers, calcium blockers, quinidine, disopyramide and lidocaine.

See also Heartbeat Irregularities

PUPIL DILATION

WHEN TO SEE YOUR DOCTOR

- One pupil is larger than the other.
- Both pupils remain dilated for more than 24 hours.

WHAT YOUR SYMPTOM IS TELLING YOU

If you've ever had a routine eye exam, you're familiar with the eyedrops that cause your pupils to open as wide as a cat's on a night stalk. The extra dilation allows the doctor to get a good look at the lens and retina inside your eyeball.

Your pupils can also widen from adrenaline medications such as epinephrine and from commercial eyedrops designed to "get the red out," according to Rick Walters, O.D., optometrist at Allentown Eye Associates in Pennsylvania. Many illegal drugs—such as marijuana—can also dilate pupils.

"In general, if both eyes are dilated, it's usually a drug-related rather than a disease-related problem," says Jason Slakter, M.D., attending surgeon in the Department of Ophthalmology at the Manhattan Eye, Ear and Throat

Hospital. The pupils will contract as the drug leaves the body, usually within a day.

If only one pupil is dilated, however, you may have Adie's syndrome, a condition in which one pupil contracts more slowly than the other in response to light. It's usually caused either by a malfunction in the mechanism that controls the dilation reflex or from a harmless inflammation of the eye nerves.

More seriously, a single dilated pupil could indicate a brain injury, stroke or tumor.

SYMPTOM RELIEF

If just one pupil is larger than the other, see the doctor immediately, says Dr. Slakter. "This is a case where a matter of an hour or two could save your life," he says.

Review your medications. If both pupils remain dilated more than a day, your physician should be able to pinpoint the medication that may be causing the problem. Be sure to let him know about any over-the-counter medicines or eye-care products that you are using.

PUS

WHEN TO SEE YOUR DOCTOR

- A sore does not stop weeping after two to three days or gets worse.
  Pus appears in deep pockets under the skin or in pustules covering a wide area of skin.
- The affected area is also red, painful, swollen, hot or discolored.
- You experience pus coming from your gums, eyes or genitals.
  See your doctor immediately if you also experience fever, chills or sweating.

WHAT YOUR SYMPTOM IS TELLING YOU

What's white, slimy, oozing and guaranteed to make the strongest stomach queasy? No, it's not your Aunt Martha's homemade mayonnaise. And it's not a Las Vegas lounge singer.

It's pus: that gross-you-out, I-think-I'm-gonna-gag substance that's made us all say *"blecchh!"* ever since our first skinned knee. What exactly *is* this awful ooze? Well, if you think it looks like death warmed over, you're exactly right.

"You're looking at a bunch of dead soldiers—casualties of a battle against infection," says Guy F. Webster, M.D., Ph.D., assistant professor of dermatology and director of the Center for Cutaneous Pharmacology at Thomas Jefferson University in Philadelphia. "When skin or other tissue is infected, the body rushes in millions of white blood cells and other products of the immune system to fight off the infection. Pus is the by-product of this confrontation—fallen white cells, rotting tissue and other debris."

This dead material is not only unsavory, it's unwelcome. "The body is trying to expel pus because it interferes with the healing process," says John M. Rabkin, M.D., assistant professor of surgery at Oregon Health Sciences University in Portland. "Not only is it an obstacle for the body repairing tissues, it's a breeding ground for any surviving bacteria that produced the infection in the first place."

Our skin normally does fine keeping infectious, pus-producing bacteria at bay. But sometimes these stubborn invaders penetrate the skin's defenses. They can sneak in through a wound or come in the form of skin disease, such as a cyst or acne. And in rarer circumstances, bacteria from an internal infection can produce pus just under the skin.

When infection sets in, pus can take two forms. One is a pustule—a self-contained, thin-walled package of visible pus popping through the outer skin. Acne is a good example, but there are a host of other infectious conditions that produce these little white volcanoes, including folliculitis (infected hair follicles) and carbuncles (infected boils).

Other times, pus forms well under the skin. Doctors call this an abscess—a deep pocket or cavity in infected tissue.

where pus collects and festers. If the abscess isn't too deep, the pus makes it's way to the surface and clears up. But if it's really deep, the abscess can grow.

"If an abscess continues to grow, it will hurt tremendously and can cause the irreversible destruction of skin or other tissue," says Kevin Ferentz, M.D., assistant professor of family medicine at the University of Maryland School of Medicine in Baltimore. For example, the pus-filled pockets formed from periodontitis—an advanced form of gum disease—can lead to the loss of teeth and bone tissue. And in extreme cases, the abscesses in an ulcerating leg wound can produce gangrene and lead to a loss of the limb.

SYMPTOM RELIEF

Pus is telling us that our white blood cells are trying to clean up the infection," says James Brand, M.D., assistant professor of family medicine at the University of Oklahoma Health Sciences Center in Oklahoma City. "The bad news is that it could mean these cells are having a long, hard fight."

Fortunately, we can give our natural infection fighters a helping hand. Multiple pustular outbreaks and deep abscesses call for a doctor's care, but here's how you can deal with minor cases.

Gently wash with a mild soap and water. The most effective thing one can do for an infection with pus is keep it clean, says Dr. Brand. No need for fancy soaps or hard scrubbings. One or two washings a day with soap and warm water are plenty to clean out bacteria and wash away accumulated pus.

Wrap it up. A bandage will absorb much of the pus from the infected area, protect it from dirt and additional injury and hold in moisture, which is vital in the healing process, according to Dr. Rabkin. There are many specialized bandages available, but a traditional adhesive bandage or gauze pad with tape works just as well. Bandages should also be changed at least three times a day.

Apply a topical antibiotic. Before bandaging, you

may want to rub on an antibiotic ointment such as
Neosporin or Polysporin or one containing the ingredient bacitracin. According to Dr. Webster, they won't
do a lot to fight the germs already inside a wound, but
they do help seal in moisture and keep additional germs
out. More stubborn infections may call for oral prescription drugs.

Apply warm, moist compresses. Wrapping a pustule or
abscess with a warm, moist cloth for 15 minutes several
times a day will gently draw pus to the surface and soften
the skin so it can naturally rupture and drain without
aggravating the infection or causing pain, says Dr. Webster.

Soak away scabs. If a scab is oozing pus, it could mean
an abscess is forming. The scab has got to go . . . but don't
rip it off. Soak it frequently in warm water and bandage it
to keep it moist. Eventually it will come off on its own.
When it does, keep the sore clean and bandaged. The pus
will drain easier and the wound will heal faster.

Have a doc get the gunk out. Deep abscesses need to be
drained, flaps of dead skin cut away and deep debris
removed.

Brush, floss and rinse with salt water. If you have gum
disease, you will have to see a dentist or periodontist for
treatment. In the meantime, brushing with a fluoride toothpaste and flossing between teeth will remove many of the
plaque bacteria causing the infection. And rinsing with salt
water can draw much of the contents out of the abscess to
prevent further damage. (For more tips on dealing with
gum disease, see Gum Problems on page 261.)

R

RASHES

- A rash develops when you take any medication.
- You also feel ill or have a fever.
- Your rash burns, stings, turns raw or becomes blistered.
- You suddenly get a bad headache, feel lethargic or have small black or purplish dots on most of your skin.
- You develop a red "bull's-eye" rash anytime after being bitten by a tick, even months later.
- More than one person in your household gets the same type of rash.
- You develop a roughly butterfly-shaped, patchy, red rash on your cheeks or over the bridge of your nose.

WHAT YOUR SYMPTOM IS TELLING YOU

It looks like a dash of red pepper on your back, a connect-the-dots picture in purple on your arm, or the constellation Orion on your forehead. It's bumpy or smooth, wet or dry, warm or cool. It itches, stings, burns or feels normal. It comes and goes or stays awhile. It's a rash.

Rashes take many different forms, but they're generally eruptions, or break-outs, on the skin, says Stuart M. Brown, M.D., clinical professor of dermatology at the University of Texas Southwestern Medical School in Dallas. The main message sent out by a rash is that your body is simply not "happy" about something. And your body can be unhappy about almost anything that is happening to it or is placed on, in or near it—from nuts that cause allergy to lethal infectious diseases.

Allergy Alert

Rashes are one of the most common symptoms of allergies, says Glenn Kline, M.D., an allergist and assistant clinical professor of pediatrics at the University of Texas at Houston. Allergies can be systemic (coursing through the body but peeking out through the skin as a rash) or localized (causing dots in specific spots). They're often caused by something you ate—eggs, milk, soybeans, fish, peanuts and wheat are the most common culprits. They can also be triggered by something you touched—the classic example being poison ivy.

There are some thoroughly modern allergic rashes out there, too: Chemicals in clothing, sunscreens, preservatives and fragrances in many cosmetics are a few common offenders, says Ivor Caro, M.D., a dermatologist and associate professor of medicine at the University of Washington School of Medicine in Seattle. You'd think a rash would pop up where an offending material touches you, but, no—nail polish and hairspray, for example, often cause rashes on the eyelids.

"One of the more interesting things right now is allergy to latex," says Dr. Kline. As more and more people don latex gloves for disease prevention, more and more skin is raising rashy ruckuses. This kind of allergy can be dangerous, says Dr. Kline, because some emergency first-aid equipment—as well as surgeon's gloves—contain latex. The last thing you want is a rash on your gallbladder or an open wound! If you're allergic to latex, or other materials, your doctor can provide a medical alert bracelet for you to wear at all times.

Rashes can also arise in reaction to antibiotics or other medications.

Infections Raise Rashes

A wide assortment of infectious diseases can announce their presence in your body with a telltale rash. These diseases include bacterial infections, such as impetigo; viral infections, such as chickenpox; and fungal and yeast infections, such as athlete's foot and some types of seborrhea. Rashes can also accompany dry skin, eczema or other skin conditions.

Parasites can also cause rashes. Scabies, for example, is caused by a mite that burrows into soft skin between the fingers, on the wrist and sometimes on the genitals or elsewhere. It causes an intensely itchy rash wherever they tunnel. (The itch may develop before the rash.) Scabies is very contagious and should be seen by a dermatologist, who can often find the microscopic mites in a skin scraping, says Dr. Caro.

SYMPTOM RELIEF

Rashes are so difficult to decipher that they're out of the realm of most self-diagnosis and over-the-counter treatment, says Leonard Swinyer, M.D., clinical professor of dermatology at the University of Utah in Salt Lake City.

Be prepared to take any stubborn unidentified rash to a dermatologist, where you will have to do a lot of talking. In order to pinpoint the reason for the rash, the doctor will ask you about the foods you eat, medications you take, your pets, home, workplace, clothing and your family's medical history, Dr. Caro explains.

If the cause of your rash is not obvious after that, the doctor may begin skin tests to see if a rash can be raised "on demand" by placing tiny amounts of various substances placed on the skin, says Dr. Kline. But until you get to the doctor, here are a few things you can try.

Call on cortisone. The first thing to try on an itchy rash is 1 percent hydrocortisone cream, such as Cortaid, says Lon Christianson, M.D., a psoriasis expert with the Dermatology Clinic Limited in Fargo, North Dakota, and spokesperson for the American Academy of Dermatology. Rub it on a mildly itchy or inflamed rash twice a day. If the rash does not show signs of healing after five or six days, see your doctor. Use cortisone only if the rash is *not* infected, says Dr. Christianson. An infected rash may be more inflamed and possibly swollen or producing pus.

Look around you. If someone else nearby is scratching away and so are you, you could have a scabies invasion. If so, a dermatologist can prescribe a medication to smite the mites.

Don't let your laundry do you. If you often get rashes, it's a good idea to cut the number of chemicals you use in your laundry. Stick with one soap or detergent and forget all those softeners and perfumes. Or baby yourself by using laundry soaps like Ivory Snow and Cheer-Free that are recommended for washing diapers and infant wear. It might also help to run your clothes through the rinse cycle twice.

Fight fungus. Fungal rashes, such as athlete's foot, jock itch and yeast infections, may be treated with an over-the-counter antifungal cream, such as Lotrimin. These conditions should be diagnosed by a doctor first, says Dr. Brown, so you know exactly what it is you're treating.

Drive away ivy. If you touch poison ivy or poison oak, very quickly wash the area and you may save yourself from a week or more of nasty rash. If you miss your chance and get an itchy, blistery rash anyway, take an oral antihistamine, like Benadryl, Dr. Kline advises. And stay away from hot water, which will make the itch worse. And *never* eat poison ivy leaves, Dr. Kline warns. This old folk "remedy," could prove fatal to sensitive individuals.

REGURGITATION

WHEN TO SEE YOUR DOCTOR

- Home remedies do not provide relief.

WHAT YOUR SYMPTOM IS TELLING YOU

Like heartburn, regurgitation is caused by acid leaking from your stomach into your esophagus—the narrow tube that connects your mouth with your stomach. Once even a little food and acid escape, it's a short, easy trip back to your throat.

People who suffer from regurgitation have an intermittent relaxation of the lower esophageal sphincter, the valve that closes off the doorway between the stomach and the esophagus. This valve opens to let food in and is supposed to stay closed while the food is digesting. But when it opens, the stomach contents can come up into the esophagus and/or mouth. Sometimes the sour-tasting mixture hitches a ride on a burp or a belch. Other times, just getting jostled, squeezed, poked or eating too much is enough to do the trick.

"This happens in everyone, but is more frequent in some—frequent enough to produce inflammation, which then leads to heartburn," says John Boyle, M.D., a gastroenterologist and chief of pediatric gastroenterology at Rainbow Babies and Childrens Hospital in Cleveland.

A condition known as Zenker's diverticulum can also sour you on your last meal, says Bruce Luxson, M.D., Ph.D., assistant professor of gastroenterology at Saint Louis University School of Medicine in Missouri. If you have Zenker's diverticulum, instead of making its way to the stomach, some of your food gets stuck in a pouch in your esophagus. If you lie down within a few hours of eating, the pouch can empty, filling the back of your mouth with food, he says. "The food never got to the stomach. It was stuck in this pouch," he explains.

SYMPTOM RELIEF

Here are a couple of ways to get rid of that sour taste at the back of your throat.

Don't lie down after a meal. A nice long nap seems tempting after a delicious meal, but you risk regurgitation if you take the snooze flat on your back. If you must catch a few Zs, choose a comfortable chair that allows you to sit partially upright. Or, better yet, stay active by going for a walk instead. That way, stomach acid will be far less likely to creep back into your esophagus, says Dr. Luxson. Because regurgitation is caused by the same things as heartburn, the same remedies work for both.

See your doctor. If none of the heartburn remedies work

for you and regurgitation continues to be a problem, your doctor should take a look at your esophagus. If you have Zenker's diverticulum, it can be corrected with surgery, says Dr. Luxson.

See also Heartburn

RESTLESS LEGS

WHEN TO SEE YOUR DOCTOR

- You frequently have leg discomfort that seriously interferes with your sleep.
- Your legs are also tingly or numb or jerk suddenly and often, with annoying crawling sensations under the skin.

WHAT YOUR SYMPTOM IS TELLING YOU

Shortly after hitting the pillow, your brain wants to drift off to Dreamland, but your legs have an irresistible urge to kick off the covers and pace the floor. It's the only way to relieve the crawling sensation deep inside them.

The night is full of floor pacers, people who are attempting to walk off the tickling-prickling-burning discomfort of restless leg syndrome. About 10 percent of the population has this condition—also called Ekbom's syndrome—which strikes at bedtime or within a half-hour of resting. Sometimes the arms and thighs get that creepy-crawly feeling, too. Both men and women get the syndrome, but pregnant women are the most likely candidates. (Their problem usually disappears soon after delivery.)

No one knows for sure what causes the uncomfortable sensations. "It's probably an abnormality in brain chemistry that may affect the nerve signals to the limbs," says Richard Allen, Ph.D., co-director of the Johns Hopkins

Sleep Disorders Center in Baltimore. The syndrome tends to run in families, he adds. It's possible that caffeine may be giving your legs the jitters. Some scientists believe that in certain people caffeine can shift the brain chemical balance, which overly excites the nerve signals to the leg muscles.

Restless legs have also been linked to an overexposure to cold, iron-deficiency anemia, nicotine, stress, fatigue and anxiety. If it's accompanied by other symptoms—tingling, numbness or cramping, for example—it could be a sign of diabetes, rheumatoid arthritis or a thyroid disorder.

In most cases, though, having restless legs is more of a nuisance than a serious health problem. The symptoms often come and go and often disappear on their own.

SYMPTOM RELIEF

In addition to floor pacing, here are other ways to settle your twitchy legs.

Slip into a warm foot bath. Warming your feet and calves will boost blood flow and also help ease a buildup of lactic acid in the muscle that can add to your misery, according to Kim Edward LeBlanc, M.D., clinical assistant professor of family medicine at the Louisiana State University School of Medicine in New Orleans. Taking a heating pad to bed is okay, he says, as long as it has a timer that automatically shuts off the heat after fifteen minutes. (Heating pads should not be used by people with diabetes, who may have nerve damage and not notice burns.)

Give those calves a rubdown. Slowly stroking your calves from ankle to knee may also stimulate blood flow and help ease jumpiness, says Dr. LeBlanc.

Massage with liniments. "It is possible that using menthol-containing topical rubs such as Ben-Gay during a massage may help suppress abnormal nerve activity," says Wayne Henning, M.D., clinical investigator of Lyons Veterans Administration Medical Center in New Jersey. At the very least, he says, the warm sensation of these rubs can distract you from the crawling sensation, allowing you to sleep.

Quell it with quinine. Taking two tablets nightly of Q-vel—an over-the-counter tablet that contains quinine and also vitamin E—seems to help settle restless legs and also any accompanying leg cramping you may have, says Dr. LeBlanc. Check with your doctor first. (For more hints and tips to alleviate muscle cramps, see page 422.)

Take aspirin. "It's unclear why it works, but taking two aspirin or Tylenol tablets at bedtime may help people with restless legs sleep better," says Thomas Meyer, M.D., associate professor of medicine at the University of Colorado in Denver.

Stay up for the late show. "People who are able to go to bed later and sleep in later don't seem to be as bothered by restless legs for some reason," says Dr. Allen. But guard against getting overly tired, he adds. Your legs may be jumpy all night.

Skip the java at supper. You'll sleep better without these stimulants, says Dr. Henning. Trying to cut down on caffeinated beverages during the day may also be worth a try, he adds.

Pass up the after-dinner brandy and cigars. Nicotine and alcohol are substances that can interfere with deep, restful sleep, says Paul Davidson, M.D., associate clinical professor of medicine at the University of California School of Medicine in San Francisco and author of *Chronic Muscle Pain Syndrome*.

Take a multivitamin/mineral supplement. A deficiency in the nutrients zinc and folate have been linked to restless legs, although the exact connection is unclear. "If restless legs runs in your family, make sure your diet includes lean meat, poultry and fish, and for extra measure take a supplement containing these nutrients," says Tucson physician Jesse Staff, M.D.

Join the daytime exercisers. A half-hour of brisk walking may help dissipate stress and calm the entire nervous system from head to toe, says Dr. Davidson.

Get a prescription medication. If these measures fail to calm your restless legs, your doctor may prescribe medications, says Dr. Henning. Possible choices include sedatives, narcotics and dopaminergic drugs. "Each has its drawbacks and should be discussed with your doctor," he says.

S

SCALP ITCHING

WHAT YOUR SYMPTOM IS TELLING YOU

There you are, scratching your head like a bluetick hound, wondering why your scalp is so doggone itchy. Muse no more, McGruff.

You may have developed a skin condition like psoriasis or seborrheic dermatitis, accompanied by a yeast that forces your skin to grow more rapidly than normal. The overabundance of skin, in turn, encourages an overgrowth of the organisms that trigger—you guessed it—itching, says Robert Rietschel, M.D., chairman of the Department of Dermatology at the Ochsner Clinic in New Orleans.

Other common head itchers: improper hair care and (yuck) head lice.

SYMPTOM RELIEF

Rather than rub yourself raw, try these treatments for itchy scalp.

Banish the bar. Never use a cake of soap to shampoo your hair, says Ron Renee, president of the Aestheticians International Association in Dallas. Not only is it harsh on hair, but it also strips the scalp of essential oils, which can lead to itching, he says.

Do the right shampoo. "You really need a pH-balanced shampoo to keep your scalp from flaking and drying, a common cause of itchy scalp," says Renee. Look for one that has a pH level between 4.5 and 5.5, he says. You can check the pH level of your favorite shampoo by using nitrozine paper test strips, which you can buy from pharmacies, he says.

Have an antihistamine. Some antihistamines used for allergies contain anti-itching ingredients that may provide temporary relief from itchy scalp, says Robert Richards, M.D., a spokesperson for the American Academy of Dermatologists with a practice in Toronto. Among the best are Benadryl and Chlor-Trimeton. Because each contains a sedative, both may be helpful with an itch that's keeping you up, he says.

Sleep on it. "If you're looking for an over-the-counter treatment for scalp scaling, there's an excellent product called Baker's P and S Liquid," says Dr. Rietschel. Apply it to the scalp at bedtime and put on a shower cap. The next morning, clean your hair with a dandruff shampoo.

Spread on some olive oil. "Olive oil does seem to have a soothing effect on some cases of dry, itchy scalp," says Dr. Rietschel. Just massage warm olive oil into your scalp and wait ten minutes before you shampoo.

Make a date with your dermatologist. "You're going to need a higher level of care if you don't begin to get substantial relief within about a week," says Dr. Rietschel.

Stopping Psoriasis

Don't get sore at psoriasis, get even—with these remedies.

Give psoriasis a scrub. Coal-tar based shampoos, while messy, seem to work best at removing the dead skin and reducing inflammation that accompanies psoriasis on the scalp, says Dr. Rietschel. "If you deal with the inflammation, then you are dealing with the itching," he says. You should see results within one to two weeks; if not, see your doctor.

Cut the itch with cortisone. If eczema- or psoriasis-induced itching continues after shampooing, reach for 1 percent hydrocortisone cream, an item available in most drugstores, says Dr. Rietschel.

Hairdos and Don'ts

It's also entirely possible that while you were trying to develop the latest hairdo, you may have committed a hair don't: You exposed your scalp to several chemicals that triggered an allergic reaction, causing inflammation and itching. Or you may simply be using the wrong kind of products to clean your hair. Consider these tips when caring for your hair.

Test your hair-care treatment. Home hair dyes often contain para-phenylenediamine, a chemical that's been linked to severe scalp itching and blistering. "Once you've had the contact, that's enough for the immunological process to run its one- to two-week course," says Dr. Rietschel. To avoid an allergic reaction, test the dye on the box as directed before using, he says.

Drop your acid perm. If you've ever experienced severe itching 48 hours or less after getting a salon perm, avoid glyceryl thioglycolate, a perm activator and common irritant. Because the chemical stays in hair even after frequent shampooing, some eczema sufferers have been forced to shave their heads to get relief. "It's really difficult to deal with," says Dr. Rietschel. "Avoid it if you can."

Liquidate Those Lice

It's not a pleasant prospect, itchy scalp *could* also be a sign that you're one of ten million Americans (mostly schoolchildren, their parents and teachers) plagued with head lice. These mustard-seed-size insects stab tiny holes in the scalp, live off blood and never, ever, dine without producing several hundred offspring.

If you suspect your child may have brought home a crop of head lice from school, you'll have to take action before the whole family starts itching, says Dr. Richards. To nix those nits:

Buy a power shampoo. A variety of prescription and over-the-counter shampoos are great at killing head lice, according to Dr. Richards. They include: Kwell, which features the ingredient gamma benzene hexachloride, and Nix, which contains permethrin. Once the lice have been killed, however, you'll need to remove their eggs by carefully combing the hair with a nit comb, says Dr. Richards. You may have to repeat the treatment several times. Any survivors won't waste time starting a new family of hungry lice.

SEEING LIGHTS

WHEN TO SEE YOUR DOCTOR

- You see "flashes of light" after you've been hit on the head or hit in the eye and they don't go away within a few seconds.
- You see flashes of light off and on for more than 20 minutes and you also feel faint.
- You have a condition or disease that predisposes you to eye problems, for example, previous eye injury, diabetes or high blood pressure.
- You also see a large number of previously unnoticed spots in your field of vision.

WHAT YOUR SYMPTOM IS TELLING YOU

If you've ever been stunned by a smack on the head, you probably know what it's like to see stars or flashing lights.

But what if you're seeing lights that shouldn't be there and you haven't been anywhere near a fist or an errant object? It most likely means that the gel-like substance in your eye called vitreous fluid is literally rubbing your eye the wrong way.

Vitreous fluid is what gives the eyeball its shape. If the gel rubs or pulls on the retina—the thin, light-sensitive membrane in the back of your eyeball that allows you to see—it can distort the image you're focusing on, creating the illusion that you're seeing flashing lights or lightning streaks in front of your eyes for a brief period.

One of the most obvious and serious causes is a tear in the retina, which can happen for many reasons, from a smack on the eye to perhaps a vigorous sneeze. The other really serious possibility is a retinal artery occlusion—a tiny clot in the central retinal artery. Flashing light symptoms should be checked by an ophthalmologist to rule out these serious possibilities.

People who suffer from migraine headaches commonly see flashes of light. In fact, it's often *the* symptom that a migraine attack is coming on.

But flashes of light can be a symptom that just about everybody will experience at some time in their life. Seeing flashes of light can be one of the many annoyances that go along with an aging body, says George L. White, Jr., Ph.D., ophthalmic researcher with the Center for Community Health at the University of Southern Mississippi in Hattiesburg. These symptoms might occur at any time but are usually experienced after the age of 40. You should get concerned if flashes of light begin to get more frequent or worsen in intensity or if they are associated with other symptoms such as vision loss, headache or dizziness, says Dr. White.

SYMPTOM RELIEF

Here's what doctors say you should—or shouldn't—do for those flashing lights.

Use your common sense. If you've been hit on the head or eye and see stars that won't go away, you should see your doctor immediately. You could have a tear to the retina that needs immediate medical attention. Retinas can be repaired with a laser or eryosurgery (cold surgery), often on an outpatient basis, says Dr. White.

Treat the headache. If you suffer from migraines, you probably already know that flashes of light are the symptoms signaling the head pain soon to come. What you may not know, though, is that this symptom can also help you head off the headache. Doctors call these flashes of light the migraine aura. The aura lasts for about 20 minutes and is not painful. What works to stop a headache varies among individuals, but some people report success with relaxation techniques and medications. (For other ways to ward off a migraine, see Headaches on page 280.)

Sit back and enjoy the show. If your doctor tells you that your light show is nothing more than a symptom of aging, there is not really anything you can do about it, says Dr. White. Nor should you be concerned about it.

SEEING SPOTS

WHEN TO SEE YOUR DOCTOR

- You suddenly see a shower of spots, flashing lights or a stationary spot accompanied by blurred vision or shadowed side vision.
- You see spots after receiving a blow to the head or eye.

WHAT YOUR SYMPTOM IS TELLING YOU

Has your line of vision been invaded by what looks like tiny black gnats swarming around you? And are you the only one who sees them? If you're getting up in years, these black specks are usually nothing to worry about. They are nothing more than harmless bits of your eyeball's inner fluid floating into view. Your doctor calls them floaters.

Floaters are common after age 50, according to Jason Slakter, M.D., attending surgeon in the Department of Ophthalmology at the Manhattan Eye, Ear and Throat Hospital.

As you age, the transparent gel-like substance inside the eyeball shrinks and separates into a clear fluid and a stringy residue. The opaque strings may float behind the lens and cast a shadow on the retina—the back of the eyeball where the image is received. This causes the sensation of dark spots, circles or squiggly lines. Near- sighted people are particularly prone to floaters, says Dr. Slakter.

More often than not, says Dr. Slakter, the spots eventually disappear on their own or your brain suppresses the image. You may not even notice them unless you're fatigued.

Even so, floaters that persist could mean you have an inflammation or infection within your eye or elsewhere in your body that is causing the problem. What's more, if you frequently experience floaters, your retina could be torn, which could threaten your sight. You should always bring persistent floaters to the attention of your doctor.

Symptom Relief

No matter what kind of spots you're seeing, there are techniques to clear them from view.

Exercise your eyeball. Floaters will vanish if you rapidly move your eyes up and down. This stirs up the eyeballs' fluid, causing the floaters to settle outside your line of vision. "It's like shaking a snow globe paperweight that stirs and then settles its fluffy contents," says Mitchell H. Friedlaender, M.D., director of corneal services in the Division of Ophthalmology at Scripps Clinic and Research Foundation in La Jolla, California, and coauthor of *20/20: A Total Guide to Improving Your Vision and Preventing Eye Disease*.

Seal the tears. If tears in the retina are causing spots— this is a diagnosis that must be made by a physician—your doctor can seal the rip with a laser light or by freezing. The procedures can be done in the doctor's office with a local anesthetic and can help prevent the retina from becoming detached.

SEIZURES

WHEN TO SEE YOUR DOCTOR

- People tell you that you lost consciousness.
- You feel disoriented and confused.
- You've lost control of your bladder or bowel.
- People tell you that you had a convulsion.
- People tell you that you engaged in bizarre behavior for several minutes.

WHAT YOUR SYMPTOM IS TELLING YOU

You might expect a person having a seizure to lose consciousness, fall to the ground, froth at the mouth and jerk his arms and legs in an uncontrolled convulsion. But not all seizures take this form.

"There are many types of seizures, some as small as blanking out for a few seconds and others as big as having a convulsion for several minutes," says Paul Gross, M.D., a neurologist at the Lahey Clinic in Burlington, Massachusetts.

A seizure is a sign that nerve cells in your brain are discharging an excessive amount of electrical impulses. That abundance of impulses momentarily disrupts normal brain activity. The effect is much like a power surge racing through your home. In your house, that electrical surge trips a circuit breaker and the lights go out. When an electrical surge happens in your brain, you may lose consciousness, lose control of your muscles or engage in odd behavior.

A seizure can be caused by infections such as meningitis or encephalitis, parasites such as tapeworm, high fever, drug and alcohol abuse, head injury, Alzheimer's disease, epilepsy, stroke or a tumor. But often there is no known cause, doctors say.

SYMPTOM RELIEF

About 60 to 80 percent of seizures are treatable with existing anti-epileptic drugs and aren't disabling," says John Marler, M.D., a neurologist at the National Institutes of Neurological Disorders and Stroke in Bethesda, Maryland. But sometimes a seizure can be a sign of serious problems in your brain and should always be discussed with your doctor as soon as possible.

Because there are few warning signs, doctors can do little to prevent a first seizure, but after the initial seizure occurs there are ways you and your doctor can prevent others from happening. Here are a few of the best methods.

Get plenty of Zs. Lack of sleep can bring out a seizure in a person who has epilepsy, says Dr. Gross. Try to get at least six to eight hours of sleep every night.

Avoid alcohol. Alcohol has a chemical effect on the brain that can trigger seizures. "The safest thing to do is not drink. But if you do drink, don't drink to excess," says Robert Slater, M.D., an assistant professor of clinical neurology at the University of Pennsylvania School of Medicine in Philadelphia. "I tell most of my patients they probably can have one or two drinks at a party without too many problems. Any more than that, you are very likely to have trouble."

Take your medication. "In this day and age, we have excellent anti-epileptic medications such as phenytoin, which if taken consistently, will prevent seizures in most cases," says C. Conrad Carter, M.D., clinical professor of neurology at the Oregon Health Sciences University in Portland. But don't stop taking the medication without consulting your physician, because even if you've been on the medication for several months, the seizures can recur if you abruptly stop taking the drug.

Leave the driving to others. Once you've had a seizure—even one—you should not drive a car until you get your doctor's okay. Laws vary, but in many states your doctor will be required to report your seizure to the state department of motor vehicles. No matter what the law in your state, you should take precautions to make sure that you are not creating a danger for yourself or others.

Don't go near the water. Swimming alone can be dangerous if you've had a seizure, because you are more likely to drown if it recurs. "I've known people who have drowned in their own bathtubs during a seizure," says Paul B. Pritchard III, M.D., chief of staff and clinical professor of neurology at the Medical University of South Carolina College of Medicine in Charleston. Always swim with a partner and make sure someone is nearby to assist you, if necessary, when you bathe.

Coming to the Rescue

Although most seizures last less than three minutes, that can seem like an eternity if you're watching a person going through a convulsion. Here's a few ways you can help the person through those crucial moments.

First, do no harm. The person having a seizure will usually fall to the ground. If you have time, try to cushion that fall. After the person is down, clear the area of solid objects such as chairs and tables. Put a towel, jacket or even your cupped hands under the head to prevent injury. Extend the head backward so that the neck is extended. This will help the person breathe.

Leave the tongue alone. It's not a good idea to try to place a stick or other object in the mouth of the person having the convulsion. Many people have the false notion that you'll help the person breathe or prevent injury to the tongue by doing that. Wrong, Dr. Carter says. "When a person goes into convulsion, the jaw muscles go into spasm and contract, forcing the teeth together. So if you stick your finger in there, you're going to get bit, and if you stick an object in their mouth, it's likely to break their teeth. So it's better to let nature run its course," he says. "Certainly it can be pretty scary to see blood coming out of someone's mouth, but remember the tongue will heal, teeth won't."

Use the recovery position. After the seizure is over, gently roll the person over on his left side. This will allow any secretions from the mouth to flow out of the body rather than back into the lungs.

SEMEN, BLOODY

WHEN TO SEE YOUR DOCTOR

- Blood appears in your semen more than three times.
- Bloody semen is accompanied by any pain in the area between your genitals and anus, or by a frequent and urgent need to urinate.
- You are more than 50 years old.

WHAT YOUR SYMPTOM IS TELLING YOU

You probably first noticed it after making love, and it scared the bejeebers out of you. But relax. There is, doctors say, no reason for immediate alarm.

Whether it appears as wispy threads of red or dyes your entire ejaculate rusty brown, blood in the semen is almost always harmless and will probably disappear on its own.

"Blood in the semen is very common. It's usually benign," says Bruce H. Blank, M.D., clinical associate professor of urology at Oregon Health Sciences University School of Medicine in Portland. "We don't find a cause in the majority of cases, and even when we *do* find a cause, it's usually not a threatening medical problem."

In other words, bloody semen is almost never serious (or, as many people first think, a sign of cancer). A minor infection can sometimes cause blood to appear in the semen, according to Dr. Blank. Occasionally, especially in older men, it's a sign of a prostate or other urological problem. In most cases, the blood disappears within three weeks.

SYMPTOM RELIEF

Here's what your doctor might do and suggest to end bloody emissions.

Leave aspirin on the shelf. Unless they're prescribed, don't take any medications that can thin the blood or prevent clotting. "Don't take aspirin, because you'll be prone to bleed more easily," Dr. Blank says. If you don't know whether medications you're currently taking fall into this category, ask your doctor or pharmacist.

Go ahead. Enjoy. There's no need to be afraid of making love, says Dr. Blank. It can't hurt you or your partner.

Get medical help. See your doctor if you still see blood in your semen after three weeks, if you feel any pain while ejaculating or urinating or if you're over 50. Whether you have a minor infection or prostatitis, the prescription is usually the same: antibiotics, probably tetracycline or doxycycline. "Since a doctor can't always determine the cause," Dr. Blank says, "the antibiotic will at least provide reassurance that a possible infection is being treated."

Prepare for a probe. During your office visit, your doctor may want to examine your prostate and perform a cystoscopy—an examination of your bladder and urethra with a small optical device. "If the blood is persistent, we have to be sure you don't have a tumor or a polyp," says E. Douglas Whitehead, M.D., a urologist, co-director of the Association for Male Sexual Dysfunction in New York City and an associate clinical professor of urology at Mount Sinai School of Medicine of the City University of New York.

SHOULDER PAIN

WHEN TO SEE YOUR DOCTOR

- You are unable to lift your arm above your head.
- You are unable to move your shoulder.
- Your shoulder feels like it has come out of its socket.

WHAT YOUR SYMPTOM IS TELLING YOU

Your shoulder is the most complex joint in your body— it's a biomechanical wonder that makes state-of-the-art robotics look like a seventh-grade science project.

But your shoulders have at least one thing in common with ordinary machinery: They can endure only so much mistreatment before they begin to malfunction. And unfortunately for you, that breakdown usually means pain.

One of the most common forms of shoulder pain is inflammation of the tendons that surround the shoulder joint. Tendinitis, as it is called, is most often caused by overuse. When you do things like saw wood or play golf, the tendons in your shoulder rub against bone, which can lead to irritation and pain, explains Robert Bennett, M.D., professor of medicine and chairman of the Division of Arthritis and Rheumatic Diseases at Oregon Health Sciences University in Portland.

Bursitis—tendinitis's compatriot in shoulder misery—is also caused by overuse. But it drops an even broader hint upon arrival: minor swelling of the bursae, soft sacs located in the joint, says Tab Blackburn, a physical therapist who's treated members of the Atlanta Braves and Houston Astros professional baseball teams and vice president of the Human Performance and Rehabilitation Centers in Columbus, Georgia.

If you feel pain in your shoulders when you lift up your arms, calcium deposits may be to blame, says Dr. Bennett. These deposits form in a tendon underneath where the shoulder blade and collarbone join. This condition is known as impingement syndrome.

And then there's the shoulder pain caused by accidents. A fall can cause a dislocated shoulder, which literally pops the upper arm out of its mooring in the shoulder joint. Breaking the fall with an arm can tear the rotator cuff— the tendons that move the arm. Without surgery, a torn rotator cuff may create lifelong shoulder problems, says Blackburn.

SYMPTOM RELIEF

Obviously, any pain caused by a fall or accident should be treated immediately by a physician. Some dislocated shoulders can be "popped" back into place by a doctor. More severe injuries sometimes require surgery.

If your pain is from overuse, the following techniques should be helpful.

Change your ways. If your shoulder is often sore after work or doing your favorite hobby, try to think of ways to give your shoulder a breather from any repetitive motions that may be causing the problem, advises Fred Allman, Jr., M.D., orthopedic surgeon and director of the Atlanta Sports Medicine Clinic. Don't quit exercising, though. If you pitch baseballs for fun, for example, give your shoulder a rest by riding a bike for a few days.

Ice is nice. At the first sign of a sore shoulder, apply an ice pack to the painful area several times a day for no more than 20 minutes, says Blackburn. Ice numbs the area and reduces swelling and inflammation.

Turn on the heat. After three days of ice treatment, provided the pain has subsided, apply a moist heating pad to the area. Use it for 20 to 30 minutes several times a day, says Blackburn. Heat increases the flow of blood, flushing the injured area. Even blasting the area with hot water during a shower is helpful, he says.

Consider trying NSAIDs. Nonsteroidal anti-inflammatory drugs (NSAIDs) won't cure your problem, but they can provide temporary relief, says Dr. Bennett. Many varieties are sold over-the-counter at pharmacies.

See your doctor. If you can't seem to shake the pain after a few days—or you're constantly reinjuring your shoulder—it's probably time to pay your doctor a visit. Your doctor might suggest ultrasound, steroids or surgery. Combined with a local anesthetic, a single steroid injection can provide relief for as long as a year, says Dr. Bennett. "It depends on how active you are afterward. If you go back and do what was provoking it, the pain will come back in just a few weeks," he says.

Some people require an operation to shave off a little bit of bone that's pressing on the tendon, says Dr. Bennett. Others might need a rotator cuff mended. But whatever your injury, make sure you get at least two opinions before allowing anyone to operate, he says.

Stretching and Strengthening

If shoulder pain seems to be a recurring problem, it's probably a good idea to condition the muscles and tendons in that area, says Dr. Bennett. Try this set of movements, known as the Super Seven. If you don't own a set of light dumbbells, you can use soup or vegetable cans.

Prone horizontal abduction. Lie on your stomach on a sturdy table or bed with your arm hanging off the side.

Hold a one-pound weight in your hand with your palm facing away from you. Now keep your arm straight and lift the weight until it's at eye level. Repeat 8 to 12 times.

Shoulder shrugs. Stand with your arms by your sides and with one-pound weights in your hands. Lift your shoulders straight up toward your ears for a two-count, then pull the shoulders back, pinching your shoulder blades together. Relax and repeat 8 to 12 times.

Supine abduction. Lie on your back and clasp your hands over your head. (Your left palm should be on top, facing your head; your right palm is underneath.) Now with your left arm, gently pull your right arm towards your left ear. Allow your right arm to resist slightly. Hold for a count of two. Relax and repeat 8 to 12 times. Then switch arms (your right palm is on top) and repeat the exercise.

Sitting dip. Sit on the edge of a sturdy chair with your hands grasping the chair at either side of you. Now try to lift yourself off the chair. Repeat 8 to 12 times.

External rotation. Lie on your left side with your right elbow against your right side and your arm flexed to a 90-degree angle. Hold a one-pound weight in your right hand and allow it to drop down across your stomach. Now, keeping your elbow tight against your side, lift the weight as high as possible. Hold for a count of two. Relax and repeat 8 to 12 times.

Shoulder abduction. Stand with a one-pound weight in each hand. Raise your arms out to the sides of your body as high as possible while rotating the palms up. Hold for a two-count. Relax and repeat 8 to 12 times.

External rotation. Lie on your stomach on a sturdy table with your shoulder and upper arm on the table and your lower arm draped over the edge. Holding a one-pound weight in your hand, lift your hand up until it's even with the table. Relax and repeat 8 to 12 times.

See also Joint Inflammation; Joint Pain

SIDE STITCH

WHEN TO SEE YOUR DOCTOR

- You have recurring pain in your side when exercising or the pain persists after you've stopped and stretched.
- If the pain radiates in to your chest, shoulder or back, see the doctor immediately.

WHAT YOUR SYMPTOM IS TELLING YOU

You're running a 10-K or dashing to catch the bus when all at once your side feels as if it's caught in a giant lobster's claw.

Anyone who pumps their legs fast while breathing rapidly can get caught in the clenches of a side stitch. A side stitch is usually a cramp in the diaphragm—the large muscle located between your lungs and abdomen that controls breathing. It's often caused when the diaphragm isn't getting enough blood during exercise. Here's how it happens.

Pumping your legs increases the pressure on your abdominal muscles, which press up against the diaphragm. At the same time, rapid breathing expands your lungs, which press down on the diaphragm. The dual pinching from above and below shuts off the flow of blood and oxygen to the diaphragm.

Without enough oxygen, muscles will go into painful spasms, according to Mona Shangold, M.D., director of the Sports Gynecology and Women's Life Cycle Center at Hahnemann University in Philadelphia and coauthor of *The Complete Sports Medicine Book for Women.*

Those who are new to exercise are most prone to side stitches. Beginners are more apt to take rapid, shallow breaths and may also push themselves before their abdominal muscles are ready to deal with the exertion. These muscles may not be strong enough to protect against the bouncing that jostles internal organs and pulls on the diaphragm.

It's also possible that food itself may add to the diaphragm's distress. A meal of less digestible, fatty food before exercising will make the stomach heavier and increase the tugging on the diaphragm.

A side stitch can sometimes be felt all the way up to the shoulder. But this kind of pain *may* signal a heart attack, especially if it persists after you've spent a few minutes stretching. And if you get a side stitch each time you exercise, you could have a problem with blood flow to the intestine.

SYMPTOM RELIEF

Often, just slowing your pace will relieve a side stitch on the spot. If not, try these methods.

Stop and blow. If you can't lie down when the stitch strikes, at least stop and press your fingers deeply into the painful spot, says Dr. Shangold. That's normally just below the ribs, on the right side. Then, purse your lips tightly and blow out as hard as you can. This should ease the tension on your diaphragm and you'll be running stitch-free, according to Dr. Shangold.

Reach for the clouds. Walking slowly with your arms raised over your head is another fast way to stretch out the tightness, according to Kim Edward LeBlanc, M.D., clinical assistant professor of family medicine at Louisiana State University School of Medicine in New Orleans. Inhale deeply as you raise your arms up, and exhale slowly as you drop them.

Become a belly breather. To stop side stitches before they start, breathe fully and deeply by pushing your abdomen out with each inhale during your workout. To get a feeling of how this is done, says running coach Owen Anderson, Ph.D., editor of *Running Research News*, lie on your back with a book on your stomach. The book should raise up with each inhale and your shoulders should not move. Belly breathing also helps strengthen the abdominal walls. "Strong abdominal muscles provide a supportive 'internal girdle' so there is less bouncing and pulling on the diaphragm," says Dr. Anderson.

Pace yourself. "Go slow when starting a new activity," says Dr. LeBlanc. "Gradually increase the intensity and duration of your workout until your breathing and body become conditioned for the increased activity."

Postpone your post-dinner workout. If you are stitch-prone, wait one to two hours after eating before you work out, says Dr. LeBlanc.

Go easy on the fat. Fatty, high-protein foods such as red meat and dairy products tend to linger longer in your stomach, says Dr. Anderson. This can create pressure and a downward tug on your diaphragm. If you must eat and run, stick to more digestible foods such as half a ripe banana.

SINUS PROBLEMS

WHEN TO SEE YOUR DOCTOR

- Your sinus pain is not helped by three to five days on over-the-counter oral decongestants.
- You also have a fever of over 101°F and a cough.
- You have a severe headache that lasts for more than a day or two.
- You develop swollen eyelids and swelling along the side of the nose.
- You have greenish or yellowish nasal discharge.
- You are also experiencing vision problems, such as blurred or double vision.
- Your sinus pain begins after underwater diving.

WHAT YOUR SYMPTOM IS TELLING YOU

Your sinuses are a collection of hollow compartments in your head, leading from your nose up behind your eyes and cheekbones into your forehead. These compartments, which regularly produce mucus, have very small openings that readily swell shut in response to irritants like cigarette smoke, colds or allergies.

Once the tiny openings of the sinuses are obstructed, the mucus they produce can't drain out. Fluids build up in the cavities, causing pressure and pain. If you are susceptible to this kind of pain, you have plenty of company—more than 32 million Americans have sinus problems.

It's easy to see why problems develop so readily. Besides being tiny and prone to swelling shut, the openings that drain your maxillary sinuses are inconveniently located. The locations, in fact, might be thought of as a "design error," says Nelson Gantz, M.D., chairman of the Department of Medicine and chief of the Infectious Diseases Division at the Polyclinic Medical Center in Harrisburg, Pennsylvania, and clinical professor of medicine at the Pennsylvania State University College of Medicine in Hershey. The openings for the maxillary sinuses behind the cheekbones, for example, are located at the top of the sinus.

"You'd have to be standing on your head in order for them to drain properly," says Dr. Gantz.

Just how sensitive are these openings? Besides closing in response to exposure to smoke and viruses, these passages may close when allergens cause the tissue to swell or from air pressure changes, such as when an airplane descends. And infections can cause a benign nasal growth called a polyp that can make a sinus problem even worse.

SYMPTOM RELIEF

Don't worry, you won't have to stand on your head to get relief from your sinus troubles.

Steam them open. Your first defense against sinus pain is steamy moisture, says Dr. Gantz. He recommends taking a hot shower twice a day to help your sinuses drain.

You can also buy a nasal steamer, or easily concoct your own, says Alexander Chester, M.D., a clinical professor of medicine at Georgetown University School of Medicine in Washington, D.C.

"Boil a pot of water, remove it from the stove, drape a towel over your head and the pot and inhale the steam for 15 minutes three times a day," Dr. Chester suggests. Make sure your face is at least 18 inches from the pot so you don't burn yourself.

Clean up your air. If it's high-pollen season, have mercy on your sinuses by keeping windows closed and letting someone else mow the grass, says Lee Smith, M.D., secretary of the American Academy of Otolaryngic Allergy, who has a private practice in Princeton, West Virginia.

Dr. Smith also suggests staying away from smokers. And consider putting a negative-ion generator in your bedroom. "These are air cleaners that really work," he says. "If you can control your exposure to toxic and stressful substances at night, you'll be in better shape during the day," he says. (For other tips on avoiding substances that bring on allergic reactions, see "Attacking the Allergies" on page 463.)

Try healthy-sinus sleep habits. "Elevate the head of your bed about six inches to help sinuses drain," Dr. Chester suggests. You can do this by placing two six-inch wooden blocks under the legs of the headboard.

A warm-steam humidifier with a few drops of eucalyptus oil added to the water will also soothe your sinuses at night, says Dr. Chester. And make sure you don't get too much sleep. Excessive sleep—significantly more than you normally need—may worsen your sinus condition because of the prone position, he says.

Keep your nose aerobic. Aerobic exercise—usually 20 minutes once or twice a day—will have a decongesting effect on your nose and sinuses, Dr. Chester says. Brisk walking will do nicely.

Consider supplements. Dr. Chester often recommends daily vitamin supplements—3,000 milligrams of vitamin C and 30 milligrams of zinc—for people who suffer from sinus problems. "We suspect that these vitamins cause shrinking of swollen tissues in the nose," he says.

Pass on the cocoa. Concentrated sweets, particularly chocolate, may cause an allergic swelling in nasal membranes, says Dr. Chester. You may want to pass on the milk, too. "Ten percent of sinus sufferers have a milk allergy," he says. "Try avoiding milk products for two weeks to see if your sinuses improve."

Help from Your Doctor

Your doctor may determine that a sinus infection—sinusitis—is the cause of your pain.

Zap the infection. Your doctor will prescribe antibiotics and oral decongestants for a sinus infection, says Randy Oppenheimer, M.D., an otolaryngologist in Encinitas, California. "I believe the combination of the two really can break the cycle," he says.

For the first few days, your doctor may also suggest an over-the-counter decongestant nasal spray like Afrin, says Dr. Oppenheimer. "Use these sprays for only two to four days," he warns. "After that, if you have to use it to breathe, the spray won't work anymore and will cause more swelling."

Get help for chronic problems, too. When your sinuses get infected over and over again, your doctor may need to evaluate you for possible nasal polyps, says Dr. Oppenheimer.

A thin fiber-optic scope allows your doctor to examine the sinus cavity, and the polyps can be removed surgically through the nose. Your doctor may also prescribe a steroid medication for a few weeks after the surgery to prevent the regrowth of the polyps.

See also Nose, Stuffy

SKIN CHAFING

WHEN TO SEE YOUR DOCTOR

- Chafed skin lasts more than two days after the original source of irritation is removed.

WHAT YOUR SYMPTOM IS TELLING YOU

You've just discovered the *perfect* exercise—walking. It's convenient, requires no equipment and lets you start at your own level. Your enthusiasm is short-lived, however. By the second day on your new walking program, your inner thighs are so red and raw that you can barely get out of bed, let alone make it around the block.

Walking isn't the only thing that can cause this problem. *Any* activity that requires skin to repeatedly rub against skin can lead to chafing. And moisture, either from sweat or rain, makes the problem worse. Some common chafing sites are the inner thighs and under the arms or breasts, says Diana Bihova, M.D., assistant clinical professor of dermatology at New York University School of Med- icine and author of *Beauty from the Inside Out*. Areas of the body that rub against clothing—under waistbands or poorly fitting bras, for example—can also chafe.

Chafing usually comes on suddenly and announces itself with a painful stinging or burning sensation, says William Dvorine, M.D., chief of the Section of Dermatology at St. Agnes Hospital in Baltimore and author of *A Dermatologist's Guide to Home Skin Treatment*. If you don't stop whatever's rubbing you the wrong way, inflamed surface skin can actually get rubbed away and the area will begin to ooze.

Anybody can experience chafing, but it's a particular problem in overweight people and in athletes—especially if their uniforms are not kept scrupulously clean.

SYMPTOM RELIEF

Chafing is a minor problem for the most part, easily treated and easily prevented. Here's what to do.

Take time out. Once your skin is chafed, you'll need to give it a chance to heal. Take a break from the activity that caused the problem. Chafing should heal in a day or two.

Slip into something slippery. In areas of repeated chafing—such as the inner thighs or groin or under the arms or breasts—you can cut down on friction by dusting on some powder, says Dr. Dvorine. Ointments—such as Vaseline, Noxzema, zinc oxide ointment and cortisone cream—can likewise help intimately close areas of skin slip past each other. "In very hairy areas, greasy applications may clog follicles and produce more irritation," says Dr. Dvorine. "So creams and lotions are better there."

Get loose. Loose-fitting cotton clothing is best for chafe-prone skin, says Dr. Bihova. Tight-fitting athletic wear should be made of natural fibers, too, because they absorb sweat and carry it away from the skin. Some high-tech exercise clothes are made from synthetic materials that "breathe," somewhat like natural fibers, says Dr. Dvorine. The key is to choose clothes that let air penetrate through the fabric and evaporate moisture.

Stop that fungus. Chafing that hangs on for more than two days after the rubbing stops may have graduated into a fungal infection. If a doctor has previously diagnosed a fungal infection, and you can recognize it when it happens again, you can use an over-the-counter antifungal medication, such as Lotrimin. "If you're not sure, though, get a medical diagnosis, because using an antifungal medication on a nonfungal problem might cause further irritation," says Dr. Dvorine.

Sweat less. If your chafing is caused by excessive sweating, you might want to confine your workouts to cooler morning and evening hours. (For other hints and tips on staying dry, see Body Odor on page 66 and Sweating on page 603 .)

SKIN CRACKING

WHEN TO SEE YOUR DOCTOR

- A crack goes all the way through the skin on your hand or foot.
- You have diabetes and develop cracked skin on your foot.
- A cracked area feels warm or sore, is swollen or red or discharges pus or fluid.
- The skin on your lower legs starts to resemble fishlike scales or alligator skin.
- Home treatments for cracking do not help after three weeks.

WHAT YOUR SYMPTOM IS TELLING YOU

Some people have a hand in everything: gardening, decorating, car repairs, cooking, cleaning. But having a hand in moisture-robbing materials like soil, solvents and soapy water can quickly leave skin chapped and cracked.

Cracked skin can look like a dried-up riverbed, and it's caused by the same thing: lack of water. It starts when water is lost from the skin surface, leaving behind layers of dry skin cells, explains Stuart M. Brown, M.D., clinical professor of dermatology at the University of Texas Southwestern Medical School in Dallas.

"Dehydrated skin is brittle, like fingernails," explains Leonard Swinyer, M.D., clinical professor of dermatology at the University of Utah in Salt Lake City. And, like fingernails, brittle skin cannot bend easily without (ouch) cracking.

Low humidity is a prime dryer. Dry air sucks moisture out of skin, as any desert dweller can attest. But home heating in any clime creates a desertlike atmosphere inside your house that can be equally dehydrating. That's why cracked skin is a particular problem in winter.

Moisture routinely does a disappearing act in the face of irritants like detergents, perfumes, lotions, rubbing alcohol and nail polish remover, Dr. Swinyer says. It makes sense to avoid household substances that cause dry, cracked skin, but many people work with moisture thieves like paints, solvents and other chemicals everyday.

Certain conditions, such as psoriasis, eczema and some allergic reactions, can also cause skin to thicken, dry and crack. Likewise, thick, dry calluses are common fissure sites, says Lon Christianson, M.D., a psoriasis expert with the Dermatology Clinic Limited in Fargo, North Dakota, and a spokesperson for the American Academy of Dermatology.

SYMPTOM RELIEF

Hands and feet are common cracking sites. But superficial cracking can occur anywhere, especially the delicate skin of shins, forearms and cheeks, says Dr. Christianson. No matter what the location, you can send those cracks packing with the right treatment.

Soak and salve. Restore moisture to mildly cracked areas by using an over-the-counter humectant, such as Lac-Hydrin Five. Humectants pull water into skin and hold it there, says Dr. Swinyer. Remember to keep bathing short—less than five minutes per day—as prolonged exposure to water removes oils from the skin and results in more dryness. If necessary, though, a dermatologist can prescribe more potent humectants.

Soften *severely* cracked skin in tepid water for five minutes, but don't use humectants on it, Dr. Swinyer cautions. "Once skin is malleable, seal in moisture immediately by covering damp skin with an ointment or lotion such as Eucerin, Vaseline or even Crisco," Dr. Swinyer suggests.

Hold it right there. Use Super Glue on small cracks that develop on fingers or other joints, says Dr. Brown. Just apply a dollop of glue directly to the open crack. It will dry in seconds and act like a cast to keep the fissure from splitting while it's healing, he explains. "Super Glue is the most incredible thing ever. It's invaluable. I've used it for about 18 years now," Dr. Brown says. "It dries in a matter of 10 to 15 seconds, and you can just go about your regular routine. You'd think it would burn like all get-out, but you don't even feel it when you put it on.

"You can even push on where that sore is split and you won't feel a thing. If it cracks again, just put another drop of Super Glue on it." You can't pull the glue off, but it will eventually fall off on its own.

Cleanse gently. Avoid hot water and use superfatted soaps or mild cleansing bars like Eucerin, Aveeno cleansing bar or Dove, advises Diana Bihova, M.D., assistant clinical professor of dermatology at New York University School of Medicine in New York City and author of *Beauty from the Inside Out*.

Or use a soap substitute, like Cetaphil skin cleanser, says Dr. Swinyer. "Cleanse with it just as you do with soap and water. Then pat more of it on—don't rub it in—and cover it with a greasy lotion to hold in the moisture," he advises.

Cover up. If your skin is prone to cracking, always wear rubber gloves when you use soapy water or chemicals for household cleaning.

Use urea or alpha-hydroxy acids. "Creams or lotions that contain urea or alpha-hydroxy acids are really good for dryness," says Dr. Bihova. "Carmol 10 or 20, Ultra Mide 25, Lac-Hydrin Five and Nutraderm 30 promote healing and can help *prevent* cracks when you use them regularly."

SKIN DISCOLORATION

WHEN TO SEE YOUR DOCTOR

- Your skin or large portions of it turns any unusual shade.
- Your natural skin pigment disappears.

WHAT YOUR SYMPTOM IS TELLING YOU

Candice always wears long sleeves, opaque stockings, a scarf around her throat, gloves and a broad-brimmed hat to shade her face. And she despises her image. She'd just love to ditch her wardrobe and join a bikini team. But a few minutes in the sun bring out her true colors: Large, lily-white patches of skin that glare starkly against the few pigmented areas that remain.

Candice has vitiligo—a common, physically harmless condition that is caused by the body's immune system "eating away" the skin's pigment. Occasionally it affects the entire body, says Leonard Swinyer, M.D., clinical professor of dermatology at the University of Utah in Salt lake City.

Not all skin color changes are quite so dramatic. A fairly common color switch is to yellow. There are several possible reasons for turning yellow. One is age. "Elderly people can develop a yellowish cast to the skin as it thins and lets the underlying fat layer show through," says Joseph G. Morelli, M.D., associate professor in the departments of dermatology and pediatrics at the University of Colorado Health Sciences Center in Denver.

If you have a package-a-day carrot habit or eat lots of foods rich in the nutrient beta-carotene, your skin might become yellowish. "Little kids often get this from eating lots of vegetable baby food," explains Robert E. Clark, M.D., Ph.D., director of the Dermatologic Surgery and Cutaneous Oncology Unit at Duke University Medical Center in Durham, North Carolina.

When an overall yellow color (jaundice) follows flulike symptoms, it can signal a serious problem, such as hepatitis, gallbladder trouble or cirrhosis of the liver. Jaundice occurs when bilirubin—a natural waste product of the body that is normally processed by the liver and excreted—backs up into the bloodstream, explains Francisco Averhoff, M.D., epidemiologist for the Hepatitis Branch of the Centers for Disease Control and Prevention in Atlanta. The toxin can give a fair-skinned person a sallow look, but it first turns the whites of the eyes yellow, regardless of skin tone.

Less commonly, reactions to certain heart medications can darken the skin or turn it a bluish shade. And on very rare occasions, a skin cancer on the surface of the body can become internalized and produce an overall color change to brown or black, says Dr. Swinyer.

SYMPTOM RELIEF

If your skin turns red from overexposure to the sun, you know you've overdone your time in the outdoors. Any other color change deserves investigation and sometimes treatment.

Light up your life; darken your skin. "A possible treatment for vitiligo is PUVA," says Martin A. Weinstock, M.D., Ph.D., director of photomedicine at Roger Williams Medical Hospital and chief of dermatology at the Veterans Affairs Medical Center in Providence, Rhode Island. A drug called psoralen (the P in PUVA) and exposure to ultraviolet-A (UVA) light, are combined in an effort to generate pigment, he explains.

Quit the rabbit food. It's the obvious solution to a beta-carotene complexion. Beta-carotene is not toxic like vitamin A (to which it converts once it's in the body). Simply taking in less beta-carotene will get rid of the yellow hue.

See a doctor. "If you have jaundice," says Dr. Averhoff, "the underlying conditions must be diagnosed and treated by a physician."

You'll also need to see your doctor to get at the root of any other color change. If a heart medication is causing a bluish color, he may be able to alter your dosage or prescribe an alternate medication.

See also Jaundice

SKIN FLAKING

WHEN TO SEE YOUR DOCTOR

- Flaking is accompanied by intense itching.
- Flaking areas have become inflamed or infected.
- You notice fishlike scaling (probably without initial itching) on your lower legs.
- Treatment you've used at home hasn't helped after three weeks.

WHAT YOUR SYMPTOM IS TELLING YOU

Dryness can stir up a flurry of flakes on most parts of your body, but it's most common on the legs and arms, where skin is thinner and more often exposed. The causes of dry, flaking skin are many.

Some people are simply born with it, says Glenn Kline, M.D., an allergist and assistant clinical professor of pediatrics at the University of Texas at Houston. But flaking is more common in older people, says Ivor Caro, M.D., a dermatologist and associate professor of medicine at the University of Washington School of Medicine in Seattle. That's because aging skin tends to be drier. At any age, dry skin is aggravated by frequent washing and bathing, especially with harsh soaps.

You may notice that at certain times of the year, dry skin is worse. Winter is prime flake season for the young and old alike, because low humidity in cold outdoor air and heated indoor air make for thirsty skin. Without enough moisture, dry skin flakes off as easily as hundred-year-old paint on the south side of a barn.

Flaking skin can also rear its scaly head in the wake of any condition that causes skin to become damaged, irritated or inflamed, such as sunburn, allergies, poison ivy, psoriasis and seborrhea.

Psoriasis is distinguished by flaking over patches of red,

inflamed skin and should be treated by a doctor, says Lon Christianson, M.D., a psoriasis expert with the Dermatology Clinic Limited of Fargo, North Dakota, and a spokesperson for the American Academy of Dermatology. This persistent skin condition usually makes its debut on elbows, knees or the scalp, but it can affect the entire body.

Seborrhea also commonly affects the scalp, usually forming yellowish, greasy scales. Eczema, a blanket name for a range of skin conditions, usually forms *dry* scales or flakes. Eczema can appear anywhere, but in adults it's most common on the hands, says Dr. Christianson. (See Dandruff on page 139.) Also, certain skin medications—Retin-A, for example—can cause skin to become inflamed, followed by peeling or flaking. "It's the body's way of shedding damaged skin after the inflammation dies down," Dr. Caro explains.

SYMPTOM RELIEF

Flaking is triggered by many conditions, yet treatment almost always comes down to this: Moisturize.

Drop the soap. Many antibacterial and deodorant soaps are too harsh for dry skin, says Dr. Kline. So, in many cases, flakes can be banished forever just by switching to a mild, soaplike substitute, such as superfatted cleansing bars. Dove is often recommended because it's less drying, says Dr. Kline. Some skin cleansers get their moisturizing power from gentle things like olive oil. But stay away from lotions with lanolin, which many people become allergic to.

Don't get rubbed the wrong way. Pat—don't rub—your skin dry after bathing to reduce the chance of irritating sensitive skin. "And always dry well after a bath or shower so that the skin isn't left damp," says Dr. Caro. "If water has a chance to evaporate, it dries skin more because it literally sucks water out of the skin, rather than just off the surface."

Seal your moisture envelope. Dry off well, then *immediately* apply a moisturizer, says Dr. Caro. There are hundreds of moisturizers to choose from. "Many of them are grease-based, which puts a waterproof layer between the

skin and air, thereby preventing moisture loss," says Dr.
Caro. Vaseline is the classic example of a pure grease ointment. Over-the-counter moisturizers, sold at most pharmacies, will help soothe your flaking skin. But if the problem
persists, ask your doctor about prescription lotions.

Wrap it up. Moisturizers may need extra help to pene-
rate and work on extremely dry, flaky skin, says Diana
Bihova, M.D., assistant clinical professor of dermatology at
New York University School of Medicine in New York City
and author of *Beauty from the Inside Out.*

If hands are very dry and show no signs of infection,
apply an ointment such as Aquaphorora 1 percent hydrocortisone cream before bed and put on plastic or vinyl
gloves, which you can buy in drugstores. Larger areas can
be covered by plastic wrap to achieve the same effect, says
Dr. Bihova.

Face facts. If face dandruff—flaking along eyebrows,
nose and hairline—shows up, treat it with 0.5 percent
hydrocortisone cream no more than once a day for a week
or two, suggests Guy F. Webster, M.D., Ph.D., assistant
professor of dermatology and director of the Center for
Cutaneous Pharmacology at Thomas Jefferson University in
Philadelphia.

SKIN ITCHING

WHEN TO SEE YOUR DOCTOR

- Your itching flares up when you take prescribed medications.
- Your itching is intense or persists more than two days,
  especially if your family history includes diabetes or
  kidney disease.

What Your Symptom Is Telling You

If only *all* itches came once every seven years....But almost everyone itches occasionally, and some people itch almost constantly.

Itching is notorious as the most common symptom of allergies, says Glenn Kline, M.D., an allergist and assistant clinical professor of pediatrics at the University of Texas at Houston. Very often, itching is a solitary symptom of allergy—at first. Only the "itchee" knows it's there because it's invisible. But scratching an allergic itch will often awaken a rash or hives.

"The really tough cases are patients who are chronically itchy but have absolutely nothing to see on the skin," says Ivor Caro, M.D., a dermatologist and associate professor of medicine at the University of Washington School of Medicine in Seattle. That's when doctors start sleuthing for possible internal causes for this maddening type of itch, such as stress or overproduction of certain hormones.

Other common causes of itches: insect bites and stings, parasites, such as chiggers and scabies (teeny mites that burrow into the skin), dry skin and damp or tight clothing.

Symptom Relief

Only kings and queens should itch, because it feels so good to scratch," Dr. Caro quotes from an ancient Chinese saying. It's okay to occasionally revel in a glorious scratch for a passing itch—like the one that nips your ankles when you peel off tight socks. But, says Dr. Kline, the agonizing rule of thumb (and thumbnail!) for scratching is a firm "Try not to." Scratching will make the itching worse and could open the skin to infection, he says. Fortunately, scratching is not the only way to deal with itches.

Cool it. Take a cool shower, Dr. Caro suggests. Or apply cool compresses: Ring a towel out in cool water and lay it over itchy areas for five to ten minutes. The evaporating water will cool and soothe the itch, he says.

Soothe it. Lotions that contain menthol or camphor—such as Prax, which is a topical anesthetic—are very cooling and soothing and tend to take itch away, says Dr. Caro.

Bathe in breakfast. A cool or lukewarm oatmeal bath will often ease all-over itching. Specially prepared, premeasured packets of powdered oats with added bath oils like Aveeno are easiest to use (and to clean up afterward). "It's very soothing and satisfying for itching that comes from dry skin," says Dr. Caro.

Don't let histamine have the upper hand. Ignore the call to scratch insect bites and stings or other allergic urgings by rubbing them with ice until the itch dies down. Then enlist oral antihistamines, such as Benadryl, Dr. Kline advises. Beware of topical antihistamines, such as Benadryl cream, though, and products whose names end in "-caine," benzocaines, for example. They can cause allergic skin reactions and may compound your problem.

Calamine is fine...at times. Calamine lotion—a famous itch beater—is best for weepy, blistery itches, such as poison ivy. But if your itch's origin is unknown or is caused by dry skin, calamine's drying action could make your itch all the more itchy, says Dr. Caro.

Stay cool. "Itching is made worse by heat," says Dr. Kline, and it could aggravate allergic reactions. A few ways to cool the heels of an intense itch: avoid hot water, sun worshipping and overheating exercise.

Keep it loose. Loose cotton clothing is the garb of choice for itch-prone people. Clothing that hugs your sensitive curves, as well as irritating fabrics like synthetics or wool, can really keep you itching. If you simply must wear wool, invest in cotton or silk underthings to keep it from getting too close for comfort.

See also Hives; Rashes

SKIN PALENESS

WHEN TO SEE YOUR DOCTOR

- You also feel weak, tired and out of breath.
- If you suddenly become pale, sweaty and have a rapid heartbeat and difficulty breathing, get to a doctor right away.

WHAT YOUR SYMPTOM IS TELLING YOU

Free-flowing blood under the skin is what gives your cheeks that rosy, glowing look of health. Slow that flow and the color fades, giving the skin a lifeless, pallid look.

Intense physical and emotional stress can interfere with the normal flow of blood under the skin. When you have an emotional shock, a severe injury or an infection or are exposed to freezing temperatures, your body responds by narrowing blood vessels in your skin and rechanneling blood to the body's center, where it raises body heat and supplies vital organs with oxygen and nutrients.

The stress of heat exhaustion—when the body becomes severely overheated—can also rob blood from your skin and turn you white as a desert sun. In this case, you'll also be sweaty and feel faint.

And you can add paleness to the host of other physical ills associated with a lifestyle that doesn't include exercise. "Sedentary people generally have less rosy complexions than more active people because their hearts are pumping less blood," says Robert A. Weiss, M.D., assistant professor of dermatology at Johns Hopkins University School of Medicine in Baltimore. "Frequent exercise may also increase the red blood cell count, delivering more oxygen to the skin."

Paleness (along with fatigue and breathlessness) is also a sign of iron-deficiency anemia. Iron helps to build the red blood cells that give blood its rich color and carry oxygen throughout the body. Iron-deficiency anemia is usually caused by heavy or persistent blood loss from menstrual periods, ulcers, gastritis, hemorrhoids, excess aspirin use and, occasionally, from bowel tumors.

In addition, lower-than-average iron stores can occur if you're pregnant, nursing a baby or skimping on iron-containing foods such as red meat.

Paleness is also a symptom of less common forms of anemia that accompany some blood disorders and chronic diseases. Some of these anemias are inherited.

Finally, paleness is one of the warning signs of a heart attack. Treat it as a medical emergency if you suddenly break out in a sweat, have a rapid heartbeat, begin panting and are very pale.

SYMPTOM RELIEF

Here's what to do if you find a ghost staring back at you from the mirror.

Find out with a serum ferritin test. A routine blood test that measures ferritin, the body's iron-storing protein, can tell you exactly how much iron your body has on hand. "It's the best way to help you spot an iron deficiency early before it progresses to full-blown anemia," says Myron Winick, M.D., professor emeritus of nutrition at Columbia University College of Physicians and Surgeons in New York City. If your ferritin is hovering around the borderline for iron deficiency, your doctor can get you on a dietary and supplemental regimen to rebuild iron stores.

Join the movers and shakers. Walking, bicycling or any exercise during which you move your arms and legs helps stimulate the formation of red blood cells and promotes better blood flow, according to John Abruzzo, M.D., professor of medicine and director of the Rheumatology and Osteoporosis Center at Thomas Jefferson University Hospital in Philadelphia. "Regular exercise may help restore that rosy glow in just a few weeks," he says.

Moisturize with fruit acids. If you're pasty-faced from a bout with an infection, forget the extra blusher. Instead, try over-the-counter lotions containing alpha-hydroxy acids made from fruit acids. "This ingredient causes a subtle inflammation, sloughing off the old cells, which makes way for fresh cells," says Dr. Weiss. "You'll get a sun-kissed look without any serious side effects."

Put your head between your knees. If you've suddenly become pale, sweaty and light-headed from overheating, bend over so that your head is lower than your heart. This helps gravity get the blood to the brain and will bring a blush to your cheeks, says Dr. Weiss. Then drink cool fluids, remove excess clothing and move to a shady spot.

SKIN PEELING

WHEN TO SEE YOUR DOCTOR

- You also have a rash.
- Your skin begins to peel soon after you begin to take a new medication.

WHAT YOUR SYMPTOM IS TELLING YOU

Your nose is peeling, your arms are peeling, your back is peeling. It's all so...unappealing.

"In general, peeling skin in and of itself is not a big problem and no harm comes of it," says Guy F. Webster, M.D., Ph.D., assistant professor of dermatology and director of the Center for Cutaneous Pharmacology at Thomas Jefferson University in Philadelphia.

Besides sunburn, common skin peelers are dryness, irritation by household chemicals and solvents, and overuse of products like Retin-A, a prescription acne and wrinkle medication that decreases the number of surface skin cells. Skin conditions like eczema or psoriasis can also make the skin peel.

"Occasionally, severe and potentially dangerous peeling of large areas is caused by a condition called TEN, or toxic epidermal necrolysis, which means toxic skin death," says Jerold Z. Kaplan, M.D., medical director of the Alta Bates Burn Center in Berkeley, California. TEN is an extremely uncommon allergic reaction to relatively common drugs, such as sulfa drugs, gout medications or penicillin, and requires hospitalization.

SYMPTOM RELIEF

When you look like a chameleon in full molt, here are a couple of things you can try.

Stop picking on you. You may hate the look of peeling skin, but you should probably resist the temptation to pick at it, Dr. Webster says. Broken skin is an invitation to infections. "And if you have a skin disease like eczema or psoriasis, peeling the skin back can damage tissue and worsen the underlying skin problem."

Get out the scissors. "If skin is hanging, the best thing is to snip it off with fine scissors so you don't pull areas that are still adherent," says Diana Bihova, M.D., assistant clinical professor of dermatology at New York University School of Medicine in New York City and coauthor of *Beauty from the Inside Out.*

Moisturize. Soothe dry, peeling skin by moisturizing it with any good moisturizing cream or lotion, suggests Dr. Kaplan. (For the lowdown on dealing with eczema and psoriasis, see Rashes on page 515.)

Take a bath. Take a cool bath or shower, suggests Dr. Webster. It will help soak away any loose flakes. For all-over peeling, a soak in an Aveeno oatmeal bath is helpful, says Dr. Bihova.

See also Skin Flaking

Skin Sores

WHEN TO SEE YOUR DOCTOR

- A sore is unusual in appearance, does not heal after two weeks or grows rapidly.
- Sores are recurring or multiplying.
- You also have fever or nausea.

WHAT YOUR SYMPTOM IS TELLING YOU

When you have a sore, you want it to go away. So does your body's immune system. It goes to work right away, sends in the cellular repair crews and—zip, zip—cleans it up. Usually.

Some sores prove to be more stubborn than others—they just hang in there and keep on coming.

Sores have hundreds of possible causes, many of which are hard to pinpoint and even harder to shake. According to William Dexter, M.D., assistant professor of clinical community and family medicine at the Dartmouth-Hitchcock Medical Center in Lebanon, New Hampshire: "When a sore rears its ugly head, it's telling you one of three things: Some kind of disease process is going on within the skin, something is going on elsewhere in the body that is being expressed through the skin or else the skin has come in contact with something it doesn't agree with."

Quite often it is the latter. The skin is a magnet for a variety of creepy crawlies—from the bites and stings of mosquitoes and bees to the burrowing and tunneling of tiny little parasites. Any of these bites and burrows can become infected, making the sores even more pronounced. And don't forget germs.

"Most of the really ugly-looking sores with pus, scabs and redness are the work of infectious microorganisms," says Guy F. Webster, M.D., Ph.D., assistant professor of dermatology and director of the Center for Cutaneous Pharmacology at Thomas Jefferson University in Philadelphia.

The most common and contagious of these are bacteria. Conditions they cause include boils, impetigo (a reddish rash on the face that forms pus-filled and crusty scabs) and folliculitis (an infected hair follicle.) Viruses are responsible for such sore-sprouting diseases as chickenpox, herpes, shingles and warts. Finally, fungi are little invaders that produce such unsavory skin conditions as athlete's foot, jock itch and ringworm.

Many skin conditions can develop sores and pustules if they get infected. Skin afflicted with dermatitis or eczema is very susceptible to secondary infections, especially if there's a break in the skin's surface (from scratching, for example).

But infectious agents aren't the only culprits that make sores. Things like age spots or cysts form benign skin growths. A precancerous lesion with the potential of becoming a true skin cancer may first appear as a tiny sore.

Deep wounds, skin breakdown and ulcerations on the surface of the body are really signs of more serious conditions deep inside. Examples are sores associated with poor circulation, diabetes, Lyme disease and AIDS.

SYMPTOM RELIEF

The secret to treating sores is to treat the cause, but in most cases, a person really doesn't have a clue whether he's dealing with a case of shingles, impetigo or bedbugs.

"There's no such thing as a general, all-purpose treatment for sores, because they have so many different causes," says Stephen M. Schleicher, M.D., clinical instructor of dermatology at Temple University Medical School and Philadelphia College of Osteopathic Medicine and co-director of The Dermatology Center in Philadelphia. "You would treat a virus much differently than you would a bacterial infection, and what works on one cause may have disastrous results if used on another."

Because improper self-medication can delay healing, treating stubborn sores should be in the hands of a doctor. In the case of minor sores, the body's natural defense system is usually sufficient to clean up lesions on its own— given time and proper care. Here's how you can help.

Keep the sore clean. "The best thing you can do for sores is to keep them as clean as possible," says Dr. Schleicher "You don't want to traumatize a sore by scrubbing i roughly. Just use gentle soap and warm water one or two times per day and pat it dry with a towel."

Keep most sores exposed and dry. "Open air on a sore will cause sores to dry up and encourage bacteria to move away," says Lawrence C. Parish, M.D., clinical professor of dermatology at Jefferson Medical College of Thomas Jefferson University in Philadelphia. "Covering up sores will encourage bacteria and other germs to breed and fester." The exceptions are large open sores that are oozing pus, blood or liquid. These should be cleaned and covered tightly with a bandage to absorb the ooze and to keep out infectious germs.

Ditch the itch. Nothing will invite infection faster than scratching an itchy sore. Oral antihistamines like Chlor-Trimeton and Benadryl reduce the urge to scratch, says Dr Dexter. So will bathing in Aveeno, a commercial colloidal bath product made from oatmeal. You can also apply a 0.5 to 1 percent hydrocortisone cream to the itchy sore, but ask your doctor first: Some infections will intensify if exposed to these medications. (For other ways to deal with skin itching, see page 553.)

Check your medicine cabinet. Some medications produce an allergic-type reaction, causing eruptions to appear all over the skin. Ask your doctor if a change in your medications is in order.

Ask your doctor about these treatments. Bacterial infections are treated with a variety of antibiotics. These include over-the-counter topical ointments like Neosporin and Polysporin and bacitracin as well as more potent oral and topical drugs like penicillin and cephalosporin. Prescription antiviral medications include acyclovir for chickenpox and shingles. Scabies respond to prescription creams like Kwell and Scabene. And over-the-counter medications like tolnaftates and miconazoles will handle most fungal infections.

Skin Tenderness

WHEN TO SEE YOUR DOCTOR

- Your tender skin is also red, scaly, flaking, peeling or blistered.
- Your skin looks sunburned, but you haven't been over-exposed to the sun.
- Your tender spots are turning a dark color.
- Your tender skin is red and warmer than the skin in the same area on the opposite side of your body.

What Your Symptom Is Telling You

If you've sun-roasted, scalded or burned yourself, chances are you're not confused about the cause of your tender skin.

But sometimes the causes of skin that feels very tender or sore to the touch are not quite so clear. For example, it might surprise you to know that your skin can get the flu. Oddly enough, viral infections of almost any kind (respiratory or intestinal) can actually make your skin hurt, along with bringing aches to your muscles and bones.

One virus that is particularly unkind to skin is *Herpes zoster,* which causes the searing pain of shingles.

Another common cause of tender skin is dryness from lack of humidity in the air, particularly in wintertime. Almost any injury that presses on or injures a nerve can make skin painfully sensitive, doctors say. If a specific area of skin bothers you after an episode of back pain, for example, there may be damage to a single segment of nerve. Diabetic neuropathy, which irritates the nerves in the skin, may also cause skin to be sore or numb to the touch.

Symptom Relief

Here's how to help tender skin become comfortable to live in again.

Soothe the flu. If the flu or another virus is making you skin sore, try aspirin to relieve the pain, says Libb Edwards, M.D., chief of dermatology at the Carolina Medical Center in Charlotte, North Carolina. (Caution Don't give aspirin to a child with flulike symptoms. Us acetaminophen products like Children's Tylenol instead Aspirin given to children under age 21 during the flu, chick enpox or any feverish period may cause Reye's syndrome, potentially fatal swelling of the brain.)

Hydrate the skin. If you suspect dryness is causing you tender skin, try this basic hydrating technique from Caroline Koblenzer, M.D., clinical associate professor o dermatology at the University of Pennsylvania i Philadelphia. Soak in a bath to let your skin absorb mois ture, then seal in the moisture with an inexpensive emol lient like white petroleum jelly or Eucerin lotion. Both ar available without prescription at pharmacies. (For othe hints and tips on dealing with dry skin, see Skin Flaking o page 551.)

Don't let shingles send you through the roof. If you painful skin is caused by shingles, a mild, over-the-counte pain reliever such as aspirin, ibuprofen or acetaminophei will help, says Charles Ellis, M.D., a professor of derma tology at the University of Michigan Medical School in Ani Arbor. But if the pain is severe, Dr. Ellis advises you to se your doctor. He may prescribe acyclovir, a drug that cai shorten the illness.

Stop the pain that persists. Skin pain can linger after ; bout of shingles, particularly in older people. Prescriptio oral cortisone can treat this problem, as can tricyclic anti depressants. (In fact, the tricyclics are good for *any* chronic nerve pain.) For long-term cases, Dr. Ellis suggests you con sider asking your doctor to refer you to a university pai clinic.

SLEEPWALKING

WHEN TO SEE YOUR DOCTOR

- Your sleepwalking becomes disruptive or potentially harmful to you or someone else.
  Sleepwalking is accompanied by repetitive, ticlike twitches of the face or arms.
- An adult begins to sleepwalk for the first time.

WHAT YOUR SYMPTOM IS TELLING YOU

Your kid looks like he's auditioning for *The Child of Frankenstein* or *The Invasion of the Midget Zombies*—he's sleepwalking again. Not to worry. "Sleepwalking is perfectly normal in children and probably perfectly normal in adults," according to Mark Mahowald, M.D., director of the Minnesota Regional Sleep Disorders Center at Hennepin County Medical Center in Minneapolis.

The best (and perhaps only) thing you can do is make sure your somnolent stroller doesn't hurt himself. Lock windows, shut basement doors and put gates across stairways. Eventually, you'll be able to relax precautions—your kid will grow out of sleepwalking just as inexplicably as he grew into it. Sleepwalking *can* begin in adulthood, however. Factors like family history, alcohol consumption and sleep deprivation can predispose someone to take a real-life stroll through the Land of Nod, researchers say.

SYMPTOM RELIEF

Back when he went to medical school, Dr. Mahowald was taught that if sleepwalkers persisted in their nocturnal nomadism through adolescence and into adulthood, a strong likelihood of a psychiatric disorder existed. "That's just flat out not true," he says. "That's a myth that continues to be promulgated. A majority of the medical profession, however, still has that attitude."

So now that you know that you don't have a psycho in the house, how do you deal with a family member doing the 2:00 a.m. two-step?

Don't wake them up. No, not because they'll go crazy or get lockjaw or because the soul will be trapped out of the body—all of these beliefs were prevalent in the past—but because there's no reason to rouse them. "If you wake them, which could be difficult to do, they'll be startled and won't know what's going on," says Neil B. Kavey, M.D., director of the Sleep Disorders Center at the Columbia Presbyterian Medical Center in New York City. "Why disorient someone?" he says. Just guide your sleepwalker safely and gently back to bed.

Take a chance on a trance. "Hypnosis is a wonderful treatment for this," says Paul Gouin, M.D., director of the Sleep Disorders Program at Ingham Medical Center in Lansing, Michigan. A few visits to a hypnotherapist should convince your subconscious mind that when you're asleep, your body should *rest*.

Reassure the roamer. Because of the misconception that sleepwalkers have psychological problems, Dr. Mahowald says, "a majority just need assurance that nothing is really wrong with them. That's the most important thing."

Ask about medication. If sleepwalking persists or presents problems or hazards, physicians sometimes prescribe medication. "We're loath to do so, though, because we're predominantly talking about children," Dr. Mahowald says. Behavioral therapies are often effective and frequently preferable, he says.

SMELL LOSS

WHEN TO SEE YOUR DOCTOR

You have not recently had a cold and your sense of smell is gone or decreased.

Your sense of smell is distorted (you are smelling strange or foul odors that are unaccounted for).

You have a cold or stuffy nose and your sense of smell has been gone for more than one week.

You lost your sense of smell following an accident or head injury.

You lose your sense of smell seasonally every year.

WHAT YOUR SYMPTOM IS TELLING YOU

Remember holding your nose as a child when a spoonful of medicine came your way? Chances are you instinctively recognized the intimate relationship between what you smell and what you taste. When your favorite foods have lost their savor, it's usually a diminished sense of smell that is to blame.

Any infection or inflammation that causes the mucous membranes lining your nose to swell prevents odor-carrying molecules in the air from reaching the smell receptors inside your nose. Colds, allergies, upper respiratory infections, a bacterial infection of the sinuses or nasal polyps can all obstruct the nasal airways and inhibit your sense of smell.

Because the tiny nerves that carry smell messages to your brain are so delicate, a hard jolt or blow to the head can tear them. (Oddly enough, it's often less damaging to the sense of smell to get popped right in the snoot—the cartilage in the nose collapses like a car's bumper, absorbing the shock before it reaches the olfactory nerves.)

Chronic exposure to some pollutants and toxic chemicals—acids, formaldehyde and particularly tobacco smoke—will cause a slowly progressing loss of smell.

Thyroid medications, seizure disorders and certain tumors can also affect the sense of smell. And some dementia-related disorders like Alzheimer's and Parkinson's disease can result in loss of smell—though loss of smell is not necessarily a sign that you are developing these conditions.

Aging, too, gradually diminishes the sense of smell. At 80, your sense of smell will work about half as well as it did when you were 30.

SYMPTOM RELIEF

Doing without the smell—and taste—of your favorite meals is only one reason to be concerned about losing your sense of smell. Odors often serve to protect you from danger. If you can't smell, then spoiled food can't give you its pungent warning. And what about a gas leak from the furnace or stove? Or the first tendrils of smoke that signal a fire?

Loss of smell is aggravating and in some instances dangerous. Fortunately, in many cases it is also reversible.

Rest and wait it out. It's not at all unusual to have your sense of smell conk out for just a day or two—when you have a cold, for example. But in most cases, it should return on its own within two or three days, says William H. Friedman, M.D., an otolaryngologist, facial plastic surgeon and director of the Park Central Institute in St. Louis. And while you're waiting, he says, make sure you get plenty of sleep.

"It usually takes three nights of very good sleep to cure a cold," he says.

Sweat it out. If your sense of smell is gone because your nose is stuffed up—from a cold or allergy, for example—mild exercise or taking a hot bath until you start to sweat can prove helpful. "Breaking a sweat will cause your nose to clear," says Dr. Friedman.

Reduce the inflammation. Ask your doctor if your reduced sense of smell is from inflammation, suggests Richard Doty, Ph.D., director of the Smell and Taste Center of the University of Pennsylvania School of Medicine in Philadelphia. An upper respiratory infection could be the culprit in this case. Your doctor may prescribe corticoseroid medication or recommend supplements containing some of the antioxidant vitamins—C, E and beta-carotene.

Arm against allergies. If your loss of smell comes regularly during hay fever season, you'll need to see an allergist, says Jordan S. Josephson, M.D., an otolaryngologist in Brooklyn. "For a day or two, the usual over-the-counter antihistamines are fine," he says. "But if it lasts more than two weeks, your allergist may recommend nasal steroid sprays or a prescription decongestant." (For more tips on allergy relief, see Nose, Runny, on page 461.)

Clear your sinuses. When sinus infection stops your sense of smell, your doctor will treat you for one to two weeks with antibiotics and a prescription decongestant, says Dr. Josephson. But avoid combination antihistamine/decongestant medicines. "It's like using buckshot to swat a fly," he says. If your sinusitis doesn't clear up in two weeks, your doctor may prescribe an extended course of antibiotics. In more severe cases, infected sinus tissue may be removed with the aid of a tiny fiber-optic telescope called an endoscope, he says. (For more tips on clearing sinuses, see Sinus Problems on page 540.)

Have polyps removed. Nasal polyps vary from small irregularities on the surface of nasal membranes to larger fluid-filled sacs, says Dr. Friedman. If caught early, they can be treated with steroids. "While these drugs have a checkered reputation from being abused, they are miraculous," he says. "They can make polyps melt away in early stages."

Polyps are also treated with antibiotics, decongestants and antihistamines, he says. If tests indicate extensive polyps, surgical removal may be necessary.

Stop smoking. Though smoking causes long-term damage to the sense of smell, the damage is partly reversible if you quit, Dr. Doty says. He has done studies that show that improvement is slow but sure.

Mask yourself. If your work or hobby exposes you to chemicals or heavy dust, wear a filter mask, says Dr. Josephson. Hardware stores sell these masks (a version of the kind surgeons wear), and using one can prevent further damage to your sense of smell.

Review your Rx. If you take thyroid medication, ask

your doctor if adjusting your prescription might help you
impaired sense of smell, suggests Dr. Doty.

Treat a tumor. Most tumors that cause problems wit
sense of smell are benign, says Dr. Friedman. Depending o
the type of tumor, treatment will be some combination o
surgery, radiation or chemotherapy. The prognosis is gen
erally good, he says.

News for Older Noses

If aging has made your sniffer insensitive, here are som
important reminders from Donald Leopold, M.D., an oto
laryngologist at Johns Hopkins University's Francis Scot
Key Medical Center in Baltimore.

Install detectors. If your sense of smell is gone, "there i
no way you will smell a fire," says Dr. Leopold. Make sur
your home has battery-powered smoke detectors that ar
working.

Rent-a-nose. Be sure to keep up your personal hygiene
whether or not you think you need it. Ask a friend to le
you know if you need a shirt change, for example. And i
you wear a fragrance, be sure to apply measured amounts

Keep careful fridge files. Without a sense of smell, yo
won't detect sour milk until it's lumpy or moldy bologn
until it's green. If you live with someone, assign them th
task of evaluating food in the refrigerator to see if it'
spoiled. If you're on your own, be sure to label foods wit
the date you bought them.

SNEEZING

WHEN TO SEE YOUR DOCTOR

- Your sneezing fits recur and aren't helped by home
  remedies or over-the-counter antihistamines.

WHAT YOUR SYMPTOM IS TELLING YOU

Here comes the ah-choo-choo train. But you'd rather not be the conductor. You'd rather stand on the platform at the station and wave good-bye as the ah-choo-choo train chugs off into the horizon.

You can, but first you have to understand what causes those nasal blasts.

A sneeze is simply the nose's response to an allergen or irritant, says Elliott Middleton, Jr., M.D., professor of medicine and pediatrics at the State University of New York at Buffalo and an allergist at Buffalo General Hospital. Sneezers are just more sensitive to one or more of the many things that fly up everybody's nostrils. Some people's noses ignore them. Other people sneeze out the irritant and get on with their lives. In people who are allergic, the body releases histamine as a response to the microscopic invaders. Besides making them sneeze up a storm, histamine afflicts them with a runny, itchy nose; nasal and chest congestion; and red, teary eyes.

Those sneeze-causing allergens include pollen, grass, mold, pet dander and dust mites, says Dr. Middleton. The most common irritants are smoke or perfume, says Susan L. Wynn, M.D., an allergist in private practice with Fort Worth Allergy and Asthma Associates in Texas.

Colds and upper respiratory infections can bring on sneezing, along with a host of other symptoms. A quick change in temperature, such as walking into an air-conditioned room from the afternoon heat, can also make you sneeze. Expectant mothers frequently complain of sneezing and stuffiness when hormonal changes produce what's called rhinitis of pregnancy. And some people are compelled to sneeze when their eyes meet up with bright sunlight.

For a clue to the cause of continued bouts of sneezing, Dr. Wynn says to take your temperature and check your nose. If you have no fever but your nose is itchy, you have an allergy. If your nose isn't itchy or if you're running a temperature, you probably have a cold or some other upper respiratory infection.

SYMPTOM RELIEF

When you start to ah...ah...ah..., don't restrain th choo. "It's bad to suppress a sneeze," Dr. Wynn say Letting that strong blast of air implode into your hea rather than explode into a hanky can blow bacteria int your sinuses or your middle ear. You also could pop you eardrums, she warns. Get on with the Gesundheits and tr these more effective ways of ending your sneezes.

Play Dick Tracy. "The major form of treatment for sneeze is to discover and avoid the perpetrator of you sneezes," says Dr. Middleton. If you're alert, you'll event ally make associations between what you breathe and whe you sneeze.

He says the sneezing can be stopped easily if your dete tive work turns up a teddy bear or a neighbor's pet cat the culprit. It's much more difficult if the criminal is as co mon as pollen.

Try an antihistamine. Despite the different names an claims, over-the-counter antihistamines all possess abou the same anti-allergy effectiveness to dry up your nose an stop the itching. All of them can also cause drowsines especially if taken with alcohol or certain other medic tions, Dr. Middleton says.

Time your dose. If you're going on a picnic and are alle gic to grass, or if you're about to begin spring cleaning an dust provokes nasty nasal outbursts, take an antihistamin *before* the pollutant sends your symptoms soaring, D Wynn recommends. "Antihistamines work better befor your body starts releasing histamines," she says.

Mask your allergy. If you have to be outside to cut th grass, rake the leaves or pull weeds, and you can't unloa the chore on someone else, wear a filter mask, Dr. Wyn says. "It won't prevent the allergens from reaching yo completely, but a mask will cut it down," she says.

Shut off the outside world. Maybe you don't have t hibernate all year round, keep yourself barricaded insid and receive provisions through the crack under the door– but you *should* keep your windows closed and turn on fan or the air-conditioning. "That way, you can create a re tively pollen-free environment that you can retreat to," Dr. Wynn says.

Reschedule your rounds. Pollen counts in the air are higher early in the day and decrease during the afternoon, Dr. Wynn points out. "Try taking your jog or running your errands later on," she says.

Expose your skin. If you can't figure out what's causing your sneezing fits or if you can't control them, visit the doctor for an allergy test, Dr. Middleton says. Skin tests are more sensitive than blood tests in determining what you're allergic to. Depending on the results and your response to medication, you may have to undergo a series of allergy shots.

SNORING

WHEN TO SEE YOUR DOCTOR

Your spouse notices your loud snoring is interrupted by pauses in breathing of about ten seconds or more, perhaps followed by gruff snorts or gasps for air.
You also complain of frequent daytime sleepiness or fall asleep during the day.
You snore and have any of the following: high blood pressure, leg swelling, problems getting an erection, memory lapses or difficulty in concentrating.

WHAT YOUR SYMPTOM IS TELLING YOU

Your snoring punctures the night with the low, distant rumble of an approaching freight train, swelling louder and louder. You—and probably anyone in hearing distance—are riding the Red-Eye Express at least as far as Tired Days Junction.

Snoring is so common, so difficult to cure and usually so

medically insignificant that doctors can be reluctant to trea
it. "Snoring may be a normal human condition," says Pau
Gouin, M.D., director of the Sleep Disorders Program a
Ingham Medical Center in Lansing, Michigan. "So man
people are snorers (men more so than women) that it'
be kind of hysterical to become overly concerned,
Occasionally, however, snoring has a darker side—slee
apnea.

"At the bottom of everything, we're looking at a stru
tural issue, at how people's throats are built," says D
Gouin. "When awake, throat muscles keep the airway ope
and unrestricted." Once asleep, muscle tone decreases an
the throat relaxes. In snorers, the tongue or the tissue o
the inside of the throat partially obstructs the smooth pa
sage of air through their windpipes. Like the sudsy slurp c
air sucked through a straw at the foamy bottom of a milk
shake, snoring is the sound made when oxygen is inhale
between the obstructing tissue.

Now take a wet paper straw and suck really hard. Th
sides of the straw, already weak and spongy, collapse, pe
mitting no air to pass. That's what happens inside th
throats of people with sleep apnea. "In the act of breathing
you're trying to suck your throat down your throat," D
Gouin explains. "In trying to overcome the partial ob
struction, you inhale harder, and the relaxed walls of th
throat fly inward and stick to each other."

A person with sleep apnea stops breathing, not just onc
or twice but as frequently as hundreds of times during th
night. All this gasping and snorting interferes with restfu
slumber, possibly straining the heart and forcing a rise i
blood pressure.

SYMPTOM RELIEF

Not every snorer has sleep apnea, doctors say. Bu
almost every person with apnea is a snorer. For both
keeping the throat unrestricted can be as difficult as maneu
vering the straw between the bubbles in the shake
"Treatment is very frustrating to deal with," says Mar

Mahowald, M.D., director of the Minnesota Regional Sleep Disorders Center at Hennepin County Medical Center in Minneapolis. "You can't predict with any certainty the degree of success."

Nonetheless, the treatments are legion, and all of them work for some people.

Round up the usual suspects. Colds, sedatives, allergies, obesity, advancing age and drinking alcohol before going to bed all can affect your nighttime respiration and all should be considered in snoring treatment. "But you can have those things—you can have all of those things—and still not be a snorer," Dr. Gouin says. Conversely, you can eliminate all of them and still rattle the rafters.

Roll over, Beethoven. If dogs can be taught to roll over, so can snorers. And when you talk about positions in bed, the best one—at least to prevent snoring—may be on the side, as relaxed tongues and throat tissue are less likely to block air. "You can teach yourself to sleep on your side with position training," says Suzan Jaffe, Ph.D., clinical director of the Sleep Program at Hollywood Medical Center in Florida.

Stay off your back. Sew a pocket for a tennis ball into the back of your pajamas between your shoulder blades, near the neck. "Within a few weeks," Dr. Jaffe says, "you will have trained yourself to sleep on your side, and you won't need the tennis ball."

If that doesn't work, ask for an elbow nudge. "It's the famous honey-turn-over technique," Dr. Gouin says. Nudging the snorer enough to turn him or her over is all that's needed in certain cases.

Become tongue-tied. Mouthpieces and other professionally fitted dental devices, which retain the tongue and form an easier passageway for air, are "enjoying a resurgence of interest," according to Dr. Gouin. While they may sometimes be effective, snorers may find them uncomfortable to wear, he says.

Just say no. Resist the urge to purchase gimmicky items that promise relief. Neck braces and molded pillows designed to stop snoring haven't been shown to be worth anything, Dr. Gouin says.

CPAP is a blue-ribbon gear. There's one exception to the no-devices tip, however. If you don't mind wearing to bed what looks a bit like skin-diving apparatus, continuous positive airway pressure (CPAP) machines are virtually guaranteed to end apnea and snoring. Upon retiring for the night, you don a small triangular nose mask that's attached by tubing to a small fan in a box that sits on your night stand. The fan sends just enough air through your nostril into your throat to keep the airways unobstructed and the night silent.

"People report feeling much better after the first night they use it," Dr. Mahowald says, "and it stops snoring too." What about the cumbersome gear? "Wearing under wear is intrusive, too," Dr. Gouin says, "and nobody thinks about that. Once it becomes standard operating procedure you don't think any more about it."

A CPAP machine, which can be obtained only from a doctor and usually only to prevent apnea, isn't cheap. Expect to pay upwards of $1,000.

Take a slice and roll the dice. To cure common snoring that is not a health threat, surgical procedures to open up the nose or remove excess tissue in the throat are iffy. Operations to straighten deviated septums (the bone and cartilage that separate your nostrils) or remove nasal polyps don't have uniform success, doctors say.

In children, however, enlarged tonsils and adenoids "are often a forerunner of things to come," Dr. Jaffe says, and removal at an early age often prevents snoring or apnea problems later in life.

One of the most complicated procedures is uvulopalatopharyngoplasty, in which the tonsils, the back of the soft palate and the uvula (that little "punching bag" in the back of the mouth) are removed. "It's like tucking up the skin of the throat," Dr. Gouin says. Again, though, success is "notoriously unpredictable."

SPEECH PROBLEMS

WHEN TO SEE YOUR DOCTOR

Your speech problems show up after an accident or head injury.

See your doctor immediately if your speech suddenly becomes garbled, slurred, thickened or unclear.

See your doctor immediately if you suddenly begin to repeat words or phrases over and over or if your words continue to come out wrong even though you know what you intend to say.

See your doctor immediately if you can't speak at all for several minutes, even though you recover the ability later.

WHAT YOUR SYMPTOM IS TELLING YOU

We all know what it's like to grope for a word now and then. You know what you want to say—you can almost *see* that word—but it just hangs there on the tip of our tongue.

Speech is the most complex function of the human brain, says Daniel Zwitman, Ph.D., a Los Angeles speech pathologist with expertise in neurological dysfunction. "In order to just say 'ahhh,' 76 muscles have to work in union," he explains. "With all the interrelationships in communication, it's easy to see how it can break down."

What can break down the ease of speech? Anything that injures the brain or the nerves controlling speech can create difficulty in finding words or in simply "getting out" what you want to say.

Garbled speech could, for example, signal a stroke or a transient ischemic attack (TIA). TIA, also known as a ministroke, is a warning that a full-blown stroke could happen in the near future. During a TIA, spasming blood vessels can clamp down hard enough to temporarily cut off blood flow to the brain's speech command center.

A migraine headache is a milder form of TIA. During migraine, you can experience a brief moment of aphasia—difficulty expressing thoughts and understanding spoken and written words.

Any injury, tumor or slowly debilitating neurological disorder or disease can damage the parts of the brain that control speech and disturb the smooth flow of words. With some conditions, such as Parkinson's disease, speech might become unintelligible—either very slow or excessively fast and repetitive.

Speech problems vary greatly, and the specific kind of difficulty you have in speaking helps experts determine where in the brain the problem lies. Normally, doctors say if your speech problems come on suddenly, they are most likely the result of a stroke. If the process has been gradual, a neurological problem or disease is more likely to be the cause.

There are simpler causes for speech problems, too. The kind of momentary lapse that we all experience now and then ("Darn it, what is that word?") is perfectly normal. It might be ordinary forgetfulness.

SYMPTOM RELIEF

When speech problems appear suddenly, don't delay. Get medical help *immediately*. If you are having a stroke, quick treatment will make a great deal of difference in your recovery. Here are a few other things to be aware of.

Treat neurological conditions. Speech symptoms from some diseases of the brain or nervous system may respond to medication, says Charles Diggs, Ph.D., director of consumer affairs for the American Speech-Language-Hearing Association in Rockville, Maryland. Parkinson's disease, for example, is often treated with drugs such as Larodopa, which is derived from dopamine, a brain chemical found to be in diminishing supply in those with the disease.

Ease a migraine. If you routinely experience migraine headaches, your doctor can prescribe ergotamine to take as soon as you feel the headache coming on, says Austin King, M.D., an otolaryngologist in Abilene, Texas. Severe migraines may be prevented with beta blockers or calcium channel agonists, he says. (For other ways to deal with migraines, see Headaches on page 280.)

Ask about speech therapy. If you've had a stroke or head trauma that affects your ability to communicate, speech therapy can help to facilitate the return of your language or your ability to speak more clearly. "The earlier you begin therapy, the better the probability you will overcome depression and get faster return of your ability to communicate," says Betty Horwitz, Ed.D., a speech pathologist in private practice in New York City.

SPUTUM DISCOLORATION

WHEN TO SEE YOUR DOCTOR

- Your phlegm is yellow, green, brown or rust-colored for more than a week.
- You also have a fever, chills, shortness of breath or pain when you inhale deeply.

WHAT YOUR SYMPTOM IS TELLING YOU

Coughing up a lot of gunk?

No exact color key exists to match mucus to malady, but if your sputum is anything other than clear or white, it means you have a viral or bacterial infection somewhere in your respiratory tract or an inflammation in your lungs, says Sally E. Wenzel, M.D., an assistant professor of medicine at the National Jewish Center for Immunology and Respiratory Medicine in Denver. The infection could be as mundane as a cold or as serious as bronchitis or pneumonia.

While yellowish, puslike phlegm usually means some

sort of mild to moderate infection, any severe irritant, such as smoking or an allergen, can also be responsible, according to Anne L. Davis, M.D., associate professor of clinical medicine in the Division of Pulmonary and Critical Care Medicine at New York University Medical Center and assistant to the director of chest service at Bellevue Hospital Center in New York City.

Some infections also can color sputum green. A brown or rusty hue to your mucus may mean an infection, or it could be old, dried blood that lingered down in your lungs for some reason, Dr. Davis says.

SYMPTOM RELIEF

If your phlegm is an abnormal color, chances are you've noticed other symptoms that are a bit more bothersome—a nasty cough, difficulty in breathing, chest congestion, a fever or an overall lousy feeling. Depending on the severity of your sickness, you'll either tough it out or you'll go to the doctor, who probably will give you a prescription for some antibiotics. A simple respiratory infection in an elderly person or someone with a chronic lung disease is more serious. As for that spectrum of sputum, there are a couple of points to keep in mind.

Make it a double. Double the amount of liquid you normally drink, Dr. Wenzel says. "In addition to the discoloration, your mucus may be thicker, and liquids will thin it out and loosen it." (See Congestion on page 125 for more suggestions on fighting phlegm.)

Cough it up. Don't take cough suppressants, says Dr. Wenzel. Your cough has a purpose: to get rid of mucus, whatever its color.

STARING

WHEN TO SEE YOUR DOCTOR

- Someone informs you that you've had a brief staring spell during which you were unresponsive and you have no memory of the episode.

WHAT YOUR SYMPTOM IS TELLING YOU

It's normal to stare if a Grace Kelly look-alike sits across from you on the bus. Or to have a vacant, out-to-lunch look when daydreaming about winning the lottery. But what if you've just been told that you've had a brief, fixed, blank stare on your face, you didn't respond to your name and worse, you remember zilch about this staring spell?

You could have had a mild type of epileptic seizure, according to Allan Krumholz, M.D., professor of neurology at the University of Maryland Medical Center in Baltimore. This type of seizure was formerly called *petit mal* but is now called absence, because people look absent-minded, he says.

When a person has an absence seizure, says Dr. Krumholz, they've momentarily lost consciousness because their brain has been taken over by abnormal electrical activity.

SYMPTOM RELIEF

If this is your first staring episode, it's important to see a doctor to identify the cause and start treatment, says Dr. Krumholz. (For more information about the kinds of things your doctor will consider, see Seizures on page 529.)

STOMACH CRAMPS

WHEN TO SEE YOUR DOCTOR

- You also have a fever or bloody stool.
- Your cramps continue for a week or more.

WHAT YOUR SYMPTOM IS TELLING YOU

Stomach cramps are the evil henchmen of your gut. They never mastermind their own crime. But they can be found doing some of the dirty work of the usual stomach bad guys—thugs like diarrhea, constipation, a viral infection, irritable bowel syndrome, diverticulosis, lactose intolerance, even food poisoning. Of course, all these digestive disorders have other symptoms. But like a siren on a police cruiser, it's the cramps that get your attention.

"Stomach cramps are usually a painful squeezing sensation that comes and goes over a span of minutes. They crescendo up and then decrease," says Bruce Luxson, M.D., Ph.D., assistant professor of gastroenterology at Saint Louis University School of Medicine in Missouri. The squeezing sensation does not always originate in your stomach, by the way. Sometimes the trouble is further down.

Take, for example, irritable bowel syndrome (IBS)—a troubling and unexplained digestive problem that can cause pain, cramps, diarrhea and constipation. What you perceive as stomach cramps are actually spasms of the intestines. "In less severe cases of IBS, you get cramps when you have the urge to go to the bathroom, and they go away after you've defecated," says Andrew H. Soll, M.D., a professor of medicine and director of the affiliated training program for gastroenterology at the University of California at Los Angeles and chief of gastroenterology at Veterans Administration Hospital.

What you put in your mouth is another common cause of stomach cramps. Lactose intolerance—the inability to digest the sugar in dairy products—affects a third of Americans and can cause cramps. Downing spoiled potato salad at your company picnic—or any other inappropriately handled food—usually leads to a bacterial battle down below called food poisoning that features cramping, vomiting and sometimes diarrhea. And not enough fiber or water are the leading causes of both constipation and diarrhea, often linked to cramping, says Dr. Luxson.

Diverticulosis is a disease characterized by small pouches filled with stool or irritating bacteria that form on the muscle wall of your small bowel. It not only causes spasms and cramping, but hemorrhaging as well, says Dr. Soll. Another medical problem—viral infection—can also cause cramps.

Stress also apparently plays a role in stomach cramps for children as well as adults, says John Boyle, M.D., a gastroenterologist and chief of pediatric gastroenterology at Rainbow Babies and Childrens Hospital in Cleveland. "It doesn't *cause* the cramps, but it can bring them on," he says.

SYMPTOM RELIEF

By eating the right foods and keeping stress under control, you can minimize the possibility of stomach cramps. Here's how.

Get wise to water. When constipation is causing stomach cramps, pour on the water. Drinking over a gallon of water a day (that's eight eight-ounce glasses) should help make you regular in no time, says Dr. Luxson. Go easy on coffee and cola drinks. Caffeine is a diuretic and can quickly deplete the body's water supply, he says.

Stay clear. When food poisoning or viral infections strike, stick with clear liquids—like water—until your distress subsides.

Limit your lactose. Gas, cramps and diarrhea will often accompany even a small glass of milk if you are lactose intolerant, says Dr. Luxson. To test whether you have this problem, eliminate all dairy products for three days and then add an eight ounce glass of skim milk to your diet.

Gradually work more dairy products, like nonfat yogurt and cheeses, into your diet. If your cramping returns at any point, you may have found your culprit. If you do find out that you're lactose intolerant, you can buy Lactaid—a product containing the digestive enzyme lactase to be taken when you consume dairy products. Lactaid is available in tablet or liquid form.

Try some Miller's bran. A quarter cup of Miller's bran or any other fiber supplement added each morning to your oatmeal may be just what the doctor ordered to end your stomach cramps. Boosting fiber can help not only to end constipation and diarrhea but also to control diverticulosis and irritable bowel syndrome, says Dr. Soll. Eating too much fiber without giving your body time to adjust, however, may actually cause more gas and diarrhea. If you get relief from the cramps, but start to suffer from gas, try adding another form of fiber, like pre-made fiber bars, to your diet, he says. (For more information on banishing constipation, see page 128.)

Relax. Because some doctors believe that many causes of cramping are linked to stress, it's important to get your stress level under control. Whether you walk three times a week for 30 minutes at a time or learn biofeedback, you should see some relief from your cramps, says Dr. Boyle. Biofeedback is a technique that teaches you to relax by using a monitor to give you "feedback" on your level of muscular tension. Ask your doctor to refer you to someone who can provide training.

See also Stomach Pain

STOMACH GURGLING

WHAT YOUR SYMPTOM IS TELLING YOU

After years of studying stomach noises, ground-breaking research has proven that your digestive system has a language all its own! Long, low rumbles that occur during midmorning, for example, have been translated as:

"Pardon us, but we've been reassessing this breakfast thing. And, well...speaking for the entire group, we're willing to compromise. If you'll make sure we're fed sometime before, oh, let's say, 9:30 a.m., we'll promise to keep quiet during your important staff meetings. If not, we'll be forced to take matters into our own intestines."

Kidding aside, doctors *do* have a word for stomach noises. It's called *borborygmi,* basically the sounds that come from your digestive system as food, air and gas move through. To get an idea what's happening down there after a meal, think of the motion of a slithering snake. Bathed in stomach acid, your food is squeezed slightly forward and slightly back through your digestive tract, helping break the meal down and absorb nutrients, and sometimes creating noise. Within four to six hours, most of the food is emptied from the stomach, says Jorge Herrera, M.D., assistant professor of medicine at the University of South Alabama College of Medicine in Mobile and member of the American Gastroenterological Association and the American College of Gastroenterology.

Whether you've eaten or not, however, every one to two hours, there's a rush of digestive juices sweeping through the digestive tract to clear out anything that remains behind, says Dr. Herrera. This can also cause gurgling sounds, he says.

An upset stomach and irritable bowel syndrome can also cause stomach noises.

SYMPTOM RELIEF

If your stomach is trying to get your attention and you're tired of the turmoil, try these tips.

Sip some warm 7-Up. Warm 7-Up or ginger ale may be just what the doctor ordered for a gurgling stomach—if the gurgles are caused by gas or air, says Thomas A. Gossel, R.Ph., Ph.D., professor of pharmacology and toxicology and associate dean of the College of Pharmacy at Ohio

Northern University in Ada. Putting soda bubbles in your belly may help encourage gas trapped in your stomach to come up as a belch, says Dr. Gossel.

Sneak a snack. You probably don't have time for a meal, but sneaking a snack should silence your stomach. "If you're in a hurry, you could eat a cracker or a piece of bread. That could stop the noises from happening," says Dr. Gossel.

Don't gulp. Ever tried to take a deep breath to stop your stomach from gurgling? You may have made the situation worse, says Dr. Gossel. "You're just taking in more air—part of the problem in the first place. So if you do take a deep breath or yawn, try not to swallow the air."

For information on irritable bowel syndrome and other digestive problems that create discomfort along with gurgling noises, see Stomach Pain below.

STOMACH PAIN

WHEN TO SEE YOUR DOCTOR

- You experience sudden, severe abdominal pain.
- Pain persists for more than four days.
- You also have rectal bleeding or weight loss.
- You experience recurring abdominal pain and diarrhea.

WHAT YOUR SYMPTOM IS TELLING YOU

If yet another hot night at José's House of Jalapeños has you moaning in a foreign language, take heart—you're probably just suffering from an old-fashioned upset stomach. In a few days (at the most) you'll be ready for another el scorcho of a meal.

But let's assume for a moment that you played it safe

and opted for rice and beans, and you still have serious, lingering tummy trouble. What's causing it?

Don't bet the dinner check, but you could be suffering from an ulcer. Characterized by lesions on the inside of your digestive tract, ulcers come in all shapes and sizes—and locations. (In fact, stomach pain that is *relieved* for a short time by eating can be a symptom of a peptic or duodenal ulcer, which is located in your intestines.) Unlike a temporary upset stomach, however, ulcers keep coming back.

And while doctors aren't exactly sure what causes ulcers (recent evidence has linked them to pesky bacteria called *Helicobacter pylori* that live in your stomach), things like taking daily doses of aspirin or drinking too many cups of coffee each day could be making your ulcer worse.

"Certain medications—like aspirin—actually block the ability of the stomach to heal itself," says Jorge Herrera, M.D., assistant professor of medicine at the University of South Alabama College of Medicine in Mobile and member of the American Gastroenterological Association and the American College of Gastroenterology.

Then again, you might not have an ulcer. You could have plain old indigestion—your stomach lining's way of letting you know that it doesn't appreciate your dinner choices. Among the most common causes: spicy and acidic foods—like José's legendary jalapeños.

Another cause of abdominal pain—irritable bowel syndrome—is the mark of an angry digestive system. No ulcers here, just intestines having trouble moving your food through your body. A telltale sign of irritable bowel syndrome is abdominal pain accompanied by diarrhea or constipation and bloating. Pain relief follows a trip to the bathroom, but the pain returns again and again.

Food poisoning is another possible pain trigger. You might have absentmindedly eaten a chicken salad sandwich that's been sitting in your refrigerator a few too many days, but your intestines will know the difference.

And then there's gas. Air swallowed during chewing, or methane produced during digestion of foods like beans, can get trapped in your digestive system and cause discomfort until it's released by belching or breaking wind.

Unfortunately, a number of digestive diseases that can bring on sudden attacks of severe abdominal pain are also fairly common. These include ulcerative colitis, Crohn's disease, gallbladder disease, appendicitis, diverticulitis and pancreatitis.

SYMPTOM RELIEF

You should see your doctor—soon—for any sharp, intense abdominal pains. The causes of sharp and recurring pain are often serious and should receive medical attention.

But there are a few things you can try on your own for a minor bout of abdominal discomfort.

Take some tea. The tannic acid in a cup of brewed tea apparently helps rid the body of some of the bacteria or chemicals that can cause stomach pain, especially if you also have diarrhea, says Thomas A. Gossel, R.Ph., Ph.D., professor of pharmacology and toxicology and associate dean of the College of Pharmacy at Ohio Northern University in Ada. "You should feel relief in about an hour or so," he says.

Try an antacid. Nearly all over-the-counter antacids contain ingredients that do a good job of neutralizing excess stomach acid, says Wendell Clarkston, M.D., an assistant professor and director of the Fellowship Training Program in Gastroenterology and Hepatology at Saint Louis University School of Medicine. (For other hints and tips on banishing stomach acid, see Heartburn on page 298.)

Banishing Ulcer Pain

Doctors may not be exactly sure what causes ulcers, but they have a good idea of how to get rid of them. Try these techniques.

Use the right medication. A variety of prescription H2 antagonists and other medications actually block the stomach's ability to produce or secrete acid, says Dr. Herrera. Research shows that these powerful drugs have a 95 to 98 percent healing rate over six to eight weeks. "I think most people should use this as their main therapy." he says.

Team up with Tagamet. Prescription-only drugs like Tagamet or Zantac actually shut off the production of the acid that provokes stomach ulcers, says William B. Ruderman, M.D., chairperson of the Department of Gastroenterology at the Cleveland Clinic– Florida in Fort Lauderdale.

Ask for an antibiotic. If you have persistent abdominal pain and diarrhea, you may need a prescription antibiotic to help knock out the bacteria that has taken up residence in your stomach lining, says Dr. Clarkston.

Sip some milk. Drinking a glass of skim milk during an ulcer attack may provide quick relief. "Milk works like an antacid. When it gets to the stomach, it neutralizes the acid and the pain will go away," says Dr. Herrera. Use caution, however: Some people who drink milk for ulcer pain report feeling even worse a short time later, says Dr. Herrera.

Eat smart. Doctors learned long ago that spicy foods, like Mexican food, or acidic delights, like pickles, don't cause ulcers. But they can make an already angry ulcer feel worse. "The ulcer tissue is more sensitive and hurts more when you eat spicy or acidic foods," says Dr. Ruderman. You don't have to stick to a bland diet, but stay away from foods that turn on the burn.

Cut the cups. Once again, there's no hard evidence that big-time coffee drinkers are going to get an ulcer, but coffee can aggravate one, says Dr. Herrera. "As a rule, we tell patients to use caffeine in moderation—maybe no more than two or three cups of caffeine-containing drinks per day."

Avoid too much aspirin. Research shows that excessive use of the active ingredient in aspirin—salicylic acid—actually wears away the lining of the stomach and causes it to bleed, says Dr. Herrera. "If you take aspirin for two to three days because you have a cold or headache, you'll be okay. But if you take it on a daily basis for more than three months or so—that's when you run into problems," he says. Ask your doctor or pharmacist to recommend alternatives that won't irritate your stomach.

Stop smoking. Nicotine damages the lining of the stomach and makes ulcers worse, says Dr. Herrera. Get professional help to quit if you have to.

Dealing with Irritable Bowel Syndrome

The bad news about irritable bowel syndrome is that it's still a bit of a mystery. The good news is that by the time you're diagnosed with it, all serious health problems have already been ruled out, says Dr. Herrera. To manage the problem, try these tips.

Don't panic. Because it's often tough to determine the cause of irritable bowel syndrome, you need to be patient while your doctor searches for an explanation. "When all the tests are negative and no one can tell you what's going on, it's natural to get worried," says Dr. Herrera.

Fill up on fiber. Not only are vegetables and whole grains loaded with nutrients, they can also help prevent constipation and tame your irritable bowel. "You just don't get enough fiber every day from hamburgers," says Dr. Clarkston. If the thought of chewing all those veggies makes you feel like a rabbit, consider one of the many over-the-counter fiber supplements. From tablets and wafers to powders that you add to juice, most are available at drugstores and supermarkets.

Cut the fat. Fatty foods also have been linked to irritable bowel syndrome, says Dr. Herrera.

Give zip the slip. Spicy foods have been known to cause their share of problems, says Dr. Herrera.

Try the elimination diet. Although not all stomach doctors agree, some gastroenterologists believe that irritable bowel syndrome may be caused by an allergy to certain foods. You can try an elimination diet to determine whether a food allergy could be contributing to your problem, says Dr. Herrera. Milk, eggs, wheat, corn, soy, peanuts, citrus fruits, colas and chocolate are some of the most common foods that cause allergic reactions. During an elimination diet, you avoid one group of foods at a time, carefully monitoring yourself for symptoms. If your symptoms disappear, you may have found the culprit.

Ask about medication. If you suffer from persistent irritable bowel syndrome, ask your doctor about antispasmodics, which prevent spasms by relaxing intestinal muscles, for use during severe episodes, says Dr. Clarkston.

STOOL, BLACK

WHAT YOUR SYMPTOM IS TELLING YOU

Your stool is black. But that's no reason for your mood to be. Maybe you've eaten a couple of helpings of your Aunt Debbie's prize-winning beets. Perhaps you've been taking iron supplements. Or you enjoyed a package of chewy black licorice. Maybe you overdid the feasting altogether and then turned to a bottle of Pepto-Bismol for relief. All four items have been known to turn stools black, says Barry Jaffin, M.D., a specialist in gastrointestinal motility disorders and a clinical instructor in the Department of Gastroenterology at Mount Sinai Hospital in New York City.

But's there also a strong likelihood that your stools are black because they contain blood. Bloody stools are a warning sign of some potentially serious digestive diseases that need medical attention. For the lowdown on bloody stools and what to do about it, see below.

STOOL, BLOODY

WHEN TO SEE YOUR DOCTOR

- See your doctor any time you see blood in your stool.

WHAT YOUR SYMPTOM IS TELLING YOU

If you had red pepper in your salad last night, there's a slight chance that it made the treacherous journey through your digestive system and emerged as red as ever.

But generally speaking, when you see something red in your stools, you don't need a medical degree to know what it is.

"If you see something that looks like blood in your stool, with rare exceptions, it's blood," says Samuel Labow, M.D., president of the American Society of Colon and Rectal Surgeons and a private practitioner in Great Neck, New York.

Perhaps the most common causes of blood in your stool or in your toilet bowl are hemorrhoids or an anal fissure, says Nicholas J. Talley, M.D., associate professor of medicine at the Mayo Clinic Medical School in Rochester, Minnesota. A hemorrhoid is a puffy little bit of tissue that's left its proper spot inside the rectum and protruded out where it's not supposed to be. Even just a little overambitious wiping or straining can make it bleed. Anal fissures are cracks in the skin surrounding the anus—also from straining.

In both cases, the blood is added to the stool on its way out. When blood is actually *in* the stool, a number of things could be responsible. If you're taking large amounts of aspirin or some other nonsteroidal anti-inflammatories for relief from arthritis, you may notice some blood in your stool, says Barry Jaffin, M.D., a specialist in gastrointestinal motility disorders and a clinical instructor in the Department of Gastroenterology at Mount Sinai Hospital in New York City. Many of these medications can irritate the stomach and small intestine and even cause ulcers, which may be painless, but *can* sometimes be bloody, he says.

Inflammatory bowel disease—a digestive disorder with no known cause—can also cause bloody stool. This condition is often accompanied by pain, says Dr. Jaffin.

Although less likely, bloody stool may also mean that you've developed a polyp or even a cancerous tumor in your colon. "Most of the small polyps don't show any signs at all, but when they get to a certain size, they bleed," says Dr. Labow. "If they are far enough up inside your colon, the blood will be on the surface of the stool and possibly mixed in the stool."

Diverticulosis can be another cause of bloody stool, although there's little doubt when you're suffering from it. Like a bulge in the side of a tire, diverticulosis is a weak spot in the colon wall that can sometimes bleed, says Dr.

Labow. When it does, the bleeding isn't something that you can ignore, he says. "You don't go to the bathroom and see a little bit of blood on the tissue, or a couple of drops of blood in the toilet bowl and say, 'Oh, that's my diverticulosis.' Diverticulosis by its nature will usually give you very, very significant bleeding. It's a hemorrhage," says Dr. Labow.

SYMPTOM RELIEF

If you had a bloody nose, you might stuff it with cotton gauze. If you cut your finger, an adhesive bandage would probably be in order. Your first line of defense against bloody stool: a phone call to your doctor.

"It's vital that you get bloody stool checked as soon as possible," says Dr. Talley.

Here are a few things you should be aware of.

Wash it down. One of the easiest ways to end the straining that can cause the hemorrhoids or anal fissures that sometimes result in bloody stool is by drinking more fluids. In fact, drinking between six and ten eight-ounce glasses of fluids—like juice or water—a day will actually help prevent constipation, says Dr. Jaffin. (For more tips on putting an end to constipation, see page 128.)

Alter your medications. If you're taking aspirin or some other anti-inflammatory painkiller for arthritis, you should discuss your medications with your doctor.

Expect tests. Once you say okay to a gut check, your doctor will probably perform a sigmoidoscopy. During this office procedure, your doctor will use the magic of fiber optics to look inside your colon for whatever might be causing the problem, says Dr. Jaffin.

STOOL, STRAINING AT

WHAT YOUR SYMPTOM IS TELLING YOU

While genius has been described as 1 percent inspiration and 99 percent perspiration, here's one case where a little *less* effort may make for a true masterpiece—and a lot fewer health problems.

That's because straining at stools—trying too hard to relieve yourself—can be downright dangerous. "You could actually get a tear right at the opening of the anal canal (called an anal fissure) when you really strain, causing pain and bright red rectal bleeding," says Samuel Labow, M.D., president of the American Society of Colon and Rectal Surgeons and a private practitioner in Great Neck, New York. "Without question, straining with a bowel movement can also make hemorrhoids swell and bleed, increasing your discomfort."

Years of excessive straining may actually push your rectum inside out, weakening your anal muscles and, ultimately, causing you to lose control of your bowel movements, says Richard Billingham, M.D., a clinical assistant professor in the Department of Surgery at the University of Washington in Seattle. "Once it has fallen out, your rectum is subject to injury even from just wiping after a bowel movement," says Dr. Billingham.

Straining can also cause a hernia, which may make it even more difficult to move your bowels, he says.

So much for why you shouldn't strain. The appropriate question at this point is, why *do* you strain? And the answer, in a word, is constipation.

SYMPTOM RELIEF

Your best bet to prevent straining is preventing yourself from becoming constipated in the first place, says Dr. Labow.

"Don't accept the fact that sitting on the toilet for 45 minutes to an hour is the way the world goes to the bathroom," says Dr. Labow. "It's not."

See also Constipation

STOOL LOOSENESS

WHAT YOUR SYMPTOM IS TELLING YOU

Doctors say there's virtually no difference between loose stools and a case of diarrhea.

"They're basically the same thing with similar causes," says Barry Jaffin, M.D., a gastrointestinal motility disorder specialist and clinical instructor in the Department of Gastroenterology at Mount Sinai Hospital in New York City.

See also Diarrhea

STOOL PALENESS

WHEN TO SEE YOUR DOCTOR

- You're also experiencing abdominal pain.
- You detect a slight yellow cast to your skin or the whites of your eyes.
- You're also losing weight.

WHAT YOUR SYMPTOM IS TELLING YOU

A consistent lack of color from this part of life's palette can be a clue that you have digestive trouble brewing.

Of course, gobbling massive amounts of applesauce, rice or other light-colored fare will cause pale stool for a day or so. But if you've noticed over a week's worth of pale stool, something else is to blame.

In a healthy gut, dark-colored bile flows from your liver into your intestines. Once there, the bile eagerly helps digest fat. It also adds color to your stool, says Barry Jaffin, M.D., a specialist in motility disorders and a clinical instructor in the Department of Gastroenterology at Mount Sinai Hospital in New York City.

If the stool isn't dark, then the proper amount of bile is not reaching the intestine. A gallstone or a growth could be blocking a bile duct, forcing bile pigment into the bloodstream. Liver disease, often caused by the hepatitis virus, can also cause pale stool, along with a considerable amount of pain. And a malfunctioning pancreas has also been linked to pale stool.

SYMPTOM RELIEF

Don't panic at the first sign of pale stool. But if your stool is pale and your urine dark for several days in a row, see your doctor, says Nicholas J. Talley, M.D., associate professor of medicine at the Mayo Clinic Medical School in Rochester, Minnesota. This is not something you can deal with on your own. Expect a battery of tests that look at your digestive system to help pinpoint the problem.

STUTTERING

WHEN TO SEE YOUR DOCTOR

- You begin stuttering for the first time as an adult.
- Periods of stuttering begin to occur more often, or talking seems to require more effort or sound strained.
- As a parent, you are worried about your child's speech.

WHAT YOUR SYMPTOM IS TELLING YOU

If you have a child who starts to stutter, the first thing to remember is that he's in illustrious company. Winston Churchill, Marilyn Monroe, Carly Simon and James Earl Jones—to mention just a few famous stutterers—each struggled with the problem.

Stuttering usually does begin in childhood, and it occurs more often in boys than girls. In fact, boys are four times as likely to stutter—and the stuttering usually begins just when kids are developing language abilities. It's normal for kids to repeat words, such as, "I want-want-want that cookie." But a child who stutters repeats *sounds* instead of words—as in "I w-w-w-want that cookie." Doctors say that a child who repeats word *sounds* more than two times is beginning to stutter.

While researchers are still uncertain about the exact causes of stuttering, they suspect there is a genetic predisposition—it tends to run in families. The child who develops persistent stuttering may be experiencing major stress in the home, or he might start stuttering when he's tremendously excited. Either cause can trigger the beginning of stuttering in a child who has inherited the tendency. But stuttering is *never* the child's fault, according to doctors, so it's essential that the child should not be blamed by parents or teachers.

In adults, the onset of temporary stuttering is very rare, and usually, it's a signal that you need a doctor's attention. The stuttering may come after a mini-stroke, called a transient ischemic attack (TIA). In rare cases, a head injury or encephalitis—inflammation of the brain—may cause someone to stutter who has never had a problem before. If you suddenly begin stuttering, consider it a warning signal and see a doctor immediately.

SYMPTOM RELIEF

The child who begins to stutter will need a speech therapist rather than a doctor. But professional therapy is only a starting point. The more that parents, teachers and friends can help, the easier things will be for child—not just in childhood, but as an adult as well. Stuttering sometimes goes away on its own, but there are many ways children can be helped to deal with it and feel more in control of their speech.

Here are some pointers on the right way to help a child who stutters.

Get professional help. The ideal time to get help from a speech therapist is when a young preschooler is beginning to stutter, but not yet fighting with it or reacting to it, says C. Woodruff Starkweather, Ph.D., professor of speech, language and hearing at Temple University in Philadelphia. "If you treat children before they enter school, it is usually completely effective," he says. The therapist is likely to tell you to bring in the child for periodic evaluations and counsel you on how to deal with the problem at home.

Listen for the meaning. "Make sure you listen closely when your child talks," advises Charles Diggs, Ph.D., director of consumer affairs for the American Speech-Language-Hearing Association in Rockville, Maryland. "And sit down and speak directly to your child. Show your child through touch that you are listening and that you care. What's important is to listen for *what* your child is trying to tell you, not the *way* it is said."

Don't be a fast talker. If your normal pace of speech is rapid, try to consciously slow down, suggests Dr. Diggs. You provide a good model for your child to follow when *he* speaks—and at the slower pace, you also give him more attention. That creates a better atmosphere for communicating with your child, according to Dr. Diggs.

Create a calm communication zone. "Be sure to give your child a period of undivided attention each day, without competition from other children," advises John Haskell, Ed.D., adjunct assistant professor of speech pathology at Columbia University Teachers College and a speech language pathologist in private practice in New York City. When there are conflicts among siblings, you may have to step in to control them and calm the other kids down. Be sure the child who stutters always gets a turn to speak.

Have a bedside chat. "Have a lot of quiet talks with your child," says Dr. Haskell. A conversation that only lasts 5 or 10 minutes is fine—but try to have these chats as frequently as possible during the week. "A daily private time with quiet, *relaxed* talk about the child's interests will help a lot," says Dr. Haskell. Talk about things that interest your child, but keep the conversation relaxed and undemanding. Or read a story aloud and talk about what's happening in the story. "But avoid asking direct questions, like 'What did you do today?' "

Banish the taboo. A child may feel as if his stutter is an unmentionable topic, just because no one *does* mention it. Parents can end this taboo by using the direct approach. "Talk about stuttering with your child," Dr. Starkweather says. "Give emotional support in words the child can understand, like 'That was sticky for you to say, wasn't it?' " If you encourage your child to talk about speech, he'll realize that he's allowed to discuss it as much as he wants to.

STY

WHEN TO SEE YOUR DOCTOR

- Your sty lasts more than a week.
- Your sty is accompanied by blurred vision.
- A hard lump (chalazion) develops on the lid itself.

WHAT YOUR SYMPTOM IS TELLING YOU

A sty is a lot like a pimple. It's swollen, red and sometimes painful, and it gives you that same sinking feeling when you look in the mirror. The only thing that distinguishes it, really, is its particularly sensitive location.

Sties are the result of an infected oil gland at the base of the eyelash. You can get more than one sty at a time or several in succession because the infection can spread from one hair follicle to others. Infection can occur, for example, when a contaminated mascara or makeup brush gives bacteria a free ride into the oily pores along the lashes. People who have super-oily skin or scalp may be sty-prone, just as they may be acne-prone, according to Kenneth Kauvar, M.D., assistant clinical professor of ophthalmology at the University of Colorado School of Medicine in Denver and author of *Eyes Only*.

SYMPTOM RELIEF

Like pimples, sties are usually harmless and disappear on their own, says Dr. Kauvar. Here's how you can help clear them up.

Drain, don't squeeze. "Popping a sty could push bacteria into your bloodstream and transport the infection to the brain," says Dr. Kauvar. Instead, drain the sty naturally and promote healing blood flow by applying a warm washcloth to your closed lid, he advises. Apply the washcloth for 15 minutes four times a day. You should notice improvement in a day or so, says Dr. Kauvar.

Take it to the doctor. If the sty worsens or remains after a week, your doctor can prescribe an antibiotic or steroid to reduce inflammation or lance the sty in a painless office procedure.

Keep a clean upper lid. As with facial acne, you need to keep your eyelids clean and oil-free, especially if you have recurrent sties, says Dr. Kauvar. "The easiest way to do this is to dip a cotton swab in diluted baby shampoo and use it to clean the base of the lashes," he says.

Take a break from eye makeup. Resume applying eye makeup only after your sty is gone. And toss the mascara you were using before the sty appeared and replace all eye makeup brushes to prevent further infection.

Ditch that dandruff. Dandruff can fall onto eyelids and trigger a sty, says Dr. Kauvar. (If dandruff is a problem, see page 139.)

SWALLOWING PROBLEMS

WHEN TO SEE YOUR DOCTOR

- You have difficulty swallowing that persists more than a day or two.
- You choke when you try to swallow.
- You also have ear pain and you are coughing up blood.

WHAT YOUR SYMPTOM IS TELLING YOU

Swallowing is one of those things you hardly think about—until you have trouble doing it.

But you think about it plenty when it hurts to swallow, eating becomes awkward because it is hard to swallow or you feel a strange sensation or "lump" in your throat.

Swallowing is as natural as breathing. Your throat muscles go through this motion hundreds of times a day both to take in food and drink and to move along the flow of saliva and mucus your body continually produces. When you swallow, the circular muscle at the upper end of the esophagus, called the sphincter, relaxes, allowing whatever has gone through your mouth and throat to pass on into your digestive system.

Since it takes relaxation of the sphincter to make this process run smoothly, it stands to reason that a body that is not relaxed as a result of tension, stress or stage fright can tighten the throat. As the saying goes: "That's hard to swallow."

Other reasons for a swallowing difficulty can be just as innocuous. Chronic irritation of the throat—particularly by dry indoor air in winter—can make it hard to swallow, especially when you first wake up. And if you're not drinking enough fluids, your throat will become dry, making swallowing uncomfortable. And difficulty swallowing is part of the package of a sore throat or the flu.

If you're a smoker, consider cigarettes the prime suspect.

If you're a smoker and your swallowing problems are also accompanied by hacking and pain, consider it a serious symptom that needs evaluation by a doctor.

Feel like you have a lump in your throat? It's quite likely the cause is acid reflux, a glitch in the digestive system in which stomach acid leaks back into the esophagus because of a sphincter muscle that doesn't always want to stay closed when it should. You can figure that acid reflux is your problem if you also have heartburn.

In rare instances, swallowing difficulty can be caused by a physical abnormality, such as a spasm of the sphincter muscle. And acid reflux can interfere with swallowing if you have an ulcer. Difficulty swallowing can sometimes be the first sign of a tumor.

SYMPTOM RELIEF

If you're a smoker and you are having trouble eating or swallowing, you should get checked out by your doctor. Also, any suspicious swallowing symptom that you cannot connect to stress, the air or your personal habits should be brought to the attention of your doctor. But for those things that you can control, here's what to do.

De-stress yourself. Stress and tension can sometimes make life itself hard to swallow. Anything that brings on relaxation—exercise, massage, meditation, yoga, deep breathing—can all release the pressure on your throat, says Michael Benninger, M.D., chairman of the Department of Otolaryngology-Head and Neck Surgery at Henry Ford Hospital in Detroit. Putting a warm compress on your throat during tense moments can also ease the uneasiness in your throat.

Humidify and hydrate. Because many swallowing problems are caused or made worse by dryness in the throat, putting extra moisture—both inside and outside the body—can be helpful, says Dr. Benninger. Most experts recommend drinking at least eight full glasses of water daily. "And check your furnace gauge," says Dr. Benninger. "You need about 35 to 40 percent humidity in the air. A bedroom humidifier will help. Though the benefits of warm and cool humdifiers are still being debated, the cool-mist models feel better to the throat."

Treat the reflux. If you suspect you have acid reflux, there are plenty of things you can do to control the condition, including cutting out caffeine, alcohol, chocolate, wine and tobacco, says Dr. Benninger. (For other tips on banishing reflux, see Heartburn on page 298.)

Examine your anatomy. Although physical abnormalities are rare, your doctor may want to put you through a few tests to rule them out, says Charles Krause, M.D., chief of medical affairs at the University of Michigan Medical Center in Ann Arbor. In one test you drink a chalky liquid containing barium so that your throat and esophagus can be x-rayed. If the cause proves to be a spasm of the esophageal sphincter muscle, the first approach would be a prescription for muscle relaxants, says Dr. Krause. Next, the muscle can be relaxed by insertion of a stretching instrument, a procedure that's usually done in the doctor's office.

"This often brings permanent relief," Dr. Krause says. In more severe cases, a surgeon can divide the sphincter muscle so it will stay relaxed.

Congenital problems and a condition called Zenker's diverticulum—in which the lining of the esophagus forms a pouch that interferes with swallowing—may also be corrected surgically.

SWEATING

WHEN TO SEE YOUR DOCTOR

- Sweat continually soaks and soils your clothes and shoes or trickles down your skin even when the room is cold.
- Sweating impacts on your career or personal life.
- You are also experiencing persistent or recurrent fever, dizziness or rapid heartbeat.
- The sweat has a color, crystallizes on the skin or causes skin irritations.

WHAT YOUR SYMPTOM IS TELLING YOU

Let's face it: We all perspire, but some people just plain *sweat*. In buckets. If you're one of them, you don't need anyone to tell you; your wet clothes are probably doing that.

Almost all sweating is triggered by heat, humidity, stress or anxiety; it's the body's means of regulating its temperature. Most excessive sweaters simply have a genetic predisposition to produce a bit more coolant in response to these normal stimuli. It's not a medical problem; their sweat glands are just more exuberant.

Sweating is a perfectly normal side effect of puberty, menstruation, menopause and other hormonal changes. Physical exertion, hot and spicy food, alcohol and smoking are other common causes of perspiration attacks.

On the more serious side, excessive sweating can occur as a result of an infection. "This can be anything from the common cold to a more serious underlying disorder, either of which can produce constant or intermittent fevers," says Hinda Greene, D.O., staff physician of internal medicine with Cleveland Clinic–Florida in Fort Lauderdale. "Sweating is the body's way of dissipating the heat of a fever."

Among the laundry list of conditions that bring on those feverish sweats is Hodgkins' disease, tuberculosis, overactive thyroid, heart disease, cancer, pneumonia, malaria and liver and kidney disease.

SYMPTOM RELIEF

If you don't want to go with the flow, the following are some doctor-recommended remedies that'll leave you high and dry.

Dress cool. "Dress in light, loose-fitting, natural fabrics like cotton to absorb perspiration and let cool air in and warm air out," says R. Kenneth Landow, M.D., clinical associate professor in the Department of Medicine and Dermatology at the University of Southern California in Los Angeles. "Man-made fibers such as rayon, nylon and polyester will not absorb perspiration or provide ventilation."

Roll out the antiperspirant. Careful. Deodorants are not antiperspirants, but a deodorant may *contain* an antiperspirant. Most over-the-counter anti-wetness products work well. "The most effective ones contain aluminum chlorohydrate or some other aluminum salt to block the ducts of the sweat glands," says Dr. Landow. "It can be applied to any affected area: the hand, foot, body, even the forehead." Stronger antiperspirants, like Drysol (aluminum chloride), have higher concentrations of these aluminum salts and are available by prescription.

Apply it, don't spray it. Sticks and roll-ons provide more protection and greater coverage than aerosols, says Selma Targovnik, M.D., staff dermatologist at Good Samaritan Medical Center in Phoenix. Dry yourself off thoroughly before applying your antiperspirant—moisture will dilute its effectiveness. If using a liquid roll-on, shake it well. The active ingredients may have settled to the bottom.

Zap your glands. "We now have a technique called iontophoresis in which we apply a weak electric current to problem areas to constrict the sweat ducts and keep sweating under control," says Stephen Z. Smith, M.D., a dermatologist in private practice and clinical instructor in the Department of Dermatology at the University of Louisville School of Medicine in Kentucky. "These devices are used at home under a physician's direction and can cost several hundred dollars." A similar device called the Drionic is available without a prescription for about $125, but it uses a much weaker current. These nonprescription devices are not as effective, but they're certainly worth a try.

Rub on some alcohol. "A little rubbing alcohol will constrict the pores and hold back sweating for several hours," says Dr. Landow. "This should only be done occasionally because excessive use of rubbing alcohol could cause severe skin drying and irritation."

Take a powder. "For some, it is sufficient to just sprinkle on a lot of powder—baby powder, cornstarch, baking soda, etc." says Dr. Landow. "It doesn't prevent sweating, but it absorbs much of the moisture and leaves you feeling drier."

Immerse yourself in water. Got a job interview and want to avoid sweaty palms or underarms? According to Dr.

Targovnik, soaking in cool water will temporarily curb your sweats. A 30-minute soak of the affected parts will shrink pores enough to provide about three hours of wetness protection.

Avoid hot, spicy foods. One reason you sweat every afternoon could be that bean burrito with extra sauce you eat for lunch. Or the soup. Or all that hot coffee. Cut back on those foods that can turn your stomach into a furnace and your body will reduce its perspiration buildup, says Dr. Smith. Finding out which foods turn up your internal thermostat may call for a little experimentation. Try eliminating suspected offenders one at a time, beginning with the most obvious: spicy foods.

Bag the booze and butts. They're not just unhealthy habits, but sweaty ones, too. "Alcohol tends to dilate the vessels in the skin, increasing your body heat, and tobacco increases your body's levels of adrenaline, both of which will make you sweat more," says Dr. Landow.

As a last resort, consider surgery. If all else fails, and you're desperate for relief, you might want to discuss three possible surgical procedures with your doctor. One is a sympathectomy, in which the nerves connected to the sweat glands are severed. The second removes the glands themselves from the affected area. And in the third, liposuction, the glands are sucked out of your skin tissue through a small tube. Dr. Landow warns that all three have risks, including scarring and nerve damage, and in many cases, sweating returns within two years.

SWELLING

WHEN TO SEE YOUR DOCTOR

- An unexplained or relatively small swelling persists for more than one day. (Larger swollen areas should be seen immediately.)
- The swelling is discolored or numb or hinders your movement.
- The swelling follows a bite from a spider, snake or insect.
- The swelling is caused by a burn that forms blisters or breaks the skin.
- See your doctor immediately if swelling occurs in your throat or neck, you have any trouble breathing or you feel dizzy or faint.

WHAT YOUR SYMPTOM IS TELLING YOU

If you've ever been laughed at, picked on or made fun of, you know how easy it is for a personal insult to make your thoughts swell up in anger. When it comes to sensitivity, however, even the most delicate of egos can't compare with our skin. It, too, gets its fair share of insults of the *physical* type—anything from the trauma of a hard blow to a bee sting to some irritant that just rubs it the wrong way. But while you may bite your tongue and let an insult roll off your back, your skin is not so willing to turn the other cheek.

Your ticked off hide has no reservations about letting the world know that it's mightily peeved and wastes no time in responding with a quick and furious comeback. But instead of lashing out and screaming with rage, the skin vents its wrath by blowing up like a balloon.

Your once-peaceful skin becomes a hotbed of activity. "Insult to the skin triggers a variety of reactions as a self-defense mechanism," says William Dexter, M.D., assistant professor of clinical community and family medicine at the

Dartmouth-Hitchcock Medical Center in Lebanon, New Hampshire. "Vessels and capillaries dilate and expand as the body tries to rush more blood to the area. Fluid can leak from these vessels and collect in the skin tissue. Cells also migrate to the site of the insult and release substances like histamines, which stimulate inflammation by attracting more cells. And the body's immune system goes into overdrive producing additional cells to fight off infection and repair damaged tissues."

What kinds of things stimulate this inflammatory process? Plenty! We've already discussed skin damage from trauma. Now imagine a more subtle sneak attack on the skin. "Anywhere there is a break in the skin, foreign agents like bacteria, fungi or viruses can invade and cause an infection called a cellulitis," says Kevin Ferentz, M.D., assistant professor of family medicine at the University of Maryland School of Medicine in Baltimore. "These can occur either at the site of entry or the invaders can migrate elsewhere throughout the skin."

Sometimes skin is hypersensitive to certain substances and mere contact is enough to send it into a tizzy. Dermatologists call this tizzy *contact dermatitis*. The resulting inflammation can be produced in two ways. An *irritant dermatitis* often results from exposure to or repeated usage of harsh soaps, detergents and other chemicals, usually on the hands. A *contact allergy* is an allergic response to anything from cosmetics to jewelry to plants like poison ivy.

The causes of *atopic dermatitis* or eczema are not so well known. This chronic, recurring eruption, accompanied by itchy, red, scaly patches, is believed to be inherited and may be related to eating certain foods.

Foods and medications can also cause some people to suddenly break out into a series of swollen, itchy skin lumps called hives or urticaria. These swollen patches, lasting minutes to hours, represent an allergic response to such drugs as aspirin and penicillin, and such foods as strawberries, tomatoes and shellfish. In it's most serious form, urticaria can develop into what is called anaphylaxis—a life-threatening emergency in which the throat and lungs swell and fill up with fluid.

SYMPTOM RELIEF

Prolonged skin swelling can lead to tissue damage, so it is important to bring it under control quickly. Try these swell-stoppers.

Chill it and raise it. Cool baths, or a bag of ice applied to the swollen area for 15 minutes at a time several times a day will encourage blood vessels to constrict, says Jeffrey S. Dover, M.D., chief of dermatology at New England Deaconess Hospital in Boston and assistant professor of dermatology at Harvard Medical School. This constriction reduces most kinds of swelling. Also, keeping the swollen area elevated will help drain fluids and bring down the inflammation.

Apply heat for cellulitis. Warm, moist towels wrapped around the area of a cellulitis infection will bring more blood to the area and help control the spread of bacteria and other infectious microbes and may bring this type of swelling under control, says Dr. Ferentz. Heat should be applied for 15 to 20 minutes at a time and can be repeated every few hours.

Cream it with hydrocortisone. Most topical medications won't help much for swelling from contact dermatitis. The lone exception is a 0.5 to 1 percent hydrocortisone cream available in drugstores. The cream will help ease minor inflammation and itching, says Lawrence C. Parish, M.D., clinical professor of dermatology at Jefferson Medical College of Thomas Jefferson University in Philadelphia. But it should not be used if there is an infection present; it will only worsen it.

Double-check your shopping list. And your wardrobe. And your accessories. If you have any new products in your home or at work that are coming in contact with your skin, they may be causing a skin allergy and need to be replaced, says Stephen M. Schleicher, M.D., clinical instructor of dermatology at Temple University Medical School and Philadelphia College of Osteopathic Medicine and co-director of The Dermatology Center in Philadelphia. "Sometimes just stopping the contact is all that's needed to stop the swelling," he says.

Wear gloves. If you come into contact with a lot of chemicals and substances that can cause irritation, like detergents or industrial oils, put on some protective outer gear like rubber gloves, boots and aprons. But be careful: Sometimes these products are treated with formaldehyde or made of latex, both of which can be irritants.

Take an antihistamine. Many good over-the-counter oral medications are available that will bring down swelling, says Dr. Dover. Among the ones he recommends are the antihistamines Chlor-Trimeton and Benadryl.

Ask about oral antibiotics. Most skin infections do not respond to topical medications and will have to be treated by taking oral antibiotics as prescribed by your doctor, says Dr. Ferentz.

Avoid aspirin and anesthetics. Aspirin is considered an anti-inflammatory drug, but it can actually worsen swelling by encouraging bleeding, says Dr. Dexter. And topical anesthetics like benzocaine will only aggravate swelling.

Avoid scratching and rubbing. Further irritation to the area will worsen the swelling. Keep your hands off and try to wear loose clothing that won't rub against the swelling, says Dr. Ferentz.

Remove stinger and clean. A stinger or any other foreign object left in the skin will continue to cause the skin to swell until it is removed. If it's sticking out of the skin, remove the stinger with tweezers then wash the wound with soap and water, suggests Dr. Ferentz. If the stinger is in deep, see your doctor to have it removed.

Treat your sting like beef. Sprinkling some Adolph's Tenderizer on a bee sting or mosquito bite can reduce some of its swelling as well as pain and itch, according to Dr. Parish.

T

TASTE LOSS

WHEN TO SEE YOUR DOCTOR

- See your doctor any time that you feel you have lost your sense of taste.

WHAT YOUR SYMPTOM IS TELLING YOU

Remember when you tried your new recipe for that delicately flavored carrot soup—how marvelously *interesting* it tasted? Thank your nose for that memory.

The taste buds on your tongue are actually quite limited—they recognize only four tastes: sweet, salty, bitter and sour. It's your *nose* that sniffs out the subtleties of flavor. (That's why you should be sure to read Smell Loss on page 567, after you've finished this chapter. The same factors that cause you to lose your sense of smell will often interfere with your sense of taste.)

In fact, 80 to 90 percent of people who think they've lost their sense of taste *haven't*—they've actually lost their sense of smell. For those other 10 to 20 percent, the problem *is* with their taste buds, and it can be caused by (hold on to your hat—we're about to throw another sense into the mix) ear infections or middle-ear surgery. That's because a major nerve for the taste buds passes through the middle ear. These ear problems don't cause an outright loss of taste sensation, but they do cause strange tastes in your mouth. (Most taste problems reduce or distort your sense of taste. It's rare for your sense of taste to vanish completely.)

A yeast (candidiasis) or fungal infection of the tongue can also play tricks with your taste buds. Poor oral hygiene, tooth infections and cavities can blunt your ability to taste.

611

And if you're using antibiotics, a mouth infection called glossitis can dull your palate.

Too little iron in your diet can lead to anemia, which can cause a tongue inflammation that interferes with your sense of taste, says James Stankiewicz, M.D., an otolaryngologist at Loyola University Medical Center in Maywood, Illinois. Researchers have also found that deficiencies in vitamin B12, folate and zinc can cause problems with taste.

And if you light up a cigarette after a dinner that's low in these nutrients, you're in double trouble: Smoking can burn out your taste buds.

People who have been through radiation therapy for cancer often report a loss of taste, as do those who've had major head injuries. Upper respiratory infections can also lead to loss of taste. And, rarely, tumors of the oral cavity, brain or brainstem can damage the sense of taste.

Symptom Relief

As with loss of smell, in many cases your loss of taste will reverse on its own or with help from your doctor. Here are ways to spice up your taste experience.

Use spice—twice. "Switch to highly spiced foods if you feel taste is a problem," suggests Donald Leopold, M.D., an otolaryngologist at Johns Hopkins University's Francis Scott Key Medical Center in Baltimore. "Make liberal use of hot, sour and bitter flavors, such as mustards, hot pepper, chilies and lemon juice for eating enjoyment."

Delight your dentist. Renew your commitment to proper oral hygiene, suggests William H. Friedman, M.D., an otolaryngologist, facial plastic surgeon and director of the Park Central Institute in St. Louis. Make a point of getting regular dental checkups, and while you're there, ask for instructions in proper brushing and flossing techniques.

Quit smoking. "Smoking itself is a very common cause of blunting of the sense of taste," Dr. Friedman says. Smoking causes inflammation, which gets worse the more you smoke. Give up the habit and your food will taste better.

Get enough vitamins and minerals. To make sure you're getting adequate amounts of vitamins and minerals—especially iron—consider taking a daily multivitamin supplement.

"Take iron supplements only as recommended by your doctor," suggests Dr. Stankiewicz. "B12 injections and prescription zinc medications are also available from your doctor." Over-the-counter zinc medications are not recommended, he says.

Wash away mouth infections. If glossitis develops while you're taking antibiotics for another infection, using a salt mouthwash can ease the assault on your taste buds.

"Use one tablespoon salt in an eight-ounce tumbler of warm water to relieve glossitis," Dr. Friedman suggests. If that doesn't do the trick, your doctor may recommend a prescription antifungal mouthwash. Prescription mouthwashes or lozenges can also clear up a yeast infection in the mouth, he says.

Give it time to heal. If you've had an ear infection, your dulled sense of taste should recover after you fully recover, says Richard Doty, Ph.D., director of the Smell and Taste Center at the University of Pennsylvania School of Medicine in Philadelphia. It just may take a while.

TEMPERATURE SENSITIVITY

WHEN TO SEE YOUR DOCTOR

- You usually feel colder or warmer than people around you.
- You feel hot for more than five days.
- You often feel tired, weak and irritable.
- You also have insomnia, brittle nails or a tremor in the fingers.
- Your weight fluctuates rapidly without changes in your diet.
- If you're a woman, you have abnormally heavy or light periods.

WHAT YOUR SYMPTOM IS TELLING YOU

Some people are just naturally more sensitive to warmth or cold than other people. If it's not a new problem, there's probably nothing wrong," says Peter Sigmann, M.D., an associate professor of internal medicine at the Medical College of Wisconsin in Milwaukee. "On the other hand, if it is a new problem, it could be a sign of anemia or a thyroid disorder."

Temperature sensitivity also could be a warning signal of a cold, any infection, menopause or a migraine.

Feeling cold is also a symptom of depression and its sad cousin, seasonal affective disorder (SAD), which afflicts people who are extremely sensitive to the reduced sunlight of winter. People who have SAD often have scrambled body temperature rhythms. "For most of us, our minimum body temperature occurs at about 3:00 a.m. But people with SAD have an altered rhythm. Their minimum temperature is usually pushed forward to around 6:00 a.m. So when they wake up, they feel very cold. Physiologically, it feels like the middle of the night to them," says David Avery, M.D., an associate professor of psychiatry and behavioral sciences at the University of Washington School of Medicine in Seattle.

SYMPTOM RELIEF

Fortunately, temperature sensitivity is usually a minor problem that is easily relieved. Here are some things you can try.

Check your temperature. Heat or cold sensitivity may be a sign of a fever. So the first thing you should do is take your temperature, Dr. Sigmann says. Take it at bedtime, when there is less chance of temperature fluctuation, he suggests. If you do have a fever, get some rest and drink plenty of liquids. (See Fever on page 219 for more tips.)

Scope out your drugs. Certain medications, like beta blockers used to treat high blood pressure, heart disease, migraines and thyroid diseases, can make your hands and feet more sensitive to cold. Ask your doctor about the side effects of the drugs you're taking and if an alternative medication would be better for you.

Brighten up your day. If you feel cold and depressed in the morning, Dr. Avery suggests you try resetting your biological clock by taking a 15- to 20-minute walk after sunrise soon after awakening, three times a week. "Morning is the best time to receive light exposure because that's when the biological clock is most easily reset," he says. "Once you reset it, you might wake up more refreshed and less temperature sensitive."

Iron it out. "Iron deficiency is the most common cause of anemia, especially among women who have heavy periods and have poor diets. If you get anemic, you may frequently feel cold," Dr. Sigmann says. To prevent anemia, eat plenty of iron-loaded foods like lean meat and turkey, tuna, broccoli and potatoes. If you are iron deficient in spite of a good diet, your doctor may want to check for intestinal problems.

Cool the fire. If you are a woman nearing the age of menopause and begin having hot flashes, ask your doctor to check your estrogen levels. If your estrogen is low, he may recommend hormone replacement therapy (HRT). (For the lowdown on HRT and other ways to deal with hot flashes, see page 316.)

Get help for your headache. "Some people complain they get cold hands or feet when they have a migraine," says John C. Rogers, M.D., M.P.H., vice chairman of the Department of Family Medicine at Baylor College of Medicine in Houston. Foods such as red wine, coffee, cheese, nuts, tea, chocolate and spicy meats often trigger migraines and should be avoided. (For other tips on dealing with a headache, see page 280.)

See your doctor. If your sensitivity to heat or cold is accompanied by any symptoms listed at the beginning of this chapter, see your doctor. You might have a serious thyroid disorder that requires medical attention. To treat your thyroid, your doctor may prescribe medication, radioactive iodine or surgery.

TESTICLE PAIN

- Pain in the testicle or scrotum is accompanied by any of the following: swelling, nausea, vomiting, abdominal pain, redness, penile discharge or difficulty in urinating.

WHAT YOUR SYMPTOM IS TELLING YOU

There's a good reason why instructors in self-defense classes show women where to aim their knees. For a man, there are few pains that match the numbing agony of a direct hit in the family jewels. But not all testicular pain has an external source. Sometimes the body itself is doing the dirty work.

The likely cause of testicular pain depends on how old you are, according to Bruce H. Blank, M.D., a clinical associate professor of urology at Oregon Health Sciences University School of Medicine in Portland. When adult males develop pain in the testicles, Dr. Blank says, they're likely to have epididymitis, a bacterial infection of the epididymis—a spaghetti-like tube coiled up behind the testicle inside the scrotum. Not only will the scrotum hurt but you probably will also feel a swelling of or lump on the epididymis.

Children and teens with testicular pain are probably suffering from torsion, a condition that develops when the testicle virtually strangles itself by spinning, somehow, on the spermatic cord to which it is attached. Almost as frequently in kids, but much less serious (though maybe no less painful), is a similar twist that develops in a body part called the appendix of the testicles or the epididymis.

Whatever spins, the cruel twist of fate usually happens spontaneously, Dr. Blank says. The child could be physically active when it occurs, or he could just awaken with it in the middle of the night.

Testicular pain can also be caused by mumps. In addition, it can have indirect causes, such as pinched nerves in the back, kidney stones or varicose-type veins in the spermatic cord.

SYMPTOM RELIEF

There's no time to lose when you're doubled up with excruciating scrotal pain, for if torsion's twisting at your testicles, you have breathing room of maybe four to six hours before the organ dies from lack of blood. And until you get to the hospital, knowing whether it's torsion of a testicle, torsion of a testicular appendage, epididymitis or a hernia doesn't help at all. They all hurt just the same, Dr. Blank says, and diagnosis can be difficult even for physicians. "Having acute scrotal pain requires you to see the doctor right away, because you could lose the testicle if it's not corrected in just a few hours."

See if a lift alleviates. A simple, though never foolproof, test may determine the cause. Elevating the swollen scrotum, either by lying down with a pillow under your rump or wearing an athletic supporter, or changing position might temporarily ease the pain of epididymitis but will worsen torsion's torture. Males with torsion also may feel nauseated or vomit.

Let the doctor give it a whirl. A physician may try to untwist the spermatic cord without surgery, Dr. Blank says, but that often is too painful. Normally, surgery is necessary. The doctor unwinds the testicle, then stitches it and its partner to the inside of the scrotum to prevent future torsion. If it's untangled without surgery, the doctor still may want to operate to affix the testes to the inside of the scrotum, Dr. Blank says.

Take some cold comfort. No surgery is necessary if the doctor finds torsion of an appendix of the testicle or epididymitis, Dr. Blank says. While still as painful, torsion of an appendage is not dangerous. Doctors usually recommend ice compresses, elevation of the scrotum and pain medication for a few weeks, although most of the pain will naturally subside over two to three days, he says. You can raise the scrotum with the lift of an athletic supporter or by lying down with a pillow tucked under your tush. If the ache lingers, surgery may be necessary.

The Germs of Pain

You'll be saved a visit to the operating room—but not the doctor's office—if epididymitis pains your privates. The bacterial or sexually transmitted infection—usually from an unknown bacteria but sometimes from chlamydia or gonorrhea—causes pain to increase gradually over hours or maybe even days. While most of the men who get the infection are sexually active, sexual intercourse isn't the only way to catch it. "Any bacteria, possibly one responsible for a urinary infection, can cause testicular pain," says E. Douglas Whitehead, M.D., a urologist, co-director of the Association for Male Sexual Dysfunction in New York City and an associate clinical professor of urology at Mount Sinai School of Medicine of the City University of New York.

Once infected, a lump will emerge inside the scrotum, which may be red and feel hot to the touch. You may have trouble urinating or you may notice a discharge from your penis.

Epididymitis isn't the medical emergency that torsion is, Dr. Blank says, but the pain probably could be enough to drive you to the doctor's office as quickly as you can get there. In addition to taking any antibiotics that are prescribed, here's what the physician may tell you to do.

Take a load off. Bed rest is just what the doctor ordered for epididymitis, Dr. Whitehead says. Raising the scrotum eases the pain.

Take a bath. Reclining in a tub of warm water "soothes the swelling and pain and stimulates blood flow," Dr. Whitehead says.

Glide some ice on the ache. Ice compresses also will help reduce the swelling and inflammation, Dr. Blank says.

Get some support. Wearing a jock strap, along with staying off your feet for a few days and applying ice, will be prescribed if mumps is causing your testicle pain, Dr. Blank adds.

TESTICLE SWELLING

WHEN TO SEE YOUR DOCTOR

- A lump or protrusion can be felt on the otherwise smooth, even surface of a testicle.
- Your testicles and scrotum look or feel swollen or larger than they normally do.

WHAT YOUR SYMPTOM IS TELLING YOU

Your average, healthy, run-of-the-mill testicle feels like a small, peeled hard-boiled egg—same shape, same texture, same firmness. But even with "swelling" the testicle itself may not change, because the most common form of swelling happens not to the testicle but to the sac that surrounds it, says E. Douglas Whitehead, M.D., a urologist, co-director of the Association for Male Sexual Dysfunction in New York City and an associate clinical professor of urology at Mount Sinai School of Medicine of the City University of New York. For reasons doctors don't understand, the sac can simply and painlessly fill up with fluid, causing a swelling that's called *hydrocele*.

Sometimes the veins in the scrotum will dilate, causing a swelling that probably won't even be recognized. The medical term for the condition is *varicocele*. "Most guys don't notice varicoceles," Dr. Whitehead says, "but it looks sort of like varicose veins." If you have a varicocele, you also may feel a sort of heaviness or dragging sensation in the scrotum.

Scrotal swelling also can result from an infection, although the swelling produced from the bacterial invasion probably will be painful. Any lump that appears on the testicle could be epididymitis, but it must, of course, be checked for cancer. Epididymitis is an infection of the epididymis—the coiled tubes that lie behind the testicles and serve to store and transport sperm cells.

Symptom Relief

Only surgery, if even necessary, can cure the various causes of testicular or scrotal swelling. For hydrocele, some doctors will drain the fluid, but most urologists will recommend surgery to alleviate the problem. Varicocele won't interfere with a normal sex life, but it may affect your ability to have children. "Most men don't need treatment for it," Dr. Whitehead says. "Only if there are fertility problems or testicular discomfort may surgery be needed."

But your testicular health isn't entirely in the urologist's hands. There is one crucial thing you can do.

Pass the testicle test. Beginning at 13 or 14 years old, males should examine their testicles at least once a month. It will help identify hydrocele or varicocele, but most important, "it's key for the earliest detection of testicular cancer," Dr. Whitehead says.

Only 2 out of 100,000 men will get cancer of the testicles, which manifests itself first as a small lump or hardened area. While without a doubt rare, it still ranks as the number one cancer in males between the ages of 15 and 35. The good news is that it's curable—if detected early enough. Survival rates, in fact, are close to 100 percent.

Perform the exam in the shower, when the scrotum is more supple and relaxed. Roll each testicle between the thumb and the first three fingers of your hand, feeling for any lumps, hardness or other irregularity, Dr. Whitehead says. Except for the epididymis, you should feel only the smooth surface of the testicles. Also be sure to note any pain or sensation of heaviness, he says.

See also Testicle Pain

THIRST

WHEN TO SEE YOUR DOCTOR

- You are experiencing severe thirst, an increased appetite and excessive urination.
- You also have excessively dry skin, lips or mouth.
- You also feel weak or fatigued.

WHAT YOUR SYMPTOM IS TELLING YOU

Thirst works something like your car's temperature light: It goes on when fluids are low.

Those fluids can get low from excessive sweating, vomiting, diarrhea, fever, hot flashes, sunburn or dieting. Even sitting for hours in the dry cabin of an airplane can cost you a pint or more of water because of evaporation from your skin and breath. Diuretics or steroid medications can also dehydrate the body.

As your fluid levels go down, your body steals water from saliva, making your mouth feel cottony and dry. If you don't replace fluids at this point, you'll start to feel tired, weak and headachy. As dehydration advances, you could experience dizziness and other severe symptoms.

It all seems so simple: Dry mouth means take a drink. The thirst signal isn't always reliable, however. If you're hiking a mountain trail in the noonday sun, you could be significantly dehydrated before the thirst sensation even begins to kick in, according to Beau Freund, Ph.D., research physiologist at the U.S. Army Research Institute of Environmental Medicine in Natick, Massachusetts.

Another type of thirst—continual thirst no matter how much you drink, along with an insatiable appetite and frequent urination—can be a sign of adult-onset (Type II) diabetes.

This is the most common form of the disease and, true to its name, it targets people over age 40. The problem is that the body has too much blood sugar (glucose). The body tries to dilute the sugar buildup in the bloodstream by pulling fluids from the cells.

SYMPTOM RELIEF

Thirst is a warning signal that should be heeded," says Dr. Freund. Here are some guidelines.

Drink before you get thirsty. You can't always rely on thirst, says Liz Applegate, Ph.D., sports nutritionist and lecturer at the University of California in Davis. That's especially true as you age, since the years tend to dull your sense of thirst. Drinking a half-cup of water every hour will control mild dehydration, she says. You'll need more, however, if you are perspiring or if the air is hot or dry. Many doctors recommend drinking eight eight-ounce glasses of water a day.

Let your urine be your guide. To guard against dehydration, you need to drink enough so that your urine is clear rather than pale or dark yellow, says Dr. Applegate. Clear urine means you have adequately hydrated your body, she says.

Keep water, water everywhere. Use visual reminders to help you remember to drink enough fluids. Keep a filled bottle of water smack in the center of the fridge, for example. Carry a portable supply of fluid for your desk and car, too.

Drink before, during and after exercise. During a workout, you can lose up to four pounds of fluid before you realize you're thirsty. "To be safe, you need to drink about a half-cup 15 minutes before exercise, then every 15 minutes throughout and following exercise," says Hinda Greene, D.O., staff physician of internal medicine with the Cleveland Clinic–Florida in Fort Lauderdale. If you're feeling weak and tired during exercise, stop and drink a few ounces of water.

For long, sweaty workouts, try sports drinks. When you exercise heavily for more than two hours, you sweat away lots of water *and* minerals, called electrolytes, that help transmit nerve signals to the muscles. "Drinking water alone is not enough to replace these particles," says Dr.

Greene. "You're better off with a sports drink." They contain salt to help you retain water, electrolytes such as potassium, and also glucose, a carbohydrate that speeds the absorption and provides energy. (If you have diabetes or high blood pressure or you're taking a prescription diuretic, ask your doctor before using these products.)

Drink hard water. Water softening removes calcium and magnesium, replacing them with sodium. This may trigger thirstiness, says Dr. Greene. If you have a water-softening system in your house, you might want to consider removing it, or at least making sure your tap water is hard.

Check your medications. Let your doctor know that you think your diuretic or steroid is making you thirsty, says Dr. Greene. A lower dose could ease symptoms.

See your doctor for a blood test. Diabetes isn't a treat-it-yourself disease. "If your blood contains high amounts of glucose, you'll need to work with your doctor to get it under control," says Richard Guthrie, M.D., professor of pediatrics at the University of Kansas School of Medicine and director of the Diabetes Center at St. Joseph's Hospital in Wichita. The American Diabetes Association recommends a supervised program that includes both diet and exercise.

THROAT, WHITE PATCHES

WHEN TO SEE YOUR DOCTOR

Any white patch in your throat stays more than seven to ten days, particularly if you smoke or chew tobacco.
• The white patches are firm, raised or painful.

WHAT YOUR SYMPTOM IS TELLING YOU

You're flossing your teeth and you notice a few white patches at the top of your throat. A cause for alarm? Probably not.

There are many causes of white patches in your throat and most of them are temporary, harmless conditions. They'll go away and so will the patches. (But if the patches linger, see your doctor.)

White patches are a common companion of many throat infections, from the painful stab of strep to a monilia or thrush infection. Your body sometimes produces soft, white debris that collects in tiny indentations in the tonsils called crypts. It may taste bad and give you bad breath. It's harmless and will usually go away over time.

Sometimes your immune system gets out of hand and mistakes the body for an enemy, leading to an "autoimmune" reaction. This type of reaction can cause a skin condition of the mouth and throat called lichen planus. It looks like white latticework and doesn't require treatment unless it becomes painful.

Another common form of white patches in the throat—particularly in people who smoke or chew tobacco—are leukoplakia. These can turn into cancer, but 80 percent of them are benign.

Another form of chewing—chewing straw or other objects picked up off the ground—can cause a fungus called actinomysis that leaves its calling card as white-looking areas at the back of the tongue and the roof of the mouth. And chewing aspirin tablets can cause white-looking burns in the mouth and throat. (In fact, *any* chemical injury can cause this problem.)

Sometimes people develop a swelling of the mouth's lining called leukoedema that shows itself as little white areas in the mouth and the throat. The cause is unknown, but it's very common and nothing to worry about.

Syphilis can also cause whitish-looking lesions in the throat that turn red after three weeks.

SYMPTOM RELIEF

There are several things you can do to clear up white patches in the throat as well as a variety of treatments your doctor can try.

Find out if it's normal. If your doctor tells you that your white patches are leukoedema, relax. It's a normal body change that doesn't need treatment, says Sanford Archer, M.D., an assistant professor of otolaryngology at the University of Kentucky in Lexington.

Don't worry about lichen planus. Charles Krause, M.D., chief of medical affairs at the University of Michigan Medical Center in Ann Arbor, says not to worry if the back of your throat looks like a rose trellis without the roses: You have lichen planus, and it's harmless. If it does become sore or irritated, your doctor can prescribe a hydrocortisone cream or lozenge.

Have your tonsils examined. If you have a lot of white stuff in your throat, don't worry about it. It's very rare that the condition becomes bothersome enough to require removal of the tonsils, says Dr. Krause.

Don't munch on straw. If you sometimes like to chew on a leaf or straw you've picked up from the ground, give up the habit and avoid the actinomysis fungus, says Charles Ford, Jr., M.D., a professor of otolaryngology at the University of Wisconsin in Madison.

Swallow your aspirin. Take an aspirin tablet the usual way—swallowed whole with water, says Dr. Archer. That way you'll avoid a possible burn to your throat.

Learn about Leukoplakia

Although leukoplakia is normally just a minor change in the appearance of the skin in your mouth or throat, it should be carefully watched by your doctor for possible precancerous changes.

Stay on the lookout. Anyone with thin leukoplakia patches should have their doctor examine them at regular intervals, says Dr. Krause. If the patches become thicker, your doctor will apply a small amount of local anesthetic and remove some of the tissue for closer examination, he says.

Put away the plug. "Chewing tobacco—as well as smoking it—is a very strong cause of leukoplakia," says Dr. Ford. Your doctor can treat leukoplakia with a month-long regimen of high doses of Vitamin A, he says. But don't try to self-treat the problem with the vitamin. Too much vitamin A can hurt you. You need a prescription.

THROAT CLEARING

WHEN TO SEE YOUR DOCTOR

- Your repeated throat clearing has persisted for a week or more.
- Clearing your throat is disturbing your sleep or affecting your speech.
- Your throat clearing has begun to cause hoarseness or pain in your throat.
- You also have trouble breathing or swallowing.

WHAT YOUR SYMPTOM IS TELLING YOU

A hem. Clearing your throat is a time-honored way to draw polite attention. Just ask Miss Manners. But you may be clearing your throat so often that it's drawing *negative* attention. Perhaps a family member is wondering if you have some kind of throat problem. It's even starting to annoy *you*.

Chances are, it's just a habit that got started when you had an upper respiratory or throat infection a while back. Even though the original secretions that produced the tickle were over, you continued to clear your throat. That repeated throat clearing has been banging your vocal cords together, and when they meet so forcefully, they swell and create the sensation that something is *still* there in your throat. Your response? Ahem-and-ahem—*more* swelling, *more* sensation, and the cycle goes on.

Another common cause of throat clearing is acid reflux —excess stomach acid that creeps up the esophagus and irritates your throat, usually while you sleep. You may have reflux even without experiencing heartburn, doctors say.

Inadequate fluid intake and smoking can also dry and irritate the throat, prompting you to clear it. A good case of stage fright can do the same thing.

Aging can also have a drying effect on mucous mem-

ranes and prompt throat clearing. And if you've undergone
adiation therapy, that may have dried your throat as well.

SYMPTOM RELIEF

There's a lot you can do to clear up a throat-clearing
problem.

Raise your fluid level. You need a crutch if you want to
quit the throat-clearing habit, says David Alessi, M.D., an
otolaryngologist in Los Angeles. And that crutch is water.
"Feel like clearing? Stop and think—drink instead. Always
carry a bottle of water with you," he says. "In three weeks,
our habit will be broken."

Hydrate for stage fright. "Warm liquids are good if
you're fighting stage fright," says Howard Levine, M.D.,
director of the Mount Sinai Nasal Sinus Center in
Cleveland. "Your mouth and throat are drier when you're
scared," he points out. Try this concoction when you need
to use your voice in front of a group: Warm water with
lemon juice and honey. "It creates humidity, coats the
throat and gives soothing relief," says Dr. Levine.

Humidify the air. In winter, when there's dry forced hot
air inside and cold dry air outside, use room humidifiers,
suggests Steven Zeitels, M.D., an otolaryngologist at the
Massachusetts Eye and Ear Infirmary in Boston. The vapor
will ease irritated throat membranes.

Swallow the problem. "Instead of clearing your throat,
do a hard swallow—an extended swallow as though you
had something in your throat," suggests Glenn Bunting, a
senior speech pathologist at the Massachusetts Eye and Ear
Infirmary. "It may alleviate the sensation that something is
there."

Try the hard stuff. Bunting recommends sucking on hard
candy to increase saliva and moisturize the throat. But
don't use menthol lozenges, he says. They may be drying.

Be gentle. Your vocal cords are very small, about the size
of a nickel, says Bonnie Raphael, Ph.D., a vocal coach for
the American Repertory Theatre in Cambridge, Massachusetts.
Imagine blowing into a tiny musical instrument, she sug-

gests. "How hard would you blow? You need to avoid overpowering the vocal mechanism and think instead of providing just a steady, gentle breeze." Here is her prescription for reducing your ahem-ing.

"The safest way to clear the throat is to sharply sniff and then swallow. If you feel you must clear the throat, then do so silently without any voice at all. The more you avoid abusing your throat, the less damage you'll do to your vocal cords," she says.

Dry up the drips. If postnasal drip from an allergy or sinusitis is the culprit, treat these underlying conditions first, suggests Dr. Levine.

Relieve reflux. "If throat clearing is occurring after meals or when you're asleep, it may be the result of reflux," says Dr. Zeitels. Try taking antacids. (For more information on how to recognize reflux and tips on how to deal with it see Heartburn on page 298 and Regurgitation on page 518.)

See also Nose, Runny; Postnasal Drip; Sinus Problems

THROAT REDNESS

WHAT YOUR SYMPTOM IS TELLING YOU

You're ahhh-ing in the mirror, maybe flossing your teeth, when you notice your throat looks quite red. It's not really sore, though.

Should you be concerned?

If there are no other symptoms accompanying your red throat, it may be only a reaction to acid reflux—stomach acid sneaking up past the esophagus, especially while you sleep (see Heartburn on page 298 and Regurgitation on page 518). Or an allergy or other inflammation of the throat may cause it to redden, says Frederick Godley, M.D., an otolaryngologist with the Harvard Community Health Plan in Providence, Rhode Island.

"Don't worry about it. A red throat without soreness will generally go away," says Robert M. Centor, M.D., professor and chairman of the Division of General Internal Medicine at the Virginia Commonwealth University/ Medical College of Virginia in Richmond.

See also Throat Soreness

THROAT SORENESS

WHEN TO SEE YOUR DOCTOR

- You also have a fever of 101°F or higher, difficulty swallowing, swollen glands in your neck or white patches on your tonsils or in the area where your tonsils used to be.
- You have been exposed either to strep throat or mononucleosis, or there is a community outbreak.
- You have a history of rheumatic fever.
- You also have a reddish, sandpaper-like rash on your trunk.
- You get sore throats frequently and haven't been to a doctor.

WHAT YOUR SYMPTOM IS TELLING YOU

When your throat is sore, it usually means that there is an inflammation somewhere between the back of your tongue and your voice box. One cause might be breathing through your mouth because of a congested nose, or some stomach acid creeping up into your esophagus. Either your own smoking or inhaling someone else's sidestream smoke can cause a sore throat, as can fumes and chemicals in the environment or exposure to a substance you're allergic to. Overly dry indoor air during the winter months can also irritate your throat and make it sore.

Your sore throat might also result from an infection, such as mononucleosis or the infamous strep throat.

SYMPTOM RELIEF

Fortunately, there's a lot you can do to soothe the soreness.

Breathe through your nose. If your nose is stuffed up, you're undoubtedly breathing through your mouth, a practice that dries out and irritates your throat. Decreasing swelling in your nasal passages so you can breathe through your nose again may clear up your sore throat, too, says Frederick Godley, M.D., an otolaryngologist with the Harvard Community Health Plan in Providence, Rhode Island. (To unstuff your nose, see Nose, Stuffy, on page 464.)

Mist away your misery. Sleep with the soothing mist of a bedroom humidifier, particularly during months when you have the heat on, to ease your sore throat pain, says Dr. Godley.

Humidify yourself, too. When you're in pain from a sore throat, drink an extra glass of water with every meal and another at bedtime, Dr. Godley advises. A well-hydrated throat is less likely to hurt.

Gargle. A salt water gargle will ease your sore throat pain. Use 1½ teaspoons salt to one quart warm water, advises Edward Mortimer, M.D., a pediatrician and epidemiologist at Case Western Reserve University in Cleveland.

Skip those smokes. Whether it's your own tobacco smoke or the passive smoke you inhale from a nearby cigarette, stay away from it, advises Robert M. Centor, M.D., professor and chairman of the Division of General Internal Medicine at the Virginia Commonwealth University/ Medical College of Virginia in Richmond. The irritants in tobacco smoke not only inflame your throat but can also lead to throat cancer, he warns.

Buy some houseplants. There is growing evidence that

umes from glues, carpets and furnishings in new buildings
an cause health problems, including sore throat, says Dr.
Godley. "Architects and contractors are now 'baking' new
buildings at 90°F for two weeks before occupancy to drive
off toxins and glue fumes," he says.

Can't put your own home or office in the oven? Keep
plants in your rooms, and be sure you have access to windows that open for fresh air, Dr. Godley advises. The plants
will absorb toxins, and fresh-air breaks will improve the climate for your throat, he says.

Heal your heartburn. Even if you don't feel the symptoms of heartburn, your sore throat may be caused by acid
reflux—stomach acid that seeps up past the esophagus and
into the throat at night. (To control the reflux see
Heartburn on page 298 and Regurgitation on page 518.)

Super Throat Soothers

No matter what the cause of your sore throat, you'll still
want relief from the pain. Try these preparations to soothe
and comfort.

Suck on lozenges. There are a lot of throat lozenges, but
all that matters is choosing the one that works for you, says
Dr. Centor. Some doctors recommend lozenges that contain
phenol, which kills surface germs in the throat while it
numbs the pain.

Get a coat for your throat. Demulcents are ingredients
containing mucilage, which coats and soothes irritated
throat membranes, says Varro E. Tyler, Ph.D., professor of
pharmacognosy at Purdue University in West Lafayette,
Indiana.

"Slippery elm bark, for example, is a good demulcent
for sore throat and has been approved by the Food and
Drug Administration as a drug," Dr. Tyler says. Look for
lozenges containing slippery elm at pharmacies or health
food stores.

While you're at the health food store, you can also pick
up some marshmallow root or mullein root to brew a
throat-coating tea, Dr. Tyler suggests. The honey you add
to the tea provides another demulcent for your throat.

Take an analgesic. Over-the-counter painkillers like acetaminophen or ibuprofen can help kill sore throat pain, says Dr. Mortimer. But if you're treating a child or young adult, avoid aspirin. In children and young adults who have the flu or chickenpox or any fever, aspirin can cause Reye's syndrome, a life-threatening neurological disease.

The Strep Steps

Even though it's common, strep throat can be tricky to diagnose, doctors say. But it's crucial to treat it, because untreated strep infections can pose a danger to your heart. That's why a persistent sore throat should be brought to the attention of your doctor.

Your doctor is likely to suspect strep throat if you have any combination of these symptoms along with your sore throat: fever, white patches on the tonsil area, swollen glands in your neck and difficulty swallowing, says Dr. Centor.

Expect a test or two. A blood test and throat swab or culture will help your doctor distinguish between the strep bacteria and a virus, says Dr. Godley, but cultures aren't foolproof. Mononucleosis, for example, may take weeks to appear in cultures. Your doctor may need to ask you to come back several times for tests.

Stay the course. The most important part of your treatment for strep, says Dr. Mortimer, is that you take your antibiotics for the full number of days prescribed, even though you may feel better after a day or two. The usual medication is a ten-day course of penicillin (or erythromycin).

The contagious part of the illness will pass 24 to 36 hours after treatment begins, but you need to continue the treatment so the infection doesn't recur.

Use caution with antibiotics. Dr. Centor adds an important caution: "Even if a bacterial infection is suspected, don't take the antibiotics amoxicillin or ampicillin for a sore throat." If you have undetected mononucleosis, these drugs may produce a rash which resembles penicillin allergy, and might result in you being falsely labeled as allergic to penicillin.

TICS AND TWITCHES

WHEN TO SEE YOUR DOCTOR

- Any tic that disrupts your life, brings pain or persists
  for more than three months should be brought to the
  attention of your doctor.

WHAT YOUR SYMPTOM IS TELLING YOU

You sure do feel conspicuous whenever you suddenly
jerk your head for no apparent reason. It's as if the
Wicked Twitch of the West has cast a spell on you.

Most tics involve simple body movements like head
jerks, shoulder shrugs, eye blinks, nose twitches and tooth
clicks.

Although adults can develop tics, most begin in childhood around the age of six, says Allan Naarden, M.D.,
clinical professor of neurology at the University of Texas
Southwestern Medical Center in Dallas. In fact, some doctors estimate that up to 10 percent of all children may have
tics. Often, the tics worsen as a child approaches puberty
and gradually subside in adulthood. In adults, tics usually
last less than a year.

Tics, on rare occasions, can be long-lasting and involve
more complex movements such as jumping, arm thrusting
or incessant touching. In addition, some people have vocal
tics. They involuntarily bark, whistle or say repeated
phrases and obscenities. These are the signs of Tourette's
syndrome, the most severe and infamous tic disorder, which
generally strikes before age 21. People with Tourette's also
may have learning disabilities and hyperactivity. Tourette's,
however, only affects 2 people in 10,000, Dr. Naarden says.

Other rare causes of tics include thyroid disease, schizophrenia, brain damage and the abuse of stimulant drugs.

Researchers suspect that many tics have a genetic link
since 30 to 50 percent of people with tics have a family

member with tics. There also is evidence that people with tics may have abnormal levels of a brain chemical called dopamine.

However, up to 15 percent of children have temporary or transient tics. These transient tics, which are not always hereditary, are especially heightened in times of stress or anxiety.

SYMPTOM RELIEF

Most people who have transient tics eventually get rid of them; transient tics often disappear within a year and are not nearly as serious as Tourette's syndrome (TS).

Medications such as haloperidol and pimozide can help control TS tics, but many doctors are reluctant to prescribe them because of possible side effects such as drowsiness, tremors and depression. In fact, doctors usually avoid treating with medication unless an individual can no longer tolerate the tics.

But even where medication is used, most doctors would prefer you try the following strategies first. These may help your doctor determine your diagnosis and help you cope with your problem.

Start writing. If you notice a tic, then start keeping a diary. That can help you answer many questions your doctor will ask to determine the cause and possible treatment. When did it start? How long does it last? What body parts are involved?

Make 'em sweat. "Many people seem to improve or appear not to mind their tics as much if they're into an exercise program," Dr. Naarden says. Any exercise, including swimming, running and walking, is helpful, but you should do it three times a week for at least 20 minutes per session.

Feed your head. Stress management methods such as yoga, deep breathing and relaxation techniques may help some people reduce the severity of their tics, says Erwin Montgomery, M.D., associate professor of neurology at the University of Arizona College of Medicine in Tucson.

Don't be too sweet. "A number of parents have told me
~~th~~at caffeine and refined sugar seem to make children's tics
~~w~~orse," Dr. Naarden says. "Since caffeine and sugar aren't
~~n~~ecessary, I suggest staying away from refined sugars and
~~ca~~ffeinated beverages."

TINGLING

WHEN TO SEE YOUR DOCTOR

You experience tingling that dramatically increases
when you sit, cough or sneeze.
Any unexplained tingling that affects an entire side of
your body or is accompanied by muscle weakness war-
rants immediate medical attention.

WHAT YOUR SYMPTOM IS TELLING YOU

~~I~~n most cases, tingling is harmless. It usually occurs after
~~you~~ pinch a nerve or press on an artery and reduce blood
~~fl~~ow in your arm or leg causing it to "fall asleep." When
~~y~~ou change body position and relieve the compression, the
~~ti~~ngling quickly goes away.

But tingling can also be a symptom of any number of
~~pr~~oblems, including anxiety, a herniated spinal disk, poor
~~b~~lood circulation, diabetes, heart disease, stroke, arthritis,
~~m~~ultiple sclerosis, carpal tunnel syndrome or a tumor.

SYMPTOM RELIEF

~~T~~ingling that happens without a detectable cause should
be brought to the attention of your doctor, says Sean
~~G~~rady, M.D., a neurosurgeon at the University of
~~W~~ashington Health Sciences Center in Seattle.

If your doctor suspects your tingling is a symptom of a

disease, he will probably perform a complete neurologic and physical examination. He also might take a blood sam ple to determine if diabetes is causing your problem.

If, however, your arm or leg has simply fallen aslee there's no need to see a doctor. The following tips should t very effective.

Give it a rubdown. Massaging the muscles in the tinglin area can usually enhance blood flow or reduce pressure o a pinched nerve and end the tingling real fast, Dr. Grad says.

Don't just sit there. Moving an arm or leg that has falle asleep will help bring blood into the area and wipe out th tingling. If you walk around or change body positions sev eral times an hour, you can prevent tingling in the fir place. By moving about, you're less likely to pinch a nerv or artery, Dr. Grady says.

Loosen up. Some people who wear tight pants or bel may experience tingling in their thighs. "Loosen the bel wear suspenders, get new pants or, better yet, if you nee to, lose weight," says Dr. Grady.

Straighten up. "One of the reasons you might be havin tingling is a disk problem in the neck or back. By slouchin you could be irritating a nerve near that disk," says Steve Mandel, M.D., clinical professor of neurology at Jefferso Medical College and an attending physician at Thoma Jefferson University Hospital in Philadelphia. "It's impo tant to maintain good body posture by standing straigh and not slumping in chairs."

See also Numbness

TOE DEFORMITY

WHEN TO SEE YOUR DOCTOR

- Your crooked or curled toes are painful.

What Your Symptom Is Telling You

Some people cross their fingers and hope for the best, but no one crosses their toes on purpose.

Crooked toes can be caused by bunions, muscular imbalances or even rheumatoid arthritis. They're also hereditary. But the most common cause of crooked toes by far is improper footwear, according to Sally Rudicel, M.D., associate chair of the Department of Orthopaedics at Albert Einstein Medical Center in Philadelphia.

Tight shoes can cause the big toe to turn toward the other toes, crowding the second toe and possibly even causing the two toes to curl. And that sometimes forces the second toe into an arched position called a hammertoe, explains Dr. Rudicel.

Shoes like high heels, which squeeze the front of the feet, have also been linked to something called mallet toe, a condition characterized by toes that curl under at the tip, says Dr. Rudicel.

Symptom Relief

Putting crooked toes back on the straight and narrow without surgery is tough. But you may improve your situation by following these tips.

Provide support. To prevent toes from curling under, try a crest pad, suggests Steve Guida, D.P.M., a podiatrist in Fort Lauderdale, Florida. A crest pad is a tapered cushion made of foam that is placed under the toes and attached to the top of the foot. You can buy crest pads at medical supply stores, he says.

Slip on some sandals. "Often, eliminating the pressure on the tops of crooked toes caused by regular shoes will end discomfort," says Patrick O'Connor, M.D., author of *Footworks: The Patient's Guide to the Foot and Ankle.*

Pick a made-to-order pair. Custom-made shoes that take crooked toes into account may also help ease pain. For best results, contact a pedorthist—a person who's skilled in creating shoes and appliances for painful foot problems, says

Charley Simpson, a certified pedorthist and former owner of Simpson Shoes in Boston.

Consider surgery. Although the last resort, surgery to replace toe joints or reduce the tension on foot tendons that are pulling toes awry may be the only way to correct your particular problem. Ask your doctor, says Dr. Guida.

See also Corns

TOENAIL DISCOLORATION

WHEN TO SEE YOUR DOCTOR

- The discoloration from your nail spreads to the surrounding tissue.

WHAT YOUR SYMPTOM IS TELLING YOU

It's really not fair to single out one particular toe for special treatment. But in a way, you already have.

Out of all ten digits, you picked this one to use as a final resting place for your errant bowling ball. Or to pound into the pavement during your morning 10-K. And now blackness has descended across your toenail like a little piece of night.

While it may be unsightly, your black toenail is caused by nothing more than dried blood collecting underneath the nail. Nothing dangerous. Nothing permanent. And with a little therapy and patience, you'll be throwing strikes (or be on the run) again in no time.

SYMPTOM RELIEF

If a blow to your toe has made the blood flow, try these tips.

Water the pain. Immediately run cold water over the injured nail, submerge it in cold water or apply an ice pack for 15 to 20 minutes. This reduces swelling, says Richard K. Scher, M.D., a professor of dermatology and nail specialist at Columbia Presbyterian Medical Center in New York City.

Give yourself a raise. Elevating your foot after a soak may also provide relief, says Mark Scioli, M.D., an orthopedic surgeon at the Center for Orthopedic Surgery in Lubbock, Texas.

Poke a hole. You can relieve painful pressure and discoloration caused by blood building up under a nail by having your doctor gently poke a small hole in it, says Dr. Scioli. You may not lose the nail, but if it does come off, it could take three to four months to grow back, he says.

Tape that toenail. Afraid you'll rip off the injured toenail while putting on socks or slacks? Carefully secure the nail by wrapping it with adhesive tape, says Patrick O'Connor, M.D., author of *Footworks: The Patient's Guide to the Foot and Ankle.*

"When I was running, at any given time I had a toenail that was coming off," says Dr. O'Connor. "So this comes from practical experience."

Check your shoes. Running in shoes that are too tight—athletic or not—can pound your toes into blackness, says Martin L. Kabongo, M.D., Ph.D., dermatology coordinator for the family practice residency program at Bon Secours Hospital in Grosse Point, Michigan. For added protection, buy running shoes with soles that cover some of the toe area, he says. You can also shield your toes from damage at work by wearing steel-toed boots, says Dr. O'Connor.

TOENAIL PAIN

WHEN TO SEE YOUR DOCTOR

- The skin surrounding your toenail is red and swollen or discharging green or yellow fluid.
- You have diabetes.

WHAT YOUR SYMPTOM IS TELLING YOU

Toenails are the Rodney Dangerfields of the anatomy. They get no respect. While Americans each year spend millions buffing, trimming and polishing their *fingernails*, toenails are fortunate to see a new pair of socks now and then.

But sometimes toenails *make* you notice them—like when they're ingrown.

"Whether you work on your feet or not, an ingrown toenail can be incapacitating," says Archie W. Bedell, M.D., Ph.D., chairman emeritus of the Department of Family Practice at Henry Ford Hospital in Detroit.

Black toenail is another possible source of toenail pain; see page 638.

SYMPTOM RELIEF

Just because an ingrown toenail has developed doesn't mean that you have to stand for it. Try these tips for relieving the pain—and the problem.

Go soak. Soaking your foot in a basin of warm water with two tablespoons of Epsom salts for 15 to 20 minutes will soften your toenail and the skin, says Dr. Bedell. Or use a solution made with water and Betadine, an over-the-counter antiseptic. (Don't use this if you have diabetes.)

Make the move. Once you've soaked your foot and carefully washed your hands, gently pull the skin away from the trapped nail. If the procedure is too painful, see your doctor for treatment, says Dr. Bedell.

Pad it. After the nail and the skin have been separated, you can plug a small piece of cotton between the nail and the skin for a few days until the nail grows out and the skin heals, says Dr. Bedell.

Or try tape. First, secure a narrow strip of adhesive tape (like Johnson & Johnson's) near the ingrown toenail and then pull the skin away from the nail and wrap the tape so it prevents the edge of the nail from digging back into the skin. You'll have to experiment a bit to make this work, but basically any wrapping technique that frees the skin and keeps it there is fine. Then apply a small amount of a topical over-the-counter liquid antiseptic, says Patrick O'Connor, M.D., author of *Footworks: The Patient's Guide to the Foot and Ankle*. Change the tape and apply the antiseptic every day until the wound heals, he says.

Or make a kind cut. Carefully trimming the nail with a pair of toenail clippers is another way to keep it from burrowing further into your flesh, says Myles Schneider, D.P.M., an Annandale, Virginia, podiatrist and coauthor of *How to Doctor Your Feet without a Doctor*. Here's how the procedure works. Once the area has been cleaned, numb it with an ice pack for five to ten minutes. Using a pair of toenail clippers, trim the offending portion of nail. Clean the entire area again with a Betadine solution. For the next three days, soak your foot once a day in a basin of warm water and two tablespoons Epsom salts. If the toe flares up again or gets red and infected, see a doctor, advises Dr. Schneider.

Be clipper correct. To avoid a recurrence, it helps to trim your toenails properly. Instead of using small rounded fingernail clippers for your toenails, invest in a pair of toenail clippers. They're broader, increasing your chances for a straighter cut, says Dr. Bedell. Avoid using small scissors.

Make straight your trim. When cutting toenails, be sure to cut them straight across (if your nails are relatively straight), says Dr. Bedell. This will prevent the nail from slowly growing astray—and under the surrounding skin—he says. If you have misshapen nails, trim the corners so they can't grow into the skin.

Buy smart shoes. Tight shoes that cramp toes can lead to ingrown toenails, says Dr. Bedell. Make sure your shoes allow plenty of room for the toes.

TONGUE PROBLEMS

WHEN TO SEE YOUR DOCTOR

- Discoloration or coating on the tongue—especially if it's white, curdlike or stringy—does not disappear with regular brushing.
- You develop a sore on the side of your tongue.

WHAT YOUR SYMPTOM IS TELLING YOU

Open your mouth, stick out your tongue and say "A-a-a-h." When a doctor tells you to do that, he's just trying to get your tongue out of the way to see down your throat. You may do it in front of the bathroom mirror if you see something weird going on—and a lot of weird things *can* show up on the tongue.

The normal tongue is a healthy coral pink and is sandpaper rough, covered with fissures, grooves and small hairlike projections called papillae. The normal tongue is also a breeding ground for all sorts of gunky growths.

"It's an incubator for bacteria and fungus of all kinds," says J. Frank Collins, D.D.S., a dentist in private practice in Jacksonville, Florida. "The grooves can get filled up with plaque and food, and then bacteria set up housekeeping there."

Bacteria may build up because of poor hygiene. And for a variety of reasons, the bacterial balance may be tipped in favor of just one species, which then flourishes, Dr. Collins explains. That's when things get weird.

The papillae, for example, can grow from their original length of just a silly millimeter or two to as long as 20 millimeters (about 3/4 inch), making it look as though your tongue has sprouted a beard. As if that weren't bad enough, Dr. Collins says, the hairs and the debris between and below them become colored—white, black, green or red, depending on the particular bacterium and foodstuffs involved.

In contrast to the hairy look, the tongue also can be too smooth. That usually happens because of a nutrition deficiency. The small papillae don't fall off, Dr. Collins explains. Rather, the inflamed tongue tissue swells and engulfs them.

Sores can also show up on the tongue. They can be benign, like canker sores, or be caused by a bite. Or they can be a bit more serious, perhaps a fever blister. Sores on the sides of the tongue are of more significant concern. While they could be any of the above, they also could be oral cancer and need to be checked out by a doctor, Dr. Collins says.

And if the papillae are missing altogether in places, a person may have what is known as geographic tongue. It sounds exotic, but is no cause for concern, according to Louis M. Abbey, D.M.D., a professor of oral pathology at Virginia Commonwealth University/Medical College of Virginia School of Dentistry in Richmond. A person with geographic tongue has smooth red patches on the tongue that seem to change location from time to time. "You see this in 20 to 30 percent of the population," he says.

Geographic tongue is *not* those little brights spots interspersed with whitish areas that are part of a healthy, pink tongue.

Geographic tongue sort of resembles a topographical map, and if you have it, someone in your family also probably has it, because it's seen in families, although no one has ever proved it's hereditary.

SYMPTOM RELIEF

If your tongue discoloration can't be tied easily to a bottle of wine, a glass of milk or a green jawbreaker, you may have acquired something that only a doctor can remedy. Here are your options.

Grab your toothbrush. Whenever you notice a discoloration or coat on your tongue, the first recourse is to use a toothbrush on it, Dr. Collins says. "If it doesn't come off with brushing, and it persists for a couple of days, then go see the dentist and ask what the problem is. If it does come off and your tongue returns to normal, just keep on brushing."

Change your prescription. Many drugs—such as Darvon and other analgesics or tetracycline and other antibiotics—change the balance of bacterial flora in the mouth, Dr. Collins says. That allows certain stronger strains to grow like dandelions in a spring lawn. If you're taking medications and your tongue changes color or begins to develop a growth, he recommends that you continue to brush your tongue regularly. And ask your doctor if you can discontinue the medication you're on or take something less likely to tint your tongue as a side effect.

Don't smoke. Tobacco use can aggravate or cause tongue problems, Dr. Abbey says. You've heard it before, but here it is again: Stop smoking.

B takes the skid off. A slick or smooth tongue usually is a sign of pernicious anemia, caused by a vitamin B12 deficiency. "It's *usually* pernicious anemia, but that's not *always* the case," Dr. Collins says. "If it's not pernicious, chances are it's some other type of anemia, maybe iron deficiency. Or it's some other blood-borne problem." Your doctor will have to diagnose the cause of slick tongue. He may treat it with a vitamin B12 shot or have you take a supplement. In the meantime make sure you eat plenty of foods high in B12, like fish, low-fat yogurt and cottage cheese.

Make sure it makes its move. Geographic tongue may cause a burning sensation in your mouth. If necessary, talk to your doctor for possible treatments. Other than that, geographic tongue is of no real concern, Dr. Abbey says, "although you and your dentist should watch to make sure it doesn't turn into something else."

Diet drinks do it. Certain foods may cause discomfort or burning for people with geographic tongue, Dr. Collins says. "I've seen some people with it who are irritated by diet drinks or spearmint oil in chewing gums," he says. You'll have to experiment with eliminating different drinks or foods from your diet to see if it eases the soreness.

Don't blame it on your teeth. If you develop a sore (painful or not) on the side of your tongue, schedule a visit with the doctor. It could be a canker sore or cold sore. But for some reason, the sides are a favorite site for oral cancer, Dr. Collins advises. "You might think it's caused by scraping against a sharp tooth, but it doesn't have anything to do with a tooth," he says. "Teeth don't usually cause sores on your tongue."

TOOTHACHE

WHEN TO SEE YOUR DOCTOR

- You feel a sharp or recurring pain in one or more teeth.
- A tooth hurts when you eat or drink something hot.
- A painful tooth suddenly stops hurting.

WHAT YOUR SYMPTOM IS TELLING YOU

In the old movies, if you had a toothache, they'd tie one end of a string to the bothersome bicuspid and the other end to a doorknob. And sooner than you could say "see ya later," the door would slam into the jamb and you were out of your jam.

Fortunately, in real life you can rely on better diagnosis and treatment. In fact, when your tooth aches, there are only a few likely causes.

Something as simple as a popcorn kernel lodged between two teeth could be causing your pain. More likely, though, the pulp inside your tooth has become infected and inflamed, according to J. Frank Collins, D.D.S., a dentist in private practice in Jacksonville, Florida. The inflammation either squeezes the tooth nerve or pushes against the periodontal ligament that holds the tooth inside your mouth, and that causes the pain, he explains.

A number of things can cause inflammation, including long-time neglect of brushing and flossing, a broken or loose filling, recent dental work, a cracked tooth or blows to the mouth. Usually the pulp darkens, and the discoloration shines through the outer layer of the tooth. The pain may rise up gradually or smack you in the face all of a sudden. It could feel like an electrical jolt, as with cracked teeth, or it may erupt and linger after you've eaten or drunk something hot or cold.

Even an old injury that you thought was relatively minor can come back to haunt you. You may never have realized that you damaged the nerve in a tooth during that fall you had when you were a kid, according to Lisa P. Germain, D.D.S., M.Sc.D., an endodontist in private practice in New Orleans. "But 30 years down the line, you could develop the symptoms." (Endodontists specialize in root canals.)

A tooth could also—on its own and with no forewarning—just decide to become inflamed, hurt and die, Dr. Germain says. "Like appendicitis, there's no way to predict when it will happen," she says, "but it's painful, and you have to have it taken care of by a dentist or orthodontist."

An overall dull ache in your teeth might be because you gnash and grind them while you sleep. And problems with how your jaw works may transfer pain to your teeth. Toothache could also be a symptom of a sinus problem. "If you can't figure out which tooth it is, it could be sinuses," says Van B. Haywood, D.M.D., an associate professor in the Department of Operative Dentistry at the University of North Carolina School of Dentistry in Chapel Hill. Because the roots of your upper teeth extend into the sinuses, any pressure up there pinches tooth nerves. "It's like sitting on your foot and it falls asleep," Dr. Haywood explains. (For more information, see Sinus Problems on page 540.)

SYMPTOM RELIEF

If you're unwilling to try the string-tied-to-the-doorknob approach for the ultimate in toothache relief, there's not much you can do other than see your dentist. Here's what to do before your appointment.

Reach for the ibuprofen. Whether the tooth is dead or not, you're still feeling inflammatory pain, Dr. Germain says. And ibuprofen is an excellent anti-inflammatory drug that you can get over-the-counter. "I prescribe 600 milligrams of Motrin (a prescription brand of ibuprofen) for my patients, and that really does help a toothache," she says. "But you could take 400 milligrams of over-the-counter ibuprofen four times a day. The dosage is different, but the drug is the same."

Save aspirin for *head*aches. Aspirin and acetaminophen don't seem to have as great an effect on tooth pain, according to Dr. Germain. You certainly don't want to try the old cure of putting an aspirin directly on the throbbing molar. "Aspirin will burn your gums and the soft tissue inside your mouth," she cautions. "Don't do it."

Don't try to ignore it. Even if the toothache goes away, it will come back and torment you with a vengeance. If you ignore a pulsating toothache and the pain eventually vanishes, that probably indicates that decay or trauma has killed the nerve, Dr. Germain says. From there it's only a short step to a pus-filled abscess. "One day you'll wake up in severe pain with a huge swelling on your face," she says. "Don't assume that when the pain is gone the tooth has healed."

Don't munch on ice. Or unpopped popcorn, either. "They're the greatest ways to crack teeth and give you a toothache—more than automobile accidents or football or anything," Dr. Haywood says. Those hard popcorn seeds can hide in a handful scooped from the bottom of the bowl, he points out, and ice puts a brittle freeze on your teeth just before you bite down.

Put aside your fear. Contrary to how horribly anguishing everyone thinks they are, today's root canals, in which the dentist or endodontist removes the damaged tooth nerve and pulp, are painless, Dr. Germain says. "We're so good at making patients numb now that it doesn't hurt any more than the regular soreness of getting a filling," Dr. Germain says. "It only takes three seconds to remove the nerve inside the tooth, and then from there, we're working in an empty space."

See also Jaw Problems; Tooth Grinding

TOOTH DISCOLORATION

WHEN TO SEE YOUR DOCTOR

- One tooth or several teeth darken or turn gray or yellowish brown.
- A tooth turns reddish pink.

WHAT YOUR SYMPTOM IS TELLING YOU

Perfectly white teeth may be just another Hollywood fantasy, but a lot of people *are* going around with teeth that could be whiter. The discoloration might be harmless and superficial, indicating nothing more than too much coffee, too much blueberry pie and too few visits to the dental hygienist. Or it might be a sign of tooth decay. It could also be the result of a pervasive (yet harmless) stain deep inside the teeth.

You might think that more brushing means whiter teeth. Not true, says Van B. Haywood, D.M.D., an associate professor in the Department of Operative Dentistry at the University of North Carolina School of Dentistry in Chapel Hill. Brushing cleans but doesn't remove stubborn stains. Scrubbing too hard and too frequently (particularly with abrasive polishes) can actually erode the white enamel covering your teeth, exposing the darker dentin beneath.

But other factors may steal the sparkle from your smile. Age is one that affects us all. Teeth quite naturally darken as you age. Over the years, the soft pinkish pulp at the core of teeth disappears, replaced by the darker dentin, Dr. Haywood says.

Age, just like blueberry pie, will alter the color of your teeth uniformly. If, though, a single tooth or a couple of teeth side by side turn darker (usually gray or yellowish brown), you probably have developed an abscess, a pus-filled infection. It is very likely that a root canal can be performed and the tooth can be saved, says Lisa P. Germain,

D.D.S., M.Sc.D., an endodontist (a specialist in root canals) in private practice in New Orleans. If left to fester, an abscess can erode the bone holding the tooth in place and the tooth may have to be pulled.

Abscesses, which blacken the pulp inside a tooth, occur either because of a blow to the mouth or advancing decay. The blow doesn't even have to be recent, Dr. Germain says. "You could have been hit when you were a child and 20 years later suffer the effects." And there may not be accompanying symptoms—like a toothache or sensitivity to hot or cold foods.

A tooth also could begin to dissolve itself without reason, a process called internal resorption. If that occurs, Dr. Haywood says, the tooth likely will appear pink or reddish.

And what if *all* your teeth are dark? Chances are they're not all decayed, says William R. Howard, D.D.S., an assistant professor of dental hygiene in the Department of Allied Health at Western Kentucky University in Bowling Green. Besides stains from food and drink, the discoloration could be caused by certain medications.

"Antibiotics, especially tetracylines, are a really big problem," he says. If taken frequently in childhood or early adolescence, as they often are for infections and acne, tetracycline will color the dentin inside your teeth gray. And that grayness will show through the enamel. Children of women who take tetracylines in the later stages of pregnancy also may have grayish teeth, Dr. Howard says.

SYMPTOM RELIEF

Some people actually choose to have root canals done to whiten their teeth, Dr. Haywood says. "That certainly is a creative way to do it, but root canals should be used only as a final resort when the health of the tooth is at stake." Here are better ways to put a white wink on your smile.

Don't flub the scrub. Use a wet soft-bristle brush and a gentle touch when you clean your teeth, Dr. Haywood recommends. And don't forget to floss. While regular hygiene only minimizes, not eliminates, tougher stains, it will keep your smile looking good because it keeps your gums healthy.

"No matter how white your teeth are," says Dr. Haywood, "when your gums look unhealthy, your smile looks unhealthy."

Find promise in pumice. The most basic whitening job available from the dentist or dental hygienist is a pumice polish, which is applied with a small rotary rubber cup. While effective against superficial coffee and tea stains, it won't lighten deeper, darker discolorations.

Ask the dentist to reach for the bleach. The best way to whiten teeth is a bleaching system you can obtain through your dentist for use at home. At the office, you'll be fitted with a mouth guard (dentists call them splints) and given a prescription bleaching gel. You squeeze a couple of drops of the gel into the guard, which you wear several weeks for an hour or two each day or while sleeping. There's a small chance that the gel, which contains carbamide peroxide, similar to hydrogen peroxide, may burn or sting soft tissue in your mouth, but the treatment is generally safe and effective. But the cost is expensive—more than $200.

"The results can be dramatic," Dr. Haywood says. Teeth stained by tetracycline don't respond as well, though. "They definitely do get lighter, but it's a lighter shade of gray," he says.

Don't try this at home. You can buy over-the-counter whitening kits, but most dentists recommend that you don't try them. The active ingredient is hydrogen peroxide or something that breaks down into hydrogen peroxide in your mouth, Dr. Howard says. Repeated use of hydrogen peroxide may speed the development of oral cancers, especially in smokers. "Some of the stronger solutions also can really burn your mouth," he says.

Another ingredient, titanium dioxide, is little more than whitewash for your teeth, Dr. Haywood says. And in informal tests he has done, the commercial home kits "couldn't get teeth white even with 60 applications in some cases."

Put a cap on it. Or a plastic bonding or a porcelain veneer. For deeply stained teeth, you may want to opt for any of these decorative coverings that your dentist can apply. With bonding, you can color just a portion or all of a tooth as well as reshape it or fill in gaps. Porcelain veneers, which cover the whole tooth, look more natural but are more expensive. Caps, the most expensive alternative, cover all surfaces of the tooth—front, back, sides and top.

TOOTH GRINDING

WHEN TO SEE YOUR DOCTOR

- You find yourself habitually gnashing your teeth together or clenching your jaw muscles as if chewing or biting something.
- Your spouse says you grind or gnash your teeth while asleep.

WHAT YOUR SYMPTOM IS TELLING YOU

Tired of the same old daily grind? Well, if you're not, your jaw probably is.

The habitual gnashing and grinding of teeth—known as bruxism—is caused by three main factors, according to Brendan C. Stack, Sr., D.D.S., an orthodontist and president of the National Capital Center for Craniofacial Pain in Vienna, Virginia, and past president of the American Academy of Head, Neck, Facial Pain and TMJ Orthopedics. Most people who have this problem simply are using their teeth to vent their stress. Others have a dislocated jaw joint that causes the jaw muscle to go into painful spasm. In some instances, Dr. Stack says, some people, usually women between the ages of 17 and 35, seem to have a slight central nervous system disorder that compels them to clench and grind.

People in certain jobs that demand very careful and

exacting precision, like watchmakers and brain surgeons, also tend to grind their teeth, according to J. Frank Collins, D.D.S., a dentist in private practice in Jacksonville, Florida. A new filling that doesn't fit the mouth quite right or is higher than the other teeth will also cause a person to grind, almost unconsciously trying to wear the filling down to the level of the other teeth.

Tooth grinding may seem like a minor annoyance, but it's important to get treatment. At the very least, habitual gnashing and clenching will give you sore jaws, says Eric Z. Shapira, D.D.S., a trustee on the national board of the Academy of General Dentistry and a dentist in private practice in Half Moon Bay, California. As you continue to grind, you may dislocate or damage the jaw joint and give yourself headaches, neck or shoulder pain and ringing in the ears. And you almost certainly will loosen your teeth and wear away their chewing surfaces. If you grind down your teeth, you can throw your whole jaw out of whack and your teeth won't align properly.

SYMPTOM RELIEF

Because many causes of bruxism must be treated by a medical professional, it's a good idea to bring this problem to the attention of your dentist. Here are a few things you can try on your own as well as a few treatments that your doctor might suggest.

Pay attention. Whenever your mouth is closed, your teeth shouldn't touch. Your upper and lower teeth should come into contact *only* when you're chewing and swallowing. Check yourself several times a day and if you find yourself clenching, relax your lower jaw.

Give your jaws a workout. If you tire your jaw muscles deliberately, Dr. Shapira says, you're less likely to clench and grind while asleep. Try his Popsicle stick workout: Place a Popsicle stick along the bottom teeth on one side of your mouth and bite down for a minute, then put it on the other side and bite down again. Add another stick and keep biting down. Keep adding sticks and switching the pile back and forth and biting until you have five sticks stacked up in your mouth.

Do the exercise two or three times a day. You'll have to keep it up for at least a month before you see some benefit, Dr. Shapira says. "You'll be fatiguing the muscles in your jaw, and they'll be so tired that you won't want to clench at night," he explains.

Get less stress. Because teeth grinding primarily is a habit in response to stress, Dr. Shapira says, you should try to unwind any way you can. Relaxation techniques, massage, gentle exercise and yoga are among the many ways you can calm down and reduce or end bruxism.

Guard your mouth at night. If you are grinding your teeth, a simple sports mouthguard, available at your local sporting goods store, can protect your teeth as you grind at night. A dentist also can make a guard that will fit your teeth precisely, Dr. Collins says.

Protect your teeth during the day. Dentists trained in jaw problems or orthodontics can fashion a specialized mouthguard that you wear out of sight all the time in the back of your mouth, Dr. Stack says. "The mouthguard includes a spacer that makes it physically impossible to clench your teeth," he explains. "The worst you can do is grind against the rubber mouthguard."

Fix the joint. For tougher cases of bruxism, specialists can, through repositioning splints or surgery, repair the dislocated joint that causes the jaw muscles to go into spasm, Dr. Stack says.

Cap the clench. If you're a serious tooth grinder and have worn down your bite considerably, your teeth may need to be capped, dentists say.

Fix the filling. If you grind your teeth because of a filling that is too high, your dentist can smooth the filling down in a brief (and painless) office visit.

TOOTH LOOSENESS

WHEN TO SEE YOUR DOCTOR

- Anytime you notice a tooth is loose.

WHAT YOUR SYMPTOM IS TELLING YOU

"Loose lips sink ships," went the saying during World War II. Loose teeth are hardly a national security risk, but they'll certainly sink your enjoyment of everything you can't sink your teeth into.

Assuming you're not a six-year-old reading this book, a loose tooth usually means you have one of two problems: Advancing periodontal disease or a blow to the jaw.

The more likely of these two causes is periodontal disease—severe deterioration of the tooth's bone foundations and gum support. "If you don't have a good attachment of the gum membrane to the bone, teeth loosen," explains Paul A. Stephens, D.D.S., a dentist in private practice in Gary, Indiana, and president of the Academy of General Dentistry. But other dental problems sometimes also cause loose teeth.

An improper bite, in which your upper and lower teeth don't align correctly, can loosen teeth, according to Samuel B. Low, D.D.S., assistant dean and director of postgraduate periodontics at the University of Florida College of Dentistry in Gainsville. And habitually gnashing and clenching your teeth—a stress-based reflex called bruxism—not only wears down the tops of teeth but also loosens them, he says. (See Tooth Grinding on page 651.)

SYMPTOM RELIEF

You can't grab a bottle of super glue and reattach your loose tooth. In fact, if the loose tooth is caused by gum disease, you might as well start mourning. Your tooth probably can't be saved. "It depends mostly on the tooth's bone and soft tissue foundation," says Timothy Durham, D.D.S., director of adult general dentistry at the University of Nebraska Medical Center in Omaha. And he adds this less-than-hopeful comment: "If enough of this foundation was lost to loosen the tooth, then options for securing it are limited."

If your tooth was loosened or knocked out in an accident, your chances of reattaching it are much better. Here's what you and the dentist can do.

Don't touch. When you notice a loose tooth, resist the urge to fiddle around with it with your fingers or tongue. That will only make its hold in your mouth more tenuous, say dentists. But if you do pull it out or if it's knocked out, says Dr. Durham, "try to get the tooth right back in there and reposition it as exactly as you can."

Rinse, but don't scrub. If the knocked-out tooth is dirty, run it under warm water, but don't scrub it, says Dr. Durham. The tooth probably will have bits of dental ligament still attached that will help in reimplanting it.

Put it under your tongue. Some people are too squeamish to reinsert a knocked-out tooth in its socket, says Dr. Durham. If that's you, then at least store it in your mouth until you get to the dentist. Put it under your tongue or in your cheek. If a knocked-out tooth is from a child, an adult can keep it in their mouth. Just don't suck on it like a lozenge, he says.

Store it in milk. For those too squeamish to keep a knocked-out tooth in their mouths, put it in a glass of milk, says Dr. Durham. That seems to work better than wrapping it in a wet tissue.

Hurry up. Get to the dentist as soon as possible. "The longer it's out of where it's supposed to be, the more likely it is that you'll lose the tooth," says Dr. Durham.

Try surgery or a brace. Gum surgery can firm up the foundation of a tooth loosened by periodontal disease, says Dr. Low. Success depends on the extent of the gum and bone loss. Sometimes the most that can be done is to hold the tooth in place with a splint attached to neighboring teeth. The tooth will never stand on its own, but at least your own tooth will be in your mouth.

TOOTH SENSITIVITY

WHEN TO SEE YOUR DOCTOR

- Pain lingers after eating or drinking any cold food.
- Your teeth feel any pain at all in response to heat.
- The sensitivity is concentrated in one tooth.
- Toothpaste for sensitive teeth doesn't help.

WHAT YOUR SYMPTOM IS TELLING YOU

No matter what flavor ice cream you choose, it always ends up tasting bittersweet—so luscious on your tongue, so painful to your teeth.

Everyone occasionally experiences fleeting pain in their teeth when they bite into something cold. That's usually because teeth have lost some of their enamel protection. And beneath the enamel lies a honeycomb of tiny, fluid-filled tunnels called dentinal tubules. These tubules lead directly to the tooth's inner core, which contains pulp—and the tooth's sensitive nerve.

Normally, saliva helps deposit calcium on the enamel to cover and protect the tubules' openings. But excessively hard brushing (especially with abrasive tooth polishes), receding gums, acidic foods and tooth grinding can all erode that protective covering, baring the ends of the tubules. Cracks in the teeth and loose fillings also expose the tubules or even the pulp itself.

Whatever the cause, once the tubules are exposed, extreme changes in temperature cause fluids inside them to flow back and forth quickly, explains J. Frank Collins, D.D.S., a dentist in private practice in Jacksonville, Florida. That movement causes the twinge in your teeth.

Eroded enamel can cause painful reactions to hot and cold food or drinks, says Lisa P. Germain, D.D.S., M.Sc.D., an endodontist in private practice in New Orleans. If you're sensitive to anything hot or if the reaction to cold either builds up slowly or lingers for more than a moment, you could have an irreversible inflammation, which can lead to an abscess—a pus-filled inflammation.

SYMPTOM RELIEF

If you've recently had dental work and are experiencing sensitivity to hot and cold, however, you shouldn't be immediately concerned, says Dr. Germain. This kind of irritation is normal and should go away within a few weeks. It means the pulp inside the tooth became slightly inflamed and needs time to return to normal. If the pain does not go away for several weeks, see your dentist, or an endodontist (root canal specialist), because the nerve in the tooth may be dying.

Otherwise, curing your teeth's sensitivity to cold can be as easy as squeezing a tube of the right toothpaste and avoiding certain foods and drinks.

Plug up touchy teeth. Toothpastes for sensitive teeth work by plugging up the tubules with strontium chloride, which, like sodium fluoride, helps draw calcium from saliva into the tubules and the enamel. To be effective, says Dr. Collins, "you have to use it frequently, and you must brush meticulously."

Do the fluoride swish. Fluoride mouthwashes also help block the tubules, Dr. Collins says.

Try ibuprofen. If you're feeling sensitivity to hot or cold after a trip to the dentist, try ibuprofen to relieve the discomfort, says Dr. Germain.

Try a gentler brushing technique. Always use a soft-bristle toothbrush, wet the brush before you apply toothpaste and never scrub very hard, recommends Van B. Haywood, D.M.D., an associate professor in the Department of Operative Dentistry at the University of North Carolina School of Dentistry in Chapel Hill. "Probably the most common cause of sensitivity is that people brush too hard with a hard-bristle brush. They wear off the enamel," he says. "They saw back and forth like they're sawing down a tree, and that's what they'll do. They'll saw a tooth right in half. You can literally saw a notch in the tooth."

Change your brushing technique. If you're like most people, you put the most effort and pressure into the beginning of your brushing and slack off by the time you've covered all your teeth. Typically, too, you start your brushing in the same spot every time. "The place you start is usually the place that's sensitive," Dr. Haywood says. "You can almost pick out the right-handers who come in complaining of sensitivity in their top left-side teeth, because that's where they start brushing."

Begin with the backs of the lower front teeth, Dr. Haywood recommends. "That's the most inaccessible spot in the mouth and where most of the tartar builds up, so you'll be putting most of your effort onto the most difficult area."

Proper brushing will also help prevent receding gums, which can contribute to tooth sensitivity.

Save the acid for chemistry class. Acidic foods and drinks—tomatoes, lemons, colas and other carbonated soft drinks—will very quickly eat the enamel off your teeth and make them much more vulnerable to sharp temperature changes, Dr. Haywood says. "Some people get a seasonal tooth sensitivity in the summer because they eat a lot of tomatoes or suck on lemons," he says. "Carbonated beverages do a lot of damage over the long haul to your teeth—but because they're so acidic they're great for bug stains on your windshield."

Stop that grinding. If your dentist says tooth grinding is causing your problem, ask him to fit you with a protective device that you can use while sleeping.

Get a spark of insensitivity. If nothing works to stop the sensitivity, your dentist might suggest a procedure called iontophoresis, in which an electrical current is used to apply protective fluoride deep within the tubules, says Dr. Haywood. The procedure can be done in the dentist's office.

See also Tooth Grinding

TREMORS

WHEN TO SEE YOUR DOCTOR

- You are experiencing a persistent tremor that is becoming more frequent and disruptive.

WHAT YOUR SYMPTOM IS TELLING YOU

Singer Jerry Lee Lewis was right. There is a whole lot of shaking going on.

"We all have tremors. But most of the time they're so minor that we don't notice them," says Allan Naarden, M.D., a clinical professor of neurology at the University of Texas Southwestern Medical Center in Dallas.

A tremor is a shaking caused by involuntary contractions of muscles. They can occur in any part of the body, but usually they affect the neck, arms or hands. Most people will have noticeable tremors only if they're under stress, extremely tired, drinking excessive caffeine or taking medications that cause shaking as a side effect, Dr. Naarden says.

Some people have recurrent, serious tremors. The two most common causes are Parkinson's disease and an often-inherited disorder known as essential tremor. You can suspect essential tremor if the shaking occurs when reaching for a cup, tying a shoe or performing some other movement. Although bothersome, essential tremor isn't necessarily anything that puts your health at risk.

Other causes of persistent tremor include alcoholism, multiple sclerosis, tumor, stroke, an overactive thyroid and Wilson's disease—a rare inherited ailment that disrupts the body's metabolism of copper.

SYMPTOM RELIEF

People with disabling tremors need medical and sometimes surgical treatment," says Joseph Jankovic, M.D., director of the Parkinson's Disease Center and Movement Disorders Clinic at Baylor College of Medicine in Houston.

Your doctor may prescribe drugs such as propranolol and primidone to control your tremors. But whether you're on medication or not, there are several ways you may be able to lessen the severity of your tremors—regardless of their cause. Here's how.

Shake the stress. If you feel tense or under stress and you find a way to relax, you may alleviate your shaking, says Erwin Montgomery, M.D., associate professor of neurology at the University of Arizona College of Medicine in Tucson. Biofeedback training, progressive muscle relaxation and other stress reduction techniques can help. Biofeedback involves using a monitor to help you learn how to let go of tension in your muscles. Ask your doctor to refer you to someone who can give you training. (For other methods of dealing with stress, see Anxiety on page 25.)

Stop after two. Caffeine can increase the intensity of your tremors. Limit yourself to two eight-ounce cups of coffee or tea each day, suggests Carroll Ramseyer, M.D., clinical professor of neurology at the University of Southern California School of Medicine in Los Angeles.

Tuck in your tremor. Getting regular amounts of adequate rest may get your tremors to snooze, too, Dr. Ramseyer says. Set a reasonable bedtime and try to get the same amount of sleep each night. Most people need at least seven to eight hours a night.

Check the medicine cabinet. Over-the-counter cold and allergy medications containing decongestants like pseudoephedrine and prescription drugs such as epinephrine—a medication used to treat asthma—also can cause tremors in some people. Make a list of your medications and ask your doctor or pharmacist if any of those drugs could be contributing to your problem.

Managing Day to Day

Tremors are not easily controlled. But just because you can't control your tremors doesn't mean they have to control you. Here are a few simple forms of therapy you can do at home that may help you remain active.

Weigh it down. Wearing one- or two-pound cuff weights around your wrist or elbow when you're eating, cleaning or doing other activities may keep your tremor temporarily in check, says Anne Ford, manager of rehabilitation services at Walter O. Boswell Memorial Hospital in Sun City, Arizona. She suggests that you only wear the weights when you're doing an activity, since prolonged use of the weights can fatigue your muscles and actually worsen your tremors. The weights are available at most sporting goods stores.

Try special utensils. Extra-heavy forks, spoons and knives may make it easier to eat. You also might consider using customized plates that have a one-inch wall on one side. The wall will prevent food from sliding and make it easier to scoop up. These utensils can be ordered at most medical and surgical supply stores.

Bear down. Right before you're going to do a task, try sitting in a chair with your hands at your side. Grasp the seat or arms of the chair with your hands palm down. Then, keeping the elbows stiff, gently push your hands down against the chair for one to two minutes. "By holding in that rigid position you might fatigue the muscles and alleviate tremors for a short time," Ford says.

U

UPPER BACK PAIN

WHEN TO SEE YOUR DOCTOR

- Your upper back pain radiates to the front of your chest, lower part of your rib cage or your abdomen.
- You have a family history of cardiovascular disease.
- You have no idea why your upper back hurts.

WHAT YOUR SYMPTOM IS TELLING YOU

Think of upper back pain as the voice of your mom. Remember her urgings not to slouch? Most of the time, that's what your upper back is trying to tell you when it hurts: *Please* stand up straight.

Poor posture can lead to weakened muscles and strained joints and ligaments, setting the stage for more upper back pain.

Overusing the muscles of the upper back can also cause pain. (If you've been painting the ceiling in your den, for example, you *know* why your back hurts.) And if you have particularly large breasts, just straining to stand up straight can cause pain in the upper back.

More serious causes of upper back pain include osteoporosis, a ruptured spinal disk and injury. Osteoporosis is a disease in which the bones become porous and fragile—so fragile, that a vertebrae can shatter, just from the spine's own weight. Rupturing a disk in the upper back is, fortunately, quite rare, but it can generate angry bolts of pain. As for injuries, a traffic accident can cause whiplash, which severely strains upper back muscles in addition to damaging the neck.

Finally, heart disease or other serious illnesses can announce themselves in the form of upper back pain.

Among the most common areas of pain are the trapezius—the large, triangular-shaped muscles of the upper back—and the shoulder blades.

SYMPTOM RELIEF

If your upper back has been troubling you and you're not sure why, it's a good idea to have your doctor look at it for diagnosis and treatment. If you have osteoporosis or heart disease, or if you've sustained an injury to your back, you definitely need to be under a doctor's care.

If your back hurts because of a mechanical problem—strain, underuse or poor posture, for example—here are a few things you can do on your own.

Handle the pain yourself. One minute of self-massage each hour in the problem area of your upper back should help provide relief for muscle spasm, says Morris Mellion, M.D., past president of the American Academy of Family Physicians and medical director of the Sports Medicine Center in Omaha, Nebraska. "Deep massage over the most exquisitely tender spot should produce results a short time later," he says. Just reach across with your hand to the opposite shoulder and rub.

Get the knead you need. Gently kneading the trapezius muscle relieves pain by stretching the area and increasing circulation, says Patrice Morency, licensed massage therapist and sports injury management specialist in Portland, Oregon, who works with Olympic hopefuls. Have a friend or spouse first knead the muscles on the left and then the right side of your upper back with the palms of their hands. They should press repeatedly and gently in the same way a cat kneads with its paws.

Elbow away pain. Another soothing massage technique for upper back pain employs the use of someone's elbow. Simply have your assistant press the point of their elbow gently into your trapezius muscle for between 15 and 30 seconds. Release, and then repeat, says Morency. Pressing on the area slows the blood supply briefly and releasing it floods the area with blood and oxygen, often allowing a muscle in spasm to relax, she explains.

Try a sports bra. Women with large breasts may experience immediate relief from upper back pain after shedding
their everyday bras for a sports bra that has better support,
says Karl B. Fields, M.D., associate professor of family
practice and director of the Sports Medicine Fellowship at
Moses Cone Memorial Hospital in Greensboro, North
Carolina.

Hold your head up. When reading at your desk, instead
of bringing your eyes—and head—to your paper, try bringing your paper to your eyes. "People are constantly using
poor body mechanics when they read," says Hubert
Rosomoff, M.D., D.Med.Sc., medical director of the
University of Miami Comprehensive Pain and Rehabilitation Center in Miami Beach. "Instead of holding their
heads erect, they tend to scrunch their heads and necks forward on their shoulders."

Hold the phone. Rather than propping the phone
between your head and shoulder—which can strain the
muscles in your upper back—hold the phone in your hand.
Or better yet, buy a headset or speaker phone, says Dr.
Rosomoff.

Improve your posture. Poor posture eliminates the natural, weight-supporting S curve of your back, often weakening the muscles of the upper back and making them
susceptible to strain, says Fred Allman, Jr., M.D., an orthopedic surgeon and director of the Atlanta Sports Medicine
Clinic. Healthy posture—chest out, stomach in, buttocks
tucked under—restores that S, making it easier on the muscles of your upper back. If you frequently suffer from upper
back pain, ask your doctor to evaluate your posture and—
if appropriate—to recommend someone who can teach you
exercises that will restore your posture.

Pump up your upper back. You never know when you're
going to wrench your upper back or suffer a whiplash
injury. But if your upper back and neck muscles are strong,
you're less likely to suffer a severe pull or tear in that area,
doctors say. "If those muscles support you, then part of that
stress is absorbed by the muscle, and not by the bone or the
ligaments or the other tissues," says Dr. Fields. You can
strengthen your upper back with this simple exercise: hold a

can of soup in each hand, keeping your arms straight by your side. Lift your shoulders straight up toward your ears for a two count, then pull the shoulders back, pinching your shoulder blades together. Relax and repeat 8 to 12 times.

See also Lower Back Pain

URINATING EXCESSIVELY

WHEN TO SEE YOUR DOCTOR

- You've cut back on liquids, and you still excrete a large volume of urine.

WHAT YOUR SYMPTOM IS TELLING YOU

So you think you urinate too much. Do you *really*?
"For the health of your bladder, you need to put out about one to two liters of urine a day," says Margaret M. Baumann, M.D., associate chief of staff for geriatrics and extended care at the Veterans Administration West Side Medical Center in Chicago. (Two liters is the amount in a family-size bottle of soda.) If you don't excrete that much, your urine will be too concentrated with wastes, she says. That can harm the lining of the bladder, leading to the formation of kidney stones or causing the bladder to contract even when it's not full.

Some prescription drugs—like diuretics for high blood pressure—can cause you to produce more urine than normal. And the one disease that can cause increased urinary output is undetected or poorly managed diabetes.

SYMPTOM RELIEF

Assuming you have no underlying medical problem, there is nothing wrong with producing a lot of urine.

If you're uncomfortable with your output, though, you might want to try some of these tips.

Measure your output. The first step in taking any action about your urine output is measuring it. To do that, over the course of a 24-hour period urinate into a soda bottle or jar calibrated for liters or quarts. (Two liters equals a little more than two quarts.) If you want a really accurate record, says Dr. Baumann, also note what and when you drink, and when you urinate.

See your doctor...maybe. "If you're producing six or more liters of urine a day," says Dr. Baumann, "you might want to get an examination to see if you're diabetic."

Put a muzzle on your guzzle. If you excrete, say, four to five liters a day, try cutting your liquid intake in half, Dr. Baumann suggests. "You won't be a healthier person by producing more than one to two liters of urine a day," she says. Besides, while generating a high volume of urine won't necessarily cause incontinence, it may contribute to it, she says.

Don't be a stranger to the restroom. What you perceive as emitting too much urine at one time may be the result of too few trips to the bathroom. If you habitually resist the urge to urinate, you'll enlarge the capacity of your bladder and may also cause a bladder infection, says Joseph M. Montella, M.D., an assistant professor and director of the Division of Urogynecology in the Department of Obstetrics and Gynecology at Jefferson Medical College of Thomas Jefferson University in Philadelphia. At the worst extreme, your bladder eventually could become so big and so out of shape that it loses its ability to contract.

To maintain a strong bladder that doesn't have an overly expanded capacity, Dr. Montella says, urinate according to a schedule, about every three to four hours, whether you feel the urge or not.

See also Incontinence

URINATING FREQUENTLY

WHEN TO SEE YOUR DOCTOR

- Frequent trips to the bathroom are still necessary even though you've cut back on liquids and bladder stimulants.
- The number of bathroom visits you need interferes with normal work, travel or sleep.
- Frequency is accompanied by an almost constant urge to urinate.
- You have pain or burning when you urinate.

WHAT YOUR SYMPTOM IS TELLING YOU

You guzzled a cup of coffee to wipe the sand from your groggy eyes when you awakened. You gulped another along with orange juice and milk before you left for work. Then there was that diet soda later that morning, along with some sips of water every time you passed the fountain. You chased down lunch with a can of soda and had another java jolt later in the afternoon as a pick-me-up. During dinner, maybe you had a large glass of milk or water. And don't forget that evening beer in front of the TV.

Do you still wonder why you go to the bathroom so often?

There's no standard for how frequently you should go to the bathroom, urinary experts say. Urinary frequency varies from person to person, even from day to day.

Kidney stimulants and bladder irritants are the most common cause of frequent urination, according to Allen D. Seftel, M.D., an assistant professor of urology at University Hospitals of Cleveland. Caffeine and alcohol top the list. That's because they are natural diuretics, making your body produce urine more quickly than it normally would. Certain medications, such as diuretics for high blood pressure, also force your body to put out more. They don't call them water pills for nothing.

Urinary tract infections (UTIs), which are extremely common, cause frequent trips to the bathroom because they irritate the kidneys, bladder or urethra. Nephritis, a potentially serious kidney disease, also causes frequent urination. The mysterious condition called interstitial cystitis that creates almost constant urinary discomfort also causes frequent urination.

Women are much more likely than men to be affected by all these ailments, which may also produce pain in the abdomen or back and a burning sensation when they urinate, Dr. Seftel says. In men, a prostate infection brings on similar symptoms. Undiagnosed or poorly controlled diabetes also causes you to urinate more often. In addition, blockages anywhere in the urinary system (like stones in the kidney or bladder) can prevent you from emptying your bladder completely, so it's filled up more quickly and you have to urinate more often. That's a particular problem for older men: An enlarged prostate can squeeze on the urethra, dam up the plumbing and cause frequent urination during the night while they're lying down.

If you're urinating more at night, it may simply be a part of aging. Aging transfers the body's production of urine to the night shift. "Older people produce two-thirds of their urine during the night and one-third during the day," notes Margaret M. Baumann, M.D., associate chief of staff for geriatrics and extended care at the Veterans Administration West Side Medical Center in Chicago. "That's the reverse of what you do when you're younger."

SYMPTOM RELIEF

If you feel no pain, burning or discomfort on your many visits to the water closet, little reason exists to worry about frequent urination. But if it's constantly inconvenient, you have a couple of options.

Don't drink like a fish. Why act like a bedouin who has just encountered his first oasis in weeks? Just cut back on your fluid intake. "The vital importance of drinking eight glasses of liquids a day has been overstated to some extent," says Dr. Baumann. "And it's not really true that you're flushing out toxins by drinking more. You won't be healthier if you produce more urine."

Build a bigger bladder. You may have to knock your knees together or jump up and down a bit at first, but you can expand the capacity of your bladder, says Joseph M. Montella, M.D., an assistant professor and director of the Division of Urogynecology in the Department of Obstetrics and Gynecology at Jefferson Medical College of Thomas Jefferson University in Philadelphia. The trick is to not give in to the urge as soon as you feel it. In fact, you actually can shrink your bladder's capacity if you give in to every slightest urge.

To practice bladder training, try staving off the urge to go for, say, 15 minutes. After a week or so, Dr. Montella says, endure a little longer, maybe another 15 minutes. Over the following weeks and months, continue to lengthen the time between urge and surge until you're going to the bathroom about every three or four hours. But don't try to get into *The Guinness Book of World Records* with an endurance record. Years of continually suppressing your urine for hours on end can lead to bladder infection and incontinence.

Don't pop that pill in the p.m. If you're taking diuretics and sleep is interrupted by frequent trips from pillow to potty, ask your doctor about changing your medication schedule, says L. Lewis Wall, M.D., Ph.D., an assistant professor of gynecology and obstetrics at Emory University School of Medicine in Atlanta. Because many drugs stimulate the urinary tract, ask your doctor whether other substitutions might help, too.

Act as if infected. If you're a woman and you frequently have UTIs, follow the tips in Urination, Burning, on page 670. Men can try the hints, too, but because they're so much less likely to contract a simple UTI, they should see a doctor.

Have your prostate checked. If you're an over-40 male and none of these techniques seem to help, you may have an enlarged prostate that interrupts the flow of urine. See a urologist for tests, Dr. Seftel says. The right medication may help alleviate your symptoms. Surgery is also a simple solution. The doctor can remove the obstruction without incisions and restore control.

See also Incontinence

URINATION, BURNING

WHEN TO SEE YOUR DOCTOR

- The burning persists for more than 24 hours after you've tried self-help remedies.
- Burning is accompanied by a discharge from your vagina or penis.
- In addition to burning, you urinate frequently, feel sudden urges to urinate or experience any flulike symptoms, fever, chills or back pain.

WHAT YOUR SYMPTOM IS TELLING YOU

Complaints of burning upon urination, often accompanied by frequent urges to urinate, send eight million women to the doctor's office every year. The usual source of the problem is a urinary tract infection (UTI). One out of every five women gets a urinary tract infection at least once a year, and of those, 15 percent contract more than three a year.

Why are women so prone to UTIs?

Both the rectum and the vagina are perfect incubators for bacteria that all too easily find their way to the nearby urethra, the exit tube for urine. And since the female urethra is not very long, it provides an easy route for the bacteria to invade the bladder, causing cystitis. The bacteria can even move farther upstream to the kidneys, causing a more serious infection called pyelonephritis.

Men have longer urethras, and the prostate gland secretes bacteria-fighting substances that provide a barrier against infections. "It's unnatural for a man to get a urinary tract infection," says John P. Long, M.D., assistant professor of urology in the Department of Urology at Tufts University New England Medical Center in Boston. "When men experience burning as they urinate, it's nothing to be trifled with."

For men, burning urination may signal a sexually transmitted disease, such as gonorrhea or chlamydia. An inflamed prostate—a condition called prostatitis—can also cause a burning sensation.

A number of other factors can cause or aggravate a burning sensation when you urinate, according to Tamara G. Bavendam, M.D., assistant professor of urology and director of female urology at the University of Washington Medical Center in Seattle. Possible irritants include spicy foods, coffee, tea, alcohol, acidic foods and beverages, chemicals in hygiene products and trauma from sex.

Yeast infections can also cause burning.

SYMPTOM RELIEF

Depending on the cause, there are a few keys to getting rid of that burning sensation. Eliminate the bacteria that cause infections or avoid the irritants. These tips will help you do just that.

Flood your bladder. At the first hint of burning, drink two eight-ounce glasses of water, recommends Kristene E. Whitmore, M.D., chief of urology at Graduate Hospital in Philadelphia, clinical associate professor of urology at the University of Pennsylvania and coauthor of *Overcoming Bladder Disorders*. Then dissolve one teaspoon baking soda in four ounces water and drink that. Then, for the next six to eight hours drink eight ounces of water every hour. Consult your doctor if the symptom is not relieved after a day.

What you're doing is diluting your bacteria-filled urinary tract and forcing yourself to urinate, rather than holding it in, which prolongs the infection. "Oftentimes, the water is enough to flush out the bacteria and make your symptoms tolerable," Dr. Whitmore says. "Sometimes that's all that's needed."

See the doctor. If the burning remains after a day, you should see the doctor. If you're experiencing the burning for the first time, you'll need to give the doctor a urine specimen to check for bacteria. The doctor also will check for a yeast infection or sexually transmitted disease. If you're a man, a prostate examination will be done.

Antibiotics in combination with the baking soda and water may rid you of the problem, but if it persists or recurs, more extensive testing will be required, Dr. Whitmore says. That could include more urine cultures, an ultrasound of your kidneys or running a scope up your urethra for a close-up look at your bladder.

Don't feed the burn. Many foods and drinks can irritate the urinary tract, either causing or aggravating the burning, Dr. Bavendam says. These include alcohol, coffee, tea, cranberry juice, chocolate, carbonated beverages, all citrus fruits, tomatoes, chili, spicy foods, vinegar, aspartame and sugar. Even decaffeinated coffee can be an irritant, Dr. Whitmore adds.

Eliminating all of these foods from your diet can ease the burning and other urinary discomforts within about ten days, according to Dr. Bavendam. Once the burning sensation is gone, you can start adding them back to your diet one at a time to see which substance (or substances) is causing a problem. As you do so, she emphasizes, drink a minimum of one quart of water throughout the day.

Ease the pain. Urinating through an inflamed urethra or letting urine touch infected or raw skin is like rubbing salt into an open wound. To ease that pain, try urinating while sitting in a tub of warm water or while standing in the shower, Dr. Bavendam suggests.

Wipe right. If you're a woman, wipe yourself from front to back after a bowel movement. Doing the reverse can more easily sweep bacteria from your rectum into your urethra.

Practice clean sex. Sex can be a significant source of burning by irritating the urethra or introducing bacteria. "Urinate after having sex," Dr. Bavendam suggests. And after you urinate, says Dr. Whitmore, wash your vagina with a hand-held showerhead or bathe it in some water with a tablespoon or so of baking soda.

Stay free of chemicals. Pay particular attention to whether soaps or hygiene products cause irritation, Dr. Bavendam says. Bubble baths, douches, deodorants and scented toilet papers all contain chemicals that can irritate your urethra or the skin surrounding it.

Dry up. In the summer, don't lounge about in a wet bathing suit, which may stimulate a vaginal yeast or bacterial infection. "Wash off the chlorine," Dr. Whitmore says. "And I tell women to carry a spare bathing suit. Change into the dry one after swimming." (For other hints on avoiding yeast infections, see Vaginal Itching on page 689.)

URINATION URGE

WHEN TO SEE YOUR DOCTOR

- Despite the strong urge, you release a relatively small amount of urine or none at all.
- Frequent urination, a burning sensation, pain or discomfort accompanies your urges to go to the bathroom.

WHAT YOUR SYMPTOM IS TELLING YOU

The urge to urinate seems as natural as sleepiness or hunger. But sometimes you feel the urge and think you're going to go—yet not much comes out, or the amount doesn't match the urgency. Usually, the reason is that something is impeding the flow or irritating the urinary tract.

In a glitch-free urinary tract, the urge to urinate comes courtesy of your bladder, the hollow, baglike muscle into which your kidneys dump urine. When the bladder fills to the brim, it wants to contract itself to empty. That sends a signal to your brain, giving you the urge to go.

But urinary tract irritants and stimulants can fool your bladder. Alcohol, and caffeine-containing beverages like coffee and tea stimulate the bladder, according to Margaret M. Baumann, M.D., associate chief of staff for geriatrics and extended care at the Veterans Administration West Side Medical Center in Chicago. "NutraSweet brand sweetener is another substance that can create a false urge, and can be terribly irritating to some people's bladders," she says.

Simple stress or anxiety can also jar the neural network into making you think you have to go to the bathroom, says Allen D. Seftel, M.D., an assistant professor of urology at University Hospitals of Cleveland.

Infections also aggravate the urinary tract and are a common cause of this symptom. Whether an infection hits the kidneys, bladder, urethra, vagina or prostate, it either stimulates the production of urine or gives you the sensation that you have to go to the bathroom, explains Dr. Seftel. Infections also can produce a burning sensation when you urinate. A poorly understood infection called interstitial cystitis also causes an almost continual urge to go to the bathroom as well as pain or discomfort.

Constipation can block the flow of urine. "The bladder and bowels are neighbors," he adds. "Sometimes you have the urge and you do have to go, but pressure from the stool obstructs the flow of urine."

Kidney stones, bladder stones and enlargement of the prostate can also block the flow of urine along the urinary tract, Dr. Seftel says. The bladder cannot empty completely because of the obstruction, which means it fills more quickly. If these conditions are left untreated, urination becomes more forced and difficult, and incontinence could result.

SYMPTOM RELIEF

You *could* give in and go—or try to—every time you feel the calling. But that can be frustrating, not to mention counterproductive, according to Joseph M. Montella, M.D., an assistant professor and director of the Division of Urogynecology in the Department of Obstetrics and Gynecology at Jefferson Medical College of Thomas Jefferson University in Philadelphia. By always urinating as soon as you sense the slightest desire, you actually can shrink the size of your bladder, he says, and you'll end up having the urges even more. Here are a few hints that might prove helpful.

When the urge hits, relax. As paradoxical as it sounds, what you don't want to do when you have a knee-banging urge to urinate is tense up. Relax instead. "I know it seems counterintuitive," says Dr. Baumann, "but since the bladder is a muscle that contracts to empty, you want to relax it to overcome the urge." When the urge hits, sit down, close your eyes and take some deep breaths. Be careful not to relax the pelvic muscles responsible for preventing a spill. Or try any of your favorite relaxation techniques. "It often seems to calm the urge in many of my patients," Dr. Baumann says. This technique works especially well when stress is responsible for the urge.

Tense your sphincter. The same signal responsible for squeezing your pelvic sphincter muscles also tells your bladder to relax, Dr. Montella says. In about a minute, the urge to urinate will subside—temporarily, of course.

Keep a diary. By keeping a record of what you eat and when you urinate, you may be able to spot the food and drinks that provoke the urge. Then you can reduce or even eliminate those irritants from your diet.

Fight off infections. Taking antibiotics for a couple of days will eliminate any infections that might be causing your urges to rush to the bathroom. Tell your doctor about your problem and ask for a checkup and urine test.

See also Incontinence

URINE, BLOODY

WHEN TO SEE YOUR DOCTOR

- See your doctor anytime you notice that your urine is tinted red or contains red streaks or clots.

WHAT YOUR SYMPTOM IS TELLING YOU

"There are no ifs, ands or buts about it. You *must* see a doctor at the first sign of blood in the urine," says Richard J. Macchia, M.D., professor and chairman of the Department of Urology at State University of New York Health Science Center at Brooklyn. "Until we prove otherwise, we assume it's caused by a tumor. The symptom is that important."

The cause usually *isn't* a tumor, of course. Extremely strenuous exercise—such as running a marathon—can cause hematuria (the medical name for bloody urine). So could a bruised kidney from a fall or an automobile accident, according to E. David Crawford, M.D., professor and chairman of the Division of Urology at the University of Colorado Health Sciences Center in Denver. In some people whose bodies lack certain enzymes, eating beets produces reddish urine that looks like blood. And certain drugs—the phenolphthalein in over-the-counter laxatives, for example—may also tint urine red.

Vigorous voiding—giving a real heave-ho to a bladderful of urine that you've been holding for a long time—can rupture small veins, says John P. Long, M.D., assistant professor of urology in the Department of Urology at Tufts University New England Medical Center in Boston. It's not very serious, but the symptom still demands that you see a doctor, he says. Infections, kidney stones, prostate problems and kidney disease also can cause blood in the urine.

The blood could appear as threadlike streaks or small clots, Dr. Long says. More likely, though, all of the urine will be discolored. "It might look like Hawaiian Punch," he says, "or cranapple juice or, more severely, tomato juice."

SYMPTOM RELIEF

Don't expect to go to the doctor, tell him you have blood in your urine and have a prescription handed to you. "It's incorrect to merely treat blood in the urine," Dr. Macchia says. "A definite diagnosis must be established, or at the very least, a tumor must be excluded." Here's what to do before getting into the examination room and what to expect once you get there.

Call a urologist. You probably should bypass your family physician and go straight to a urologist or urogynecologist, Dr. Long says. Because of the tests involved, that's where you'll end up anyway. The only exception, he says, might be for a woman with a history of cystitis, a urinary tract infection (UTI). (UTIs are discussed in detail in Urination, Burning on page 670.)

Track the flow. If you can, before you get to the doctor, note the exact color of your urine and when the discoloration appears. That can provide an important clue to where the problem originates.

A smoky or darker red color urine may indicate an infection or a kidney problem, Dr. Crawford says. If all the urine is a bloodier red, it could be a kidney or bladder problem. If an initial stream of red clears, it may mean a prostate or urethra problem in men or a urethra problem in women. (The urethra is a tube through which urine passes from the bladder.) Clots or threads of blood in an otherwise normal stream of urine could signal bleeding in the upper urinary tract or bladder, Dr. Crawford says.

Prepare for probes. Expect to be subjected to a whole battery of tests until doctors find the cause of the bleeding. "We'll investigate upstairs and downstairs, from the kidneys down to the opening of the urethra," Dr. Crawford says. Tests may include urine cultures, a kidney x-ray and a cystoscopy, in which a tiny viewing instrument is inserted into the urethra and snaked through the urinary tract.

URINE, DISCOLORED

WHEN TO SEE YOUR DOCTOR

- Your urine is tinted red or contains red streaks.
- Your urine is cloudy or milky and foul-smelling.

WHAT YOUR SYMPTOM IS TELLING YOU

With just a couple of exceptions, urine usually is clear or a delicately tinged yellow, with a slight hint of ammonia odor. A change from this norm is sometimes cause for concern.

A red or pinkish color, for example, may indicate bleeding somewhere in your urinary tract, and that needs immediate attention. Cloudy or milky urine suggests a bladder infection or kidney stone, says E. David Crawford, M.D., professor and chairman of the Division of Urology at the University of Colorado Health Sciences Center in Denver. A foul odor may accompany the infection-caused cloudiness. And apart from any particular color change, diabetics with poor blood sugar control may have urine with a slightly fruity scent.

Anything else reflects what you're eating or drinking, urologists say. Beets may mimic the presence of blood, as can the phenolphthalein found in over-the-counter laxatives. Beta-carotene supplements may color urine slightly yellow or orange, while vitamin B6 may evoke a distinctive smell. Urine turns green with a foul odor after you eat asparagus. The drug Risanpin, an antibiotic usually prescribed for tuberculosis or staph infections, can turn urine a shade of blue or green. And some diagnostic drugs will paint your urine a peculiar hue, but they're prescribed for that express purpose.

Very yellow urine means you're dehydrated and not drinking enough water. Chronic dehydration, with urine that's almost constantly a concentrated yellow—even when you don't think you're all that thirsty—can lead to kidney stones, Dr. Crawford cautions.

"If you exercise and are sweating a lot, your urine will be a very concentrated yellow when you urinate several hours later," he says. "But if you just had 15 beers, your urine will be much clearer. You're not going to be able to tell it from water."

SYMPTOM RELIEF

Though you shouldn't be drinking 15 beers to achieve the goal, your urine always should be almost colorless. There's only one thing to do.

Pay attention. All you have to do is notice the color of your urine, says Richard J. Macchia, M.D., professor and chairman of the Department of Urology at the State University of New York Health Science Center at Brooklyn. When it turns intensely yellow, it means the body is eliminating highly concentrated liquid waste. It's too concentrated, actually. You should start drinking more juices and water.

Don't count your glasses. We've all heard that we should be drinking eight to ten glasses of water a day. That's a good rule of thumb, but the amount of liquids a person actually needs varies depending on age, gender, exercise, weight and even the weather, says Dr. Macchia. "Try to stay away from numbers," he says. "If your urine is very yellow, you're not drinking enough. Drink, drink and drink until it becomes clear—and keep it clear."

Don't ignore red. Red urine could mean that your urine contains blood. Take this warning seriously.

See also Urine, Bloody

URINE, DRIBBLING

- Dribbling advances from a couple of drops after urination to a leak that's difficult to control.
- You are also experiencing genital discomfort, a burning sensation when you urinate or frequent urges to urinate.

WHAT YOUR SYMPTOM IS TELLING YOU

Basketball players are supposed to dribble. You're not.

Unfortunately, some people do dribble a little—a little urine, that is. But they shouldn't worry. If it's not more than a few drops, it usually isn't a sign of a serious health problem. And it's often easy to correct.

Before we proceed, let's define what dribbling *isn't*. We're not talking about incontinence, the outright inability to control your bladder. By dribbling, we mean that little extra urine that almost inevitably seems to trickle out after you have deliberately tried to stop the flow or those little wet spots you unexpectedly feel in your underwear.

A couple of built-in obstacles interfere with the flow of urine from the bladder through the urethra and out of the body, according to Kevin Pranikoff, M.D., associate professor of urology at the State University of New York at Buffalo. In men, urine has a tendency to pool in the bulbus urethra, the widest part of the urethra near the base of the penis.

In women, urine also might pool in the urethra, but more commonly, female anatomy creates the potential for pooling outside the urethra, according to Tamara G. Bavendam, M.D., assistant professor of urology and director of female urology at the University of Washington Medical Center in Seattle. The labia may trap some escaping urine, damming it up into the vagina. In girls, the hymen may block urine. And in women of any age, other folds of pelvic skin, even in women who aren't especially overweight, may interfere with a free flow. "Depending on the woman, there may be several inches of skin from the opening of the urethra to the outside of the body," Dr. Bavendam says.

Poor form can compound the natural obstacles, according to Dr. Pranikoff. Men constrict the flow of urine when they expose their penises over the top of their pants or underwear instead of through their fly. And women obstruct the flow when they don't pull their panty hose down far enough to allow them to spread their legs. The result: A little urine may pool in the vagina and leak out later.

But even with exquisite urinary etiquette, if you have lax pelvic floor muscles, you'll be at a disadvantage in trying to internally clamp off the urethra and halt the flow of urine. If the muscle weakening is minor, you'll probably dribble a bit. Should the weakening continue and urinary control become more difficult and less successful, you may be on your way to developing a form of incontinence (see page 321). "If the cause is weak muscles, dribbling is sort of an intermediary step between full control and incontinence," according to Richard J. Macchia, M.D., professor and chairman of the Department of Urology at the State University of New York Health Science Center at Brooklyn.

Aging is a prime cause of muscular weakening for both men and women, but giving birth and going through menopause increase the likelihood of women losing some control over their pelvic muscles. Men have a slight advantage in this regard thanks to their prostates. The gland, which surrounds the urethra below the bladder like a doughnut, grows as a man ages, Dr. Macchia explains. If the enlargement is otherwise benign and not great enough to cause a significant obstruction, the prostate squeezes on the urethra only lightly, compensating for any loss in pelvic muscle tone that could lead to leaking.

But before women start to develop prostate envy, they—and all the men—should know that an inflammation of the gland, called prostatitis, can produce a discharge that could be mistaken for dribbling, Dr. Macchia says. It'll also cause a burning sensation upon urination and a frequent need to go to the bathroom. The bacterial infection that results in prostatitis can hit men at any age, but younger men are especially prone to the problem.

Besides the pelvic weakening associated with giving birth and advancing through menopause, women have an additional concern that can lead to dribbling. Sometimes a small pocket, called a diverticulum, forms on the walls of the female urethra. This pocket can collect some urine that later drips out, Dr. Macchia says. The diverticulum often remains completely harmless. But if the dribbling becomes excessive or if the pocket enlarges, breaks or becomes infected, he says, the diverticulum may have to be surgically removed.

SYMPTOM RELIEF

Ending wet spots could be as simple as learning better bathroom form or strengthening the muscles in your pelvis, say urologists. Try these tips before seeing your doctor.

Nudge out what's left. "Men should learn to milk their urethra," says Dr. Pranikoff. First, urinate through your fly, not over the top of your pants or that constrictive elastic band around the top of your shorts. When finished, with one hand apply some gentle pressure behind the scrotum to coax out any remaining urine from the bulbus urethra.

Sit back, sit wide. For women, urinating with your legs wide apart helps prevent any urine from pooling in the vagina or the urethra. Leaning forward also helps, Dr. Pranikoff says.

Give it a squeeze. Kegel exercises can help you strengthen the muscles in the pelvis and gain better control even if you do have an enlarged prostate. And they're simple to do. The muscles you want to strengthen are the ones you use to start and stop the flow of urine. Squeeze and slowly release those muscles several times. Urologists recommend that you practice this action until you can contract those muscles 50 times in a row several times a day. (For more on Kegels, see Incontinence on page 321.)

See also Incontinence

V

VAGINAL BULGE

You feel an unusual heaviness or pressure inside your vagina.
You feel something protruding from the vaginal opening.

WHAT YOUR SYMPTOM IS TELLING YOU

Chances are, if you have a vaginal bulge, you've also had children, maybe several of them, says David Soper, M.D., a gynecologist at the Virginia Commonwealth University/Medical College of Virginia in Richmond. Over the years, gravity, childbirth and the tissue-thinning processes of menopause can weaken the ligaments and muscle supports that hold your pelvic organs in place. And when the organs begin to drift downward, the condition is called prolapse.

It's a very gradual process, and though a bulge inside your vagina feels very scary, it's not dangerous. It's just very uncomfortable, it can interfere with sexual intercourse and it's hard to live with, says David Chapin, M.D., a gynecologist and instructor in obstetrics, gynecology and reproductive medicine at Harvard Medical School and director of gynecology at Beth Israel Hospital in Boston.

The vagina begins to turn inside out, and depending on the location and degree of prolapse, the bladder, rectum and uterus may come along with it. Most commonly, the bulge is the front wall of the vagina that has given way, says Dr. Chapin. The sensation is something like feeling an egg at the opening of the vagina, he says. The bulge or protrusion can get as big as a fist, or even the size of a grapefruit.

Sometimes a prolapse can make it hard to retain urine when you sneeze, laugh or cough. And if the rectum has "fallen," you may have problems passing stool.

SYMPTOM RELIEF

There are several solutions to the problems of prolapse, and your doctor can help you determine which is right for you.

Befriend that fiber. Although it won't correct the prolapse, eating a high-fiber diet to keep stool soft will make moving your bowels easier, says Roger Smith, M.D., a professor of obstetrics and gynecology at the Medical College of Georgia Hospital and Clinics in Augusta. He recommends lots of fruits and vegetables, with a fiber supplement like Metamucil or Citrucel as needed.

Make multiple "rest stops." Your bladder will be less likely to leak from the pressure of the prolapse if you keep it empty, Dr. Smith says. Remind yourself to urinate regularly, even if you don't feel the urge.

Let it be. If your prolapse is mild enough that it's not causing major problems, it may be appropriate to simply leave it alone, Dr. Chapin says. Talk it over with your doctor.

Repair the foundations. Your doctor may advise you to have surgery for your prolapse. It would involve repairing the front and back walls of the vagina. If the uterus is involved, your doctor may recommend a vaginal hysterectomy, which removes the uterus without an abdominal incision.

Wear a pessary. If surgery is not an option for you, your doctor may prescribe a pessary—a plastic or rubber diaphragm-like device worn inside the vagina to hold up the collapsing structures. Pessaries must be changed every few months, and though they may cause odor and small ulcerations of the vaginal lining, they are safe to use, Dr. Chapin says.

VAGINAL DISCHARGE

WHEN TO SEE YOUR DOCTOR

- Your discharge is accompanied by severe itching.
- Your discharge is cheesy, yellow or greenish.
- Your discharge has a strong fishy or yeasty odor.

WHAT YOUR SYMPTOM IS TELLING YOU

A small amount of discharge is just the normal moisture your vagina produces to keep you comfortable. Even a heavy discharge, caused by cervical mucus production, is normal in some women and harmless, says Eva Arkin, M.D., chief of gynecology at Scottish Rite Hospital and obstetrician and gynecologist with Atlanta Women's Specialists.

But what if your discharge *doesn't* feel normal? What if it is accompanied by itching? You probably have a vaginal infection, and that's a true cause for concern.

One of the most common vaginal infections is *Candida albicans* or *Monilia,* commonly known as a yeast infection. The classic discharge of a yeast infection has a sort of cottage-cheesy texture and is associated with intense itching. Sometimes a yeast infection results from taking a course of antibiotics for another infection in your body.

Bacterial infections (some of which are sexually transmitted) are caused by organisms like gardnerella, chlamydia or gonorrhea and are usually associated with a yellowish discharge that often has a fishy odor. In addition to discharge and itching, you may also feel burning sensations.

A watery, frothy, greenish yellow discharge may be a symptom of trichomoniasis, an infection that's often passed back and forth between partners. Although 35 years ago it was the most common vaginal infection, these days it's relatively rare.

SYMPTOM RELIEF

Wondering if you should play detective with your own discharge? Most doctors say no. Discharges can be deceptive, and you may even have a combination of two types of infection, each of which will need appropriate medication. Your doctor will take a sample of the discharge and examine it under the microscope for a specific diagnosis.

For a look at medical treatments and home remedies for the vaginal infections that cause most itchy discharge, see Vaginal Itching on page 689. And to keep that discharge from returning, here are a few basic reminders.

Don't douche. Douching can actually be a dangerous way to deal with vaginal discharge, says David Eschenbach, M.D., professor and chief of the Division of Gynecology at the University of Washington School of Medicine in Seattle. Douching can drive infectious material or the douche preservatives up through the cervix into the uterus or change the bacteria in the vagina and cause pelvic inflammatory disease (PID), he says.

Let your powder take a powder. Though it may feel good, using talcum powder or cornstarch to dry up a discharge is also ill advised, Dr. Eschenbach says. Over time, the tiny particles move from the vagina into the uterus and end up near the ovaries. Eventually, these deposits may be a factor in the development of ovarian cancer.

Count on condoms. It's difficult for doctors to pinpoint the cause of most bacterial vaginal infections, but one obvious possibility is frequent sex with multiple partners. Using condoms consistently can prevent the transmission of many of these infections, says Patti Jayne Ross, M.D., an associate professor in the Department of Obstetrics and Gynecology at the University of Texas Medical School at Houston. But you should refrain from even protected intercourse until your infection clears up.

VAGINAL DRYNESS

WHEN TO SEE YOUR DOCTOR

You are approaching the age of menopause.
Vaginal dryness is accompanied by itching.

WHAT YOUR SYMPTOM IS TELLING YOU

Many women of all ages run into vaginal dryness now and then. But common or not, a dry vagina feels uncomfortable and can make sex downright painful.

The amount of vaginal lubrication varies from woman to woman, with a wide range of normal, says Theresa Crenshaw, M.D., a sex therapy specialist and author of *Bedside Manners*. The fluid itself is clear and relatively odorless. Apart from its gentle blessing when you're sexually aroused, you may not take much notice of your vaginal fluid most of the time. But when it's *absent*, you may start to feel dry as a desert.

Vaginal dryness can have a variety of causes. Your sensitive vaginal chemistry may be reacting to another kind of chemistry—in harsh alkaline soaps, for example. Or you may be drying up as part of an allergic response to perfumes or dyes. As you get closer to the years of menopause, lowered estrogen levels may also cause dryness of the vagina. And certain skin conditions may interfere with vaginal lubrication.

SYMPTOM RELIEF

Here's how to get that gentle lubrication flowing again.

Scrutinize your soap. "The vagina wasn't designed to be sterile," says John Grossman, M.D., a gynecologist at George Washington University Hospital and Medical Center in Washington, D.C. "It has its own biologically normal, natural method of bacterial control—mainly by maintaining a natural level of acidity (pH of 4 to 4.5)."

His advice? "Use a superfatted hypoallergenic soap with no dyes or fragrances—one that is nonalkaline and pH balanced."

Avoid those allergens. If your dryness is a reaction to a substance that you are allergic to—an allergen—you may have to do a little detection to pinpoint the culprits. Two common allergens are the fragrances and dyes in laundry detergent and toilet paper, Dr. Grossman says.

Toss out the designer-patterned and perfumed paper in favor of a soft, white, unscented variety, he suggests. If laundry detergent seems to be a problem, you may not need to switch brands. Just send your underwear through a second rinse cycle. You might also try switching to white cotton underpants.

Learn where you lubricate. It's normal for some women not to lubricate copiously when they're sexually aroused. It's also possible to lubricate without realizing it, says Dr. Crenshaw. If you're lying on your back, the moisture may pool in the back of your vagina, too far away to make sexual intercourse comfortable. The solution? Before intercourse, try dipping a finger into the vagina and drawing some of the lubrication out to coat the dry surface, she suggests.

Try a healthy substitute. If your dryness is only occasional, use a water-based lubricant like K-Y Jelly or Surgilube during sexual intercourse, says Roger Smith, M.D., a professor of obstetrics and gynecology at the Medical College of Georgia Hospital and Clinics in Augusta.

"Avoid Vaseline and oils," he says. "They tend to plug up pores, and if you're using a condom, the oil-based products will eat holes in it."

Although K-Y and Surgilube are fine for occasional dryness, Dr. Smith recommends Replens for safe and continuous relief. Replens contains a special molecule that draws water into vaginal tissues. After using it daily for about a week, you should be able to decrease your usage to two to three times a week, as needed, he says.

Check with your doctor. Your doctor may determine that a dermatologic problem is causing your vaginal dryness, Dr. Grossman says. A wide range of skin conditions an cause vaginal dryness. Your doctor may take a tiny tissue sample and treat you with a prescription cream or antibiotic, he says.

Harness help from your honey. The nicest advice may be this: When you have sex on a regular basis, you naturally make more lubrication, says Mary Beard, M.D., an assistant clinical professor in the Department of Obstetrics and Gynecology at the University of Utah Latter Day Saints Hospital in Salt Lake City. Continuing sexual activity is an important help in holding back the thinning and drying effects of menopause on vaginal tissues, she says.

Ask about hormones. If you have reached menopause and your vaginal dryness just won't let up, you may want to discuss hormone replacement therapy with your doctor, says Dr. Beard.

The dryness, thinning and tenderness of vaginal tissues after menopause can be relieved by estrogen, which you can take orally, by using a transdermal patch or by inserting a vaginal cream.

VAGINAL ITCHING

WHEN TO SEE YOUR DOCTOR

- Itching persists more than three days, doesn't respond to home remedies or is getting progressively worse.

WHAT YOUR SYMPTOM IS TELLING YOU

Unless you spend your summers at a nudist camp, your private parts are often covered in three or four layers of material—perhaps a pantiliner, panties, a pair of snug-fitting pantyhose and your coolest Calvin Kleins.

So what is that warm, moist part of you doing under all those layers?

It's itching! And it's driving you nuts.

Vaginal itching can come from something as simple as trapping bacteria for too long under too many layers of too-tight clothes. All that warmth and moisture provide perfect conditions for incubating infections.

In fact, itching can be the unwelcome calling card of a wide variety of infections, ranging from bacterial vaginitis to yeast (also called *Candida albicans* or *Monilia*) and trichomoniasis.

The itching can also signal an allergy to a chemical in soap, deodorant or dye, or may simply be a sign of thinning vaginal tissues in women approaching menopause.

SYMPTOM RELIEF

Let's take a soothing look at how to banish that infernal itching.

Sitz in some salt. Several forms of vaginitis will often respond to a simple home remedy—the saline sitz bath. Here's the recipe from Gideon Panter, M.D., a gynecologist in New York City.

Dissolve a half-cup table salt in a shallow tub of warm water. In the tub, insert your finger into your vagina to let the warm salt water in, then remove your finger and relax for 10 to 15 minutes. Two or three consecutive nights of sitz baths should ease the itch, if yours is home treatable, Dr. Panter says.

Abstain for the duration. Don't have sexual intercourse until your itching has cleared up, Dr. Panter says. If the organism that set up its itchy housekeeping in your vagina was transmitted by your partner, there's no sense in reexposing yourself to trouble. Take a few days to show love in other ways, he suggests.

Consider the condom. Condoms provide wonderful protection against both unwanted pregnancy and sexually transmitted disease. If condom use always seems to be followed by a bout of vaginal itching, however, it's possible that an allergy to the condom's latex rubber, powder coating or lubricant could be the problem.

Try this simple home patch test from Bruce Katz, M.D., dermatologist and assistant clinical professor of dermatology at Columbia University College of Physicians and Surgeons in New York City. Tape an inner-side piece cut from a fresh condom to one arm, and an outer-side piece to the other arm. Leave both pieces in place for 48 hours, and keep the areas dry. If both arms react, you're allergic to the rubber. If only the arm with the inside of the condom taped to it gets itchy or rashy, you're allergic to the powder. If only the arm with the outside piece reacts, you're allergic to the lubricant.

Does this mean you should avoid using condoms? Absolutely not, says Dr. Katz. Their role in reducing infection risk is too critical. Instead, have your partner use two—lambskin over latex if you are allergic to rubber, or reverse the order if the powder is the problem. Why not just switch to lambskin? Lambskin on its own can't protect against some organisms, including the virus that causes AIDS. Dr. Katz says a nonlatex condom should be on the market shortly, which will solve the problem entirely.

Ask your doctor. You'll need your doctor's help to determine which type of infection is causing your itching. If you've been diagnosed with yeast infections in the past, and are very familiar with the specific symptoms, call your doctor for a prescription, recommends R. Don Gambrell, Jr., M.D., clinical professor of endocrinology and obstetrics and gynecology at the Medical College of Georgia Hospital and Clinics in Augusta. Your doctor will prescribe antifungal medications such as Vagistat, Nystatin or Monistat.

Trichomoniasis is treated with the prescription antibiotic Flagyl. Bacterial infections call for antibacterial agents—either sulfa drugs or, if you're allergic to sulfa, with Betadine antiseptic, an over-the-counter product, says Dr. Gambrell.

"And be sure to have your doctor test you for the human papilloma virus (HPV)," recommends Jessica L. Thomasson, M.D., a gynecologist at Columbia Medical Center in Milwaukee. This virus, which causes genital warts, is an important and frequently overlooked cause of vaginal itching, she says.

Get help for menopause symptoms. If you're approach ing menopause, ask your doctor about treatments for itch ing caused by changes that are taking place in the vagina Hormone replacement therapy is an option, but you shoul also ask about prescription hormonal creams for th vagina.

Bag the douche and powder. Douching not only won help to relieve itching or vaginitis, it may be dangerou: says David Eschenbach, M.D., professor and chief of th Division of Gynecology at the University of Washingto School of Medicine in Seattle. Douching may drive infec tious material up through the cervix and cause pelvi inflammatory disease, he says.

The use of talcum powder or cornstarch is questionabl too, Dr. Eschenbach says. Over time, the tiny particles ma collect near the ovaries and increase ovarian cancer risk.

Defeating the Yeast Beast

Fortunately for women who suffer from recurrent yeas infections, these infections respond well to treatment. An there's plenty of prevention available, too.

Cut down on sugar. Sugar feeds yeast, so cut back o high-sugar foods, advises Marjorie Crandall, Ph.D., microbiologist, candida researcher, and founder of Yeas Consulting Services in Torrance, California.

See what C can do. Take 500 milligrams of vitamin (twice a day, recommends Eva Arkin, M.D., chief of gyne cology at Scottish Rite Hospital and obstetrician and gyne cologist with Atlanta Women's Specialists. Vitamin (increases the acidity of the vagina, creating a yeast unfriendly environment, she says.

Blow it away. After a shower or bath, blow-dry the vagi nal area, Dr. Arkin suggests. Yeast needs moisture to sur vive. Set your blow dryer on cool, and position the dryer si to eight inches from the vaginal area.

Try another sort of sitz. Another type of sitz bath work well to fend off yeast infections, says Dr. Arkin. Once month after your menstrual cycle, add three tablespoons o boric acid to six inches of water in a pan large enough to s in. While you're roosting in your roaster for five to ten minutes, the yeast is in retreat.

Lay on the lactobacillus. A cup-a-day habit of yogurt with active *Lactobacillus acidophilus* cultures will reduce your likelihood of yeast infections, a study from Long Island Jewish Medical Center shows. Health food stores are your best bet for "live" natural yogurt. (You *eat* the yogurt, by the way; you don't douche with it.) Lactobacillus is also available in powder and capsule forms at health food stores.

Take the scratch test. If your yeast infections persist, you may be allergic to Candida, and allergy shots of Candida extract can help prevent further problems. Ask your doctor to refer you to a board-certified allergist for skin testing, Dr. Crandall recommends.

Yank yeast from your diet. If you test positive, Dr. Crandall suggests avoiding allergic reactions to Candida by avoiding foods and beverages containing yeast and molds, at least until you have received the allergy shots for about six months. Look out for the following yeast and mold troublemakers: bread, pizza, English muffins, bagels, croissants, raised doughnuts, beer, wine, liquor, apple cider, moldy cheeses, cider or wine vinegar, pickles, grapes, berries, cantaloupe, fruit juices, brown sugar, sprouts, mushrooms, yeast extract, vitamins derived from yeast, smoked meats and fish and leftovers.

Prime your prescription. If you know you get frequent yeast infections, then ask for anti-yeast medication whenever your doctor puts you on antibiotics, Dr. Crandall suggests. (Antibiotics taken for other infections kill off both friendly and unfriendly bacteria in the vagina, clearing the way for an overgrowth of yeast.)

Plan your prevention. Any vaginal irritation can pave the way for yeast infection, says Dr. Crandall. That's why it helps to avoid any vagina/chemical contact, including perfumes, colored toilet paper, dyed underpants, deodorants and commercial sexual lubricants. Dr. Crandall recommends unscented mineral oil or vegetable oil as a nonirritating lubricant alternative. (These cannot be used with condoms or a diaphragm, however.)

To prevent yeast flare-ups, she suggests laundering your clothes with unscented detergent, avoiding fabric softeners and wearing loose-fitting cotton clothing, white cotton underwear and no pantyhose.

VARICOSE VEINS

WHEN TO SEE YOUR DOCTOR

- You also have persistent leg aches, cramping or itching.
- You also have ankle swelling or are bleeding from a vein.

WHAT YOUR SYMPTOM IS TELLING YOU

Those blue lines on your thighs are starting to look like interstates. And the ugly bulges surrounding them make them look like they're under construction.

If your legs are a road atlas in 3-D, you probably have varicose veins.

"Twenty percent of adult Americans have varicose veins. The majority are women whose mothers had them, too," says John Hallett, M.D., associate professor of vascular surgery at the Mayo Medical School in Rochester, Minnesota.

Varicose veins develop when a vein wall weakens and stretches. That weakening affects the small valves within each vein that keeps the blood flowing toward the heart. As a result, the blood is trapped in the vein—and the vein bulges. The pooled blood can also flood the tinier "spider veins" located near the skin's surface.

Varicose veins not only look bad, they can *feel* bad. In severe cases, the backed-up blood can make legs that have spent too much time walking around the mall or standing at the stove feel like they're made of lead. Your legs might also itch or cramp during the night.

Women are four times more likely than men to have varicose veins, possibly because the female hormones estrogen and progesterone weaken the vein walls in some way, says Dr. Hallett. Typically, protruding veins debut in pregnancy, when the hormone surge increases blood volume, he says. The veins overstretch, pop out and may never shrink back. Birth control pills and estrogen replacement therapy can also contribute to bulging veins.

The problem can worsen with prolonged sitting or standing, excess weight, constipation or tight clothing. If not controlled, the purple bumpiness can increase with age as veins further lose elasticity.

Varicose veins aren't usually a sign of a severe health problem, says Dr. Hallett. One exception is when varicose veins develop as a result of damage to deep veins in your legs from an injury, a blood clot, inflammation or a circulatory problem such as phlebitis.

SYMPTOM RELIEF

If you have varicose veins, you can't make them go away, short of having them surgically removed (which is an option). But there is plenty you can do to ease the discomfort and embarrassment.

Pump, pump, pump your legs. A 20-minute daily walk contracts the calf muscles and will help move blood out of the vein, says Robert A. Weiss, M.D., assistant professor of dermatology at Johns Hopkins University School of Medicine in Baltimore. "On long car trips, stop briefly every couple of hours and walk around your car," says Dr. Weiss. Circle your desk a few times at work or stroll up the airplane aisle on long flights. If you're stuck sitting in a lecture hall, tighten and release your calf muscles repeatedly. This immediately empties stagnant blood out of veins.

Put your feet up. Elevating your legs above the level of your heart for 15 minutes daily helps the blood move back toward your heart, says Dr. Weiss.

Cross your ankles, not your knees. "A crossed-knee position sets up a roadblock to blood flow," says Mitchel

Goldman, M.D., assistant clinical professor of dermatology at the University of California, San Diego, School of Medicine.

Graduate to compressed support hose. "If you have swollen veins, wearing regular support hose could make them worse," says Dr. Goldman. "Support that's evenly distributed basically acts as a tourniquet, aggravating the vein." Instead, you should wear graduated compression stockings that are tightest at the ankle and looser as they go up the leg.

"If you put them on in bed before you stand up in the morning, the stockings help hold in the veins and drive blood back to the heart," says Dr. Goldman. What's more, wearing graduated compression stockings during pregnancy can actually prevent varicose veins from forming. Many medical supply stores and some drugstores now carry fashionable, sheer panty hose and below-the-knee hose that are graduated. These must be prescribed by a physician.

Ditch your girdle. Any clothing that cuts off circulation in the calf or thighs, such as skin-tight pants and tight knee socks, can worsen blood pooling, says Dr. Goldman.

Avoid high heels. High heels keep calf muscles contracted and put extra stress on leg veins, says Dr. Weiss. "If you must wear spikes, slip them off periodically and pump your calves," he says.

Lose pounds. The more weight you carry around, the more pressure is put on leg veins, says Dr. Hallett.

Trade fatty foods for fiber. If you want to know what's causing your bulging veins, look at what you're putting in your belly, says Glenn Geelhoed, M.D., professor of surgery at George Washington University in Washington, D.C. "A modern diet that's generally low in fiber and high in fats, sugar and salt causes constipation and increases abdominal pressure. This forces more blood into the lower extremities," he says. "In countries where high-fiber diets are the norm, varicose veins are virtually unknown."

Dr. Geelhoed's advice: Adopt a high-fiber diet packed with fruits, vegetables and grains. This will help bulk up and soften your stool and may reduce pressure in the veins.

Give your veins a shot. Smaller varicose veins can be removed with an office procedure called sclerotherapy. A solution is injected into the vein, which irritates the lining, causing it to contract and shrivel. Eventually, the vein closes down entirely and the scar tissue it leaves behind is reabsorbed into your body. But sclerotherapy is not a cure, says Dr. Hallett. Additional veins can start to bulge, which may require additional injections.

Consider surgery. In severe cases, you may need surgery to partially or totally remove a bulging vein. Treatment with a laser can help erase the smallest spiders. "You should talk to a dermatologist or vascular surgeon who specializes in treating varicose veins to discuss your options," says Dr. Hallett.

VISION, BLURRY

WHEN TO SEE YOUR DOCTOR

- Your vision becomes blurred at any distance, whether or not you wear glasses or contact lenses.

WHAT YOUR SYMPTOM IS TELLING YOU

You hold the menu close, then at arm's length. But the words are so blurry, you can't tell if the entrée is "pasta" or "potpie."

Around age 40, most adults are blindsided by one of the body's more discouraging developments: fuzzy vision. It occurs when the lens of the eye loses some of its flexibility and can't focus sharply on near objects, particularly the newspaper, maps or other fine print.

Middle-aged people tend to develop this form of farsightedness—called presbyopia—even if they already wear corrective lenses for other vision problems, according to

Mitchell H. Friedlaender, M.D., director of corneal services in the Division of Ophthalmology at the Scripps Clinic and Research Foundation in La Jolla, California, and coauthor of *20/20: A Total Guide to Improving Your Vision and Preventing Eye Disease*. "Presbyopia progresses until about age 65," he says.

But that's not the only reason you may not be seeing clearly. You can have 20/20 vision and still become bleary-eyed if your eyes are glued to a computer screen for many hours. Smog, dust and pollen can also irritate your eyes and fuzz your view. And contacts that are not properly cared for or are wearing out can also distort your vision. So can eyes irritated by infections.

Blurred vision can also be the first sign of a serious eye condition, such as cataracts, glaucoma or macular degeneration. Sometimes conditions not directly related to the eyes can affect vision. These include diabetes, pregnancy, anemia and kidney and nerve diseases.

SYMPTOM RELIEF

Because blurry vision has the potential of leading to serious eye disease—and blindness—you should have your eyes examined by an ophthalmologist, an M.D. trained to treat eye disorders. If your problem turns out to be age-related farsightedness (most likely), here's what you can do.

Try reading glasses. Off-the-rack reading glasses may be all you need, says Dr. Friedlaender. Try on the pair with the lowest magnifying power, then stand about 14 inches away from the rack and read the printing on it. If you have trouble, try glasses with more power. To check for distortion, hold the glasses at arm's length and focus on an object with strong vertical and horizontal lines, such as a door. Move the glasses up, down and sideways. If the lines waver, choose another pair. If these don't work, you'll have to ask your eye doctor about prescription reading glasses or bifocals.

Trick your brain with two lenses. Your ophthamologist may suggest fitting you with two contact lenses, with one eye measured for far vision and the other measured for close vision, says Dr. Friedlaender. With these "monovision" lenses, the brain automatically focuses the eyes. The contacts work without reading glasses or bifocals.

Consider computer glasses. Regular reading glasses that focus at about 18 inches may not help you see the video display terminal (VDT), which is normally farther away, says Dr. Friedlaender. A weaker reading prescription for this distance can solve VDT blurriness.

Check out lubricant drops. If your exam doesn't reveal any abnormalities, often the cause of cloudy vision is as mundane as dry air, or overworn or dirty contact lenses, says Jason Slakter, M.D., attending surgeon in the Department of Ophthalmology at the Manhattan Eye, Ear and Throat Hospital. If that's the case, a number of over-the-counter lubricants may help defuzz the view. If your contact lenses are causing your problem, he adds, be sure to remove, clean and disinfect your lenses each night, using only the commercial products recommended for your lenses. Nightly removal and cleaning will help guard against the haziness produced by protein deposit buildup on the lenses.

Discuss glasses for cataracts. Even if your exam reveals cataracts—thickened spots (what doctors call opacities) in the lens that sometimes occur after age 50—all you may need is an adjustment in your eyeglass prescription. "A brand-new prescription may provide the clarity you need to perform daily functions," says Dr. Slakter. If over time the opacities further obscure your vision, you can have the cloudy lens surgically removed and a new lens implanted, he adds.

Don't skip a single drop. When you have glaucoma, pressure builds up inside the eye—pressure that can explode into blindness. If you've been diagnosed with this disease, you'll need to use eyedrops every day to relieve that pressure, says Dr. Slakter. Don't forget! The pressure rises each day you fail to take your medicine.

Consider a telescope transplant. That may sound odd, but it's one of the treatments for macular degeneration, a condition in which one of the eye's most crucial parts slowly breaks apart, leading to dimmer and dimmer vision.

Another solution for macular degeneration is magnifying lenses. "These low-vision aids can make the difference between being able to read and not being able to read," says Dr. Friedlaender.

See also Vision Loss

VISION LOSS

WHEN TO SEE YOUR DOCTOR

- Any degree of vision loss should be seen by a doctor.

WHAT YOUR SYMPTOM IS TELLING YOU

For many of us, wearing glasses or contacts to correct less-than-perfect vision is as much a part of our everyday wardrobe as underwear.

More than ten million Americans, however, have some degree of visual impairment that can't be completely corrected with glasses.

The list of sight stealers is long and varied, with Father Time at the head of the list. As the years pass, the lens inside the eyes can gradually thicken and become opaque with cataracts, leading to cloudy spots, blurriness, blinding halos around lights and poor night vision.

Time can also take a toll on the macula—the part of the eye responsible for straight-ahead vision. In fact, a lifetime of sun exposure and other factors that break down the blood vessels and tissues that nourish the macula is responsible for most vision loss that occurs past age 60. This wear-and-tear process—called macular degeneration—gradually shrivels the macula and affects the straight-ahead vision needed to see fine detail. People with macular degeneration often find that words look broken and bunched up. Blank holes appear on street signs and in the fine print on food labels. Straight-lined objects like door frames take on a wavy, warped look.

Other causes of vision loss include tears in the retina and eye diseases such as glaucoma and diabetic retinopathy. In glaucoma, fluid builds up inside the eyes, and the increasing pressure damages the optic (eye) nerves. Diabetic retinopathy is a complication of diabetes that damages the blood vessels in the retina.

A sudden and often temporary loss of vision may occur from an injury to the eye, a stroke or even a migraine headache.

SYMPTOM RELIEF

Once your ophthalmologist has diagnosed your vision problem and prescribed treatment, here's what you can do to make the most of your remaining vision.

Shed lots of light on the subject. "An ideal reading lamp should have a 60- to 100-watt coated light bulb to reduce glare enclosed in a reflective interior to intensify the light," says Amalia Miranda, M.D., director of the Low Vision Clinic and clinical instructor of ophthalmology at the Oklahoma University Health Sciences Center in Oklahoma City. High-intensity halogen lights are super bright but also hot. It's better to use them with a dimmer adjustment, she says.

Bring the world closer. Magnifiers in all shapes, sizes and strengths can restore your ability to read and enjoy your surroundings, according to Eleanor Faye, M.D., an ophthalmologic surgeon at the Manhattan Eye, Ear and Throat Hospital. A hand-held magnifier, for example, can help you read books and food labels. And special glasses with built-in telescopic-type lenses can help you read street signs or watch your grandson make a touchdown.

Blow up your books. If you can afford the investment, a special closed-circuit TV (read/write machine) can magnify your books on a TV screen up to 60 times their normal size. Large-print publications and books on tape are cheaper alternatives. A simple, yellow plastic sheet over a book page can make words pop up and give contrast, according to Lorraine Marchi, founder and executive director of the National Association for Visually Handicapped (NAVH) in New York City. Other useful low-vision aids include large telephone dials and high-contrast watch faces. For more information about these products, write to NAVH, 22 West 21st Street, New York, NY 10010.

Sight Preservers

The following sight-sparing measures may help slow, reverse or perhaps even halt vision loss.

Become a fruit-and-vegetable fan. "Before I began advising patients about proper nutrition, I was only doing half my job in helping them keep their eyes healthy," says Dr. Faye. Her advice: Eat fruits, vegetables and other foods rich in zinc and vitamins C, E and A and beta-carotene (it converts to A in the body). "Ample evidence shows that these so-called antioxidants may counteract the sun-related oxygen damage to the eye's cells and slow down age-related vision loss," says Dr. Faye.

Consider supplements for the eyes. For good measure, take a commercial eye supplement featuring the prime antioxidants mentioned above. "My patients report improved well-being after taking these nutrients and many demonstrated improved vision," says Dr. Faye. Preliminary studies confirm her findings. In a study from the University of Utah, for example, researchers gave daily doses of antioxidant supplements to 192 people with macular degeneration. Another 61 people received no treatment. After six months, a third of the first group scored better on vision tests. Other studies show cataract risk is also reduced in multivitamin users.

Wear blue blockers and a sombrero. Amber-tinted sunglasses may help block out blue light, a component of sunlight that may contribute to age-related vision loss over prolonged periods, says Dr. Miranda. These sunglasses reduce glare and improve contrast, while offering protection from the harmful ultraviolet (UV) rays of the sun, she says. Top your head with a wide-brimmed hat and you have good protection from sun damage to eyes.

Quit smoking. Researchers from Harvard Medical School found that compared with people who never smoked, people who smoke 20 or more cigarettes per day had about twice the risk of cataracts.

Watch for wavy doorways. One way to keep alert to any vision loss from macular degeneration is to regularly test yourself by looking at straight-line objects such as window frames, says Matthew Farber, M.D., an ophthalmologist in private practice in Fort Wayne, Indiana. Let your doctor know if any lines appear distorted, wavy, faded, missing or shimmery, as if seen through heat waves on a highway.

Don't delay—remove the haze. If cataracts are interfering with your vision, a surgeon can remove the cloudy lens. Clear vision is then possible with the help of a lens implant or special glasses or contacts. Your eyes will remain sun-sensitive, however. "For people who have had cataract surgery, blue-blocking sunglasses and a wide-brimmed hat are recommended," says Dr. Miranda. The latest implants have a special coating to protect against UV rays.

Look into laser surgery. Ultra-powerful high-beam laser light can seal or dissolve eye tissues and halt certain disease-caused vision loss, according to Dr. Faye. In the case of macular degeneration, a laser can sometimes repair leaking areas of the macula. This allows the retina to heal and can slow down the disease, says Dr. Faye. In some types of glaucoma, lasers can make small openings in the iris to relieve built-up pressure.

Winning against Glaucoma

Early on, glaucoma doesn't have any symptoms, but as optic nerve damage progresses, peripheral vision gets blanked out, making it seem as though you're looking through a tube. Besides laser surgery, here's more ammunition for controlling glaucoma.

Get an annual eye exam after age 35. This is especially important if glaucoma runs in your family or if you're nearsighted or have diabetes. It's also important for black people, who are more susceptible to glaucoma.

Make eyedrops a daily habit. If you have glaucoma, you'll need to take eye-pressure-controlling medicine faithfully and correctly, says James McGroarty, M.D., associate clinical professor of ophthalmology at State University of New York Health Sciences Center in Brooklyn. Each time you insert the drops, close your eye for 60 seconds. That way you won't lose any of the medicine.

Jump on your two-wheeler. Drops are the traditional way to control glaucoma. But studies show that when people with raised eye pressure used a stationary bike for 30 minutes three times weekly for ten weeks, they reduced their eye pressure. In fact, the exercise worked as well as anti-glaucoma drugs. "Elevated eye pressure in glaucoma is similar to high blood pressure in heart disease," says Linn Goldberg, M.D., associate professor of medicine at the Oregon Health Sciences University in Portland. "If you control the pressure, you can in many instances help prevent or control the disease."

Follow-up studies showed that the exercise effects were long-lasting, but that the pressure went back up to former levels once the exercise stopped. Do *not* stop taking anti-glaucoma medications on your own, warns Dr. Goldberg. If you want to try exercise as an alternative, you'll need to work with your doctor to create a program suitable for you and to monitor the pressure in your eyes, he says.

VOICE LOSS

WHEN TO SEE YOUR DOCTOR

- Your loss of voice persists longer than two weeks.
- You lose your voice after an accident or injury to your head or neck.
- If you suddenly lose your voice for no apparent reason, see a doctor immediately.

WHAT YOUR SYMPTOM IS TELLING YOU

The good news is that if you think you've lost your voice, chances are you haven't *really* lost it. What's more likely is that you have some degree of hoarseness, and there's plenty of help for that.

How do you tell? Try to cough or clear your throat. If you can do that, you are actually vocalizing. Though your voice may be unreliable at the moment, even severely hoarse—it's just mislaid, not lost entirely.

Doctors say that complete aphonia—loss of the ability to speak—is extremely rare. When it does happen, it may be the result of emotional or psychological stress.

It is possible for your voice to give out entirely after abusing it—rooting too loudly at a football game, for example. You can also lose your voice for a time after a prolonged episode of laryngitis (inflammation of the vocal cords). Straining to talk through laryngitis can actually tire the muscles you use for speech to the point where they just quit working for awhile.

Although it's very unusual, a tumor in the chest or lung can injure the nerves leading to the vocal cords, causing loss of the ability to speak. An accident or head or neck injury might also injure these nerves. And losing your ability to speak can be a sign of a stroke.

SYMPTOM RELIEF

Resting your voice and drinking plenty of fluids can help ease a lost voice. But anything that helps a hoarse voice can also help one that's faded away.

See also Hoarseness

VOMITING

WHEN TO SEE YOUR DOCTOR

- You've been vomiting periodically for more than 24 hours.

WHAT YOUR SYMPTOM IS TELLING YOU

What does a gallon of lukewarm brew have in common with a trip on the twist-o-rama at the county fair? Unfortunately for you and the vomit control center in your brain, plenty.

While primarily charged with monitoring your bloodstream and digestive system for toxins, your vomit control center is also plugged into something called your *chemoreceptor trigger zone*. This area in your brain keeps tabs on your equilibrium and your senses of smell, taste and sight.

The not-so-pretty result of this collaboration: The tiniest drop of poison can have the same effect on your system as watching a televised surgical procedure (in technicolor).

"Vomiting is actually an extremely complex act," says Jorge Herrera, M.D., assistant professor of medicine at the University of South Alabama College of Medicine in Mobile and member of the American Gastroenterological Association and the American College of Gastroenterology. "But with the right stimulus, you are almost unable to prevent yourself from doing it."

Of course, there are other causes of vomiting besides overindulgence, poisoning and motion sickness. Perhaps the most common: A stomach virus can fool your ever-vigilant vomit center into thinking that you need to throw up, says William B. Ruderman, M.D., chairperson of the Department of Gastroenterology at the Cleveland Clinic–Florida in Fort Lauderdale. (Throwing up won't do anything to eliminate the virus.)

Other causes of vomiting include severe chronic ulcers, gallstones, the early stages of pregnancy and chemotherapy.

SYMPTOM RELIEF

If nausea has set in and vomiting seems inevitable, here's what you can do.

Go with the flow. While vomiting is not the most pleasant experience in the world, you can actually *prolong* your discomfort by trying to avoid it. "The best thing is just to stay home and try to go through it, and most of the time you'll stop getting sick within 12 to 24 hours," says Dr. Herrera. "If the vomiting isn't gone by then, that's the time to seek help."

Boost your beverage intake. You lose a lot of fluids by vomiting, and that can make you dehydrated. You'll need to replenish them a short time after vomiting by sipping a glass or two of water, de-fizzed soda or even a sports drink, says Dr. Herrera.

Steer clear of diet drinks that don't contain sugar, however. Sugar assists in absorbing water, says Dr. Ruderman. If you vomit again right after beginning to drink, give yourself a break for a couple of hours and try again when the nausea has subsided.

Avoid eating. Consider solid foods off-limits until you have stopped vomiting for at least six hours, says Dr. Herrera. And when you do return to the dinner table, don't try to make up for lost time. "I don't think you should have a big burger or anything like that," he says. "You should slowly go back to your regular diet, but start with things like rice, toast, bananas—stuff that's bland but nutritious. By the second day you could probably eat anything that you want," he says.

Say no to dairy. Unless you're willing to suffer from diarrhea after vomiting, it's probably best to avoid dairy products for the next few days, says Dr. Herrera. Vomiting, particularly if from a viral illness, can temporarily diminish your ability to digest the sugar in milk, he says.

Think pink. Taking an over-the-counter stomach soother

like Pepto-Bismol may actually help settle your stomach, says Dr. Ruderman.

Have an antacid. Ulcer-related vomiting will sometimes stop if you use an over-the-counter antacid, says Dr. Ruderman.

Chew it over. Chewing gum, long a remedy for middle ear pain during airline flights, may also help reduce air sickness and thereby prevent vomiting, says Mark Babyatsky, M.D., a gastroenterology specialist at Harvard Medical School.

Get serious. For severe cases of vomiting—like those caused by some cancer treatments—your doctor may prescribe an anti-nausea drug like Compazine or Reglan, says Dr. Babyatsky.

See also Nausea

W

WALKING DIFFICULTY

WHEN TO SEE YOUR DOCTOR

- You experience changes in the way you walk—including any difficulty negotiating turns or climbing stairs.
- You also have feelings of numbness, pain, unsteadiness, twitching, muscle stiffness or muscle weakness.
- You frequently fall, stumble or bump into objects.
- You also feel that your muscles seem to be wasting away.

WHAT YOUR SYMPTOM IS TELLING YOU

Throughout the stages of your life, your walking style may change distinctly. You start off with stumbling baby steps. You plod through the awkwardness of adolescence. In later years, you may cautiously amble along with the help of a cane or walker. But for most of your life, you walk along with confidence, fluidity and ease. So when you find yourself losing control of this fundamental function, it's cause for concern.

Walking involves a harmonious cooperation among your muscles, bones, eyes and inner ears. Coordinating this effort are your brain and central nervous system, says Steven Mandel, M.D., clinical professor of neurology at Jefferson Medical College and an attending physician at Thomas Jefferson University Hospital in Philadelphia. "A problem anywhere in this network can produce shuffling, foot dragging, jerking motions or difficulty bending joints," he explains.

The eyes and inner ears are obvious places to look for problems. Elderly people who are losing their vision may have difficulty walking, and anyone with an inner ear infection could experience balance problems that interfere with walking. (For more information, see Earache on page 164.)

The central nervous system is also a likely spot. Medications, such as sedatives, can affect the central nervous system and create walking problems, says Dr. Mandel. So could alcohol or drug abuse.

Poor nutrition could conceivably be at the heart of the problem as well, particularly in the elderly. "Vitamin B12 deficiency often produces numbness in the extremities and a disturbed sense of balance, which leads to gait changes," says Lawrence Z. Stern, M.D., professor of neurology and director of the Muscular Dystrophy Association's Mycio F. Delgado Clinic for Neuromuscular Disorders at the University of Arizona Health Sciences Center in Tucson.

Finally, almost any disease or condition that affects the nerves or muscles can produce walking problems. The condition could be something as treatable as a herniated disk in the lower back. Among the more serious diseases affecting the gait are amyotrophic lateral sclerosis (Lou Gehrig's disease), multiple sclerosis, muscular dystrophy and Parkinson's disease.

"Diabetes often produces a loss of sensation in both feet," says Peter Cavanagh, Ph.D., director of the Center for Locomotion Studies at Pennsylvania State University in University Park. "Many people with diabetes lose the ability to tell where their legs are in relation to the floor and develop an unsteady stance and gait."

SYMPTOM RELIEF

A gait abnormality is cause for concern at any age. If these tips don't help, see a physician. Because so many conditions could be responsible, you should expect a battery of tests to diagnose the problem.

Have your medications checked. List all medications you are currently taking—both prescription and over-the-counter. Then ask your doctor whether any alterations in your medications are appropriate.

Keep your eyes forward. "You're much steadier when

you're looking forward than when you're head is tilted back or to the side," says Dr. Cavanagh. "Try keeping your head level and square to your shoulders and place objects at eye level so you don't have to crane your neck."

Have your vision checked. Clear vision and depth perception are extremely important factors in walking. "If you can't see the floor clearly, you will walk with an awkward, apprehensive gait," says Dr. Mandel. (For more hints on dealing with vision problems, see Night Blindness on page 451; Vision, Blurry, on page 697 and Vision Loss on page 700.)

Stripe your walls. Many hospitals and institutions whose patients have walking difficulties paint vertical stripes on the walls, according to Dr. Cavanagh. The vertical stripes give people better stabilization of gaze than blank walls or horizontal stripes and have been shown to reduce falls and injuries.

See also Balance Problems

WARTS

WHEN TO SEE YOUR DOCTOR

- Your wart is disfiguring or prevents normal functioning (as on a fingertip).
- The wart is painful, bleeding or changes shape or color.
- Your wart has grown larger than a pencil eraser.
- You're not positive it's a wart.

WHAT YOUR SYMPTOM IS TELLING YOU

Let's try on a few of the good old myths about warts. Myth number one—you can get them from handling frogs. Nope. But warts *can* be transmitted from one person to another.

Well, how about Tom Sawyer's famous remedy? Rub your wart with potato or swing a dead cat over your head and bury it, and sooner or later, the wart vanishes. That's more like it. The dead cat isn't exactly a cure, but it will work as often as any other folk remedy, doctors say. The answer to these mysterious treatments is that two-thirds of all warts will vanish on their own within a year.

But how did you get it to begin with?

There are some 60 subtypes of the human papilloma virus on the surface of the skin that can cause warts. We're all exposed to wart viruses every day, by touching someone who has a wart or touching something they've touched. There's no clear explanation for why one individual either has warts or is wart-free. Some of us are just more susceptible than others. Warts are as individual as the viruses that produce them, but there are some basic types.

Common warts, often seen on the hands of children, are thick and rough. *Flat* warts are usually smooth bumps that are skin-colored and flat-topped. These warts are most often found on the hands or face, or on the lower legs of women who shave. *Plantar* warts are found on the bottom of the foot and *palmar* warts on the palm of the hand. And *filiforme* warts look like little groups of fingers or bristles protruding from the skin.

Genital warts are called *condyloma* and can lead to more serious health problems if left untreated.

SYMPTOM RELIEF

Most wart treatments destroy or irritate the wart tissue until your body starts up an immune response to the virus. If your warts are numerous or bothersome enough, here's how your doctor can help.

Give them the acid test. Acids are often used to destroy wart tissue, says Libby Edwards, M.D., chief of dermatology at Carolinas Medical Center in Charlotte, North Carolina. Your doctor can prescribe a solution for you to drip on the wart daily for a month or two. The acids are often a combination of salicylic acid and lactic acid. They can also be applied to the wart by covering it with a plaster—an adhesive piece of fabric with medicine on the sticky side.

Freeze them away. Another common wart cure is freezing with liquid nitrogen. This method has about an 80 percent success rate, says Stephen Webster, M.D., a dermatologist in Lacrosse, Wisconsin. This treatment is somewhat painful, but it's also the fastest way to eliminate a wart.

Another chemical doctors use to fight warts is a chemotherapy agent called bleomycin. "It's injected right into the wart and makes the wart go away," says J. Michael Maloney, M.D., a dermatologist in private practice in Denver. Be aware that in cases where the wart is on a finger, bleomycin may cause scarring that can affect the regrowth of the fingernail, he adds.

Slash and burn. If your warts don't give up after other kinds of treatment, they can be directly removed. After applying a local anesthetic, your doctor can cauterize warts with an electric needle, cut them out surgically or vaporize them with a laser. The disadvantage of these treatments is potential scarring.

Do-It-Yourself Wart Removal

If you don't feel your warts are serious enough for a trip to the doctor, or you just want to try for a cure on your own, here are a few things you can try.

Do the drip. You can use the same acids your doctor would prescribe, but in milder strengths, says Dr. Maloney. Acid-containing over-the-counter remedies like Compound W or various wart plasters will work just as well as the doctor's solutions. "It's slow, but it works," he says. (Do not use over-the-counter products on genital warts.)

Hypnotize them. It may sound weird, but it can work. Research has shown that 20 to 50 percent of people who can deeply relax and give themselves hypnotic suggestions can eliminate their warts. "It doesn't matter whether you think you are hypnotizable," says Nicholas Spanos, Ph.D., a professor of psychology at Carleton University in Ottawa, Ontario. "What makes the suggestions work is your ability to *vividly imagine* your warts flaking off and growing smaller, and your skin feeling warm and tingling as it heals."

Research results indicate that self-hypnosis is even more effective on warts than salicylic acid, Dr. Spanos says.

WATER RETENTION

WHEN TO SEE YOUR DOCTOR

- Swelling in your extremities or abdomen persists for a week and your skin dents when you poke it.
- If you're pregnant and experience sudden swelling in your legs or elsewhere, see your doctor immediately.

WHAT YOUR SYMPTOM IS TELLING YOU

Your fingers are so puffy, you need soap to pry off your rings. Your legs are so swollen, your socks leave a rosy ring around your calves. Zippers aren't budging. Buttons are popping.

These are a few clues that your body is retaining more than its usual amount of water—a symptom doctors call edema.

Normally, your body's cells are bathed in water. There's water inside the cells and a certain amount of water around the cells. The amount of water—both inside and outside the cells—is regulated by hormones, sodium and the kidneys.

When there's too much sodium in your body—from eating a high-salt diet, for example—your blood becomes saltier and water is drawn from your cells to dilute it. Thirst prompts you to drink more water.

Steroid medications can also cause puffiness. These drugs cause the kidneys to hold on to sodium.

Some people's bodies seem to retain water for no apparent reason, according to Charles Tifft, M.D., associate professor of medicine at Boston University School of Medicine. The puffiness may come and go in cycles, he says, and may be related to hormone fluctuations. It can affect both men and women. In women it usually occurs in the week or so before menstruation. During this time, the surge in estrogen triggers the production of aldosterone. This hormone makes the kidneys retain water, which tends to collect in the breasts and abdomen. Some women gain several pounds during this time. Other women simply experience a shift in the distribution in water with no weight gain. Slacks and blouses often fit more snugly, however.

Water retention also occurs among women past menopause who take estrogen replacement hormones.

In late pregnancy, many women find that their legs feel like heavy water balloons. That's because the enlarging abdomen presses on the vein that returns fluids back to the heart. Fluids then pool in the legs.

In some cases, water retention signals something more serious. If your skin remains plump or your finger leaves an indentation when you poke your skin, you may have a problem with your heart, kidneys, liver or thyroid.

SYMPTOM RELIEF

If you're often puffy, the following steps may bring relief.

Skip the junk food. Too much sodium in your blood can waterlog the tissues, so reducing your salt intake makes sense, says Dr. Tifft. Besides avoiding obviously salty fries, pepperoni pizza and convenience foods, cut down on foods containing hidden salt. These include some salad dressings, cereals and canned soups. Become a label reader.

Get your feet pumping. Walking, bicycling and tennis are all activities that help pump out water and other fluids that can pool in your legs and ankles, according to Susan Lark, M.D., director of the PMS and Menopause Self-Help Center in Los Altos, California, and author of *Premenstrual Syndrome Self-Help Book* and *Menopause Self-Help Book*.

Take the load off your legs. If you have swollen calves, elevate your legs for a few minutes each day, says Dr. Lark.

Lie on the floor on your back facing a wall with your legs raised and your buttocks and hips as close to the wall as possible. Your legs should be touching the wall and extended in a wide "V" formation. Breathe easily. Hold the position for five minutes. If you're pregnant, lie on your side with your feet propped up on a stack of pillows.

Ask about your medications. Give your doctor a list of all medications you are currently taking—both prescription and over-the-counter—and ask whether any alterations are appropriate. Switching to lower-dose estrogen in your hormone replacement therapy, for example, could reduce fluid retention, says Dr. Lark. If you're taking steroids, be sure to let your doctor know about your water-retention problem.

Dig deeper for clues. If you continue to have general swelling despite these measures, you may need a blood pressure check and also kidney and liver function tests, says Dr. Tifft. If tests reveal that your problem is caused by high blood pressure, you may be given a diuretic, such as hydrocholothiazide. These drugs force your kidneys to pump water and sodium out of the tissues into the urine, thus reducing blood volume and lowering pressure. Initially, these drugs can easily drain away two pounds or more of fluid daily, but this effect tends to wear away with time. Diuretics, however, are not "casual weight-loss tools," says Dr. Tifft. "They have potent side effects and need to be closely monitored and carefully prescribed. You don't take them to lose a quick five pounds so you can fit into a dress."

Help for Premenstrual Swelling

If water retention plagues you on a monthly basis, here are several things that might prove helpful.

Pass up drugstore diuretics. Some over-the-counter medications intended to relieve menstrual cramp pain also claim to help eliminate premenstrual water weight. Some of these products contain caffeine, which may work as a diuretic, according to Candace Brown, Pharm.D., associate professor of pharmacy and psychiatry at the University of Tennessee in Memphis. "The down side to caffeine, however, is that it also promotes breast pain and tenderness as well as irritability," says Dr. Brown.

Have some herbal tea. Parsley or uva-ursi tea can help flush out excess water without any harmful side effects, according to Dr. Lark. You can find these teas in most health foods stores, she adds.

Check out vitamin B6. Taking up to 250 milligrams of vitamin B6 daily helps reduce premenstrual water retention, says Dr. Lark. This nutrient also reduces fluid buildup caused by hormone replacement therapy during menopause. Vitamin B6, however, can be toxic in higher doses and should only be taken under the supervision of a doctor. Ask your doctor whether a vitamin B6 supplement is appropriate for you.

Try calcium. Researchers at the New York Metropolitan Hospital found that a daily calcium supplement provided relief from premenstrual water retention in three-fourths of the women who took it. "Your best bet is to take a 500-milligram chewable tablet twice daily at breakfast and dinner," says Susan Thys-Jacobs, M.D., assistant professor of medicine at Mount Sinai Hospital in New York City. Ask your doctor whether these supplements might prove helpful in your case.

WEIGHT GAIN

WHEN TO SEE YOUR DOCTOR

- Your weight gain is sudden or starts after you begin taking a new medication.
- You also have insomnia or feel weak and depressed.
- You also urinate more at night or have a history of heart problems or chest pain.

What Your Symptom Is Telling You

You probably haven't gone from Twiggy to Roseanne overnight, but you have noticed a new snugness in your favorite jeans and a tug around the tummy in that tee shirt.

While fluctuations of a pound or two from day to day are normal, a steady increase in weight (actually, in fat) is not.

The most common cause of weight gain is excess fat intake and too little exercise. "It's difficult to gain weight except by eating fat," says Donald S. Robertson, M.D., medical director of Southwest Bariatric Nutrition Center in Scottsdale, Arizona, and coauthor of *The Snowbird Diet*.

A small percentage of overweight people appear to have a genetic knack for gaining weight. "We're not talking about everybody," says Richard L. Atkinson, M.D., associate chief of staff for research and development at the Veterans Affairs Hospital in Hampton, Virginia, and professor of medicine at Eastern Virginia Medical School in Norfolk. "Those who are seriously obese by say 50 or 100 pounds over their ideal body weight may have a metabolic alteration predisposing them to store calories as fat."

As you age, your metabolism gradually slows, making it easier for pounds to stick, says Dr. Atkinson. To complicate the problem, many older people are less active than when they were younger, yet continue to eat the same amount of food.

People who quit smoking often gain some weight because nicotine is no longer artificially stimulating their metabolism and because they tend to eat instead of smoke, says G. Michael Steelman, M.D., vice president of the American Society of Bariatric Physicians, who is in private practice in Oklahoma City.

And strict dieting can also make you gain weight. When you restrict calories too much, your body thinks it's starving and slows down your metabolism. When you begin eating again, it doesn't shift completely back into normal, and you put on the pounds more easily, explains Dr. Steelman.

Some medical problems can trigger weight gain. An underactive thyroid, although not a cause of significant weight gain, slows the metabolism, allowing calories to be stored more easily as fat. People with diabetes who begin taking insulin may notice an increase in weight. And, in rare instances, hormonal disturbances that cause an over-production of insulin or cortisol in the body also cause weight gain.

As a side effect, some medications can stimulate the appetite, slow the metabolism or allow calories to be stored more easily as fat. Women taking birth control pills or estrogen replacement therapy probably will notice a weight gain of about five pounds or so, says Dr. Robertson. Any glucocorticoids, such as prednisone for arthritis, can also be a problem. And Elavil, an antidepressant, is "a nasty one for inducing weight gain," says Dr. Atkinson. "Antiseizure drugs, anxiety drugs, schizophrenia drugs—many that affect mood and emotion—can also cause weight gain," he adds.

In fact, mental health itself influences body weight. While many people with depression curb eating and lose weight, some people eat and gain weight, according to Dr. Atkinson.

Not all weight gain can be attributed to the body storing away extra fat. Extra pounds could also be the result of fluid retention from kidney, liver or heart disease. Even before your ankles begin to swell, Dr. Atkinson says, you easily could gain five or ten pounds from retaining fluid.

SYMPTOM RELIEF

Some of the causes of weight gain—like fluid retention and drug side effects—are medical problems and need the attention of your doctor. As for the everyday problem of overweight, there's a lot more to be said about it than we can give you in a few tips. But the basics are, well, basic. The body doesn't *want* to be fat anymore than it wants to be sick. Weight loss *will* happen if you stick to these few principles.

Cut fat. While a little fat is necessary to metabolize some nutrients and to manufacture hormones, it should comprise no more than between 20 and 30 percent of your total daily calories, Dr. Robertson says. "Learn where the fat is and eliminate it." Current nutritional guidelines recommend that most of your diet consist of whole grains, fruits and vegetables. Cut back on the amounts of meat and dairy products that you eat, and use butter, margarine, oils and oily salad dressings sparingly.

Get moving. To burn calories that have already been stored as fat and to ensure that your body won't become a fat silo, you must work out regularly. "It doesn't have to be extremely vigorous," Dr. Robertson says. "You can walk two to three miles a day at a pace of one mile in 15 minutes, or you could do 15 minutes of aerobics followed by 15 minutes of light weight lifting." If 15-minute miles are too vigorous for you, start slowly. Take a half-hour to walk around the block if you have to. The idea is to get yourself moving and do it on a regular basis.

Exercise, by the way, will also help you deal with depression, which could be contributing to overeating. (For other ways to deal with depression, see page 144.)

Make more muscle. Don't shun lifting weights for fear of developing too much muscle or because you're too old, Dr. Robertson says. "The more muscle mass you have, the higher your metabolic rate and the more calories you'll burn at rest," he says. "That's true even into your eighties and nineties." If the idea of lifting weights intimidates you, talk to your doctor about getting some resistance exercise that's appropriate for your level of fitness. He might be able to recommend a local program that can get you started safely.

Commit to the change. Preventing fat formation requires a *lifelong* lifestyle change in favor of physical activity and healthy eating, Dr. Atkinson says. Don't think of exercise and watching what you eat as a temporary measure to help you lose weight. Realize from the start that these are activities for the rest of your life.

See also Water Retention

WEIGHT LOSS

WHEN TO SEE YOUR DOCTOR

- You're not *trying* to lose weight.
- You're trying to lose weight and *suddenly* lose more than ten pounds.

WHAT YOUR SYMPTOM IS TELLING YOU

Sounds like a dream symptom—weight loss. No plump paunch, no sagging bottom. *("Whatever it is, Doc, I don't want to be cured, because I'm looking great in my swimsuit.")*

Hold off on that delight for just a minute. Unintentional, unexplained weight loss is a serious symptom, according to Richard L. Atkinson, M.D., associate chief of staff for research and development at the Veterans Affairs Hospital in Hampton, Virginia, and professor of medicine at Eastern Virginia Medical School in Norfolk. "You need to see your doctor for a checkup," he says. "And that's particularly true if you're attempting to lose weight and you lose a lot of weight very suddenly. You may be mistaking a serious disease for success in dieting."

The only time weight loss isn't a serious symptom is if you have truly altered your lifestyle—adopting a nutritious, low-fat diet and maintaining a regular schedule of exercise and physical activity—and the weight loss is gradual.

A lot of health problems can result in sudden, unexplained weight loss. Any condition in which you lose your appetite for an extended period of time—a chronic illness like cancer, for example—can strip you of pounds. One of the most common of these anti-appetite diseases is a chronic infection. (AIDS and tuberculosis are two of the worst appetite assassins.)

Some glandular diseases make you hungrier—but also eat up your body. An overactive thyroid speeds up your metabolism, causing weight loss (and sweating, tremors, weak muscles and nervousness). In diabetes—a disease of the pancreas gland that ruins the body's ability to regulate blood sugar, a main source of fuel—the body burns off fat trying to meet its energy needs.

Some diseases of old age—Parkinson's and Alzheimer's —can steal pounds. In Alzheimer's, people can simply forget to eat. And older people often lose weight just because they're getting old—their metabolism slows, their taste sensations become dull and appetite itself can decrease, says Donald S. Robertson, M.D., medical director of Southwest Bariatric Nutrition Center in Scottsdale, Arizona, and coauthor of *The Snowbird Diet.*

But it's not only physical illness that causes weight loss. Mental illness can affect appetite, too. Some people with depression are disinterested in eating and lose weight, says Dr. Robertson. And anorexia—a psychological disorder in which a person eats almost nothing because of a distorted perception of their body—also leads to rapid, excessive weight loss.

SYMPTOM RELIEF

Unwanted or unintended weight loss is not a problem that can be solved by eating—it's probably a symptom of a serious disease, and you need to see your doctor. Here's what might turn up and what your doctor might suggest.

Treating TB. Tuberculosis isn't a death sentence—it's very treatable. Antibiotics can knock it out, says Dr. Atkinson, but you must stick with your treatment, which lasts months.

Calming an overactive thyroid. Doctors treat an overactive thyroid with medication, surgery or with a dose of radioactive iodine, which destroys part of the gland, says Dr. Atkinson. After your treatment you may have to take thyroid pills, which will provide normal amounts of thyroid hormone.

Disciplining diabetes. If your doctor diagnoses diabetes, you'll need a personal program of diet, exercise and medication (taken either orally or by injection) to regulate it.

Detecting cancer. The sooner cancer is detected, the better the chances of a cure, says Dr. Atkinson. Treatment may include surgery, radiation or chemotherapy.

WHEEZING

WHEN TO SEE YOUR DOCTOR

- Wheezing is accompanied by shortness of breath, fast breathing or coughing up phlegm.
- You have a history of heart problems or chest pain, or your feet and legs are swollen.
- You have not been previously diagnosed with asthma.
- You have asthma and need to use your bronchodilator every four hours or more to prevent wheezing bouts.

WHAT YOUR SYMPTOM IS TELLING YOU

Wheezing is the hallmark of asthma, an extreme sensitivity of the lungs that causes inflammation and constriction of the airways. "The airway walls are narrow from swelling and inflammation," says Michael S. Sherman, M.D., an assistant professor and medical director of the Department of Pulmonary Services in the Division of Allergy, Critical Care and Pulmonary Medicine at Hahneman University Hospital in Philadelphia. "The muscles also contract, squeezing the airways even more." That double dose of constriction also causes shortness of breath.

People with asthma don't go about with a constant wheeze. The constriction needs a trigger—but when your airways are supersensitive, it's a *hair*-trigger, according to Susan R. Wynn, M.D., an allergist in private practice with Fort Worth Allergy and Asthma Associates in Texas.

"Anything you can smell—fumes, cigarette smoke, perfume, even those little potpourris—can trigger wheezing in someone with asthma," she says. So can a long workout, which dries bronchial tissue and constricts the smooth muscles in the lungs. Add to the list allergies, infections and emotional stress.

But all that wheezes is not asthma. Infections as innocuous as a cold or as virulent as pneumonia can clog airways with mucus and cause wheezing in people *without* a history of asthma, says Dr. Sherman. The excess production of mucus from chronic bronchitis also constricts airways and produces a nasty wheeze (along with shortness of breath and rapid breathing). And wheezing is also a symptom of emphysema.

Asthma, emphysema and chronic bronchitis usually cause wheezing on the exhale. A wheeze or noise upon inhaling is usually caused by an obstruction in the *upper* part of the respiratory tract, according to Charles P. Felton, M.D., chief of pulmonary medicine at Harlem Hospital Center and a clinical professor of medicine at Columbia University College of Physicians and Surgeons in New York City.

In fact, any infection or swelling of the larynx or trachea can produce noisy breathing, called stridor, Dr. Felton says. So can inhaling an object—choking on a chicken bone or having food go down the wrong pipe. "Whatever the situation, stridor is always cause for alarm and needs immediate medical attention," he says.

And sometimes wheezing's main cause isn't a problem in the respiratory tract, upper or lower. A poorly functioning heart can't pump blood effectively through the lungs, which then fill up with fluid. The airways can narrow from fluid, causing a wheeze. "Additionally, when you inhale, the air hits the water, making almost a gurgling sound that doctors call 'rale' or 'crackle,' " says Dr. Sherman. How do you know if your wheeze is caused by a heart problem? Swelling in the feet or legs may be present.

SYMPTOM RELIEF

If you're wheezing, you're not just whistling Dixie. "It's pretty serious stuff," says Dr. Wynn. If you haven't already been diagnosed with asthma and you don't have a cold, you should visit a doctor or the hospital emergency room, especially if the wheeze or rattle occurs when inhaling. Here are a few tips to make your life a little less wheezier.

Cough it away. If your wheeze disappears after a few coughs clear away some mucus, you probably have a cold or some other viral infection, says Dr. Sherman. A key to its severity will be the color of your mucus. Yellow is usually a sign of infection, and you may need a prescription for an antibiotic. If the mucus is clear or white, try some of the remedies in Coughing on page 133 and Sneezing on page 570. Those tips also will be helpful in dealing with asthma.

Give your lungs a wake-up call. Drinking two cups of caffeinated coffee can ease the wheeze of an asthma episode, according to Dr. Wynn. And if you're on your way to the doctor's office because of a bout of wheezing with an unknown cause, she says that it wouldn't hurt to drink a can of cola or a cup of coffee to see if it provides some relief.

Reduce lung inflammation. A couple of prescription drugs are particularly helpful for treating asthma-induced wheezing. The antihistamine cromolyn sodium or inhaled corticosteroids are now seen as the primary medications to reduce the inflammation that narrows airways in the lungs, doctors say. "You won't notice immediate relief," Dr. Wynn says. "It's more of a gradual improvement, but over time, the corticosteroids help reduce the inflammation and irritation of whatever is triggering the asthma."

Breathe with a bronchs accent. Prescription medications that dilate the bronchial tubes—bronchodilators like albuterol and metaproterenol—immediately relax airway muscles in the midst of an asthma flare-up, Dr. Sherman says. Bronchodilators also are more useful than corticosteroids to expand the airways of people with emphysema or chronic bronchitis.

Know the plan for an attack. Make sure your physician helps you to understand precisely what medications to take when your asthma flares up, Dr. Wynn says. "It'll be different for everybody," she says. "If you get a bout of wheezing, you'll know what to do and won't panic."

Leave the rest on the shelf. Because of side effects like high blood pressure, a rapid pulse and heart palpitations, doctors don't look too favorably on using over-the-counter preparations to treat wheeze sprees. If you know you have asthma and you have no other alternative at the time, you could take a puff of something like Primatene Mist that contains epinephrine.

If you have not been diagnosed with asthma, don't treat yourself with OTC drugs. "Don't waste your time with any of that," Dr. Sherman says. "You don't know what's causing the wheeze, and time could be of the essence. See your doctor."

WORMS

WHEN TO SEE YOUR DOCTOR

- See your doctor any time you see worms or worm eggs in your stool or in your bedclothes.

WHAT YOUR SYMPTOM IS TELLING YOU

Generally, worms announce their presence inside your body through symptoms like persistent abdominal pain, anal itching or diarrhea. But certain kinds of worms occasionally show up outside the body.

"It's rare to see them in the United States because our sanitation is good and our nutrition is good," says William B. Ruderman, M.D., chairperson of the Department of Gastroenterology at the Cleveland Clinic–Florida in Fort Lauderdale.

But what if you *do* (shudder) actually see one either in your stool or (double shudder) find one in bed with you in the morning?

SYMPTOM RELIEF

Well, if worms do show up, they've done you a big favor, because now that you know they're there, you can easily wipe them out. Here's what to do.

Capture it. As unpleasant as it may sound, capture either the worm or the infected stool, place it in a plastic bag or other sealed container, and take it to your doctor for analysis, says Jorge Herrera, M.D., assistant professor of medicine at the University of South Alabama College of Medicine in Mobile and member of the American Gastroenterological Association and the American College of Gastroenterology. "That would tell us exactly what kind of worm it is and what kind of treatment you'll need," he says.

Treatment is always in the form of the appropriate anti-worm medication. Vermox, one of the strongest prescription anti-worm medications on the market, for example, is so effective it can wipe out most cases with one tablet, says Dr. Herrera. "Just to make sure, I'll prescribe it to the whole family for three days, and that's usually the end of it," he says.

Set a tape trap. If you think you've seen or felt a worm but aren't sure, you can set a pinworm trap with adhesive tape rolled into a cylinder, sticky side out. Just before bed, place the tape on either of your buttocks near your anus. When the worm crawls out to lay its eggs, the eggs or even the worm may get stuck to the tape. In the morning, save the tape (and the worm, if there is one), and take it to your doctor to have it analyzed, says Dr. Ruderman. (This is a good technique to use on children who complain about wigglies in their bottoms at night.)

Wash those sheets. If you or your children are being treated for worms, thoroughly (and immediately!) wash your bed linen and pillowcases in hot water to kill any worm eggs that may be clinging to the sheets. "Pinworms are very contagious," says Dr. Ruderman. "The eggs can be in the bed sheet and passed from one person to another."

And your hands. Ever work in the dirt and then eat lunch without washing your hands? You may be introducing worms into you own body. Worm eggs and larvae can

get under your fingernails when you've been working outside, says Dr. Herrera.

Stop thumb—and finger—sucking. Tiny fingers that
have been playing in the sandbox should not make their
way into your child's mouth, says Dr. Herrera.

Keep your shoes on. Because some worms called ascaris
can actually penetrate the skin, it's best to keep your shoes
on when walking on soil or grass, says Dr. Herrera.

Eat only well-cooked pork, beef and fish. Some worms
that live in pigs, beef cattle and fish can actually end up
making their home inside you if larvae living in the meat
isn't killed during cooking, says Mark Babyatsky, M.D., a
gastroenterology specialist at Harvard Medical School.

WRIST PAIN

WHEN TO SEE YOUR DOCTOR

- Significant wrist pain persists for more than a day.
- There is also weakness or numbness in the hand.
- You've had an accident recently, your wrist looks
  deformed and you're unable to move it.
- You also hear clicking, popping or grinding noises.

WHAT YOUR SYMPTOM IS TELLING YOU

You're the neighborhood seamstress, the one person
everyone thinks of when they need bridesmaid's
dresses. You can do wonders concealing everyone's worst
faults—wide hips, big tummy, skinny legs and all.

But lately, you're having trouble concealing one of your
own anatomical sore points. It's your aching wrist, accompanied by pins and needles—figuratively speaking, of
course—in your fingers. After a day of pinking away at
eight bridesmaid's dresses, your wrist and hand feel almost
divorced from the rest of your arm.

Inside your wrist is a small compartment, a framework of bone and ligament called the carpal tunnel. The median nerve and tendons pass through this narrow passageway on the way to your hands and fingers. If the tendons of your wrist are abused in any way, perhaps through repeated forceful movements—like bending and twisting as you scissor through a diaphanous mass of tulle—they can become irritated and inflamed, and swell up. In time, the tendons start to close in on the nerve, and before you know it, you feel a tingling, followed by decreased sensation and then numbness in your thumb, index and long fingers. You can lose coordination and strength and may even feel discomfort. This injury is called carpal tunnel syndrome, and it is the bane of anyone who uses their hands to perform the same motion over and over again.

This feeling of pins and needles, often accompanied by pain, is a dead giveaway. "You decide how hard you're gripping something by the pressure you sense in your fingers," explains Scott Barnhart, M.D., director of the Occupational Medicine Clinic at Harborview Medical Center in Seattle. "So if you lose that sensation, your perception may be that you aren't able to grab things as tightly."

Another clue might come your way in the dead of the night. You may be awakened by tingling and burning in your hand. Inflamed tendons retain fluid and can cause nocturnal discomfort. During sleep, when your arm is relaxed, the fluid has difficulty circulating properly and builds up pressure in the area, says Steven Bogard, lead physical therapist for the Mayo Clinic Hand Center in Rochester, Minnesota. "Once awake, if people shake their hands, it feels better," he says. "This relieves the built-up fluid pressure and thus the associated aching sensations." Your wrist is vulnerable to this kind of injury from overuse, but water retention during pregnancy can also cause swollen tissues and carpal tunnel syndrome, Bogard says.

Injuries such as dislocations or broken bones can also cause wrist pain. In fact, it's even possible to break your wrist and not know it at first. The pain and throbbing only later become noticeable, and you may also notice a clicking or grinding sound coming from the joint.

SYMPTOM RELIEF

Barring serious injury—which, of course, your doctor should tend to immediately—here's how to get a handle on wrist pain.

Do no further harm. Protecting your wrist from further damage is often the first step in healing it. So if you're pretty sure why your wrist is starting to hurt—for example, you've been tapping away at the computer keyboard on an all-nighter—ease up. If you can't stop completely—for example, if typing is your job—some physicians recommend that you alternate the typing with your other work duties. Modify your work habits, if you can. Take frequent breaks, and try to keep your hands and wrists in a straight line, *not* bent up or down. The doctor may prescribe splints as a gentle reminder, though many people only wear them at night.

Chill out. Using an ice pack on the pain may be helpful, says Bogard. Apply mineral oil to the skin where the pack will be placed. Put a damp towel over the oil and place the ice pack on the towel. Cover the pack with added towels for insulation. Leave the pack in place for 10 to 20 minutes, he advises. Check your skin every 5 to 10 minutes. If the skin turns white or blue (which would indicate a potential for frostbite), remove the ice pack immediately.

Take your shots. In more painful cases, the doctor may inject cortisone directly into the carpal canal to reduce the pain and swelling.

Search for the source. To tell exactly where the injury has occurred and whether there is any nerve damage, your doctor may recommend a procedure called an electromyelogram (EMG). During this test your physician will measure the condition of your muscles in the injured area by inserting needles with electrodes into the muscles and reading the electrical signals. This helps to locate where the nerve is injured and the extent of the damage. This isn't necessary for everybody, but it may be called for if the location of your injury isn't readily apparent.

Consider surgery, when necessary. In more serious carpal tunnel syndrome cases, surgery may be required to relieve the pressure against the nerve and blood vessels. This is outpatient surgery—you're in and out in a day. It usually requires only a local anesthetic, says David Rempel, M.D., an assistant professor of medicine at the University of California, San Francisco, and a biomedical engineer. "The doctor makes an incision into the wrist and palm, and cuts the tight ligament or band that forms the 'roof' of the carpal tunnel. That releases pressure," says Dr. Rempel. "A second version of that surgery is performed with an endoscope—a tube about the thickness of your little finger. A small incision is made in the wrist or palm, and a tiny knife, like a switchblade at the end of the tube, can cut the ligament from inside your wrist. This surgery is surprisingly effective at relieving the symptoms."

See also Joint Inflammation; Joint Pain

INDEX

Abdomen. *See* Stomach *entries*
Abdominal muscles, 408, 539
Abscesses, 512–13
    draining, 391, 514
    tooth discoloration from,
        648–49
    treatment, 513–14
Absence seizures, 581
Accutane (Rx), for acne, 497–98
Acetaminophen
    clotting and, 55
    night sweats and, 458
    nosebleed and, 471
    symptoms treated with
        ankle swelling, 24
        bruises, 95
        earache, 166
        fever and chills, 116, 117,
            221
        headaches, 284
        joint pain, 348
        knee pain, 360
        muscle spasms, 431
        osteoarthritis, 223
        restless legs, 522
        shingles, 564
        skin tenderness, 564
    toothache and, 647
Ache all over, 1–3, 73, 74. *See
    also* Fibromyalgia
    breastfeeding and, 73, 74
Achilles tendon injury, 19, 20
Acidic foods
    canker sores and, 108
    cold sores and, 122
    tooth sensitivity from, 658
Acid reflux. *See* Gastric (acid)
    reflux
Acids, for warts, 712-13
Acne. *See* Pimples
Actifed, 324
Actinomysis, 624, 625
Acupressure, for motion sickness,
    443
Acyclovir (Rx), 122, 562, 564
ADHD, 318–20
Adie's syndrome, 571

Advil. *See* Ibuprofen, symptoms
    treated with
Afrin, 543
Afternoon slump, 3–6
Age spots, 7–8
Aging
    appetite loss from, 30
    hearing loss from, 289–90
    memory loss and, 242
    seeing lights from, 527
    seeing spots from, 528
    smell loss and, 568, 570
    tooth discoloration from, 648
    urinating frequently and, 668
    vision problems from,
        697–98, 699, 700
Air, swallowing, 98–99, 586,
    587
Airplane travel. *See* Flying
Albuterol (Rx), 725
Alcohol, rubbing
    for body odor, 68
    chills and, 117
    for sweating, 457, 605
Alcohol, symptoms from
    drinking
    afternoon slump, 6
    anxiety, 26
    bad breath, 42
    balance problems, 44
    chest pain, 115
    cold hands and feet, 278
    depression, 144, 145
    dizziness, 154
    flushing, 225
    headaches, 282
    heartbeat irregularities, 297
    heartburn, 300
    hoarseness, 313
    low blood pressure, 506
    postnasal drip, 501
    seizures, 531
    stuffy nose, 467
    sweating, 458, 606
Allergy symptoms. *See also*
    Sneezing
    blisters, 61